Solved Papers
OPHTHALMOLOGY
for PG Students

Solved Papers OPHTHALMOLOGY for PG Students

(A must for MS, DNB & DO)

Editor

Smiti Rani Srivastava
MBBS (Hons) MS MRCS FRCS (Glasgow)
Professor and Head
Department of Ophthalmology
Institute of Post Graduate Medical Education & Research
and SSKM Hospital
Kolkata, West Bengal, India

Foreword

Asim Kumar Ghosh

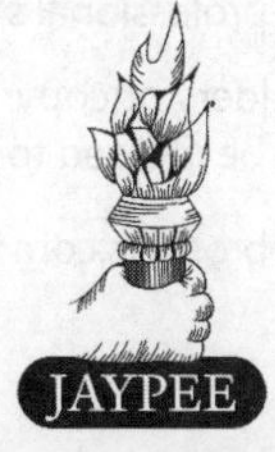

JAYPEE BROTHERS MEDICAL PUBLISHERS
The Health Sciences Publisher
New Delhi | London

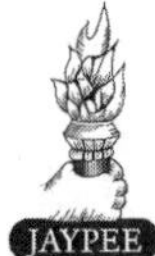

Jaypee Brothers Medical Publishers (P) Ltd

Headquarters
EMCA House, 23/23-B
Ansari Road, Daryaganj
New Delhi 110 002, India
Landline: +91-11-23272143, +91-11-23272703
+91-11-23282021, +91-11-23245672
e-mail: jaypee@jaypeebrothers.com

Corporate Office
4838/24, Ansari Road, Daryaganj
New Delhi 110 002, India
Phone: +91-11-43574357
Fax: +91-11-43574314
e-mail: jaypee@jaypeebrothers.com

Overseas Office
JP Medical Ltd.
83, Victoria Street, London
SW1H 0HW (UK)
Phone: +44-20 3170 8910
e-mail: info@jpmedpub.com

EU GPSR Authorised Representative
Logos Europe, 9 rue Nicolas Poussin
17000, La Rochelle, France
Phone: +33 (0) 6 67 93 73 78
e-mail: contact@logoseurope.eu

Website: www.jaypeebrothers.com
Website: www.jaypeedigital.com

Inquiries for bulk sales may be solicited at: jaypee@jaypeebrothers.com

Solved Papers Ophthalmology for PG Students

First Edition: **2025**

Reprint: **2026**

ISBN: 978-93-6616-230-0

Printed at: Samrat Offset Pvt. Ltd.

Dedicated to my students.

Contributors

Anchal Mitra MS DNB FICO FMRF
Consultant
Department of Pediatric Ophthalmology and Cataract
Disha Eye Hospital
Kolkata, West Bengal, India

Arpita De DO MS DNB
Assistant Professor
Department of Ophthalmology
Institute of Post Graduate Medical Education & Research
and SSKM Hospital
Kolkata, West Bengal, India

Arun Kumar Singh DO DNB
Consultant Ophthalmologist
Department of Comprehensive Ophthalmology
Siliguri Greater Lions Eye Hospital
Siliguri, West Bengal, India

Ayantika Das DNB
Fellow
Department of Vitreoretina
Susrut Eye Foundation and Research Centre
Kolkata, West Bengal, India

Bratatee Roy MS DNB
Fellow
Department of Vitreoretina
Susrut Eye Foundation and Research Centre
Kolkata, West Bengal, India

Debleena Mitra DO DNB
Consultant
Department of Vitreoretina
Susrut Eye Foundation and Research Centre
Kolkata, West Bengal, India

Ekta Bharti MS
Assistant Professor
Department of Ophthalmology
Barasat Government Medical College and Hospital
Barasat, West Bengal, India

Erum Hayet
MS DNB FICO FMRF (Pediatric Ophthalmology, Strabismus, Neuro-ophthalmology)
Ex-Senior Resident
Department of Ophthalmology
Regional Institute of Ophthalmology
Kolkata, West Bengal, India

Koustav Bhunia MS
Senior Resident
Department of Ophthalmology
College of Medicine and Sagor Dutta Hospital
Kolkata, West Bengal, India

Kshitiz Kumar MS FRCS FAICO (Retina)
Visiting Vitreoretina Consultant
Department of Ophthalmology
Institute of Post Graduate Medical Education & Research
and SSKM Hospital, Kolkata
Director and Consultant
Ikshana Eye Care
Kolkata, West Bengal, India

Mariam MS
Senior Resident
Department of Ophthalmology
Institute of Post Graduate Medical Education & Research
and SSKM Hospital
Kolkata, West Bengal, India

Niranjan Karthik MS FICO FCO
Consultant
Department of Ophthalmology
Nirmal's Eye Hospital
Tambaram, Tamil Nadu, India

Oindrila Chakraborty MS DNB
Senior Resident
Department of Ophthalmology
Institute of Post Graduate Medical Education & Research
and SSKM Hospital
Kolkata, West Bengal, India

Prabrisha Banerjee
DO DNB FMRF (Oculoplasty)
Senior Resident
Department of Ophthalmology
All India Institute of Medical Sciences
Kalyani, West Bengal, India

Prateek Nishant
MD DNB MBA MNAMS
Assistant Professor and Consultant
Department of Ophthalmology
Akhand Jyoti Eye Hospital
Saran, Bihar, India

Puja Chowdhury DO
Senior Resident
Department of Ophthalmology
Institute of Post Graduate Medical Education & Research
and SSKM Hospital
Kolkata, West Bengal, India

Rajkumari Bigyabati MS
Assistant Professor
Department of Ophthalmology
Jawaharlal Nehru Institute of Medical Sciences
Imphal, Manipur, India

Rituparna Ghosh DO DNB
Senior Resident
Department of Ophthalmology
Institute of Post Graduate Medical Education & Research
and SSKM Hospital
Kolkata, West Bengal, India

Rituparna Sarkar MS
Senior Resident
Department of Ophthalmology
Institute of Post Graduate Medical Education & Research
and SSKM Hospital
Kolkata, West Bengal, India

Rupak Roy MS FMRF
Deputy Medical Director
Department of Vitreoretina
Sankara Nethralaya
Kolkata, West Bengal, India

Sandip Samaddar MS
Associate Professor
Department of Ophthalmology
Burdwan Medical College and Hospital
Purba Burdwan, West Bengal, India

Sangeeta Roy MD (AIIMS) FICO
Visiting Vitreoretina Consultant
Department of Ophthalmology
Institute of Post Graduate Medical
Education & Research
and SSKM Hospital
Director and Consultant
Global Eye Hospital
Kolkata, West Bengal, India

Shashwat Bhattacharyya MS FRCS
Associate Professor
Department of Ophthalmology
Institute of Post Graduate Medical
Education & Research
and SSKM Hospital
Kolkata, West Bengal, India

Sinjita Dutta MD
Associate Professor
Department of Community Medicine
Institute of Post Graduate Medical
Education & Research
and SSKM Hospital
Kolkata, West Bengal, India

Smiti Rani Srivastava
MBBS (Hons) MS MRCS FRCS (Glasgow)
Professor and Head
Department of Ophthalmology
Institute of Post Graduate Medical
Education & Research
and SSKM Hospital
Kolkata, West Bengal, India

Sony Sinha MS
Additional Professor
Department of Ophthalmology
All India Institute of Medical Sciences
Patna, Bihar, India

Soumava Mandal
DO DNB MNAMS FVRS
Senior Consultant and Head
Department of Ophthalmology
Susrut Eye Foundation and Research Centre
Kolkata, West Bengal, India

Soumyajit Guha MS
Senior Resident
Department of Ophthalmology
Barasat Government Medical College
and Hospital
Barasat, West Bengal, India

Suman Mukherjee MS
Professor
Department of Ophthalmology
College of Medicine and Sagor Dutta
Hospital
Kolkata, West Bengal, India.

Tanweesha Chakraborty MS DNB
Senior Resident
Department of Ophthalmology
Institute of Post Graduate Medical
Education & Research
and SSKM Hospital
Kolkata, West Bengal, India

Tiyasha Koner MS
Senior Resident
Department of Ophthalmology
Institute of Post Graduate Medical
Education & Research
and SSKM Hospital
Kolkata, West Bengal, India

Foreword

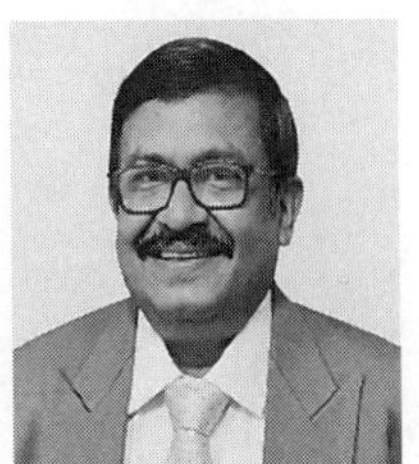

The field of ophthalmology is ever-evolving. In residency, students should be thorough with the foundational principles as well as the recent advancements. This book, *Solved Papers Ophthalmology for PG Students*, has been especially designed to serve as a valuable resource in this endeavor. It provides a collection of MS/DNB/DO questions of the last 5 years in the form of comprehensive text for those appearing for the final MS/DNB/DO examinations, meticulously solved and explained by experts in the field. This is a good book for revising before appearing for the final examinations.

Dr Smiti Rani Srivastava, Professor and Head, Department of Ophthalmology, Institute of Post Graduate Medical Education & Research (IPGMER) and SSKM Hospital, Kolkata, West Bengal, India, is a woman of many hats. From being a master in phaco surgery to an excellent teacher, she has received endless accolades for her contribution in improving the ophthalmology department at IPGMER. Although she specializes in pediatric ophthalmology, she takes a keen interest in vitreoretinal surgery. She also has numerous publications in national and international journals to her credit.

I am hopeful that her book will be a great help for all the exam-going residents in ophthalmology. My best wishes.

Asim Kumar Ghosh
Director
Regional Institute of Ophthalmology
Medical College Hospital Campus
Kolkata, West Bengal, India

Preface

This textbook, *Solved Papers Ophthalmology for PG Students*, offers a structured and comprehensive approach to learning by providing a collection of solved test papers of the last 5 years of DO, MS, and DNB examinations. Each solved paper has been carefully selected and analyzed to ensure that it reflects the core knowledge required for success in examinations and clinical practice. The answers are written in a clear and concise manner, in point form, making them easy to memorize before the examinations. Schematic diagrams and flowcharts have been added as necessary with an emphasis on logical reasoning and evidence-based practice. This compilation of questions will be of utmost benefit to the residents in their preparation for university examinations by helping them understand, remember, and represent them in the answers within the limited time of the examination.

I am hopeful that this book will be helpful for both theory and practical examinations in terms of the content provided.

I have tried my best to minimize errors in the text as this book was completed in a duration of 6 months. I look forward to suggestions as well as criticisms as I believe it will help me improve the subsequent editions.

Smiti Rani Srivastava
drsmiti_srivastava@rediffmail.com

Acknowledgments

Writing a book is rarely a solitary pursuit. It's a journey interwoven with the support, encouragement and expertise of many. First and foremost, I extend my heartfelt gratitude to the Almighty for giving me this opportunity. I take this moment to thank all my teachers of MBBS and MS, especially Prof Dr S K pal my guide and Prof. Dr Asim Kumar Ghosh, Director, RIO Kolkata, for making me who I am. This initial spark ignited the flame that fueled this project, guiding me through countless hours of research, writing and revision.

I would like to thank Prof Dr Manimoy Bandopandhyay, Director, IPGME&R for encouraging me in my academic endeavors and being a constant source of inspiration.

To my family, words seem insufficient to express my appreciation. Your unwavering belief in me and your understanding when I was away working on the book are invaluable.

To my dear friends and colleagues, Dr Rupak Roy, Prof Dr Suman Mukherjee, Prof Dr Sony Sinha, Dr Sangeeta Roy, Dr Kshitiz Kumar, Dr Sandip Samaddar, Dr Rajkumari Bigyabati and Dr Prabrisha Banerjee, thank you. This book would not have been possible without your expertise and contribution.

I am deeply indebted to the countless authors, researchers and scholars whose work provided the foundation for my own. Their published works, their online resources and their archival materials have been invaluable to my research.

I would like to acknowledge all those residents who have contributed chapters for this book. My heartfelt thanks to my residents— Dr Tanweesha, Dr Oindrila, Dr Rituparna Ghosh, Dr Ravi Prakash & Dr Imran.

I would also like to thank my resident Dr Rituparna Sarkar for her all efforts to complete this book. Without her support, it would be impossible to compile the book on time.

To the team of M/s Jaypee Brothers Medical Publishers Pvt Ltd., New Delhi, Sabyasachi Hazra, Associate Director (Publishing); Bikram Sardar, Commissioning Editor and Somoshri Banerji, Development Editor, thank you for your keen eye, your insightful suggestions and your commitment to making this manuscript the best it could be.

Finally, to you, the reader, thank you for picking up this book. I hope you find your answers within the pages.

This book is a culmination of months of hard work and dedication. It is a testament to the power of collaboration, the importance of support. I am deeply grateful to everyone who played a role in bringing this book to life.

Smiti Rani Srivastava

Contents

1. **Anatomy and Physiology** 1
Arpita De, Tanweesha Chakraborty, Oindrila Chakraborty, Tiyasha Koner

2. **Optics and Refraction** 34
Arpita De, Tanweesha Chakraborty, Oindrila Chakraborty, Mariam

3. **Eyelid** 97
Prabrisha Banerjee, Koustav Bhunia

4. **Orbit** 115
Prabrisha Banerjee, Puja Chowdhury, Koustav Bhunia

5. **Lacrimal Apparatus** 131
Shashwat Bhattacharyya, Puja Chowdhury

6. **Conjunctiva** 141
Smiti Rani Srivastava, Rituparna Ghosh

7. **Dry Eye** 157
Smiti Rani Srivastava, Rituparna Ghosh, Puja Chowdhury

8. **Episclera and Sclera** 165
Smiti Rani Srivastava, Rituparna Ghosh

9. **Cornea** 170
Sony Sinha, Smiti Rani Srivastava

10. **Refractive Surgery** 183
Prateek Nishant, Sony Sinha

11. **Lens** 189
Smiti Rani Srivastava, Rituparna Ghosh, Erum Hayet

12. **Glaucoma** 219
Sandip Samaddar, Niranjan Karthik, Rituparna Ghosh, Arun Kumar Singh

13. **Uvea** 271
Sangeeta Roy, Smiti Rani Srivastava

14. **Ocular Tumors** 290
Rituparna Ghosh, Rituparna Sarkar

15. **Diseases of the Retina** 299
Rupak Roy, Soumava Mandal, Sangeeta Roy, Ekta Bharti

16. **Retinal Detachment** 312
Soumava Mandal, Rupak Roy, Sangeeta Roy, Debleena Mitra

17. **Vitreous Disorders** 327
Soumava Mandal, Rupak Roy, Ekta Bharti, Ayantika Das

18. Diseases of Macula......334
Rupak Roy, Kshitiz Kumar, Soumava Mandal, Sangeeta Roy, Ekta Bharti, Bratatee Roy

19. Strabismus......367
Suman Mukherjee, Anchal Mitra, Erum Hayet

20. Neuro-Ophthalmology......386
Suman Mukherjee, Soumyajit Guha, Rituparna Sarkar, Tiyasha Koner

21. Ocular Injuries......412
Rajkumari Bigyabati

22. Community Ophthalmology......446
Sinjita Dutta

23. Ocular Therapeutics and Laser......460
Shashwat Bhattacharyya, Tanweesha Chakraborty, Oindrila Chakraborty

24. Ocular Manifestations of Systemic Diseases......482
Smiti Rani Srivastava, Rajkumari Bigyabati, Rituparna Sarkar

25. Miscellaneous......499
Smiti Rani Srivastava, Rituparna Ghosh, Rituparna Sarkar

Index......*525*

Plate 1

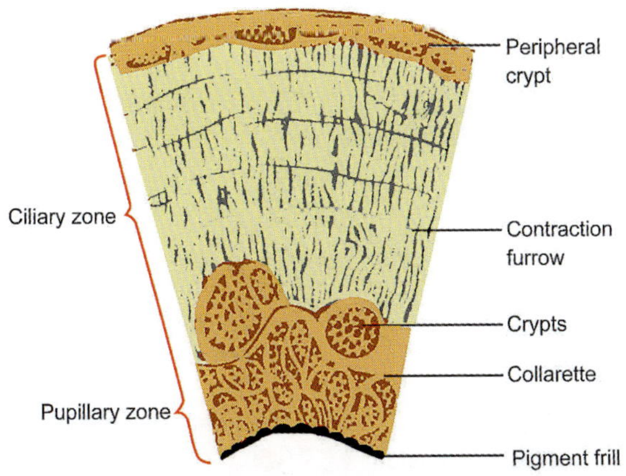

Fig. 6: Microscopic structure of iris ***(Chapter 1)***.

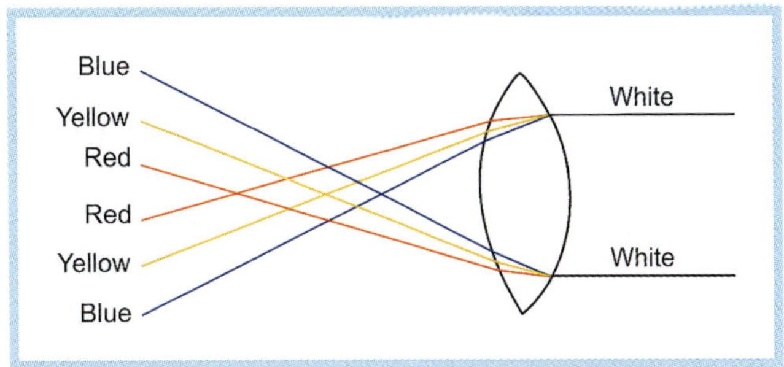

Fig. 4: Chromatic aberration ***(Chapter 2)***.

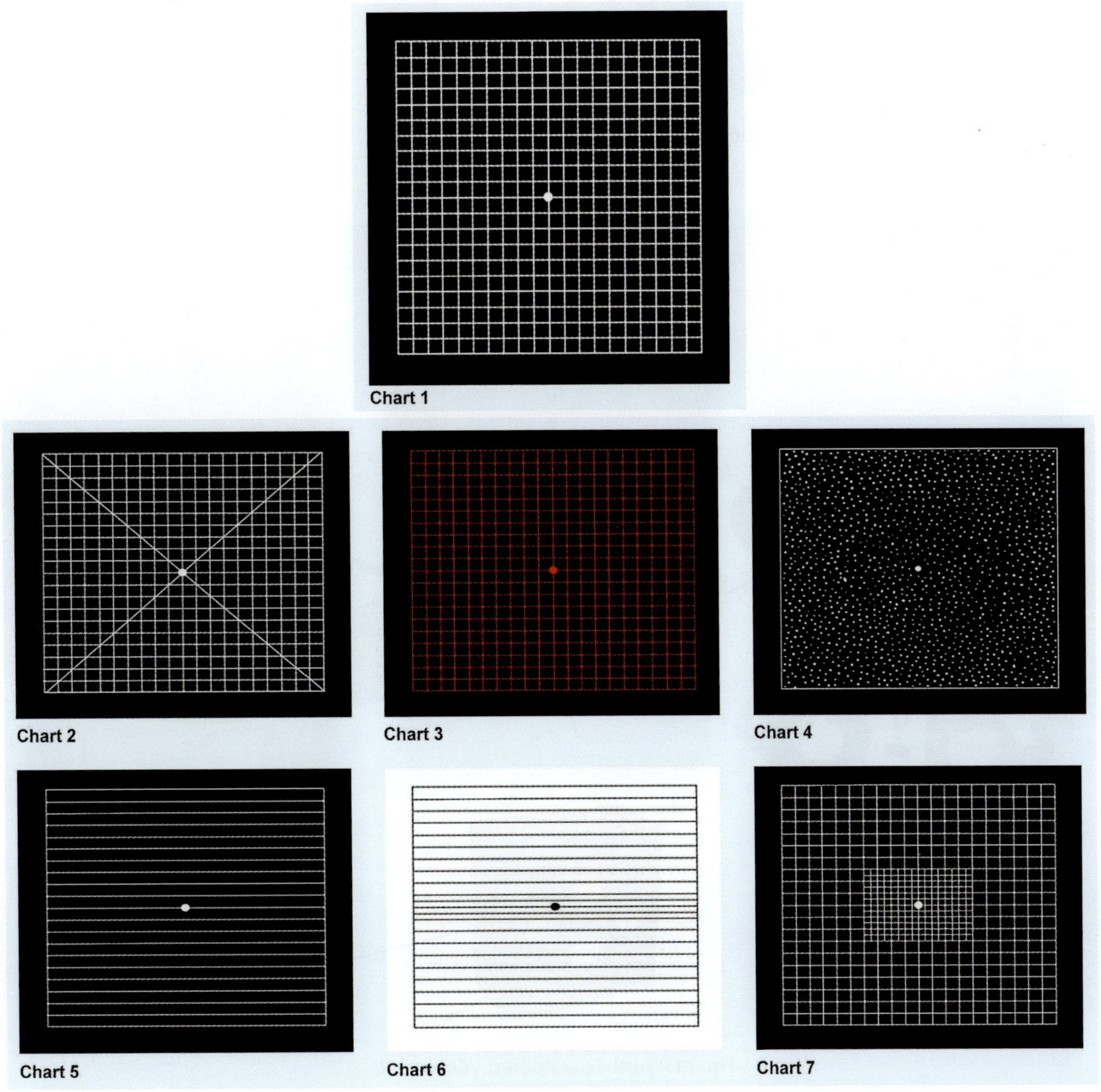

Chart 1

Chart 2

Chart 3

Chart 4

Chart 5

Chart 6

Chart 7

Fig. 7: Amsler grid ***(Chapter 2)***.

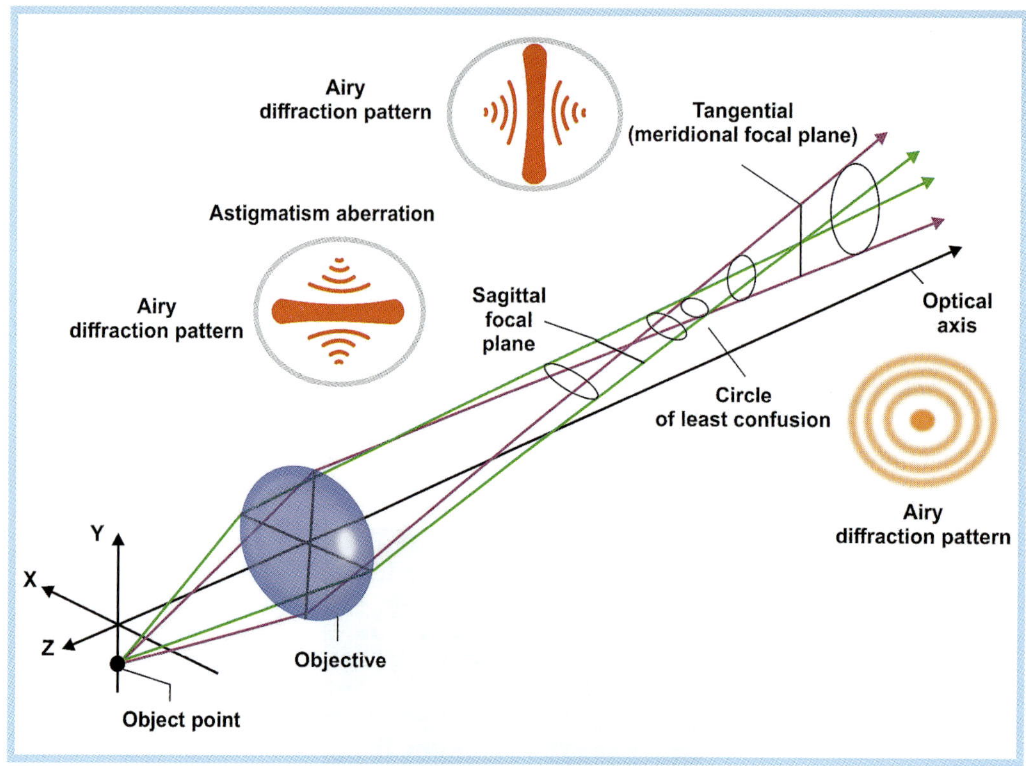

Fig. 8: Sturm's conoid. ***(Chapter 2)***

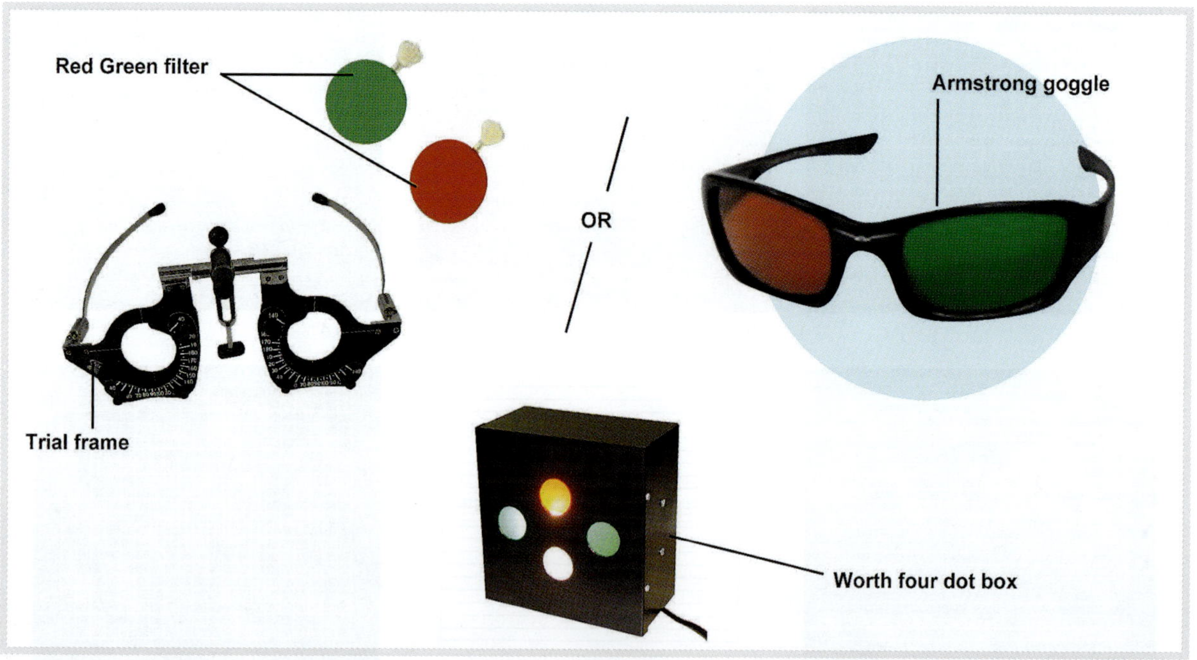

Fig. 11: Worth Four dot test. ***(Chapter 2)***

Plate 3

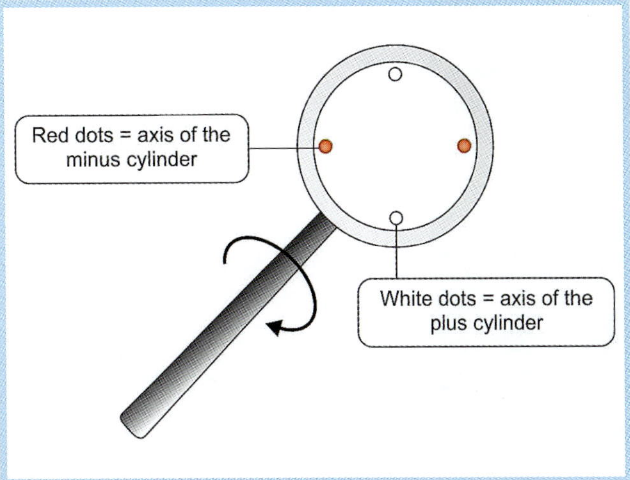

Fig. 13: The principal meridians are marked in the periphery. A handle is attached between the two marked axes. ***(Chapter 2)***

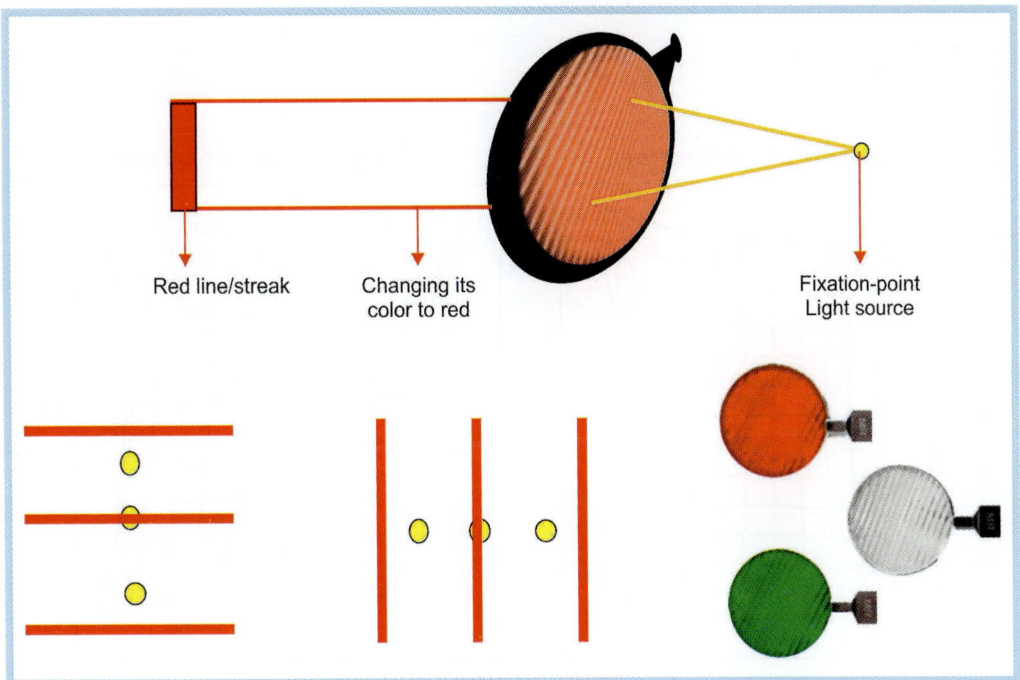

Fig. 14: The working of Maddox rod ***(Chapter 2)***.

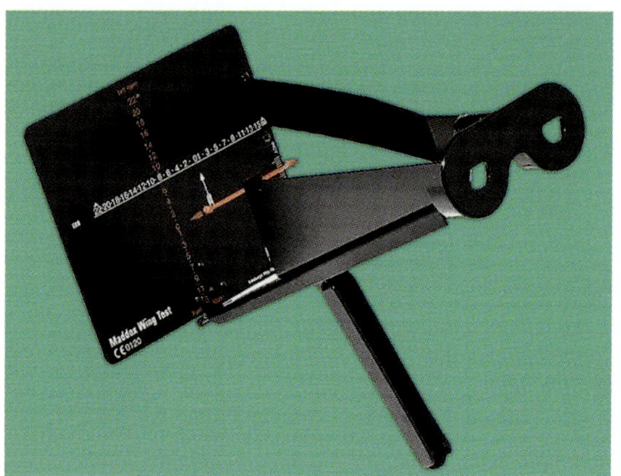

Fig. 15: Maddox wing *(Chapter 2)*.

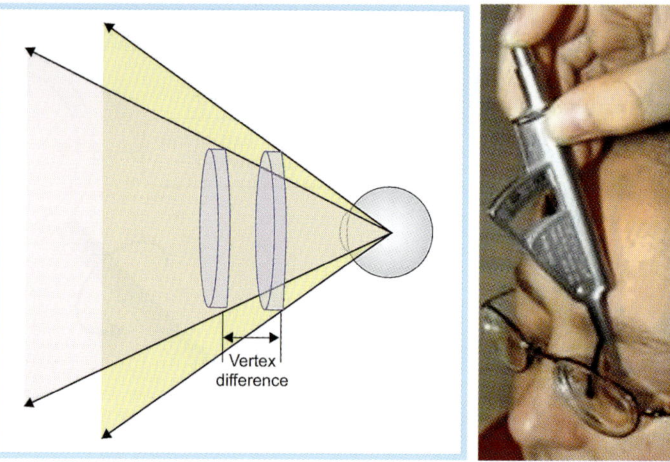

Fig. 21: Short vertex distance *(Chapter 2)*.

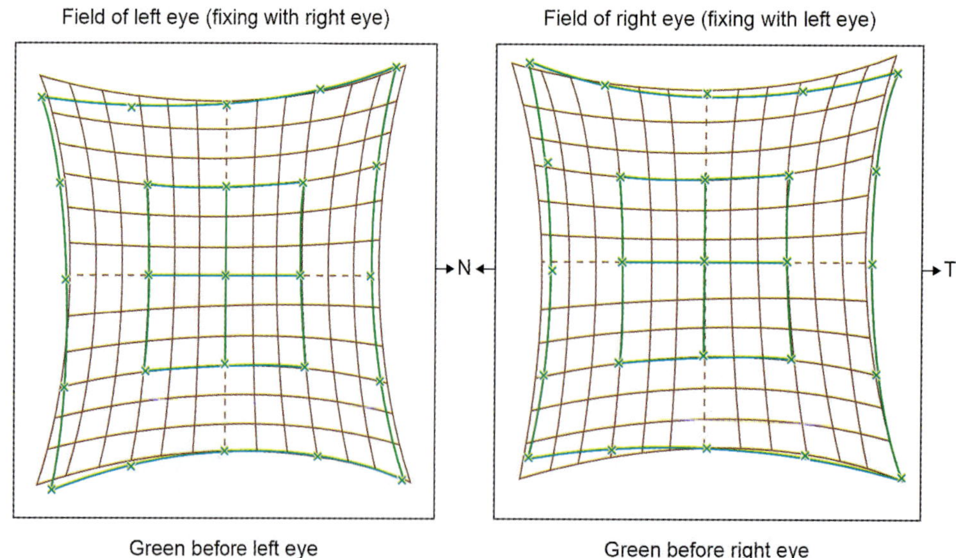

Fig. 42: Hess chart *(Chapter 2)*.

Plate 5

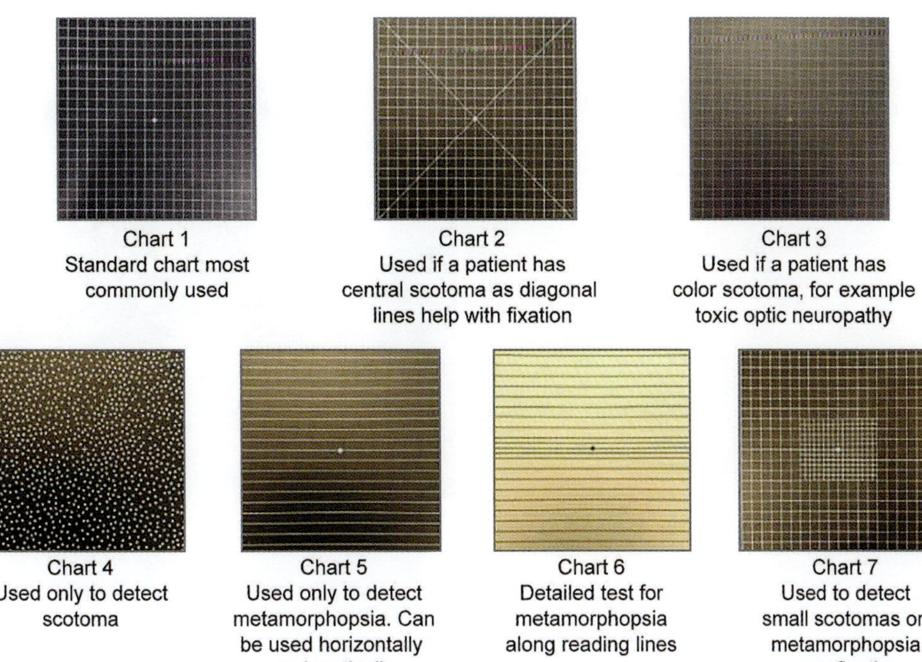

Fig. 43: Types of Amsler grid test ***(Chapter 2)***.

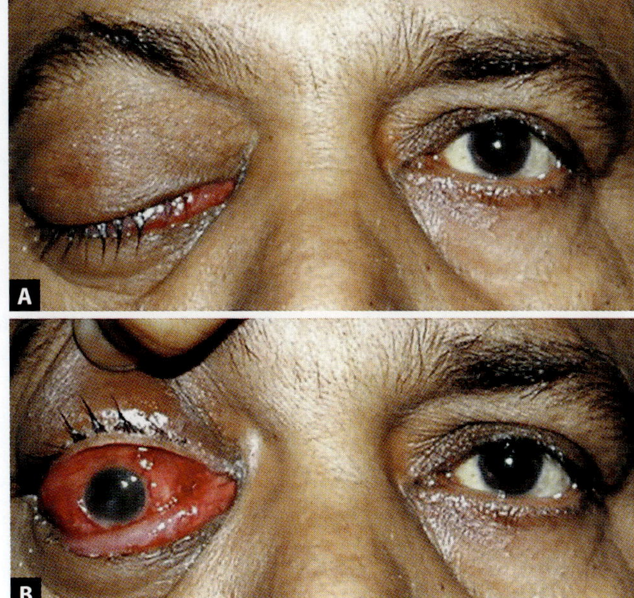

Figs. 1A and B: A 50-year-old male presenting with right eye orbital cellulitis ***(Chapter 4)***.

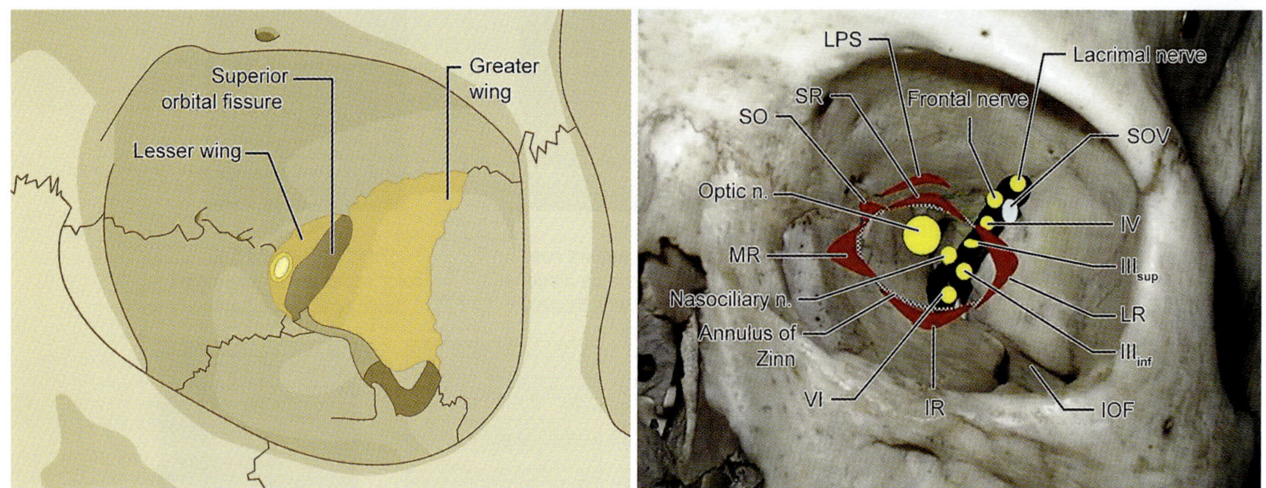

Fig. 4: Anatomy of the orbital apex ***(Chapter 4)***.

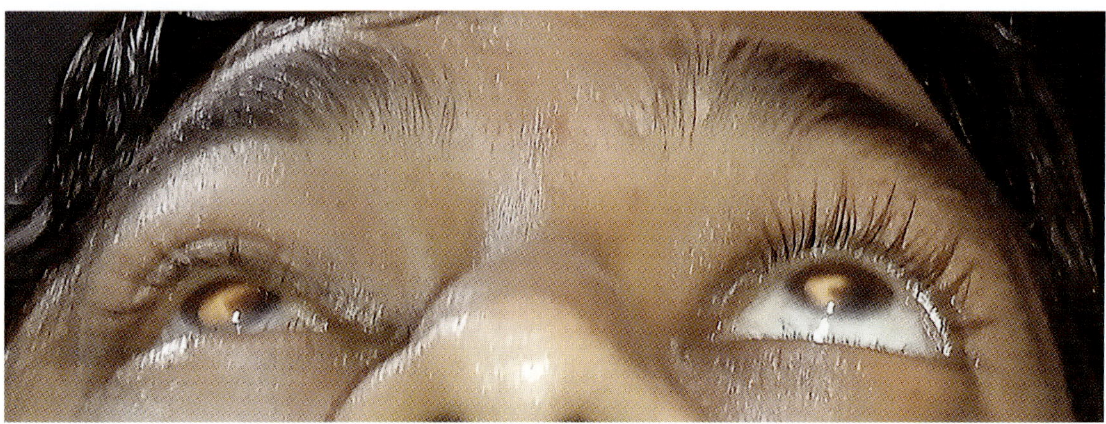

Fig. 9: A 35-year-old male presented with right eye enophthalmos due to orbital floor fracture. ***(Chapter 4)***

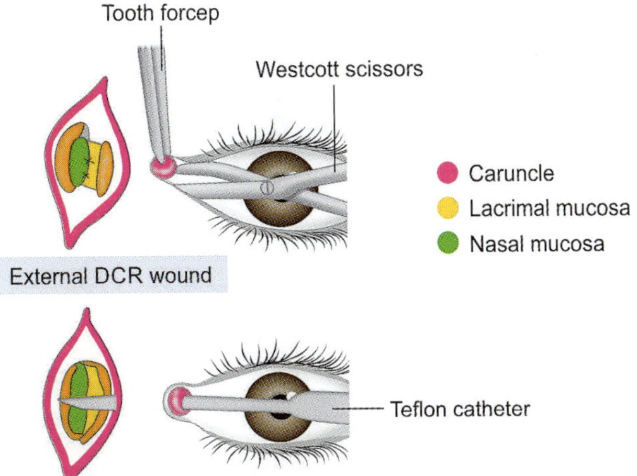

Fig. 3: Conjunctiva-DCR ***(Chapter 5)***.

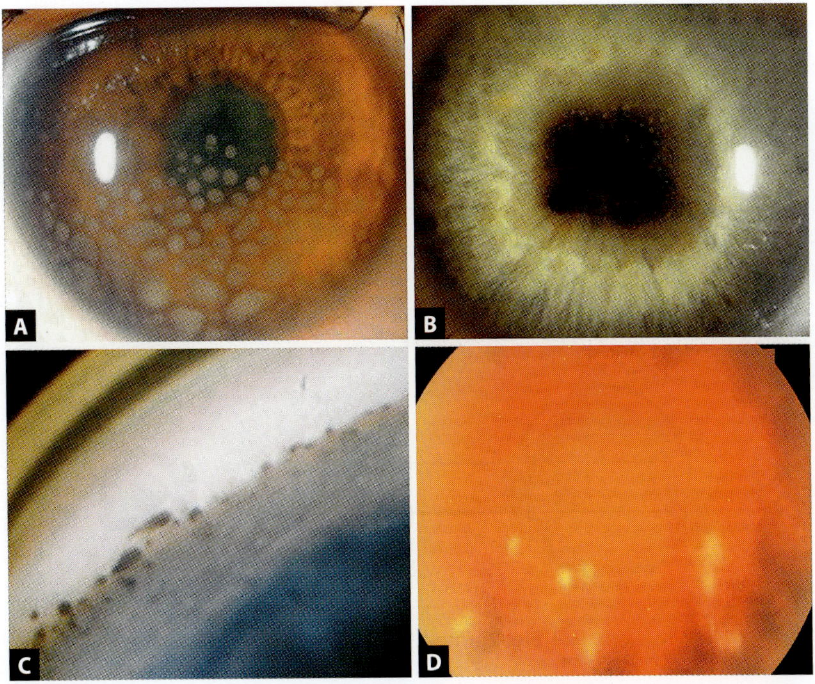

Figs. 2A to D: Ocular sarcoidosis: (A) Very large granulomatous "mutton fat" keratic precipitates; (B) Large iris nodules; (C) Nodular involvement of the trabecular meshwork; and (D) Snowballs ***(Chapter 13)***.

Plate 8

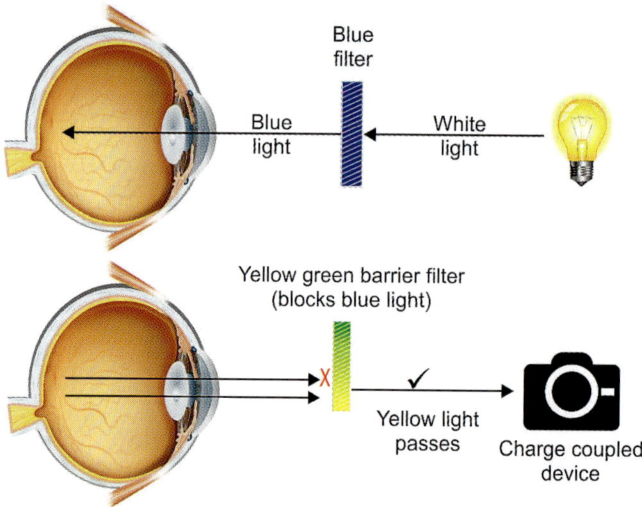

Fig. 1: Schematic diagram showing the principle of fundus fluorescein angiography (FFA) ***(Chapter 18)***.

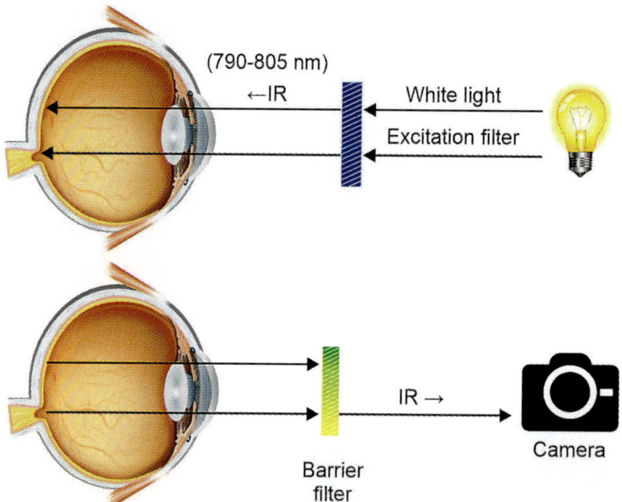

Fig. 2: Filters. ***(Chapter 18)***.

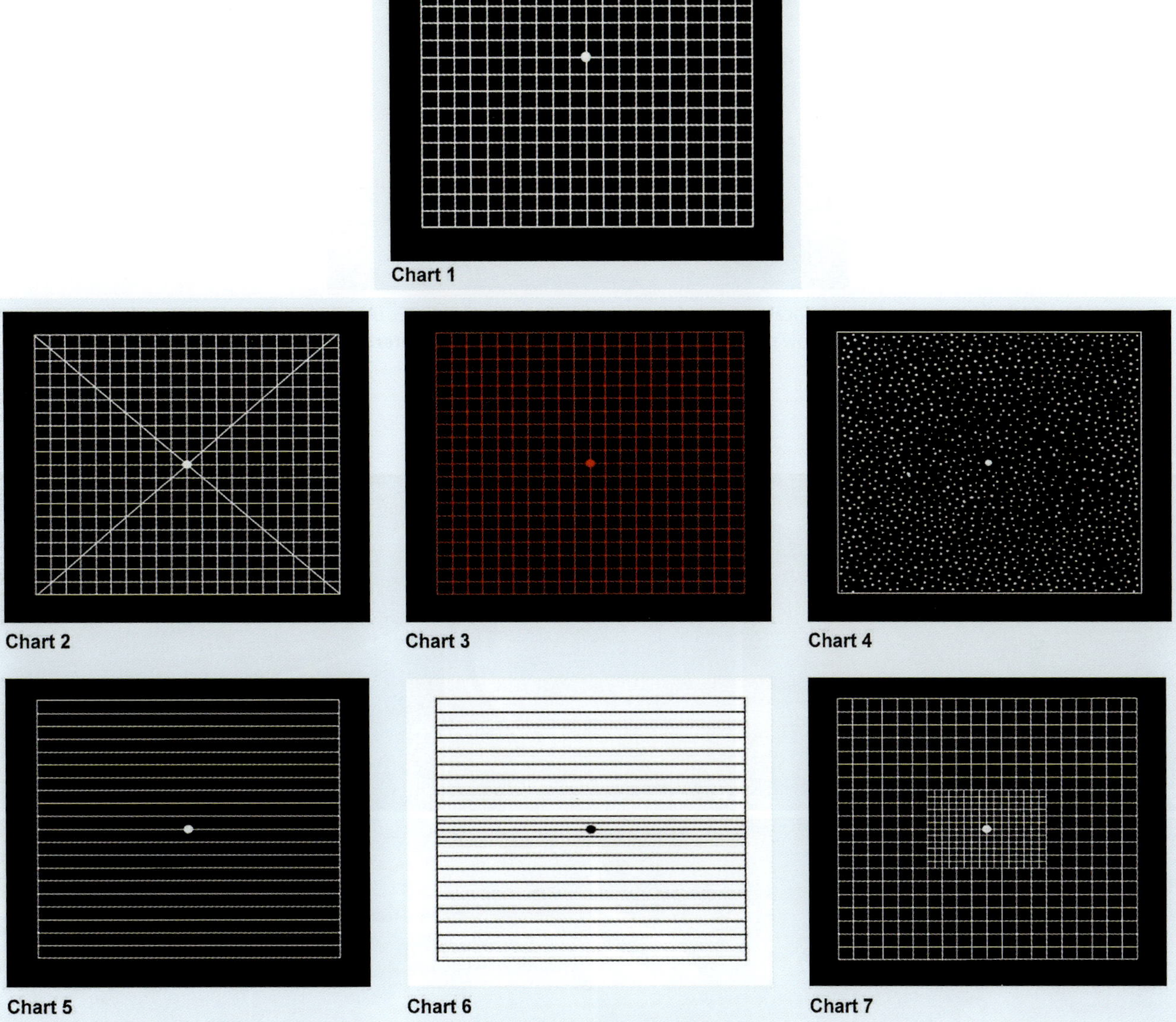

Fig. 3: Amsler grid ***(Chapter 18)***.

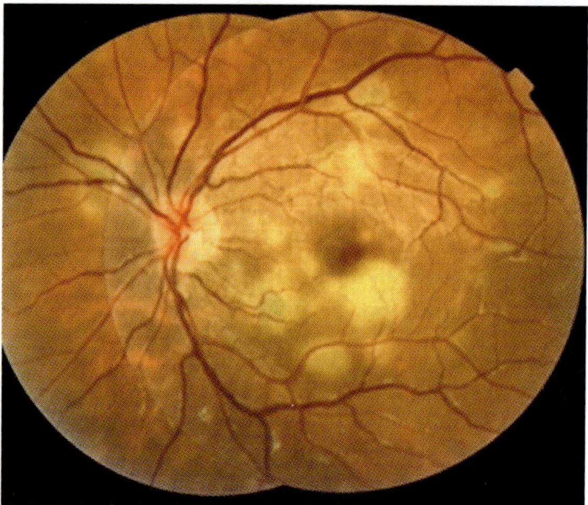

Fig. 10A: Acute posterior multifocal placoid pigment epitheliopathy (APMPPE). (A) Fundus photo shows multiple yellow placoid lesions in the posterior pole ***(Chapter 18)***.

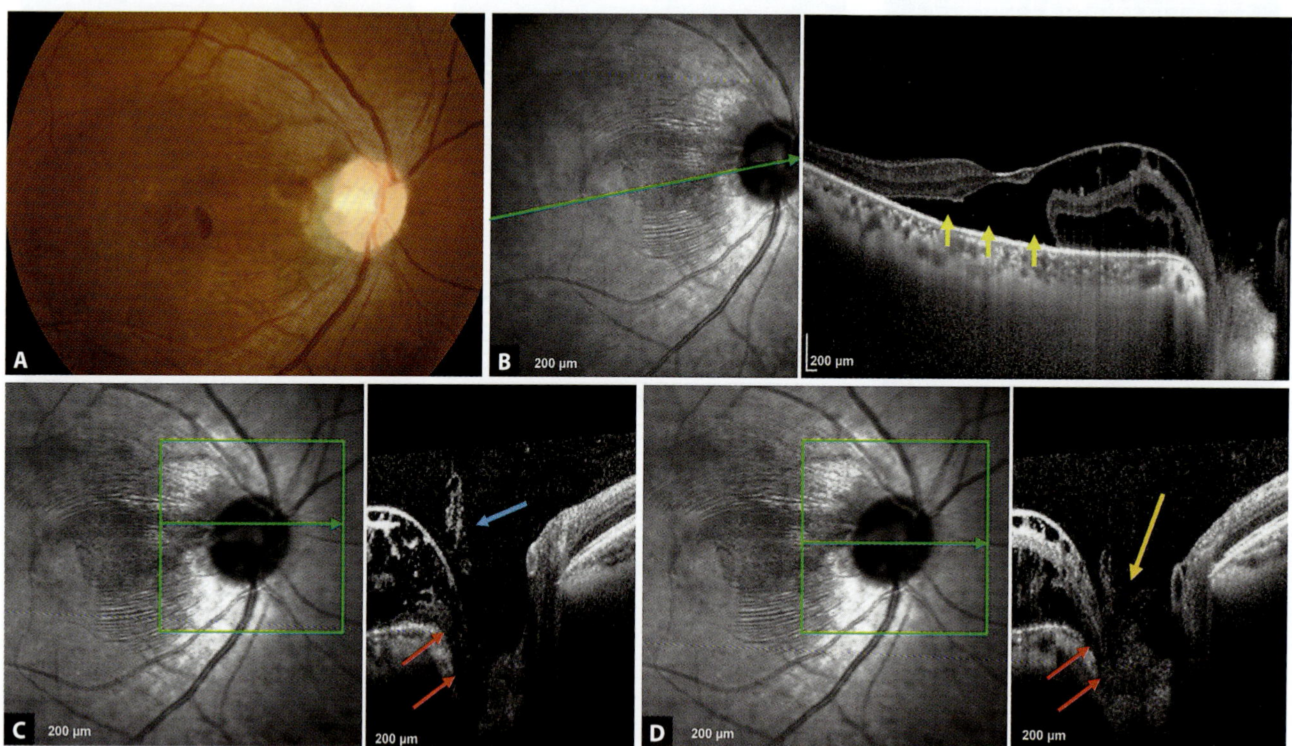

Figs. 14A to D: Preoperative images. (A) Digital fundus photograph of right eye showing macular neurosensory detachment with a pseudohole and greyish yellow double optic disc pits in the temporal segment; (B) Confocal scanning laser ophthalmoscope (cSLO) image of macula and optic disc showing the same; spectral domain optical coherence tomography (SD—OCT) along the green line shows schisis—detachment (yellow arrows), outer layer hole, retinoschisis of inner, middle and outer retina; (C) cSLO and SD—OCT images of superior pit show communication between perineural and intraretinal spaces (red arrows) and a hyperreflective membrane or glial tissue overlying the pit (blue arrow); (D) cSLO and SD—OCT images of inferior pit show communication between perineural and intraretinal spaces (red arrows) and a glial tissue overlying the pit (orange arrow). ***(Chapter 18)***.

Plate 11

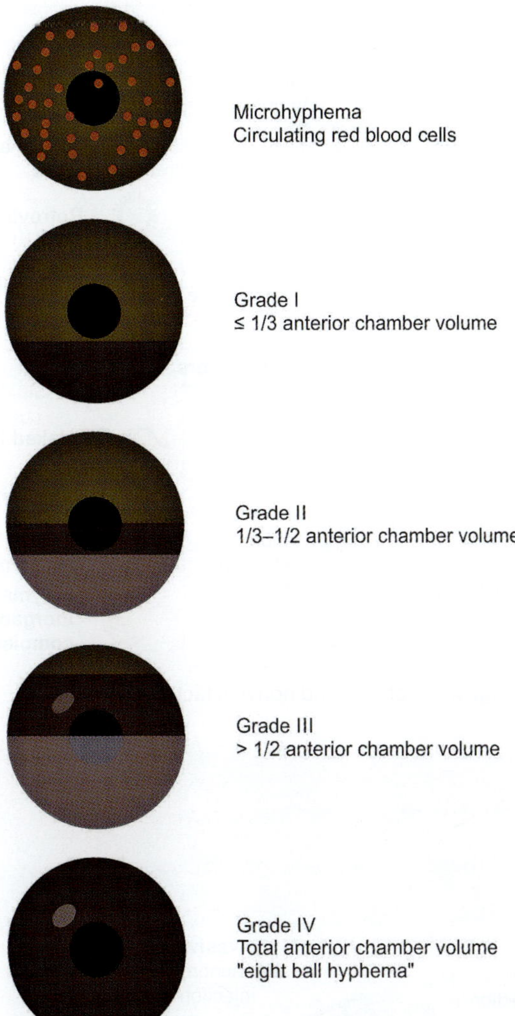

Fig. 1: Grading of hyphema ***(Chapter 25)***.

Plate 12

Viral vectors

- Many have tissue-specific tropisms
- Improved specificity over non-viral vectors
- Robust transduction

- May induce inflammatory response
- Risk of insertional mutagenesis, oncogenesis, and genotoxicity
- Expensive to produce
- Limited payload size

Adenovirus
Adeno-associated virus
Retrovirus
Lentivirus

Non-viral vectors

- Non-toxic
- Biodegradable
- Lower risk of toxicity and immunogenicity

- Low specificity
- More prone to aggregation
- Less stable than viral vectors

Naked DNA
Liposome
Niosome
Polymers and inorganic complexes

Fig. 6: List of viral and nonviral factors ***(Chapter 25)***.

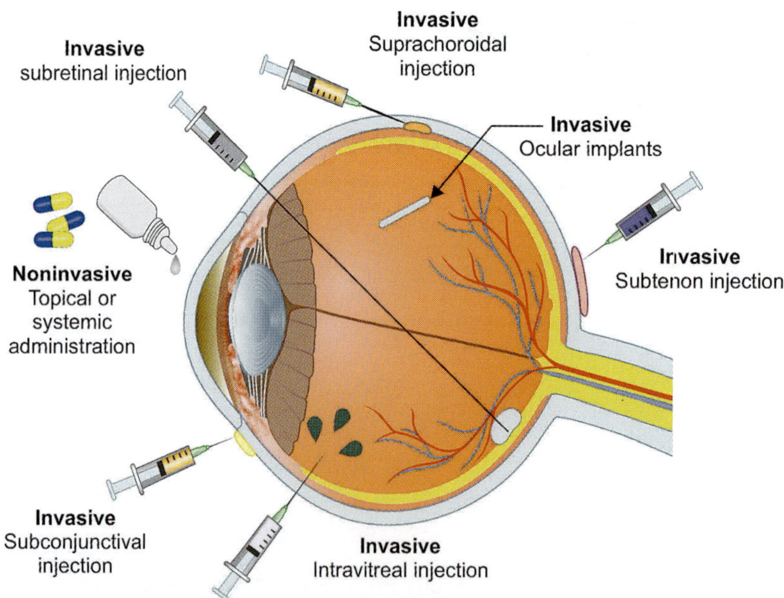

Fig. 7: Route of administration of gene therapy ***(Chapter 25)***.

CHAPTER

Anatomy and Physiology

Arpita De, Tanweesha Chakraborty, Oindrila Chakraborty, Tiyasha Koner

QUESTIONS

1. **Describe in brief the embryological steps of eyeball formation.** **(10) (WBUHS MS 2023)**
2. **Corneal endothelium—short note.** **(5) (WBUHS DO, 2015 2019)**
3. **Histological structure of cornea—short note.** **(5) (WBUHS MS 2020)**
4. **Corneal nerve supply—short note.** **(5) (BHU MS 2021)**
5. **Anatomy of limbus and applied importance—short note.** **(5) (TNMGRMU 2015, WBUHS 2020)**
6. **How is corneal transparency maintained? How can this be prolonged after death?** **(10) (MS WBUHS 2023)**
7. **Angle of anterior chamber of eye.** **(10) (WBUHS MS 2023, 2024)**
8. **Briefly describe the formation of aqueous humor and its outflow.** **(10) (WBUHS MS 2015)**
9. **Write briefly on blood aqueous barrier.** **(10) (TN MGRMU MS 2020)**
10. **Discuss the factors influencing intraocular pressure.** **(10) (WBUHS MS 2018)**
11. **Elaborate the macroscopic and microscopic structure of iris.** **(10) (WBUHS 2022)**
12. **Discuss in brief the various types of tonometry.** **(10) (TN MGRMU 2017)**
13. **Describe the blood supply of uveal tissue.** **(10) (MS 2020)**
14. **Short note on ciliary zonules.** **(5) (TN MGRMU 2021)**
15. **What is blood retinal barrier?** **(5) (TN MGRMU 2018)**
16. **Write a short note on Rods and cones.** **(5) (TN MGRMU 2018)**
17. **Retinal pigment epithelium- short note.** **(5) (WBUHS DO 2014)**
18. **Describe the pupillary pathway and discuss in detail abnormal pupillary reactions** **(10) (WBUHS MS 2019)**
19. **Write a short note on Grades of binocular vision.** **(5) (TNMGRMU, WBUHS MS 2023)**
20. **Write a short note on Depth perception.** **(5) (TN MGRMU 2015)**
21. **Write a short note on Anomalous retinal correspondence.** **(5) (WBUHS DO 2019)**
22. **Write a short note on Panum's area.** **(5) (WBUHS MS, 2014 2024)**
23. **Describe in brief: Anatomy of lacrimal gland.** **(5) (TN MGRMU 2018)**
24. **Write in brief about Tear Film and its functions.** **(10) (WBUHS MS 2021)**
25. **Describe the different muscles and ligaments attached to eyelids and their function.** **(5+5) (WBUHS MS 2021)**
26. **Write a short note on Lower lid retractors.** **(5) (TN MGRMU, WBUHS MS 2015)**
27. **Write a short note on central retinal artery—its course and branches.** **(5) (TN MGRMU, WBUHS MS 2016)**
28. **Write a short note on choriocapillaris.** **(5) (WBUHS MS 2019)**

29. Write a short note on posterior ciliary arteries. **(5) (WBUHS MS 2018)**

30. Describe with diagram the blood supply of optic nerve head. **(10) (WBUHS MS 2022)**

What is the blood supply of different parts of optic nerve? Support with a diagram. **(10) (WBUHS MS 2019)**

31. Describe the anatomy of cavernous sinus and its applied importance. **(4+6) (WBUHS MS 2023)**

Relations of cavernous sinus. **(5) (WBUHS MS 2020)**

32. Describe in brief about bones forming wall of orbit. **(10) (TNMGRMU 2018, WBUHS MS 2019)**

33. Draw a labeled diagram of posterior surface of eye with details of structure present. **(10) (WBUHS MS 2018)**

34. Draw a diagram showing the superior orbital fissure and the structures passing through it. **(10) (WBUHS DO 2020)**

35. Elaborate the boundaries and contents of Surgical spaces of orbit. **(10) (WBUHS MS 2024/DO 2019)**

1. Describe in brief the embryological steps of eyeball formation. (10) (WBUHS MS 2023)

The development of the eye starts in a 22-day-old embryo bearing eight pairs of somites and is around 2 mm in length. The following structures are involved in the formation of the eyeball and ocular adnexa **(Fig. 1)**.

- Outgrowth from prosencephalon called *optic vesicle.*
- Specialized area of surface ectoderm, known as *lens placode* and the surrounding ectoderm
- *Mesoderm* surrounding the optic vesicle
- *Visceral mesoderm* of maxillary process

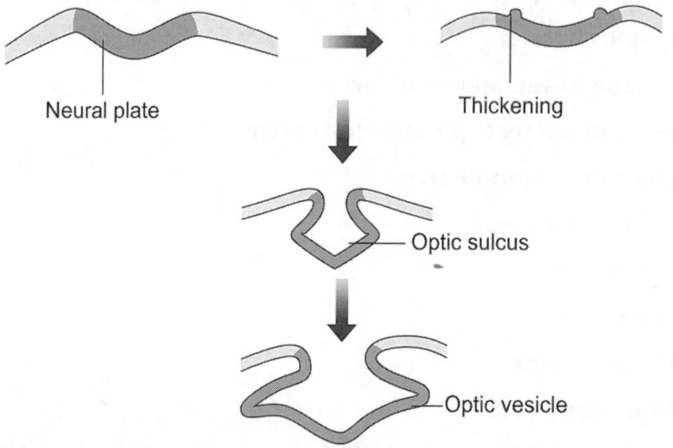

Fig. 1: Schematic diagram showing the formation of optic vesicle.

Formation of Optic Vesicle

- At around 3 weeks of gestation, the area of neural plate destined to form prosencephalon develops thickenings on either side, that is later depressed to form the *optic sulcus.*
- The optic sulcus deepens and the walls of the prosencephalon bulge outwards to form the *optic vesicle.*
- The proximal part of the optic vesicle is constricted to form the *optic stalk.*

Formation of Lens Vesicle

- At around 4 weeks of gestation, the surface ectoderm lying in relation to the optic vesicle becomes thickened to form *lens placode.*
- As the optic vesicle transitions into optic cup, the lens placode gets depressed and seeps in beneath the surface to form *lens vesicle.*

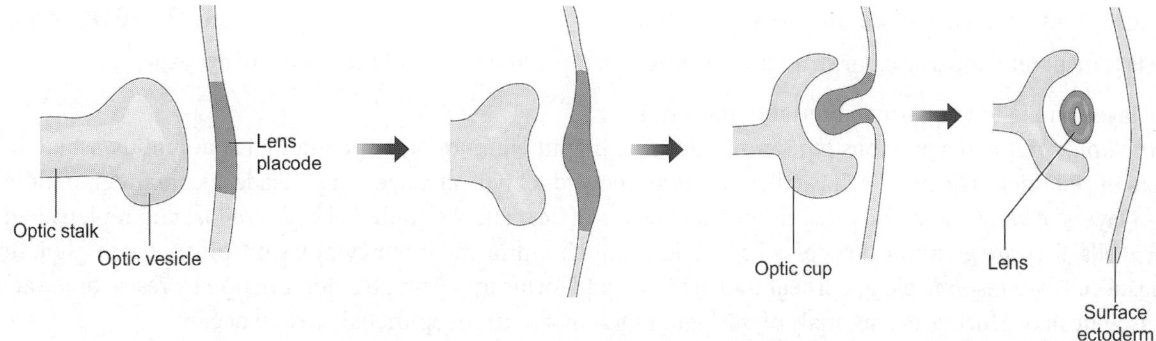

Fig. 2: The conversion of optic vesicle into optic cup.

Formation of Optic Cup

- The conversion of optic vesicle into optic cup **(Fig. 2)** develops due to the differential growth of the walls of the vesicle. The margins of the optic cup grow over the upper and lateral sides of the lens to enclose it.
- The walls of the optic cup do not grow inferiorly, leading to formation of the choroidal fissure.
- This choroidal fissure is generally closed by 6 weeks of gestation.
- Most of the ocular structures are present in the eye by 7 weeks of gestation.
- The retina and the different parts of the uvea are formed from the inner and outer layers of the optic cup.

Mesenchymal Structures

The mesenchyme around the eyeball develops the hyaloid system of vessels and other vascular structures. The corresponding vascular mesenchyme forms the iridopupillary membrane that later on forms the iris.

Applied Anatomy

Failure of closure of the choroidal fissure results in formation of colobomas of varying severity.

2. Corneal endothelium—short note. (5) (WBUHS DO 2015, 2019)

It is the innermost layer of cornea, having single layer of hexagonal cells. The endothelial cells are attached with Descemet's membrane by hemidesmosomes and laterally to each other by tight junctional complexes. This linkage is calcium dependent and helps to maintain endothelial cells integrity from anterior chamber of eye. Endothelial cells also have active pump mechanism, which is involved in active secretion and protein synthesis.

Due to presence of huge number of mitochondria, ribosome, endoplasmic reticulum and Golgi bodies, endothelial cells have high metabolic activity.

Normal endothelial cell density is around 6000 cells/mm^2 at birth and cell count falls about 26 % in first year of life. In young adult, this cell count is 2400-3000 cells/mm^2. This cell count is done by specular microscopy. Any defect in dying cells is filled by residual cells enlargement (polymegathism) **(Fig. 3)**.

When this cell count falls below 500 cells/mm^2, corneal decompensation starts, which results in pump failure and ultimately corneal edema occurs.

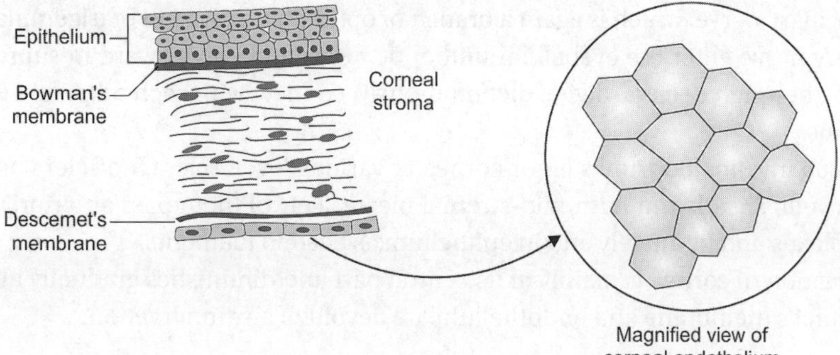

Fig. 3: Cross-section of corneal endothelium with its magnified view (inset).

3. Histological structure of cornea—short note. (5) (WBUHS MS 2020)

Cornea is transparent and avascular structure forming anterior 1/6th of outer fibrous coat of eyeball.

Corneal layers are followings from anterior to posterior:

a. *Epithelium:* Stratified squamous type, continuous with epithelium of bulbar conjunctiva at limbus, where it is 5-6 layers of cell thick. The basal cell is taller columnar polygonal type arranged in palisade-like manner, middle layer is 2-3 layers of wing /umbrella cells, superficial layer is of flat cells. As epithelial cells are lost and replenished from basal cells, they are germinal layer of cells with few mitochondria and other cytoplasmic organelles. Tight junctions of basal cells are responsible to corneal transparency and forms important barrier function by restricting water and electrolytic flow. During any anomaly of this tight junction, recurrent epithelial erosion occurs.
b. Bowman's layer-acellular, condensed collagen consisting superficial part of stroma and once destroyed never regenerate.
c. *Stroma:* It is of 90% of total corneal thickness containing collagen embedded in hydrated matrix of proteoglycans with keratocytes, macrophages, histiocytes and lymphocytes. 200-250 lamellae arranged in parallel layers to each other and to the corneal plane and continuous with scleral lamellae at limbus. In anterior 1/3 part of stroma they arranged obliquely, whereas in posterior 2/3 part, they are at right angle to each other.
d. *Dua's layer:* Pre-Descemet's layer, discovered by Harminder Dua in 2005, has high tensile strength with compact collagen lamella type I and VI and abundant elastin, only 10*um* thick (range 6-16) and almost acellular. This layer has utmost important in anterior and posterior lamellar corneal transplant surgery like pre-Descemet's endothelial keratoplasty, Fogla's mini DALK, DALK -triple, suture management of acute hydrops. This layer is also very important in pathology and clinical signs of several corneal infections, dystrophies and keratoconus due to its high elastin content.
e. *Descemet's membrane:* Homogenous layer, basement membrane of endothelium, composed of collagen and glycoprotein (no visible elastic fiber). Its thickness varies with age starting 3 *um* at birth to 40 *um* at elder life. This layer is resistant to chemicals, trauma and infection and can regenerate when destroyed. Peripherally it ends at anterior limit of trabecular meshwork as Schwalbe's line and appears as wart like excrescences (Hassel Henle bodies). On electron microscopical examination this layer can be divided into vertical banded anterior 1/3 and amorphous, granular posterior 2/3 regions.
f. Endothelium-single layer, hexagonal, flat mosaic type cell (6000 cell/mm^2 at birth) and it falls by 26% in first year of life and 2400-3000 cell/mm^2 in adulthood. These cells are counted by specular microscopy. When one cell dies, remaining cells fill in the gap by enlarging (polymegathism). When more than 75% cells are lost, corneal endothelial decompensation occurs. Endothelial cells are attached to Descemet's membrane by hemidesmosomes and laterally to each other by calcium dependent tight junctions, which accounts for barrier action. Endothelium has active pump mechanism, abundant mitochondria, ribosome, endoplasmic reticulum and other organelles.

4. Corneal nerve supply—short note. (5) (BHU MS 2021)

Cornea is highly sensitive structure and rich in sensory innervation. The main nerve supplying cornea is long ciliary nerve, branches of nasociliary nerve, which is again a branch of ophthalmic division of trigeminal nerve.

Long and short ciliary nerve enter the eyeball around optic nerve and run forward in suprachoroidal space. After reaching close to limbus, they pierce sclera, divide dichotomously, connect with each other and with conjunctival nerve to form pericorneal plexus.

From this plexus 60-80 myelinated trunks enter cornea at various level, sclera, episclera and conjunctiva. Within stroma they lose their myelin sheath and form mid-stromal plexus. Few of them pass anteriorly to form sub-epithelial plexus, intra-epithelial plexus and ultimately end in epithelium as beaded filaments.

This extensive innervation of cornea is mainly at its central part and diminishes gradually in periphery. But central posterior cornea, Descemet's membrane and endothelium are devoid of any innervation.

5. Anatomy of limbus and applied importance—short note. (5) (TNMGRMU 2015, WBUHS 2020)

- This is a circumcorneal transitional zone between conjunctiva and cornea/sclera and cornea.
- At the conjunctivo-corneal junction, stroma ends but epithelium becomes 10-12 layers thick, irregularly arranged, contain melanin pigments and continue with that of cornea.
- At the sclerocorneal junction, transparent corneal lamellae become continuous with opaque fibers of sclera.
- Surgical limbus is 2 mm wide circumcorneal zone and is characterized by anterior limbal border, mid limbal line and posterior limbal border.
- *Anterior limbal border:* It is anterior boundary of surgical limbus and overlies the termination of Bowman's membrane.
- *Mid-limbal line:* It overlies the termination of Descemet's membrane.
- *Posterior limbal border:* It is posterior boundary of surgical limbus. It is 1mm posterior to mid limbal line and overlies the scleral spur.
- *Blue limbal zone:* As the insertion of conjunctiva and Tenon's capsule into cornea varies in different quadrants, the extent of this zone also varies (1 mm superiorly, 0.8 mm inferiorly, 0.4 mm nasally and temporally). Behind this zone lies mid limbal line.
- *White limbal zone:* It is between mid limbal line and posterior limbal border. It overlies the trabecular meshwork and extent of this zone is constant in all zones.

Applied Anatomy
- More anterior incision in limbus causes Descemet's stripping and astigmatism.
- More posterior incision in limbus causes injury to trabecular meshwork, excessive bleeding and hyphema.
- So mid limbal incision is mostly preferred, which corresponds to Schwalbe's line.
- Damage to limbal stem cells result in limbal stem cell deficiency (LSCD) which is characterized by pannus formation, conjunctivalization of cornea and loss of vision. LSCDs can be classified into partial and total LSCDs.

6. How is corneal transparency maintained? How can this be prolonged after death? (10) (MS WBUHS, 2023)

The cornea forms the anterior $1/6^{th}$ of the anterior portion of the eye and is a principle refracting medium, maintaining a healthy barrier between the eye and environment. The epithelium of the cornea provides barrier to tear borne pathogens while the endothelium is responsible for maintaining hydration and clarity of the corneal stroma.

1. Stromal structure—corneal stroma consists of long, thin, striated type 1 collagen which are laid in parallel and equally placed. The fibrils are so arranged that adjacent layers lie at acute angle sot each other. The fibrils are filled in between with proteoglycans and other ground substances like glycosaminoglycans. These are responsible for water holding capacity of the stroma.
2. Control of corneal hydration—the cornea is optically transparent as the stroma lies in a dehydrated state to counter the swelling pressure. Both the corneal cell layers are permeable to solutes but resistant to electrolytes. In the epithelium, squamous cells provide barrier to ion flow as it has tight junctions.
3. Endothelial fluid pump-this helps to transfer fluid from the corneal stroma to the aqueous via an active transport mechanism.
4. Epithelial transport properties—the epithelium actively transports chloride in the secretory direction out while sodium is transported inside leading to outward transport of solute and fluid.
5. Endothelial transport properties.
6. Intraocular pressure—the IOP doesn't have much effect on corneal hydration when it is within normal range. If IOP is more than 50mmHg and there is stromal swelling from endothelial dysfunction, high IOP will cause epithelial edema and loss of transparency.

In order to prolong transparency after death, the following needs to be done:

1. The donor cornea to be packed in ice to keep it within 2-8 degrees Celsius without freezing.
2. Corneas to be preserved for a maximum of 14 days in a solution containing chondroitin sulfate, antioxidants, energy sources and nutritive substances
3. The eye is preserved through organ culture or cryopreservation to ensure the viability of endothelium till the time of transplant. In Organ culture, the tissue can be used 7 days after retrieval. The eye is rinsed in saline, placed in povidone iodine solution and kept in Eagle's minimum essential medium. In cryopreservation, the tissue is stored at temperatures below -80 degrees. Such corneas can be used months later.

7. Angle of anterior chamber of eye. (10) (WBUHS MS 2023, 2024)

Anterior chamber of eye is bounded anteriorly by corneal endothelium and posteriorly by anterior iris surface and part of ciliary body. Depth of anterior chamber is about 3 mm in normal adult and contains 0.25 ml aqueous humor. Anterior chamber of eye is connected with posterior chamber of eye through pupil and angle of anterior chamber is examined by an instrument, called gonioscope.

By gonioscopic examination, following angle structures are visualized from posterior to anterior **(Fig. 4)**.

1. Ciliary band-Most posterior grey or dark brown band like structure, formed by anterior most part of ciliary body between scleral spur and iris insertion.
2. Scleral spur- White band attached posteriorly to ciliary body and corneoscleral meshwork anteriorly.
3. Trabecular meshwork- Pigmented tan to dark brown color band anterior to scleral spur.
4. Schwalbe's line -Anterior structure and fine ridge in front of trabecular meshwork formed by prominent Descemet's membrane. It lies in the plane of posterior corneal surface and 15-20% cases it may be hypertrophied and form a glistening ridge into anterior chamber called posterior embryotoxon.

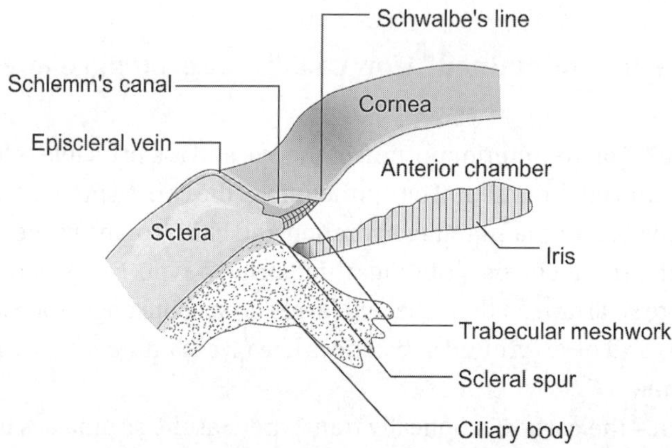

Fig. 4: Schematic diagram of the angle of the anterior chamber.

Trabecular meshwork is sieve-like structure, bridges the scleral sulcus and ultimately drain into Schlemm's canal. It is of 3 portions-

1. Uveal meshwork—innermost 2-3 layered cord like part of trabecular meshwork and extends from root of iris to Schwalbe's line.
2. Corneoscleral meshwork—middle part of trabecular meshwork and extends from scleral spur to scleral sulcus. Holes are progressively smaller than uveal meshwork.
3. Juxtacanalicular meshwork—outermost part of trabecular meshwork and extends from corneoscleral meshwork to Schlemm's canal. Inner wall of Schlemm's canal forms outer endothelial layer of juxtacanalicular meshwork and inner endothelial layer of juxtacanalicular meshwork continues as endothelium of corneoscleral meshwork.

Schlemm's canal: Endothelial lined oval shaped canal situated in scleral sulcus. Inner wall of endothelial cells are spindle shaped and vacuolated, whereas outer wall of endothelial cells are smooth and through numerous pores they are connected to collector channels, intrascleral aqueous vessels, 25-35 in number and ultimately drain into episcleral veins through direct system or indirect system through interconnecting venous plexuses.

Episcleral veins: Ultimately drain into cavernous sinus via anterior ciliary and superior ophthalmic veins.

Gonioscopic grading of angle of anterior chamber-

Shaffer's system:

Grade 4 - 35°-45° width, wide open, from Schwalbe's line to ciliary body.

Grade 3 - 20°-35° width, open, from Schwalbe's line to scleral spur.

Grade 2 - 20° width, moderately narrow, from Schwalbe's line to trabecular meshwork.

Grade 1 - 10° width, very narrow, only Schwalbe's line.

Grade 0 - 0° width, closed, no structure is seen.

8. Briefly describe the formation of aqueous humor and its outflow. (10) (WBUHS MS 2015)

Three mechanisms namely diffusion, ultrafiltration and secretion play a part in aqueous production at different levels.

1. *Diffusion:* Diffusion is a biophysical process by which molecules of a gas or solution distribute themselves uniformly by motion of its particles from areas of high concentration to areas of low concentration.
   By Fick's law of diffusion:
   Rate of movement= K (C1-C2)
   C1 = Concentration of substance on side with higher concentration
   C2 = Concentration of substance on side with lower concentration
   K = Constant which depends on nature and permeability of membrane, nature of solute and solvent, temperature.
2. *Ultrafiltration:* When a solution of protein and salt is separated from plain water or a less concentrated salt solution by a membrane permeable to salt and water and not to proteins, there will be a net movement of water on the protein side by diffusion and a movement of salt away from the protein side. The process is called Dialysis.
   Ultrafiltration refers to occurrence of dialysis under hydrostatic pressure.
3. *Secretion (active transfer):* Secretion implies an active process that selectively transport some substances across the cell membrane and substances can be moved across a concentration gradient in a direction opposite to passive mechanism.

Steps of Aqueous Formation

1. *Formation of stromal pool:* By ultrafiltration, most substances pass easily from the capillaries of the ciliary processes across the stroma.
2. *Active transport of stromal filtrates:* The tight junctions between the non-pigmented epithelial cells create part of blood-aqueous barrier.
   We can observe presence of these things:
   Abundant Na^+-K^+ active ATPase, presence of more mitochondria, higher adenylyl cyclase activity, higher specific activity for glycolytic enzymes, preferential incorporation of labeled sulfate into macromolecules.
   The basolateral membranes of the pigmented epithelial cells contain numerous Na^+ ion dependent co-transporters and exchangers and carbonic anhydrase activity is also present in these cells.
   The net effect of these ion transport system is a low level of Na^+ in both epithelial layers, high level of ascorbate and K^+ and control of intracellular pH.
   - *Sodium:* Approximately 70% found in posterior chamber is actively transported by a specific secretory pump. The active transport is ATPase dependent.
   - *Chloride:* A smaller percentage of chloride ion is actively transported and this appears to be dependent upon the presence of sodium as well as pH.
   - *Potassium:* Is transported by secretion and diffusion
   - *Ascorbic acid:* Secreted against large concentration gradient.

- *Amino acids:* Secreted by 3 carriers.
- *Bicarbonate:* Its formation is catalyzed by carbonic anhydrase

3. *Passive transport across non-pigmented ciliary epithelium:* To maintain the balance of osmotic and electrical forces water chloride and other small plasma constituents move into the posterior chamber by ultrafiltration and diffusion. Sodium is primarily responsible for movement of water into the posterior chamber and its secretion is a major factor in the formation of aqueous.

Aqueous Outflow

Aqueous flows from posterior chamber into anterior chamber through the pupil against physiologic resistance. From anterior chamber aqueous drained out by 2 routes: uveoscleral outflow (unconventional) and trabecular outflow(conventional).

1. Uveoscleral outflow:
   - It is responsible for 10-25% of total aqueous outflow.
   - Aqueous → ciliary body → suprachoroidal space → venous circulation of ciliary body, sclera & orbit
   - Matrix metalloproteinase 1 (MMP-1) plays a role in this outflow.
   - Uveoscleral outflow is possible owing to the fact that pressure in the suprachoroid is 2-4 mm of Hg lower than in anterior chamber; this can be reversed after trabeculectomy and lead to choroidal effusion.
2. Trabecular outflow:
   - Trabecular outflow is the main outlet for aqueous from the anterior chamber. Approximately 75-90% of the total aqueous is drained via this route.
   - Aqueous → Trabecular meshwork [uveal meshwork → corneoscleral meshwork → juxtacanalicular meshwork] → Schlemm's canal → collector channels → episcleral veins
   - Trabecular meshwork endothelial cells have special characteristics, active phagocytic properties, high level of cytoskeletal actin, lower levels of microtubules, contain vimentin and desmin, these are specialized both for endocytic transport of water and solutes and contractility.
   - Energy metabolism in trabecular meshwork is glycolytic
   - Transport water by activation of a water channel protein aquaporin.
   - These cells have high levels of surface tissue plasminogen activator, helps in maintaining patency and reducing resistance of outflow passages.
   - Trabecular meshwork cells have receptors for epinephrine, glucocorticoids, both induce the expression of trabecular meshwork inducible glucocorticoid response protein (TIGR). Steroid inhibit prostaglandin synthesis. Mutation in TIGR gene have found in glaucoma.
   - Trabecular meshwork cells contain free radical and hydrogen peroxide detoxifying enzymes.

   Mechanisms of aqueous transport across inner wall of Schlemm's canal<collector channel and episcleral veins:
   1. *Passive filter mechanisms:* Leaky endothelial cells, Sonderman's channels, contractile microfilaments, pores in endothelial cells, giant vacuole system
   2. *Aqueous outflow active pump mechanisms:* Oscillatory pressure transients, trabecular meshwork aqueous valve mechanisms.

9. Write briefly on blood aqueous barrier. (10) (TN MGRMU MS 2020)

It is the anterior blood ocular barrier, which controls passage of water soluble molecules more than lipid soluble molecules during transit through capillary walls.

It is formed by tight junctions between cells of inner non-pigmented epithelium of ciliary body and iris capillary endothelial cells (non-fenestrated).

Blood aqueous barrier also controls the composition of aqueous humor.

Blood aqueous barrier is not absolute and can be disturbed by following reasons-

- Ocular trauma like intraocular surgery, corneal abrasion, injury to iris, alkali burn, application of ocular irritant
- Following X-ray and atomic radiation

- Intraocular infection, ocular inflammation
- Drugs like histamine, prostaglandin, melano-stimulating hormone, cholinesterase inhibitor, cholinergic drugs.

With breakdown of this barrier, protein appears in aqueous to make an equilibrium to those of plasma. This is called plasmoid aqueous and it creates Tyndall effect during slit lamp microscopic anterior segment evaluation and ionic composition of the aqueous approaches that of simple dialysate of plasma.

Blood-aqueous barrier is formed by the tight junctions (zonula occludens and the zonula adherens) between the cells of inner non-pigmented epithelium of the ciliary body and the non-fenestrated endothelium of the iris capillaries. Blood aqueous barrier is a part of blood-ocular barrier, it prevents movement of substances from plasma to aqueous humor.

Clinical Applications

1. Hyperosmotic agents like mannitol, penetrate the eye poorly because of this barrier, but are distributed fairly widely in extracellular spaces of the body. Thus, water is drawn from the cells and the ocular fluids (vitreous more than aqueous), resulting in a fall in the intraocular pressure.
2. Ocular penetration of systemically administered antibiotics, only LMW drugs such as chloramphenicol can cross this barrier. Very poor passage is allowed to large size molecules such as penicillin, erythromycin. Out of borderline molecular weight drugs, those with high lipid solubility can pass easily, e.g., sulfonamides.

Breakdown of the Blood-aqueous Barrier

The barrier is fragile. Certain conditions which can disturb the blood-aqueous barrier are listed below:

A. Ocular trauma
   1. Mechanical:
      - Paracentesis
      - Corneal abrasion
      - Intraocular surgery
   2. Physical
      - X-rays
      - Atomic radiation
   3. Chemical
      - Alkali
      - Irritants, e.g., nitrogen, mustard

B. Pathophysiological factors
   1. Vascular dilatation
   2. Corneal and intraocular infections
   3. Intraocular inflammations
   4. Prostaglandin
   5. Anterior segment ischemia

C. Pharmacological:
   1. Melatonin stimulating hormone
   2. Cholinergic drugs
   3. Cholinesterase inhibitors
   4. Plasma hyperosmolarity

Effects of Breakdown of Blood-aqueous Barrier on Aqueous Composition

1. With the breakdown of this barrier, substances such as proteins, that are normally almost excluded from penetration, appear in the aqueous humor in measurable amounts. Thus proteins and antibodies in the aqueous equilibrate with those in plasma to form plasmoid aqueous (secondary aqueous)
2. The ionic composition of aqueous approaches that of simple dialysate of plasma.
3. The rate of penetration of smaller molecule such as sucrose or para-amino-hippurate (PAH) are increased greatly.
4. Fibrinogen appears in the aqueous, which may allow the aqueous to clot **(Fig. 5)**.

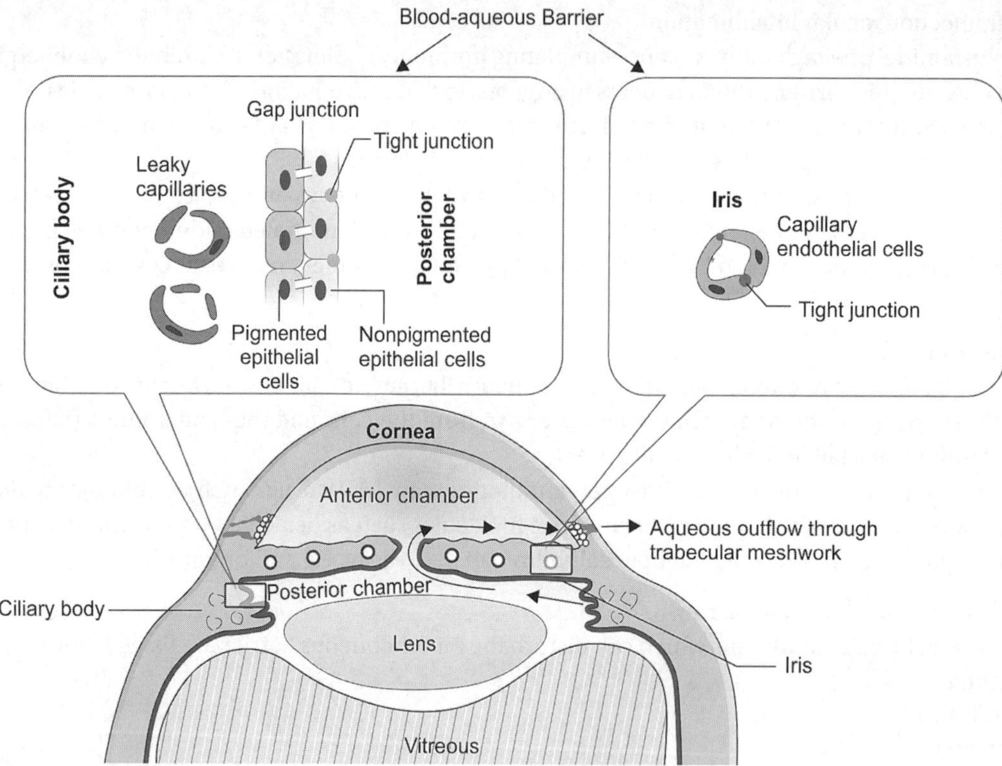

Fig. 5: Blood aqueous barrier.

10. Discuss the factors influencing intraocular pressure. (10) (WBUHS MS 2018)

The intraocular pressure (IOP) refers to the pressure exerted by intraocular contents on the coats of the eyeball. The normal level of IOP is essentially maintained by a dynamic equilibrium between the aqueous humor formation, aqueous humor outflow and episcleral venous pressure. There are some factors causing long-term changes in IOP and some factors causing short term changes in IOP.

A. Factors causing long-term changes in IOP
   1. *Heredity:* Relations of patients with primary open-angle glaucoma tend to have higher IOP.
   2. *Age:* After the age of 40, there occurs a slight increase in the mean IOP due to age related reduction in aqueous outflow, despite concomitant reduction in the aqueous production.
   3. *Sex:* IOP is equal between the sexes in ages of 20-40 years, increase in mean IOP with the age is greater in females than males.
   4. *Race:* Though population-based studies in different ethnic groups do not show significant differences in mean IOP, the race may occasionally influence IOP distribution.
   5. *Refraction:* Myopes tend to have slightly higher IOP as compared to emmetropes.

B. Factors causing short-term changes in IOP:
   1. *Arterial blood pressure:* The IOP is generally not affected by physiological changes in the arterial blood pressure, however sudden large swings may affect the IOP accordingly.
   2. *Systemic venous pressure (SVP):* Changes in SVP can cause a profound effect on IOP by affecting ipsilateral venous pressure for about 1 mm Hg rise in episcleral venous pressure(EVP) raises the IOP by 0.8 mm Hg. Common clinical conditions in which EVP is raised include external pressure of jugular veins, compression of superior vena cava by tumor, cavernous sinus thrombosis and neoplasms, inflammatory changes at the apex of the orbit.

3. *Mechanical pressure on the globe:* From outside pressure on globe initially raises the IOP by indentation but after some time due to acceleration of aqueous outflow, the IOP returns to normal and by prolonged pressure decreases below the initial levels. This forms the basis of ocular massage to lower the IOP.
4. *Plasma osmolarity:* When the total concentration of solute molecules in blood exceeds the water from eye (vitreous and perhaps aqueous also) is withdrawn, lowering the IOP. This effect is used clinically to lower IOP by use of hyperosmotic agents like mannitol. When the concentration of solutes is lower than the ocular fluids, water will enter the eye from plasma and raise the IOP, this forms the basis of water drinking test used as provocative test for glaucoma.
5. *Blood pH:* Systemic acidosis lowers the IOP by inducing carbonic anhydrase inhibition.
6. *Diurnal variation in IOP:* There are 4 types of diurnal variation curves:
   Falling type—maximal at 6-8 a.m. followed by a continuous decline (most common)
   Rising type—maximal at 4-6 p.m.
   Double variation type—with 2 peaks at 9-11 a.m. and 6 p.m.
   Flat type—with no variation.
   A diurnal variation in IOP more than 8 mm Hg is considered pathognomonic of glaucoma.
7. *Seasonal variation:* IOP with the highest pressure recorded in winter and lowest in summer.
8. *Systemic hyperthermia:* A drop in body temperature will cause a decrease in the IOP, probably by inhibition of aqueous secretion and IOP will rise with the increase in body temperature.
9. *Effect of general anaesthesia on IOP:* Some facts about the effect of general anaesthesia on IOP are as below:
   a. Acute changes in the volume of blood present in the eye due to increase in venous pressure as a result of bucking on endotracheal tube, hypertension occurring during laryngoscopy and intubation under general anaesthesia may cause a temporary increase in IOP.
   b. *Hypercapnia and hypoxia:* These will produce increase in IOP due to changes in volume of blood in the eye.
   c. *Drugs:* Diazepam, pentazocine, pethidine produce a decrease in IOP. Thiopentone sodium reduces IOP and so do most of the gaseous and volatile agents except nitrous oxide. Ketamine transiently raise the IOP when given intravenously. Suxamethonium is a notorious drug and cause rise in IOP.
10. *Effects of drugs on IOP:* Alcohol, systemic vasodilators have been reported to lower the IOP. Tobacco smoking, caffeine, LSD and corticosteroids may raise the IOP.
11. *Blockage of the circulation of aqueous:* Block may occur at 2 places
    a. At the pupil where the flow of fluid from posterior to anterior chamber may be impeded
    b. At the angle of the anterior chamber.

11. Elaborate the macroscopic and microscopic structure of iris. (10) (WBUHS 2022)

Iris is the anterior most part of uveal tissue and works like a diaphragm of a camera with a central aperture known as pupil. Macroscopic structure of iris: It can be better described under the following subdivisions.

- Anterior surface
- Posterior surface

Anterior Surface of Iris

It can be divided into 2 zones: The peripherally placed ciliary zone and the centrally placed pupillary zone, by the presence of a zigzag line known as collarette that is the remnant of the attachment of the pupillary membrane. The *collarette* is the thickest region of the iris and lies 2mm away from the pupillary margin.

Ciliary Zone

This area is characterized by radial streaks, crypts and contraction furrows. Radial streaks cover the underlying iris vessels. Crypts are depressions where the superficial part of iris is missing. They are preferred sites for creating a laser peripheral iridotomy. Contraction furrows are present concentric to the collarette.

Pupillary Zone

It is a relatively smooth zone with pigmented pupillary frill present at the pupillary margin, which is a remnant of anterior extent of the optic cup.

Posterior Surface of Iris

It is darker in color compared to the anterior surface. It is characterized by Schwalbe's contraction folds, Schwalbe's structural furrows and circular furrows.

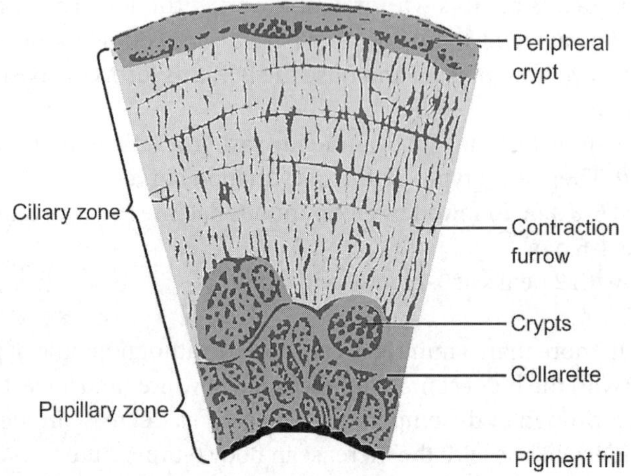

Fig. 6: Microscopic structure of iris. *(For Color version, See Color Plate 1)*

Microscopic structure of iris **(Fig. 6):**

Microscopically, the iris can be divided into 4 layers.

- Anterior limiting layer
- Iris stroma
- Anterior epithelial layer
- Posterior pigmented epithelial layer

Anterior Limiting Layer

It consists of melanocytes and fibroblasts and is the anterior most condensed part of the iris stroma.

Iris Stroma

- It is made up of collagenous network with intervening mucopolysaccharide ground substance in which is embedded the sphincter and dilator pupillae muscles, vessels and nerves.
- Sphincter pupillae lies in the pupillary zone whereas dilator pupillae lies in the posterior part of ciliary zone.

Anterior Epithelial Layer

It is the non-pigmented layer and is the anterior extension of the pigment epithelium of retina and ciliary body **(Fig. 7)**.

Posterior Pigmented Epithelial Layer

The sensory retina on approaching the ora serrata gives out and anterior extension which is the non-pigmented layer of ciliary body, that in turn continues as the posterior pigmented epithelial layer. It is derived from the inner layer of the optic cup and becomes continuous with the anterior pigmented epithelial layer at the pupillary margin.

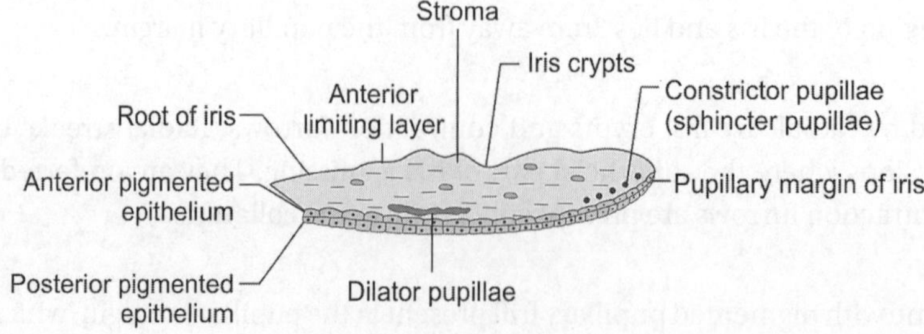

Fig. 7: Cross-section of iris.

12. Discuss in brief the various types of tonometry. (10) (TN MGRMU 2017)

Tonometry is a procedure performed to determine intraocular pressure.

Types of Tonometry

1. *Digital tonometry*
   Principle – Compressibility of ocular coat is estimated by sense of fluctuations perceived on palpitation
   Limitation – subjective, not accurate
2. Indentation tonometry –Based on the fundamental fact that weight/force will indent soft eye more than hard eye
   Prototype
   - Schiotz tonometer

   Principle: By applying standard weight via plunger, cornea is indented in a truncated cone shape in an amount which is indirectly proportional to the pressure in the eye causing volume displacement and globe distension.
   Friedenwald conversion table use to convert scale reading into IOP
   Advantages:
   - Easy to use
   - Cost effective
   - Portable

   Limitation: Depends on scleral rigidity
3. *Applanation:*
   Fixed area with variable force:
   Goldmann applanation tonometer
   Gold standard
   Slit lamp mounted
   Principle: Based on the modified Imbert-Fick principle, states that the pressure inside an ideal, dry, thin-walled sphere equals the force necessary to flatten its surface divided by the area of flattening ($p = f/a$)
   Fixed area and variable force
   Diameter – 3.06 mm
   Area – 7.35 mm^2
   Limitation: Depends on center corneal thickness
   Average CCT—520 micrometer
   Correction factor—0.7 mm Hg for every 10 micrometer
   Perkins tonometer
   Consist of biprism
   Advantages: Portable
   Uses:
   - Children
   - Bed ridden cases
   - In operative theater

   Mackay Marg tonometer
   Use plunger to applanate cornea and IOP recorded electronically
   Fixed applanation diameter 5 mm
   Used in:
   - Scarred cornea
   - Irregular cornea
   - Edematous cornea

   Tonopen tonometer
   Footplate flatten the cornea
   Microprocessor analyze the waveform internally and record IOP electronically

Used in:
- Children
- Scarred cornea
- Irregular cornea
- Over bandage contact lens

Noncontact tonometer

Principle: Puff of room air directed over patient's cornea, when intensity of light is at its peak, cornea is presumed to be flattened, time from internal reference point to the point of corneal flattening is measured and converted to IOP.

Limitation: Underestimation of IOP with increase in intraocular pressure, 3 readings should be taken to estimate IOP

Advantages:
- Use in screening
- No contamination
- Less chance of abrasion
- Can be operated by nonmedical personnel
- No anesthesia required

Rebound tonometer

Principle: Consist of two coaxial coils which propel magnetized probe towards cornea, when probe hits the cornea, the ball and wire decelerate the deceleration is more rapid if the IOP is high and slower if the IOP is low. The speed of deceleration is measured and is converted into IOP.

Advantages: Handheld, Portable

Disadvantages: Costly, not very accurate

Pneumatic tonometer

Cornea flattened by a jet of air within a small chamber

Uses:
- Deformed cornea
- Edematous cornea
- Irregular cornea
- Continuous IOP monitoring.

Newer Tonometry Techniques

Pascal dynamic contour tonometer

Measured IOP is independent of corneal thickness and rigidity

Principle: Based on contour matching instead of applanation

Tip contain hollow miniature pressure sensor in its center which influence by changes in corneal curvature, when contour of the cornea and tonometer matched then the pressure at surface of the eye is equal to the pressure inside the eye.

It also measures Ocular pulse amplitude

Advantages: Less influence by central corneal. Thickness and corneal biomechanics

Uses: Postcorneal refractive surgery

Ocular Response Analyzer

- Analyze corneal biomechanical property
- Use a column of air as the applanation force
- The difference in the pressures at the two applanation points is a measure of the corneal elasticity and uses electrooptical system to monitor corneal deformation

Contact Lens Sensor

- *Use:* 24 hours IOP monitoring
- Small change in ocular circumference, measured at corneoscleral junction corresponds to change in IOP and volume.
- 1 mm Hg changes in IOP correspond to approximately 3 micrometer in radius of curvature of cornea.

13. Describe the blood supply of uveal tissue. (10) (MS 2020)

Arterial Supply of Uveal Tissue

The uveal tissue is supplied by 3 sets of arteries -

- *Short posterior ciliary arteries:* Arising from the ophthalmic artery by 2 trunks, they subdivide into 10–20 branches and pierce the sclera around optic nerve to supply the choroid.
- *Long posterior ciliary arteries:* They are 2 in number, branch out from the ophthalmic artery to pierce the sclera on either side of the optic nerve obliquely, traversing in the suprachoroidal space to reach the ciliary muscle, on the anterior aspect of which it meets with the anterior ciliary arteries to form the major arterial circle.
- *Anterior ciliary arteries* ***(Fig. 8)****:* The muscular branches of ophthalmic artery traverse anteriorly to form the anterior ciliary arteries. These arteries are 7 in number: 2 each from the arteries of superior rectus, inferior rectus and medial rectus muscles and one from that of lateral rectus muscle. The arteries pass anteriorly and join long posterior ciliary arteries to form the major arterial circle.

Venous Drainage of the Uveal Tissue

Blood from the uveal tissue is carried by the following set of veins:

- *Anterior ciliary veins:* They drain the area of the ciliary muscle and join the corresponding muscular veins.
- *Smaller veins from the sclera:* They carry blood mainly from the sclera and correspond to scleral branches of short ciliary arteries.
- *Venae verticosae:* These are 4 in number and pierce the sclera obliquely on each side of the superior and inferior recti muscles respectively, around 6 mm behind the equator of the globe. They drain blood from whole of the choroid and also receive anterior tributaries from the iris, ciliary processes, ciliary muscle and anterior aspect of the choroid.

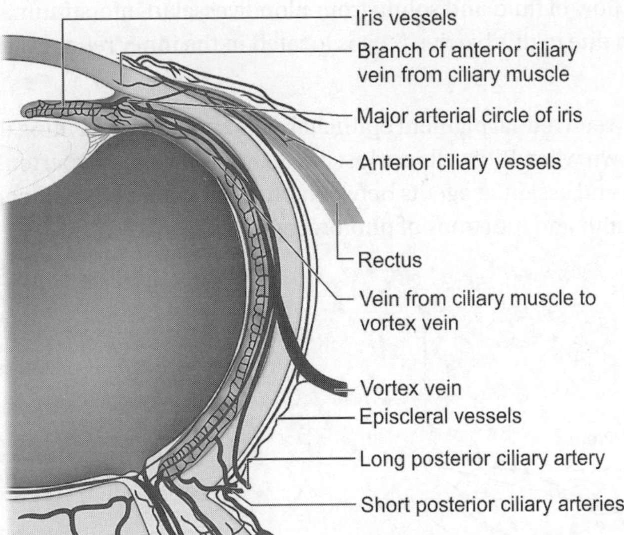

Fig. 8: Blood supply of uveal tissue.

Source: Khurana AK. Anatomy and Physiology of Eye, 3rd edition. Amsterdam: Elsevier; 2013. Chapter 3, p. 70.

14. Short note on ciliary zonules. (5) (TN MGRMU 2021)

It is triangular in shape, forward continuation of choroid at ora serrata, and iris is attached at its middle part. The anterior part having finger like processes is called pars plicata and posterior smooth part is called pars plana (5 mm wide temporally and 3 mm nasally). The anterior side of triangle forms part of angle of anterior and posterior chamber.

Microscopically the ciliary body consists of 5 layers.

1. Supraciliary lamina-Outermost condensed part and posteriorly it is continuous with suprachoroidal lamina and anteriorly with anterior limiting membrane of iris.

2. Stroma of ciliary body-made of collagens and fibroblasts with ciliary muscle with longitudinal, circular and radial fiber, vessel, nerve, pigment cells and vascular stroma.
3. Layer of pigmented epithelium-forward continuation of RPE and further continues anteriorly as anterior pigment epithelium of iris.
4. Layer of nonpigmented epithelium-forward continuation of sensory retina and further continues anteriorly as posterior pigment epithelium of iris.
5. Internal limiting membrane-forward continuation of internal limiting membrane of retina.

Ultrastructure of ciliary process:
1. Capillary network-lined by thin endothelium with fenestrae, mural cells, pericytes.
2. Stroma-ground substance consists of mucopolysaccharides, proteins, collagen, wandering cells.
3. Two layers of epithelium-outer pigmented and inner nonpigmented epithelium. Tight junctions between cells of this layer create part of blood aqueous barrier.

15. What is blood retinal barrier? (5) (TN MGRMU 2018)

It is a selective barrier that controls passage of molecules, ions, water and cells between blood and retina. It is highly specialized physiological barrier crucial for maintaining unique and tightly regulated environment of retina. It selectively allows glucose, O_2 while restricting other harmful agents. These selective permeability and physical blockade is by intercellular tight junctions to create an optical neural homeostasis. It is of 2 types-inner and outer **(Fig. 9)**.

Inner Blood Retinal Barrier

Retinal capillary endothelial cells form blood retinal barrier, as they are closely bound to each other by intercellular tight junctions of zonula occludens and these along with pericytes, mural cells astrocytes and macroglial foot processes in normal condition prevent free flow of fluid and solute from blood vessel to interstitium. Absence of fluorescein leakage from these capillaries also seen due to this barrier. So it is located in the inner retinal vasculature.

Outer Blood Retinal Barrier

It consists of tight junctions between retinal pigment epithelial cells and thus preventing the leakage of fluid from choroid to retina. This barrier breaks down when RPE cells are lost due to ischemia as in hypertensive choroidopathy. It regulates the transport of nutrients, ions and essential agents between photoreceptor cells and choroidal vasculature and plays a vital role in maintaining the health and functions of photoreceptor cells.

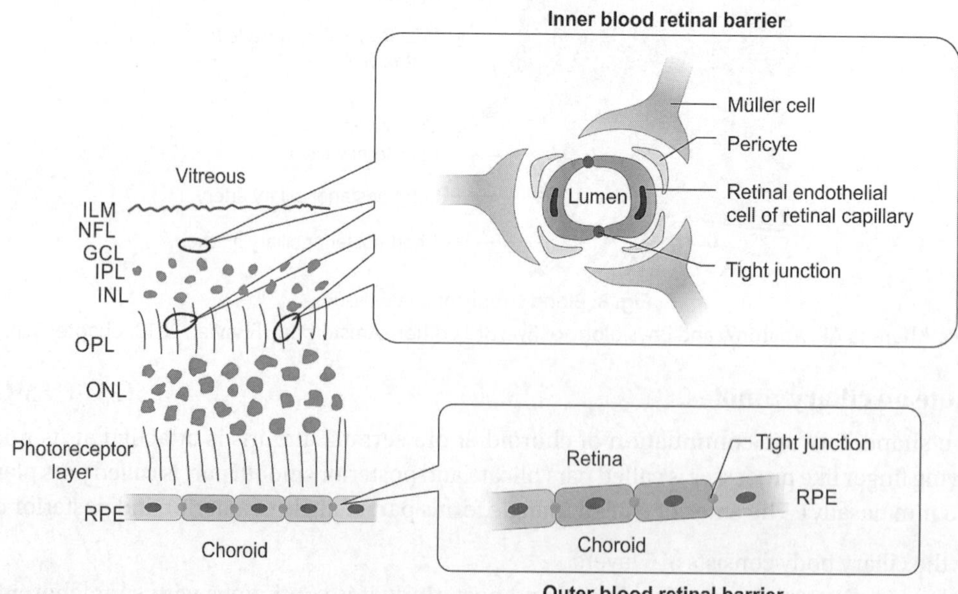

Fig. 9: Blood retinal barrier.

16. Write a short note on Rods and cones. (5) (TN MGRMU 2018)

1. Rods and cones are the end organs of vision which transform light energy to visual impulse.
2. Number of rods, 120 million while there are 6.5 million cones
3. *Distribution:* The rods are absent in the fovea but a large number is present 5-6 mm from the fovea. They are maximum below the optic disc and their numbers decrease towards the periphery. The cones are present in the fovea, their number falls outside the foveal zone with more cones in the nasal retina than temporal.
4. *Rods:* Each rod is 40-60 μm long. They have an outer segment which is cylindrical and contains the visual pigment rhodopsin. There are numerous lipid protein lamellar discs in stacks and surrounded by cell membrane. The inner segment has 2 regions- ellipsoid and myoid. Ellipsoid contains mitochondria while myoid contains glycogen and organelles. Rod inner segment ends as the inner rod fiber, terminal end of which is dilated as a bulb, called rod spherule.
5. *Cones:* Each cone cell is 40-80 μm long. The outer segment is conical and contains pigment iodopsin. The lamellar discs are similar to rods but narrower. Cone inner segment is similar to rod but the ellipsoid zone contains large number of mitochondria. The inner segment is continuous with its nucleus and lies in outer nuclear layer. Cones end as cone foot/ cone pedicle.

   There are three types of cons: red, blue, green

17. Retinal pigment epithelium- short note. (5) (WBUHS DO 2014)

It is the outer most layer of retina, consisting single layer of hexagonal cells. It is firmly attached to Bruch's membrane and loosely attached to layers of rod and cones. The potential space between RPE and sensory retina is called subretinal space. Fluid collection within this space called subretinal fluid and separation between these two layers is called retinal detachment.

RPE cells are connected to each other by tight junctions, zonulae occludens and zonulae adherens. RPE cells are also responsible for foveal dark color, as they become more taller and pigmented at fovea. The RPE cells appear dark brown due to their melanin content, that reduces damage to retina and internal nerves from ultraviolet light.

RPE cells have major functions in our visual system. These are:

1. Renewal and recycling of Vitamin A, which is important for photoreceptor function.
2. Maintain outer blood-retinal barrier and the integrity of subretinal space by RPE pump mechanism, that helps to clear out any fluid.
3. Transport of important nutrients and metabolites through blood-retinal barrier.
4. Mechanical support to photoreceptors.
5. Pigment in RPE has optical function by absorbing light.
6. Phagocytic action.
7. It prevents oxidative damage by reducing excessive accumulation of reactive oxygen species (ROS) and consequent oxidative damage.

Alterations in the RPE layer may affect vision and lead to a variety of retinopathies, such as - retinitis pigments, age related macular degeneration, Stargardt's disease, etc.

18. Describe the pupillary pathway and discuss in detail abnormal pupillary reactions (10) (WBUHS MS 2019)

As light is shone in one eye, both the pupils constrict. Constriction of the pupil over which light is shore is part of the direct light reflex. The pupil of the other eye that constricts in response to the light is part of the consensual light reflex.

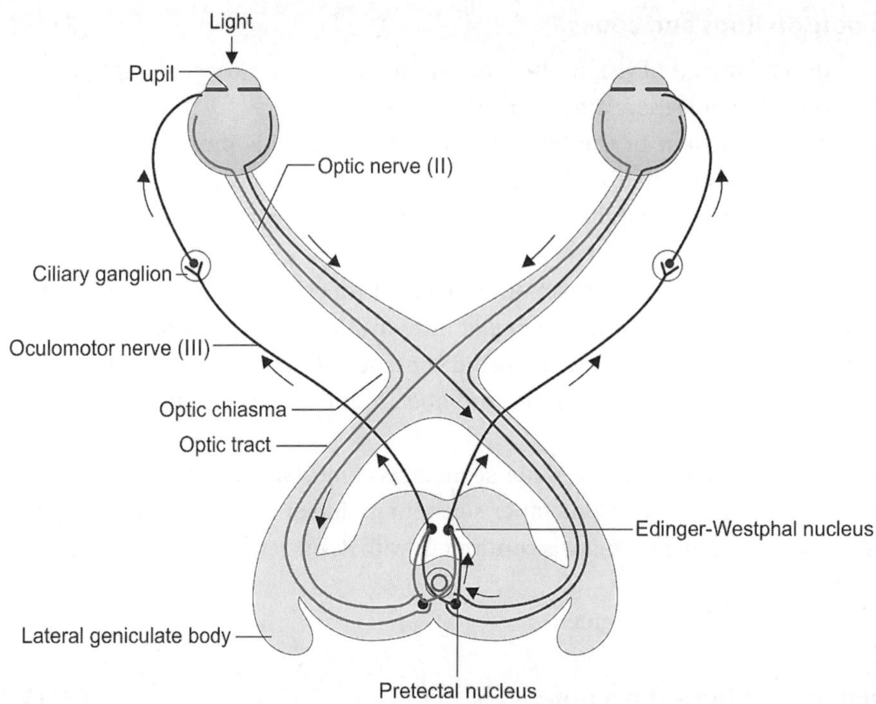

Fig. 10: Pupillary light reflex pathway.

Pupillary Light Reflex Pathway

The *afferent fibers* begin at the retina and relay to the midbrain. Rods and cones are stimulated as light falls on retina, the stimulus is then transmitted to the ganglion cells and travel along the optic nerve to the chiasma.

Fibers of the nasal retinae decussate and travel along the opposite optic tract to terminate in the contralateral pretectal nucleus, while fibers of the temporal retinae remain uncrossed and travel along the optic tract of the same side to terminate in the ipsilateral pretectal nucleus.

Internuncial fibers connect each pretectal nucleus with Edinger–Westphal nucleus of *both* the sides.

Parasympathetic fibers from the Edinger–Westphal nucleus in the midbrain constitute the *efferent fibers*. These then travel along the inferior division of the oculomotor nerve and relay into the ciliary ganglion, via nerve to inferior oblique. The post ganglionic nerves travel along the short ciliary nerves to innovate the sphincter pupillae.

Abnormal Pupillary Reflexes (Fig. 10)

Afferent Pathway Defects

Total afferent pathway defect: Complete optic nerve or retinal lesion leads to complete blindness on the affected side. There is absence of direct light reflex on the affected side and loss of consensual light reflex of the normal side. When the normal eye is stimulated, both the pupils constrict normally.

Relative afferent pupillary defect: It is a paradoxical reaction of pupil to light, which is caused by an incomplete optic nerve lesion or severe retinal disease. It is tested by swinging flashlight test.

Wernicke's hemianopic pupil: It is caused by an optic tract lesion, where nasal fibers from contralateral eye and temporal fibers from ipsilateral eye are affected.

Efferent Pathway Defects

Causes of Efferent Pupillary Defects

- Brainstem lesions
- Fascicular third nerve lesions
- Lesions of the ciliary ganglion

- Damage to iris tissue
- Pharmacological mydriasis

Tonic pupil: Damage to the ciliary ganglion or short ciliary nerves results in a dilated pupil devoid of light reflex, near reflex being slow and tonic and paresis of accommodation.

Argyll Robertson pupil: Lesion at the level of tectum i.e., rostral midbrain near Sylvian fissure results in light near dissociation where pupillary light reflex is absent but accommodation reflex is present.

19. Write a short note on Grades of binocular vision. (5) (TNMGRMU, WBUHS MS 2023)

Binocular single vision (BSV) is characterized by ability to fuse the images from the two eyes and to perceive binocular depths. BSV can be graded on the synaptophore as below **(Fig. 11)**.

First grade (simultaneous perception) is tested by introducing two dissimilar but not mutually antagonistic pictures, such as a bird and cage.

The subject is then asked to put the bird into the cage by moving the arm of synaptophore.

If the two pictures cannot be seen simultaneously, then suppression is present.

Some retinal rivalry will occur although one picture is smaller than other, so that while the small one is seen foveally, the larger one is seen parafoveally.

Larger macular and paramacular slides are used if foveal slides cannot be superimposed.

Second grade (fusion). If simultaneous perception slide can be superimposed then the test proceeds to the second grade, which is the ability of the two eyes to produce a composite picture (sensory fusion) from two similar pictures, each of which is incomplete in one small detail.

The classic example is two rabbits, one lacking a tail and the other lacking a bunch of flowers. If fusion is present, one rabbit complete with tail and flowers will be seen.

The range of fusion (motor fusion) is then tested by moving the arms of synoptophores so that the eyes have to converge and diverge in order to maintain fusion.

The presence of simple fusion without any range is of little value in everyday life.

Third grade (stereopsis) is the ability to obtain an impression of depth by superimposition of two pictures of the same object which have taken from slightly different angles. The classic example is a bucket, which should be appreciated in three dimension.

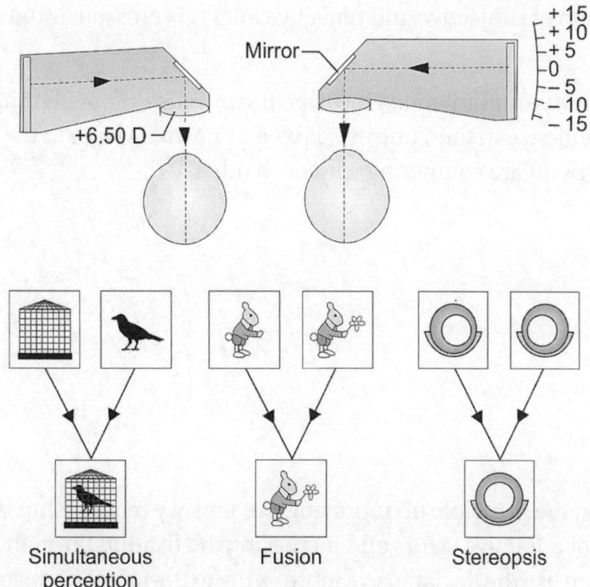

Fig. 11: Grades of Binocular vision.

Source: Jack K, Salmon JF. Kanski's Clinical Ophthalmology, 9th edition. Amsterdam: Elsevier; 2019. Chapter 18, p. 716.

20. Write a short note on Depth perception. (5) (TN MGRMU 2015)

Depth perception is the ability to see things in 3 dimensions and to judge the distance of objects.

i. Binocular vision-for accurate depth perception, there should be binocular vision. In a process called convergence, our eyes see an object from 2 angles and the brain processes them as a single image.
ii. Monocular vision- even with 1 eye depth can be perceived as Motion parallax- as one moves, the objects closer appear to move faster than those away. This helps the brain judge the distance.
iii. Accommodation- the change in the shape of the lens to focus on objects at different distances, also aides in depth perception.
iv. Stereopsis-the ability of the visual cortex to process 2 different images into a single image with depth.
v. Convergence- the inward movement of the eye when focusing on closer objects provides a cue for depth perception.

Depth perception gets impaired due to eye conditions like blurry vision, strabismus, amblyopia.

21. Write a short note on Anomalous retinal correspondence. (5) (WBUHS DO 2019)

Anomalous retinal correspondence (ARC) is a condition that occurs when light from a point in focus hits the fovea of one eye and an extra-foveal point of the other eye. Under normal circumstance, if the same image stimulates 2 non similar points on the retina, there should be diplopia. But in ARC, with time, the foveal and extra-foveal points of the respective eyes coordinate to produce a single image. This is a motor adaptation of the eyes to prevent diploma.

Etiology

The cause of ARC is due to foveal misalignment which is primarily due to strabismus. In terms of prevalence, as the angle of deviation of the eye in strabismus increases, the presence of ARC decreases. It is seen more commonly in esotropia than in exotropia.
Types of ARC depends on the objective and subjective angles of the anomaly.

Objective angle: It is the motor deviation, the angle of deviation that can be observed on the patient.

Subjective angle: It signifies the sensory deviation, the angle that patient perceives while adjusting the knobs of the synaptophore.

i. *Harmonious:* Objective angle = subjective angle
ii. *Unharmonious:* Objective angle > subjective angle.
iii. *Paradoxical:* If the localization of subjective and objective angles is crossed or uncrossed.

Clinical Features

Patient presents with strabismus without diplopia. However, it can cause binocular diplopia if a patient presents with normal and anomalous correspondence in the same eye as well as normal vision in the other eye. In this case, the fovea of both eyes and the extra-foveal point are competing with each other.

Diagnostic Procedures

i. Worth 4-dot test
ii. Bagolini striated glasses
iii. Cover test
iv. Synaptophore
v. Red filter test
vi. After image test

Treatment

The treatment modalities work on the principle of improving the sensory relationship between the two foveas and each retina. These include correction of refractive errors and increasing the fixation through the fovea of the deviated eye.

i. Occlusion of the normal eye to use the deviated eye more as the extra-foveal corresponding point is in the peripheral retina, there is suppression between the periphery and fovea. It reduces the use of the extra-foveal retinal spot and increases the use of actual fovea.

ii. Prisms—direct light into the fovea and can be used for small deviations.
iii. Using red filter on the deviated eye to stimulate the cones in the fovea increasing its use.
iv. Amblyoscope
v. Use of botulinum toxin is a newer therapy- it is injected in the extraocular muscles of the eye to correct deviation.

22. Write a short note on Panum's area. (5) (WBUHS MS 2014, 2024)

Panum's fusional area is a concept that allows for single binocular vision about the point of fixation even when corresponding retinal points are not being stimulated.

An image on the retina of one eye can be fused with a similar image on the retina of the other eye even though disparity in the retinal image exists.

Panum's fusional area is needed for stereopsis, as it defines the zone of stereovision. If images do not fall in the Panum's area, then diplopia results. Size of the Panum's area increases with retinal eccentricity. At fovea, it is 6-10 degrees of an arc.

Retinal element in one eye corresponds not only with a single point in the other but with an elliptical area surrounding the exactly corresponding point.

The objects within this area are seen as single images. The objects farther away are seen with uncrossed disparity, and the objects closer to the viewer are seen with crossed disparity **(Fig. 12)**.

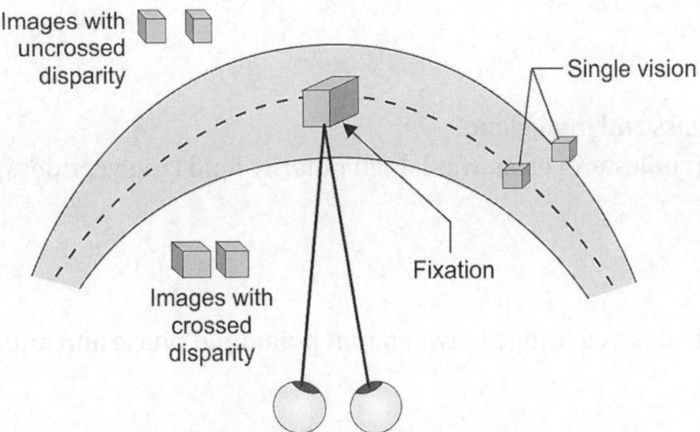

Fig. 12: Panum's fusional area.

23. Describe in brief: Anatomy of lacrimal gland. (5) (TN MGRMU 2018)

Lacrimal gland is a branched tubuloalveolar gland, supplied by lacrimal artery, a branch of ophthalmic artery. Main and accessory lacrimal glands of Krause, Wolfring comprise the structures related with formation of tear and its drainage through lacrimal puncta, canaliculi, lacrimal sac and nasolacrimal duct **(Fig. 13)**.

Main lacrimal gland lies in the lacrimal fossa in the lateral part of orbital roof at the orbital plate of frontal bone. The lacrimal gland is divided into superior orbital and inferior palpebral part by aponeurosis of levator muscle.

Orbital part of lacrimal gland has superior surface that lies in contact with periorbita of frontal bone, inferior surface that lies in contact with LPS muscle, sharp anterior border that is with contact with septum orbitale, round posterior border that is contact with orbital pad of fat, lateral end that is in contact with lateral rectus and medial end that is related to LPS.

Palpebral part of lacrimal gland is about 1/3rd size of orbital part and it is separated from orbital part by LPS, which lies superiorly.

About 10-12 ducts of lacrimal gland open in the lateral part of superior fornix.

Applied anatomy: As all the lacrimal ducts pass through palpebral part of gland, excision of this part alone can lead to deficiency of tear film.

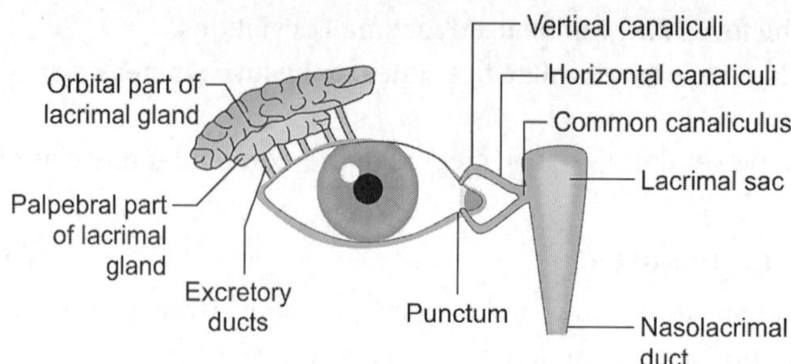

Fig. 13: Anatomy of lacrimal gland.

24. Write in brief about Tear Film and its functions. (10) (WBUHS MS 2021)

Main role of lacrimal system is to establish and maintain continuous tear film over ocular surface for high quality refractive surface and well-being of cornea and conjunctival epithelium.

Layer of tear Film: It consist of three layers

1. Outer lipid layer
2. Intermediate aqueous layer
3. Inner mucin layer

Lipid Layer

- Outer most layer
- 0.1 to 0.2 μm thickness
- Secreted by - meibomian, zeiss and moll gland.
- Content -low polarity lipid (cholesterol ester, wax), high polarity lipid (triglycerides, phospholipid)

Function

- Prevent overflow of tear
- Prevent evaporation
- Act as surfactant layer which acts as a bridge between non polar lipid phase and aqueous mucinous phase

Aqueous Layer

- Middle layer
- 8 μm in thickness
- Form main bulk of tear film
- Thin layer over cornea and conjunctiva
- Secreted by—main and accessory lacrimal gland of Krause and Wolfring
- *Content:* Protein, glycoprotein, urea, glucose, enzymes, inorganic salt, immunoglobulin A and lactoferrin.
- Buffering capacity is due to bicarbonate ions

Function

- Provide oxygen to corneal epithelium
- Washes away debris and irritant
- Antibacterial activity by lysozyme and betalysin

Mucus Layer

- Innermost layer
- Secreted mainly by conjunctival goblet cell
- 0.02 to 0.04 μm thickness
- Mucin exist as a network distributed in aqueous body of tear film
- Glycocalyx hold the mucin to corneal surface also emanate as transmembrane molecule into the aqueous and are anchored at the cell membrane

Function

- Play vital role in stability of tear film
- Convert hydrophobic to hydrophilic corneal epithelium
- Lubricate Ocular and palpebral surface
- Provide slippery coating over foreign body, thus protect against abrasive effect of such particles
- Absorbs various organic compound in tear.

Function of Tear Film

1. To make cornea a smooth optical surface
2. Keep conjunctiva and cornea moist and prevent from drying
3. Flush out debris and noxious irritant
4. Antibacterial properties owing to presence of - lysozyme, lactoferrin, beta lysine, immunoglobulin and other proteins
5. Lubricant for preocular surface and lid and prevent friction while blinking
6. Transfer oxygen from air to cornea
7. Provide pathway for white blood cells in case of injury

25. Describe the different muscles and ligaments attached to eyelids and their function.

(5+5) (WBUHS MS 2021)

From outside inwards each eyelid consists of following layers **(Fig. 14)**

- Skin
- Layer of subcutaneous areolar tissue
- Layer of striated muscle
- Submuscular areolar tissue
- Fibrous layer
- Layer of nonstriated muscle
- Conjunctiva

Layer of striated muscle: This layer consists of—

a. Orbicularis muscle
b. Levator muscle (in upper eyelid)

Orbicularis oculi muscle can be divided into 2 parts - orbital and palpebral.

Orbital part forms the most peripheral fibers of orbicularis oculi which arise from anterior part of medial palpebral ligament (MPL) and upper orbital margin medial to supraorbital notch, maxillary process of frontal bone, frontal process of maxilla and lower orbital margin medial to infraorbital foramen. From this origin, muscle fiber sweep superiorly and inferiorly and meet at lateral palpebral raphe. At the upper eyelid orbicularis joins with the fiber of frontalis and gets inserted at the skin of eyebrow. Upper medial fibers of orbital part passes to skin of the medial part of eye brow, known as musculus superciliaris. In lower part, medial and lateral peripheral fibers of orbital part attached to the skin of cheek, known as musculus malaris.

Palpebral parts also divided into preseptal and pretarsal portions. Preseptal fibers arise from lacrimal fascia, posterior lacrimal crest (deep head), anterior part of MPL (superficial head), which passes superiorly and inferiorly in front of orbital septum and unite at the lateral palpebral raphe.

Pretarsal fibers arises from lacrimal fascia and posterior lacrimal crest (deep head) and MPL (superficial head). The fibers pass laterally above and below the upper and lower tarsus to join laterally to form lateral canthal tendon, which is inserted at the lateral orbital tubercle of Whitnall.

Fibers of pretarsal which arise from lacrimal fascia and upper part of posterior lacrimal crest helping in tear drainage are called pars lacrimalis (Horner's muscle). Fibers of pretarsal which run along lid margin are called pars ciliaris (muscle of Riolan).

Orbital part of orbicularis oculi helps in forced closure of eyelids and palpebral part of orbicularis oculi helps in gentle closure of eyelids.

Orbicularis oculi muscle is supplied by branches of facial nerve.

Levator palpebrae superioris muscle- Arises at the orbital apex from under surface of lesser wing of sphenoid above annulus of Zinn, intermingled with origin of superior rectus muscle.

LPS has flat ribbon like belly, it passes forward below orbital roof slight nasally, above superior rectus and widens as it extend forward and descends vertically up to the septum orbitale. Ultimately it fans out into glistening tendon, i.e., aponeurosis and forms lateral and medial horns.

Medial horn passes over reflected tendon of superior oblique and fuses with upper border of medial canthal tendon. Thicker lateral horn dividing lacrimal gland into orbital and palpebral parts insert into lateral canthal tendon.

LPS aponeurosis passes through septum orbitale and runs forward and downward up to superior border of tarsus. Fibers of LPS are inserted into pretarsal skin of eyelid forming superior lid fold. Few fibers of muscle insert onto anterior surface of tarsus, 3-4 mm below superior border of tarsus and also attached to superior conjunctival fornix.

Fleshy part of LPS is 40 mm long and aponeurosis part of LPS is 15 mm long. Fleshy part of LPS runs horizontally and aponeurosis part of LPS runs vertically and direction changing occur at the level of superior transverse ligament of Whitnall (check ligament of LPS).

Superior transverse ligament of Whitnall (check ligament of LPS) is condensation of superior sheath of levator joined by sheath of reflected tendon of superior oblique and its thickened orbital fascia which extends from trochlear pulley to orbital lobe of lacrimal gland. LPS acts as upper lid elevator. LPS muscle is supplied by a branch of superior division of oculomotor nerve.

Applied anatomy: Injury to Whitnall ligament leads to failure of ptosis surgery.

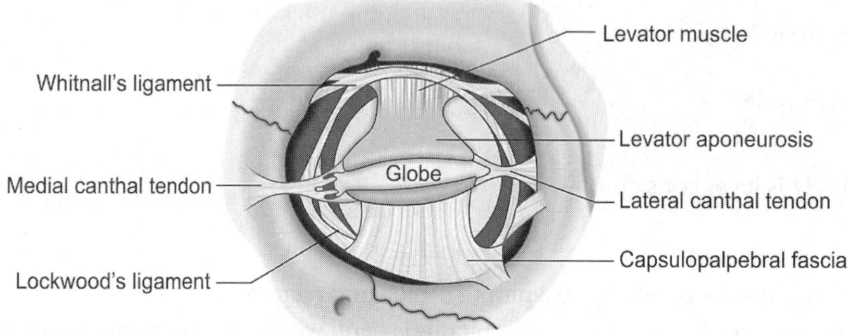

Fig. 14: Ligaments of the eyelid.

26. Write a short note on Lower lid retractors. (5) (TN MGRMU, WBUHS MS 2015)

These are system of muscles and tissues that depress the lower eyelid. These are mainly capsulopalpebral fascia and inferior tarsal muscle, which are analogous to levator aponeurosis and Muller's muscle in upper eye lid.

Capsulopalpebral fascia originates as capsulopalpebral head of inferior rectus muscle, divides and encircles the inferior oblique muscle, fuses with it and joins to form Lockwood ligament.

Inferior tarsal muscle, also known as inferior palpebral muscle runs between capsulopalpebral fascia and conjunctiva which starts at Lockwood ligament and extends to inferior conjunctival fornix with insertion to inferior tarsal border and ultimately to orbital septum. As it is innervated by sympathetic nerve, Horner's syndrome or sympathetic disruption causes inverse or reverse ptosis of lower eyelid.

Retraction of lower eyelid usually presents with dry eye and exposure keratopathy. Lower eyelid retractors depress eyelid in downgaze and maintain tarsal plate in upright position.

Applied anatomy: Conditions where lower lid eyelid retractors are lost, reconstructions are needed, cartilage replaces lower lid fascia, so lid will not move down with down gaze and so walking downstairs or reading may be troublesome and require adjustment i.e., cosmetic blepharoplasty may be needed.

27. Write a short note on central retinal artery—its course and branches. (5) (TN MGRMU, WBUHS MS 2016)

It is a major artery that supplies blood to retina and surface of optic nerve. It is an end artery with wavy course, arise from ophthalmic artery close to optic foramen with closely adherent to dura.

10-15 mm behind eye, it bends upwards along with inferomedial aspect of nerve, pierce dura and arachnoid to enter subarachnoid space.

Within subarachnoid space, it bends forwards and upwards at right angle and invaginates pia to reach center of nerve, surrounded with pial vessels and sympathetic nerve plexuses (nerve of Tiedemann).

In the center of optic nerve, artery with vein in its temporal side runs anteriorly to pierce lamina cribrosa. In the optic nerve head, it lies superficially and nasally, covered with glial tissue (meniscus of Kuhnt), divided into superior and inferior branch, which again subdivided into temporal and nasal branch at or near optic disc margin.

In the retina all these branches divide dichotomously as they proceed towards ora serrata, where they end without anastomosis.

28. Write a short note on choriocapillaris. (5) (WBUHS MS 2019)

It is a rich capillary network, which is freely anastomosing, highly permeable and mainly nourishes RPE and outer retinal layers. These capillaries are fenestrated and consists of endothelial cells joined by zonulae occludentes.

The choroidal vasculature can be divided into two categories: choriocapillaris and large caliber veins and arteries (Sattler's layer and Haller's layer).

These capillaries receive most of their blood from medium and large vessels from stroma. These capillaries are divided into non-overlapping lobules and not in free anastomosis. Endothelial cells are lined by basement membrane containing pericytes.

These capillaries are of large caliber so that 2-3 RBC s can pass through these at a time, whereas RBC s pass in single file in other capillaries.

Choriocapillaris have the following important functions.

1. Sustaining the photoreceptors
2. Filtering out waste products produced by outer retinal layers
3. Regulating the temperature of the macula

Applied anatomy: Choriocapillaris are densest in the subfoveal region and this can be measured as subfoveal choroidal thickness in ED-OCT, which may be altered in diseases such as diabetic retinopathy.

29. Write a short note on posterior ciliary arteries. (5) (WBUHS MS 2018)

These arteries mainly supply uveal tract. There are mainly 2 types of posterior ciliary arteries.

1. *Short posterior ciliary arteries:* They arise in two trunks from main ophthalmic artery. Each trunk is divided into 10-20 branches which pierce sclera around optic nerve to supply choroid in segmental manner.
2. *Long posterior ciliary arteries:* These are two, mainly nasal and temporal. They pierce sclera obliquely on medial and lateral side of optic nerve, running through suprachoroidal space to ciliary muscle. At anterior end of ciliary muscle, they anastomose with each other and with anterior ciliary arteries to form major arterial circle to supply uveal tract.

30. Describe with diagram the blood supply of optic nerve head. (10) (WBUHS MS 2022)

What is the blood supply of different parts of optic nerve? Support with a diagram. (10) (WBUHS MS 2019)

The optic nerve begins as a continuation of axons of ganglion cells from the optic disc and extends up to the optic chiasma where the nerves of both the sides meet and continue as optic tract.

Morphologically and embryologically, the optic nerve is synonymous to a sensory white matter tract of the brain due to the following features:

- It is an outgrowth of the brain

- It is not covered by neurilemma and does not regenerate when cut
- It is surrounded by meninges

Parts of Optic Nerve

- *Intraocular* part
  - Surface nerve fiber layer
  - Prelaminar region
  - Lamina cribrosa
  - Retrolaminar region
- *Intraorbital* part
- *Intracanalicular* part
- *Intracranial* part

Intraocular Part

Surface Nerve Fiber Layer

Essentially composed of nerve fibers coming from retina that converge at the optic disc. The internal limiting membrane of Elschnig is a thin layer of astrocytes covering the optic disc, separating it from vitreous.

Prelaminar Region

Composed of neurons and a significantly higher quantity of astrocytes. A layer of astrocytes surrounding this part separates it from the choroid.

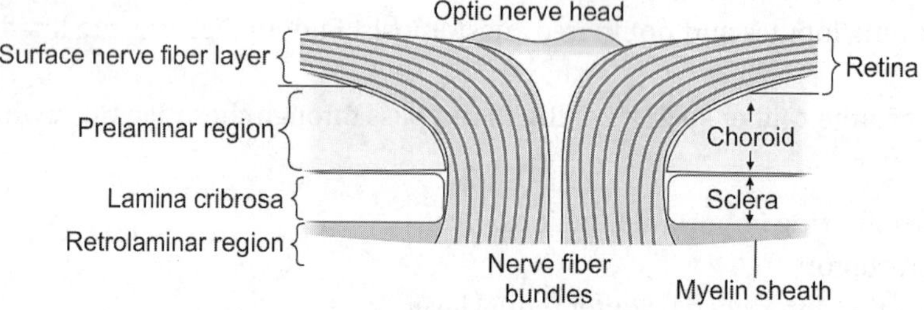

Fig. 15: Blood supply of optic nerve head.

Lamina Cribrosa

It is a sieve-like tissue made up of fenestrated sheets of scleral connective tissue lined by glial tissue all around.

Retrolaminar Region

There is a significant decrease in astrocytes in this area and the oligodendrocytes provide the myelin sheath to it. Addition of myelin sheath increases the diameter of the optic nerve as it passes through the sclera.

Blood Supply of Optic Nerve (Fig. 15)

Intraocular Part

- *Surface nerve fiber layer:* Capillaries derived from retinal arterioles that anastomose with the vessels of prelaminar region and central retinal artery of retina.
- *Prelaminar region:* Vessels from the short posterior ciliary arteries
- *Lamina cribrosa region:* Vessels derived from short posterior ciliary arteries and arterial circle of Zinn-Haller.
- *Retrolaminar region:* Supplied by both ciliary and retinal circulation. The central retinal artery provides centripetal and centrifugal branches.

Intraorbital Part

Supplied by two system of vessels—periaxial and axial system

Periaxial system: Vessels derived from the following arteries derived from the internal carotid artery: ophthalmic artery, lacrimal artery, central retinal artery of retina, long and short posterior ciliary arteries.

Axial system: Vessels derived from central retinal artery of retina before it pierces optic nerve.

Intracanalicular Part

It is supplied by a periaxial system of vessels formed by the pial plexus supplied by ophthalmic artery.

Intracranial Part

It is supplied by periaxial system of vessels made up of the pial plexus supplied by—

- Branches from internal carotid artery
- Branches from anterior cerebral artery
- Small recurrent branches from ophthalmic artery
- Small branches from anterior communicating artery

31. Describe the anatomy of cavernous sinus and its applied importance. (4+6) (WBUHS MS 2023)

Relations of cavernous sinus. (5) (WBUHS MS 2020)

Inside the middle cranial fossa on either side of body of the sphenoid bone lies a large venous space known as the cavernous sinus that gives passage to various important structures of the orbit.

Formation

Formed by the joining of the superior and inferior ophthalmic veins as they pass through the superior orbital fissure.

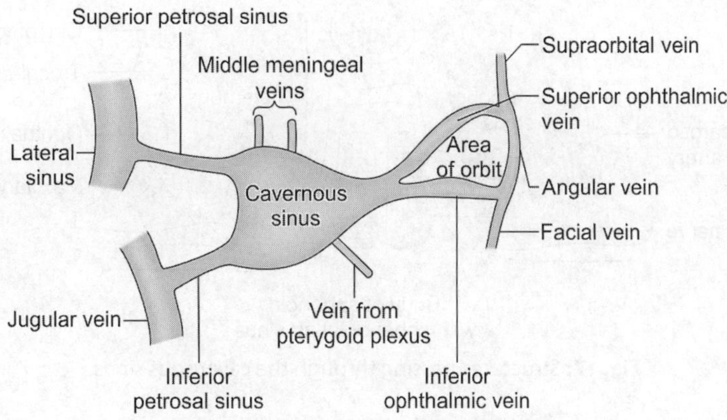

Fig. 16: Relations of the cavernous sinus.

Drainage

Blood from cavernous sinus drains into the superior and inferior petrosal sinus which in turn drain into the lateral sinus and internal jugular vein respectively.

Relations of the cavernous sinus **(Fig. 16)**:

Anteriorly

Superior and inferior ophthalmic veins; superior orbital fissure and apex of the orbit

Posteriorly

Superior and inferior petrosal sinus draining into the lateral sinus and the internal jugular vein respectively; apex of petrous temporal

Superiorly

Optic tract, internal carotid artery and anterior perforated substance

Inferiorly

Foramen lacerum and junction of body and greater wing of sphenoid bone

Medially

Pituitary gland and sphenoidal air cells

Laterally

Temporal Lobe with Uncus

Structures in the lateral wall of cavernous sinus (from above downwards) **(Fig. 17)**:

- *Oculomotor nerve:* Divide into superior and inferior divisions that exit through superior orbital fissure
- *Trochlear nerve:* Crosses superficial to third nerve and exits through superior orbital fissure
- *Ophthalmic nerve:* It is the first division of the trigeminal nerve that further subdivides into lacrimal, frontal and nasociliary nerves
- *Maxillary nerve:* Second division of trigeminal nerve that passes through foremen rotundum

Structures Passing Through the Center of Cavernous Sinus

- *Internal carotid artery:* With the sympathetic plexus around it
- *Abducent nerve:* Inferolateral to the artery.

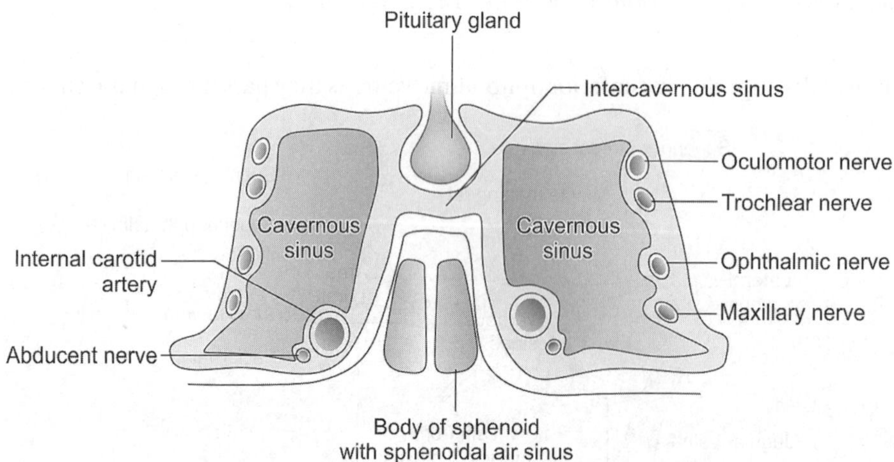

Fig. 17: Structures passing through the cavernous sinus.

Applied Importance of Cavernous Sinus

- As all the venous channels in relation to the sinus are valveless, any foci of infection in the drainage basin of the concerned vein draining superficial areas of the face and orbit may pass directly into the cranial cavity without much resistance.
- Any lesion of the cavernous sinus may lead to total ophthalmoplegia due to the presence of important cranial nerves (those supplying the orbit) in the lateral wall and inside the sinus.

32. Describe in brief about bones forming wall of orbit. (10) (TNMGRMU 2018, WBUHS MS 2019)

Each orbit is formed by following bones, e.g., frontal, ethmoid, lacrimal, palatine, maxilla, zygomatic and sphenoid to cover two quadrangular truncated pyramids situated between anterior cranial fossa above and maxillary sinuses below. It has four walls-medial, lateral, roof and floor which meet with each other at different angles of orbit.

Medial Wall of Orbit

Quadrilateral shaped, thinnest wall of orbit, formed by frontal process of maxilla, lacrimal bone, orbital plate of ethmoid and body of sphenoid. Lacrimal sac resides at the anterior part of this wall in lacrimal fossa, medial to it lie anterior ethmoid sinus in upper part and medial meatus of nose in lower part. Lacrimal fossa is bounded by anterior and posterior lacrimal crest formed by maxillary and lacrimal bone respectively.

Behind posterior lacrimal crest following structures seen:

Horner's muscle, septum orbitale, check ligament of medial rectus.

Medial to medial wall following structures seen-

Anterior ethmoidal air sinus, middle meatus of nose, middle and posterior ethmoid sinuses and sphenoidal air sinus.

Orbital surface of medial wall is related to superior oblique muscle in upper part, medial rectus muscle in middle part, and in between two-anterior ethmoidal nerve, posterior ethmoidal nerve, infratrochlear nerve, terminal branch of ophthalmic artery.

Applied anatomy: Ethmoid sinus is closely related to this wall resulting for ethmoiditis following orbital cellulitis in children and hemorrhage due to trauma during surgery to ethmoid is also common through this wall.

Inferior Wall of Orbit (Floor)

Triangular shaped, shortest wall of orbit, formed by orbital surface of maxilla medially, orbital surface of zygomatic laterally and palatine posteriorly and posteriorly this wall is separated from lateral wall by inferior orbital fissure which opens at infraorbital foramen transmitting infraorbital nerve, infraorbital artery and infraorbital vein. Below this wall lie maxillary air sinus and palatine air cells and inferior rectus muscle, inferior oblique muscle, nerve to inferior oblique muscle lie above this wall.

Applied anatomy: Blow out fracture occurs in this wall. For tumors of maxilla, inferior orbitotomy (antral approach) is done.

Lateral Wall of Orbit

Triangular shaped, strongest wall, formed anteriorly by zygomatic and posteriorly by greater wing of sphenoid. Posteriorly on this wall reside bony projection, spina recti lateralis, from which lateral rectus muscle originates. Anteriorly on this wall lie lateral orbital tubercle from which check ligament of lateral rectus and suspensory ligament of eyeball arises. Lateral wall separates roof of orbit by superior orbital fissure and floor by inferior orbital fissure.

Applied anatomy: For retrobulbar tumors palpation is done through this wall as anterior half of globe is not covered by bone laterally. Due to less number of foramina (except zygomatic-temporal vessels) lateral wall orbitotomy is mostly preferred. In Kronlein's operation, zygomatico-sphenoid suture is to be identified through this wall.

Roof or Vault of Orbit (Fig. 18)

Triangular shaped, thin wall, formed by mainly orbital plate of frontal bone and lesser wing of sphenoid partly. Lacrimal fossa with lacrimal gland resides in the anterolateral part of roof with suspensory ligament of lacrimal gland and trochlear fossa resides at the junction of roof and medial wall containing fovea for pulley of sup oblique muscle.

Frontal lobe of cerebrum with meninges lie above roof of the orbit and periorbita, frontal nerve, levator palpebral superioris, superior rectus, superior oblique, trochlear nerve and lacrimal gland seen below the roof.

Ant and post ethmoidal canals lie at the junction of roof and medial wall. Superior orbital fissure lies at the junction of roof and lateral wall.

Applied anatomy: As this wall is thin and periorbita can be easily peeled away, sharp objects can easily enter through this wall into frontal lobe of brain. Transfrontal orbitotomy preferred through roof, as this wall is devoid of major vessels and nerves.

Base of Orbit

This is actually anterior opened end of orbit, bounded by orbital margins giving attachment to septum orbitale.

Apex of Orbit

Posterior closed end of orbit, where all four walls converge, having optic canal and superior orbital fissure situated in the sphenoid bone, where body, greater wing and lesser wing meet each other.

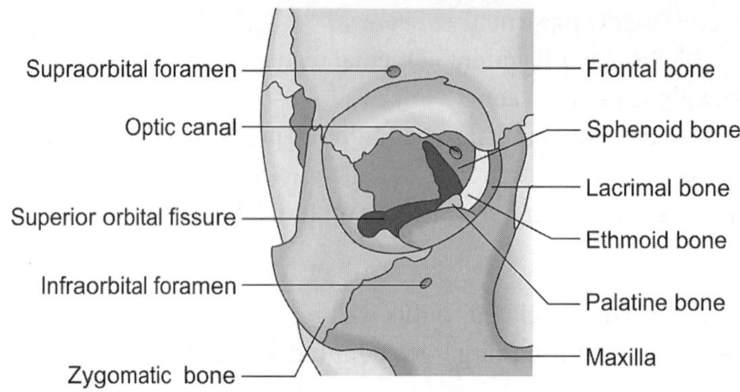

Fig. 18: Bones of the orbit.

33. Draw a labeled diagram of posterior surface of eye with details of structure present.

(10) (WBUHS MS 2018)

The structures present in the posterior surface of the eyeball are as follows:

- *Optic nerve with its meninges:* The optic nerve can be divided into four parts on the basis of location, namely- intraocular, intra orbital, intracanalicular and intracranial. The part of the optic nerve in relation to the posterior aspect of the globe is the intra orbital part. The myelin sheath of the nerve in this region is supplied by oligodendrocytes. The dural sheath of the optic nerve is continuous with that of the brain.
- *Central retinal artery inside the substance of optic nerve:* The central retinal artery enters the optic nerve by piercing its meningeal sheath inferiorly 10 mm behind the globe and goes on forwards to supply the retina and the superficial nerve fiber layer of the intraocular part of the optic nerve.
- *Ciliary nerves:* These are the long and short ciliary nerves, that pierce the sclera around the optic nerve, Short ciliary nerves arise from the ciliary ganglion, which are postganglionic and have sensory as well as motor component. However, the long ciliary nerves arise from the nasociliary branch of the Vth nerve, which are solely sensory in nature.
- *Short posterior ciliary arteries:* They arise by two trunks from the ophthalmic artery and are subdivided into 10–12 branches that pierce sclera around the optic nerve and supply the choroid.
- *Long posterior ciliary arteries:* These arteries pierce the sclera on either side of the optic nerve and pass forwards in the suprachoroidal space to anastomose with the anterior ciliary arteries and form the major arterial circle.
- *Vortex veins* ***(Fig. 19)****:* These are 4 in number and leave the globe 6 mm behind the equator 1 on each side of the superior and inferior recti muscles, draining blood from the choroid and ciliary body. They possess an ampuliform dilatation as they leave the globe and drain blood into the superior and inferior ophthalmic veins.
- *Attachment of superior oblique muscle:* The insertion of the superior oblique muscle lies at the upper and posterior part of the sclera. The reflected tendon of the superior oblique muscle gets inserted into the globe along an oblique insertion line aiding in cyclotorsion.
- *Attachment of inferior oblique muscle:* The inferior oblique muscle arising from the orbital plate of maxilla, gets inserted into the globe at the lower and posterior aspect of the sclera. it is the smallest among all the ocular muscles. The insertion line is curved and is in close relation to the macula.

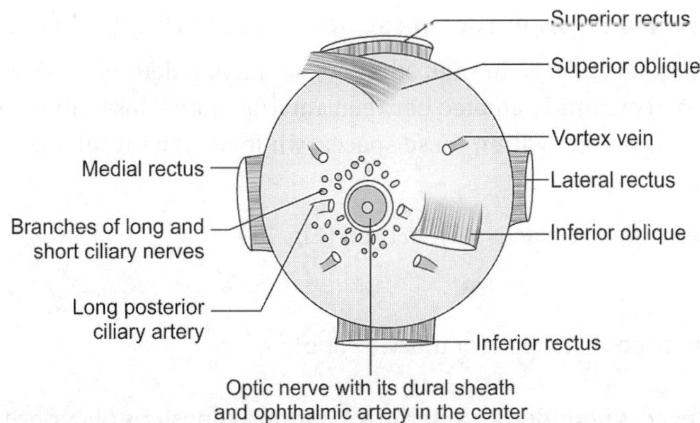

Fig. 19: Structures passing through the posterior surface of eyeball.

34. Draw a diagram showing the superior orbital fissure and the structures passing through it.

(10) (WBUHS DO 2020)

This important aperture lies at the junction of roof with lateral wall of orbit, more precisely it is surrounded by lesser and greater wing of sphenoid **(Fig. 20)**. It is comma shaped and it is situated at the apex of orbit lateral to optic foramen.

This fissure is divided by common tendinous ring into 3 parts, e.g., (a) upper and lateral, (b) middle and (c) lower and medial.

From this common tendinous ring recti muscles originate.

From (a) upper and lateral part of superior orbital fissure following structures pass-

- Nerve branches of ophthalmic division of trigeminal (lacrimal, frontal), trochlear.
- Vein-superior ophthalmic vein
- Artery-recurrent branch of ophthalmic artery

From (b) middle part (within tendinous ring) of superior orbital fissure following structures pass-

Nerve-superior and inferior divisions of oculomotor nerve, nasociliary branch of ophthalmic division of trigeminal nerve, abducent nerve

From (c) lower and medial part of superior orbital fissure following structures pass-

Vein- inferior ophthalmic vein

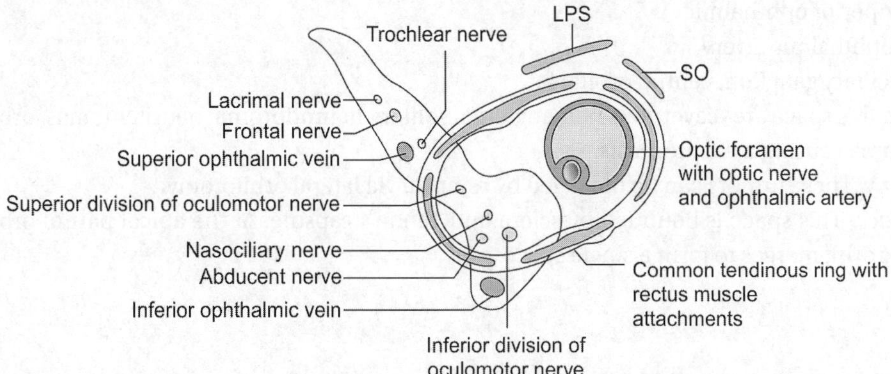

Fig. 20: Superior orbital fissure.

35. Elaborate the boundaries and contents of Surgical spaces of orbit. (10) (WBUHS MS 2024/DO 2019)

Each orbit is formed by following bones, e.g., frontal, ethmoid, lacrimal, palatine, maxilla, zygomatic and sphenoid to cover two quadrangular truncated pyramids situated between anterior cranial fossa above and maxillary sinuses below.

Benign orbital tumors tend to remain within these spaces, while malignant tumors infiltrate the walls of orbit to encroach outside these spaces.

From surgical point of view, four surgical spaces seen in orbit **(Fig. 21)**.

a. Subperiosteal space
b. Peripheral space (anterior space)
c. Central space (posterior or retrobulbar space or muscle cone)
d. Sub-Tenon's space

a. *Subperiosteal space:* This space is bounded by anteriorly by strong adhesions of periorbita to orbital rim. This space is between orbital bones and periorbita.

   Tumors arise in this space are—dermoid cyst, epidermoid cyst, mucocele, subperiosteal abscess, myeloma, hematoma, osteoma, fibrous tumor.

   Applied anatomy: As bony tumors separate thicker periorbita from bones which ultimately acts as barrier to stop intraocular infiltration.

b. *Peripheral space (anterior space):* This space is bounded by anteriorly by septum orbitale, peripherally by periorbita and four extraocular muscles with their intermuscular septa enclosing following structures-
   1. Muscles like superior oblique, inferior oblique, levator palpebrae superioris.
   2. Nerves like lacrimal, frontal, trochlear, anterior ethmoidal, posterior ethmoidal.
   3. Veins like superior and inferior ophthalmic
   4. Others like peripheral orbital fats, lacrimal gland, half of the lacrimal sac.

   Tumors arise in this space are—malignant lymphoma, capillary hemangioma, pseudotumors, lacrimal gland tumors, causing eccentric proptosis.

   Applied anatomy: These tumors can be managed by removal via anterior orbitotomy, sometimes via lateral orbitotomy.

c. *Central space (posterior or retrobulbar space or muscle cone):* This space is bounded by anteriorly by Tenon's capsule, peripherally in anterior part by extraocular rectus muscle with intermuscular septa and in posterior part this space is continuous with peripheral orbital space enclosing following structures-
   1. Nerves like optic nerve with meninges, superior and inferior divisions of oculomotor, abducent, nasociliary.
   2. Veins like superior ophthalmic
   3. Artery like ophthalmic artery
   4. Others like ciliary ganglion, central orbital fat.

   Tumors arise in this space are -cavernous hemangioma, solitary neurofibroma, neurilemomas, orbital meningioma, optic nerve glioma causing axial proptosis.

   Applied anatomy: These tumors can be managed by removal via lateral orbitotomy.

d. *Sub-Tenon's space:* This space is bounded by sclera and Tenon's capsule. At the apical part of orbit peripheral and central space of orbit merges to form a single space.

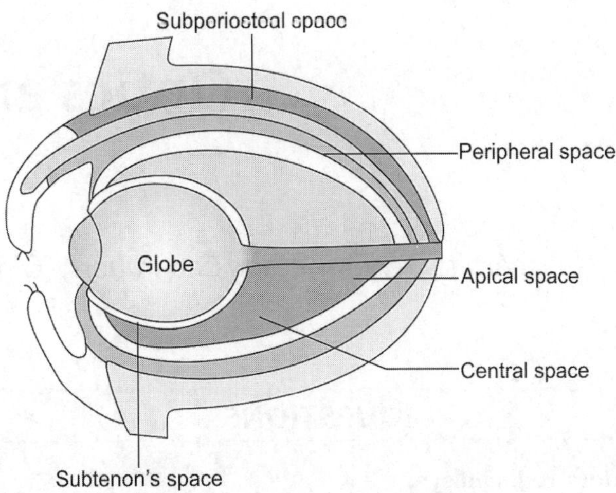

Fig. 21: Surgical spaces of the orbit.

SUGGESTED READING

1. Brar VS. AAO 2020-2021 BCSC Section 2: Fundamentals and Principles of Ophthalmology. San Francisco: American Academy of Ophthalmology; 2020.
2. Khurana AK. Anatomy and Physiology of Eye, 3rd edition. New Delhi: CBS Publishers and Distributors. 2017.
3. Sihota R, Tandon R. Parsons' Diseases of the Eye, 23rd edition. New Delhi: Elsevier India; 2019.

CHAPTER

Optics and Refraction

Arpita De, Tanweesha Chakraborty, Oindrila Chakraborty, Mariam

QUESTIONS

1. **Write a short note on Donders' reduced eye.** **(5) (BHU MS 2019)**
2. **Listing's reduced eye—explain with diagram.** **(10) (WBUHS MS 2018)**
3. **Describe different types of optical aberrations.** **(10) (WBUHS MS 2017)**
4. **Write a short note on Stiles-Crawford phenomena.** **(5) (BHU MS 2018)**
5. **Write a short note on ETDRS chart.** **(5) (BHU MS 2016)**
6. **Discuss the LogMAR chart—short note.** **(5) (TN MGRMU MS 2016)**
7. **Describe in brief about macular function tests.** **(10) (WBUHS MS 2020)**
8. **What are the theories of color vision? Describe the methods of evaluation of color vision.** **(10) (WBUHS MS 2022)**
9. **Write a short note on Contrast Sensitivity test.** **(5) (BHU MS 2015, WBUHS MS 2023)**
10. **Write a note on Measurement of visual acuity in infants.** **(10) (TN MGRMU MS 2019)**
11. **Write a short note on Sturm's conoid.** **(5) (TN MGRMU 2015)**
12. **What is hypermetropia? Define types and management of it.** **(10) (WBUHS MS 2016)**
13. **High Myopia—discuss the different types of optical correction.** **(10) (WBUHS MS 2018)**
14. **Discuss about pathological myopia and its refractive challenges.** **(10) (DNB 2018)**
15. **Astigmatism—discuss the types, signs and symptoms, investigations, and management.** **(10) (TN MGRMU MS 2014, DNB)**
16. **Discuss anisometropia.** **(10) (TNMGRMU MS 2018)**
17. **Write a short note on Aniseikonia.** **(5) (BHU MS 2021)**
18. **Describe briefly Worth Four dot test.** **(5) (TN MGRMU MS 2018)**
19. **Discuss about accommodation and its anomalies.** **(10) (BHU MS 2015)**
20. **Write a note on Convergence insufficiency.** **(10) (TNH MGRMU MS 2017)**
21. **Discuss about the management of Presbyopia.** **(10) (WBUHS MS 2023)**
22. **Write short note on Jackson Cross Cylinder.** **(5) (TN MGRMU MS 2019)**
23. **Write a short note on Maddox rod.** **(5) (TN MGRMU MS 2022)**
24. **Discuss Maddox Wing test.** **(10) (TNMGRMU MS 2022)**
25. **Write briefly regarding the principles of retinoscopy and the correct procedure of performing retinoscopy.** **(10) (WBUHS MS 2014)**
26. **Discuss the different principles of automated refraction** **(10) (WBUHS MS 2020)**

27. **Discuss about the merits and demerits of each of subjective and objective refraction—short note.** **(5) (WBUHS DO)**
28. **Write a short note on Back Vertex distance.** **(5) (TNMGRMU 2016)**
29. **Bifocals—short note.** **(5) (TNMGRMU MS 2018)**
30. **Write a short note on Optics of prisms and its clinical use.** **(10) (BHU MS 2014)**
31. **Discuss the uses of contact lenses in ophthalmology.** **(10) (TN MGRMU MS)**
32. **Write a short note on Optical biometry.** **(5) (TN MGRMU MS 2020)**
33. **Discuss the various intraocular lens power calculations, its merits and demerits.** **(5) (TN MGRMU 2020)**
34. **Write a short note on Trifocals lens.** **(5) (TN MGRMU MS 2015)**
35. **Write short note on low vision aids.** **(5) (BHU MS 2021)**
36. **Explain the working principle of synoptophore and its clinical role.** **(10) (TN MGRMU 2015)**
37. **Gonioscopes—types, techniques, structures visible and its clinical importance.** **(10) (WBUHS MS 2023, DO 2016, 2017)**
38. **Describe the technique, uses, and contraindications of specular microscopy.** **(10) (WBUHS MS 2017)**
39. **Explain confocal laser microscopy with diagram.** **(5) (TN MGRMU MS 2022)**
40. **Discuss optical principle and working of direct ophthalmoscope.** **(10) (WBUHS MS 2014)**
41. **Describe with diagram the optical principle of indirect ophthalmoscope.** **(10) (WBUHS MS 2016)**
42. **Write a short note on EOG.** **(5) (TN MGRMU 2015)**
43. **Write a short note on electroretinogram.** **(5) (TN MGRMU MS 2022)**
44. **Write a short note on visual evoked potential (VEP).** **(5) (TN MGRMU MS 2018)**
45. **Write a short note on Cover Test.** **(5) (BHU MS 2020)**
46. **Write a short note on Hess Chart.** **(5) (TN MGRMU MS 2021)**
47. **Discuss about Amsler Grid in brief.** **(10) (BHU MS 2015)**
48. **Write a short note on Titmus fly test.** **(5) (TN MGRMU MS 2017)**

1. Write a short note on Donders' reduced eye. (5) (BHU MS 2019)

The reduced eye is an idealized model of optics of human eye that replaces severe refractile bodies of the eye by an ideal air/water interface surface and converts six cardinal points into three cardinal points.

The six cardinal points are:
Two principle foci: Parallel rays come to focus at a point for a given lens or point from where diverging rays passing through the refracting surface become parallel

Two principle points: Points at which principle planes meet optical axis. *Principle planes* are planes at which emergent and incident rays meet when extrapolated.

Two nodal points: Points at which all refraction take place

When medium on both sides of the refracting object are same then principle points coincide with modal points.

Donders' Reduced Eye (Fig. 1)
Donders converted the cardinal data that was used in Listing's reduced eye into round figures, so that they can be remembered easily.

The following approximations have been made for convenience.
1. Principle point (P) lies 2 mm behind the cornea
2. Nodal point (N) is situated 5 mm behind the plane
3. Anterior focal length (F_1) is 15 mm
4. Posterior focal length (F_2) is 20 mm
5. Refractile index is 1.336
6. Total power is +60 D

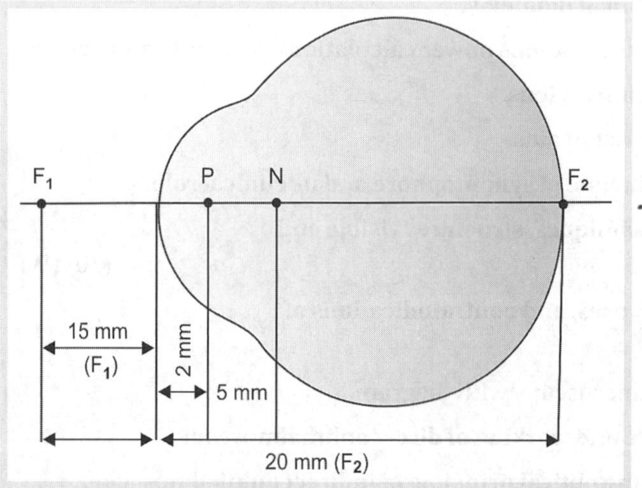

Fig. 1: Donders' reduced eye.
Source: Khurana AK. Optics and Refraction of Eye, 3rd edition. Amsterdam: Elsevier; 2013. Chapter 1, p. 35

2. Listing's reduced eye—explain with diagram. (10) (WBUHS MS 2018)

Many mathematical models of the eye's optical system are based on careful calculations and approximations. Although the first mathematical model of eye given by Gullstrand was very accurate, this model is cumbersome for most clinical calculations and hence simpler models developed further. As the principle points of the cornea and lens are fairly close to each other, a single intermediate point can substitute for them. The nodal points of the cornea and lens can be combined into a single nodal point located 17.0 mm in front of the retina. In this way, we can treat the eye like it were a single refracting element, an ideal sphere separating two media of different refractive indices: 1.000 for air and 1.333 for the eye. This simplified model of the Gullstrand schematic eye is known as the Reduced schematic eye.

One such example is Listing's reduced eye **(Fig. 2)**. The simplified data of this eye are as follows:
- Principle point (P) lies 1.5 mm behind the anterior corneal surface, which represents vertex of single refracting surface of radius of curvature being 5.7 mm
- Nodal point (N) is located 7.2 mm behind the anterior corneal surface
- Anterior focal point 15.7 mm anterior to anterior corneal surface
- Posterior focal point that is on the retina is 24.13 mm behind the anterior corneal surface
- Anterior focal length is 17.2 mm, while the posterior focal length is 22.63 mm
- Uniform refractive index is set to be 1.336
- Total Dioptric power is +58.2D.

The power of the eye is calculated as follows using the anterior focal length:

F = Refractive index of air/anterior focal length in meters
= 1*1,000/17.2 = 58.2

Using the posterior focal length, the power is determined as:

F = Refractive index of vitreous/posterior focal length in meters

= 1.336*1,000/22.9 = 58.20

So, the first focal length in air is optically equivalent to the second focal length inside the eye, which makes the reduced eye to be optically equivalent to Gullstrand's schematic eye, when rounding off liberties are applied.

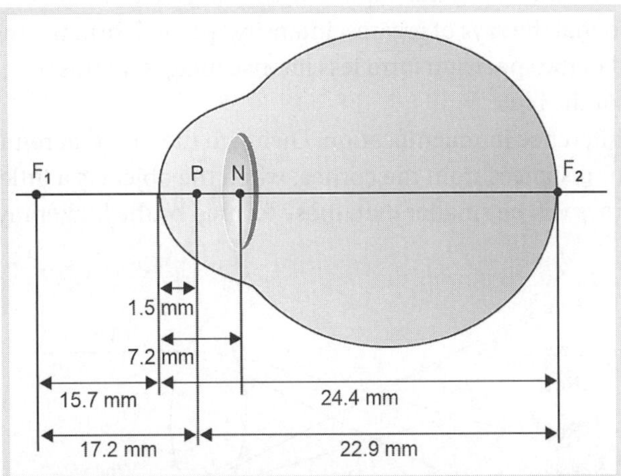

Fig. 2: Listing's reduced eye.

Source: Khurana AK. Optics and Refraction of Eye, 3rd edition. Amsterdam: Elsevier; 2013. Chapter 1, p. 35.

3. Describe different types of optical aberrations. (10) (WBUHS MS 2017)

The optical aberrations of the human eye are essentially the physiological optical defects. The accuracy with which any optical apparatus is able to form a clearly defined image is called its resolving power, which is thus an index of the efficiency of the system. The eye by no means is a perfect optical instrument, but its abilities of accommodation, adaptation, and retinal definition and differentiation render it unique.

Optical Aberrations of the Eye

1. ***Figure 3** shows diffraction of light:*

   When a wave of light travels through space, the sides of the wave tend to bend or deviate. This effect is markedly increased in a narrow wave, such as the one which passes through the pupillary aperture. The image formed, therefore, after passing through a converging lens, is not a mathematical point but a series of concentric rings of light with a bright spot at the center. The smaller the size of pupil, more is the diffraction.

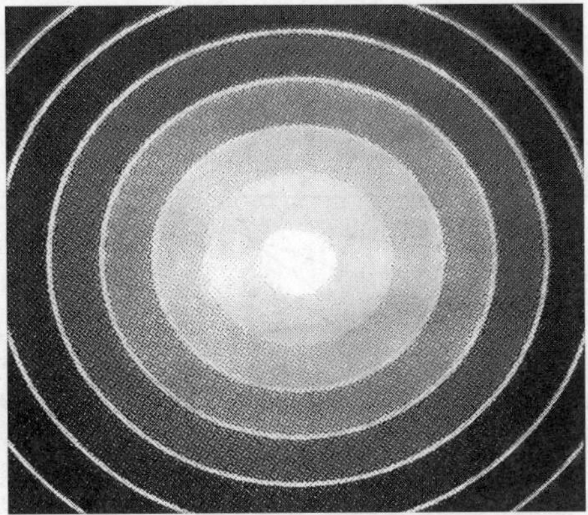

Fig. 3: Diffraction of light.

Source: Khurana AK. Optics and Refraction of Eye, 3rd edition. Amsterdam: Elsevier; 2013. Chapter 1, p. 37.

2. *Chromatic aberration* ***(Fig. 4):***
White light is composed of rays of different wavelength which when separately taken, form various colors of the spectrum. The shorter waves are retarded more when passing through a refractive medium, and hence they are more acutely bent than the longer wavelengths and hence come to focus on a point in front of the longer wavelengths. This phenomenon is "dispersion of light". This to a certain extent reduces the definition of the retinal image, but the amount is small; it increases with the size of the pupil. But, the effect to a certain extent is neutralized by the fact that the eye is normally focused so that the rays of greatest intensity (yellow) form the most sharply defined image, while the other waves on either end of the spectrum form less intense images. In this way, the eye is hypermetropic for the red wavelength and myopic for the blue.

   There is also chromatic difference in magnification. Owing to the unequal refraction of light, light rays not only are images formed at different distances from the cornea, when the object is a little to the side of the optic axis, the images produced by shorter rays will be smaller than those formed by the longer rays.

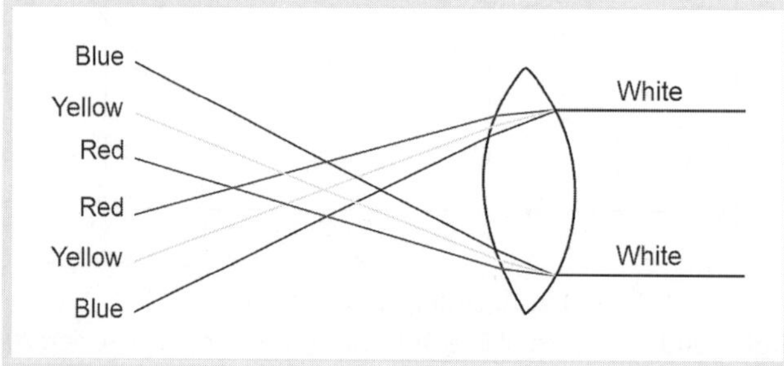

Fig. 4: Chromatic aberration. *(For Color version, See Color Plate 1)*

3. *Spherical aberration* ***(Fig. 5):***
The periphery of an optical lens has a higher refractive power than the central part of the lens, so the peripheral rays are brought to focus more quickly than the central rays. Image definition again suffers. It is, however, little evident in the eye unless the pupil is widely dilated, for in ordinary state the peripheral rays are cut by the iris. In any event, the effect of spherical aberration are somewhat neutralized by the fact that the central portions of the crystalline lens have greater density and are arranged in layers of greater curvature than the peripheral. Even when the pupil is dilated, the error is to some extent reduced by the corneal curvature.

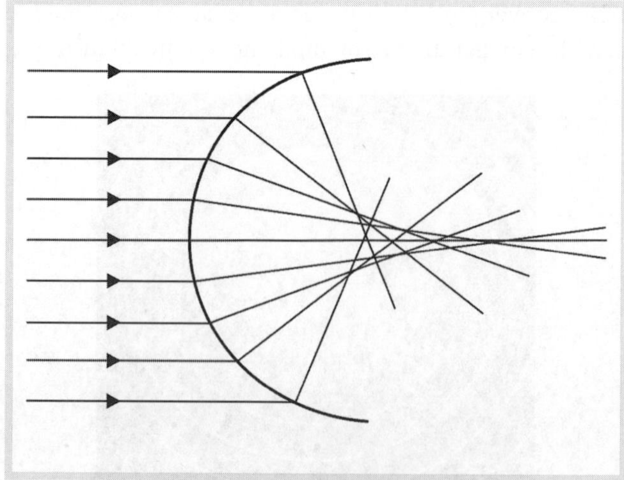

Fig. 5: Spherical aberration.
Source: Khurana AK. Optics and Refraction of Eye, 3rd edition. Amsterdam: Elsevier; 2013. Chapter 1, p. 38.

4. *Decentering:*
   The formation of an ideal image would demand that the refractive surfaces in the optical system of eye are perfectly centered. The centering of the eye is never perfect but the deviations are so small, that they are functionally negligible. As per Tscherning, usual defect is that the center of curvature of cornea is 0.25 mm below the axis of the lens.
5. *Peripheral aberrations*:
   Some optical considerations combine to make the images formed in the peripheral part of the retina less clearly defined than those in central area. Some important phenomena of this are: *coma, oblique aberration, and distortion of image.* They are usually functionally negligible. The curve of the retina has a significant effect on the efficiency of the peripheral vision and calculation shows that a very close approximation has been adopted.

The functional efficiency of the eye is greatly augmented by sacrificing the definition of marginal images to some extent in order to have the best possible condition for the central image.

4. Write a short note on Stiles-Crawford phenomena. (5) (BHU MS 2018)

Stiles-Crawford Phenomenon

- A unique directional sensitivity of the human eye is known as Stiles-Crawford phenomenon.
- According to this phenomenon, a beam of light transmitted through the peripheral region of the pupil is not perceived to be as bright as through the center of the pupil. The cone photoreceptors act as optical fibers that effectively capture light and transmit signals when they are illuminated along their axes, and they also tend to point toward the pupillary plane.
- It acts as a natural mechanism to negate the effect of spherical aberration of the human eye, among other mechanisms.

Some of the other natural mechanisms to combat aberrations of the human eye are:

I. Cutting off of peripheral rays of light by the iris
II. Higher refractive index of core of the lens nucleus than peripheral cortex
III. Reduced sensitivity of peripheral retina to light rays

5. Write a short note on ETDRS chart. (5) (BHU MS 2016)

The ETDRS chart has been introduced as a standardized visual acuity (VA) testing chart for the Early Treatment of Diabetic Retinopathy Study (ETDRS). It uses 14 lines of 5 Sloan letter optotypes in each line in logarithmic progression. The space between lines and letters is proportionally equal keeping the effect of contour interaction constant. The threshold VA corresponds to the line in which 3 out of 5 optotypes were correctly identified. Alternatively, a by-letter scoring system (–0.02 logMAR credited for each letter correctly read) can be used. The testing distance can be varied; the corresponding visual acuity can be read easily from the chart. The chart is mounted on a box that is backlit by fluorescent tubes. For repeated measurements, the chart itself can be exchanged, providing different letters for different eyes.

Charts are used in a standard light box with a background illumination of approximately 150 cd/m^2. Standard chart testing distance is *four meters*; however, shorter distances may be used when vision is severely impaired. ETDRS results can be converted to Snellen fractions, another common measure of visual acuity, in which the numerator indicates the distance at which the chart was read, and the denominator the distance at which a person may discern letters of a particular size. A larger denominator indicates worsening vision. ETDRS letters range from 58.18 to 2.92 mm in height, corresponding to Snellen visual acuity fractions of 20/200 to 20/10, respectively. Further, letter size increases geometrically and equivalently in every line by a factor of 1.2589 (or 0.1 log unit), moving up the chart. Scoring for ETDRS charts is designed to produce a logarithmic score [logarithmic minimal angle of resolution (logMAR)], suitable for statistical analysis, in which individual letters score 0.02 log units.

ETDRS charts may reliably identify changes in visual acuity of two lines (10 letters) or more, but not changes of one line (five letters) or fewer. The reliability of ETDRS charts depends on the baseline visual acuity. For eyes with acuity better than 20/100, a change in visual acuity of five or more letters has a greater than 90% probability of being a real change, while for eyes worse than 20/100, a change of 10 or more letters is required for the same reliability. A loss or gain of three lines (15 letters) is considered a moderate degree of change and is commonly used as an outcome in clinical trials. For macular edema, the FDA recommends a mean change of 15 letters or more on an ETDRS chart, or a statistically significant difference in the proportion of patients with a greater than or equal to 15-letter change in visual acuity as clinically relevant outcome measures in trials of interventions.

6. Discuss the LogMAR chart—short note. (5) (TN MGRMU MS 2016)

LogMAR Chart (Fig. 6)

The logMAR chart has been designed to enable more accurate estimates of visual acuity as compared to other acuity charts.

Each line of the logMAR chart comprises the same number of test letters (effectively standardizing the test across letter size).

The Sloan font is used (Sloan letters are approximately equally legible one from another); letter size from line to line varies logarithmically, as does the spacing between lines (making the chart easy to use at nonstandard viewing distances).

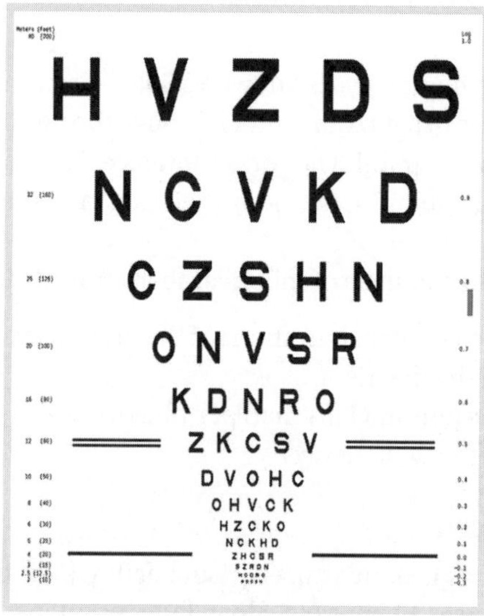

Fig. 6: LogMAR chart.

The chart comprises rows of letters and is used to estimate the visual acuity. It is particularly recommended in a research setting. Visual acuity is scored with reference to the logarithm of the Minimal Angle of Resolution. An observer who can resolve details as small as 1 minute of visual angle scores logMAR 0, as the base-10 logarithm of 1 is 0.

Relation Between Snellen's Chart and Log MAR Chart

A Snellen's score of 6/6 indicates that an observer can resolve details as small as 1 minute of visual angle, corresponding to logMAR 0 (since the base-10 logarithm of 1 is 0). Each letter has a score value of 0.02 log units. Since, there are 5 letters per line, the total score for a line on the logMAR chart represents a change of 0.1 log units. The formula used in calculating the score:

$$\text{LogMAR VA} = 0.1 + \text{LogMAR value of the best line read} - 0.02 \times (\text{no. of optotypes read})$$

Zero logMAR indicates standard vision. Positive valves indicate poor vision, and negative values indicate good vision.

7. Describe in brief about macular function tests. (10) (WBUHS MS 2020)

Macular Function Tests (MFT)

- Required for diagnosing as well as for following up of macular diseases and for evaluating the potential macular function in eye with opaque media such as cataract and dense vitreous hemorrhage.
- Indicated in as a prelude to surgery, in order to provide a preoperative prognosis for the condition.
- Not all macular function tests need to be performed on all occasions. Some like VA assessment and papillary evaluation are assessed in all patients.

MFT: Classified into 2 category (a) depending on technique (b) depending on ocular media

a. *Depending on technique:*

(1) Psychophysical test (2) Electrophysiological test

- Subjective test - Objective test
- VA, CV, photostress test - ERG, EOG, VEP
- Amsler grid, two-point discrimination test
- Entopic imagery, Maddox Rod test

b. *Depending on ocular media:*

(1) With clear media (2) With opaque media

- VA, CV, photostress test, Amsler grid—Laser interferometry
- Two-point discrimination test—PAM, ERG, EOG, VEP
- Microperimetry, FFA, OCT—Entopic phenomenon

Psychological tests: It is subjective test—

(A) *Visual acuity test (VA)*

(1) Distant VA— by Snellen VA chart, logMAR charts (Bailey–Lovie charts), the ETDRS chart (calibrated for 4 m), computer chart

- Distant VA is directly related to minimum angle of separations between 2 objects that allow them to be perceived as distinct.

(2) *Near VA:* It can be sensitive indicator of the presence of macular disease.

- Done by near vision charts (including logMAR and ETDRS vision), test type book.
- In patient with macular disease, VA is frequently worse when the patient looks through a pinhole.

(B) *Color vision testing:* Color vision depends on three populations of retinal cones, each with a specific peak sensitivity: blue (tritan), green (deutan), and red (protan). Normal color perception requires all these primary colors to match those within the spectrum.

- Acquired macular disease tends to produce blue-yellow defects, and optic nerve lesions
- Produce red-green defects.
- CV done by the Ishihara test, the City University test, the Hardy–Rand–Rittler test, the Farnsworth–Munsell 100 hue test.

(C) *Photostress test:* It can differentiate visual loss caused by macular disease from that caused by an optic nerve lesion.

- Similar to dark adaptation test
- BCVA distant is determined and ask to fixate on light of a Pen torch or an IDO held about 3 cm away for about 10 seconds, then photostress recovery time (PSRT) is measured by time taken to read any three letters of pre-test acuity line. The test is performed on the other, presumably normal eye and results are compared.
- In a patient with macular lesion, the PSRT will be longer (50 seconds or more) as compared with the normal eye. Whereas in a patient with an optic nerve lesion, there will be no difference.

(D) *Amsler grid:* Developed by Marc Amsler **(Fig. 7)**

- Is a grid of horizontal and vertical lines used to monitor a person's central visual field.
- There are 7 charts, each consisting of a 10 cm outer square.
- Tech: pupils should not be dilated, and in order to avoid a photo stress effect, eye should not yet have examined on the slit lamp.
- The chart should be well illuminated and held at a comfortable reading distance, optimally around 33 cm.
- The patient may be provided with a recording sheet and pen and asked to draw any anomalies.

Chart 1: Standard grid,

- White lines on a black background and a central white dot on which the patient fixate
- 400 small squares, each squares measures 5 mm

- Held 30 cm from the patient, each squares subtends 1 degree on retina
- When patient cannot see the central white spot, this indicates a scotoma.

Chart 2: Has diagonal lines which help maintain central fixation. This helps then point out the limits of scotoma.

Chart 3: Has red lines on black background

- Helpful in detecting color scotoma.

Chart 4: This chart comprises random dots only

- Used to differentiate scotoma from metamorphopsia

Chart 5: Has horizontal lines

- Helps to detect metamorphopsia along specific meridian.

Chart 6: Similar to Chart 5, but has white background and central lines are oriented closer for detailed evaluation.

Chart 7: Has fine central grid

- Each square subtends on angle of half a degree when the chart is held at 30 cm from patient.

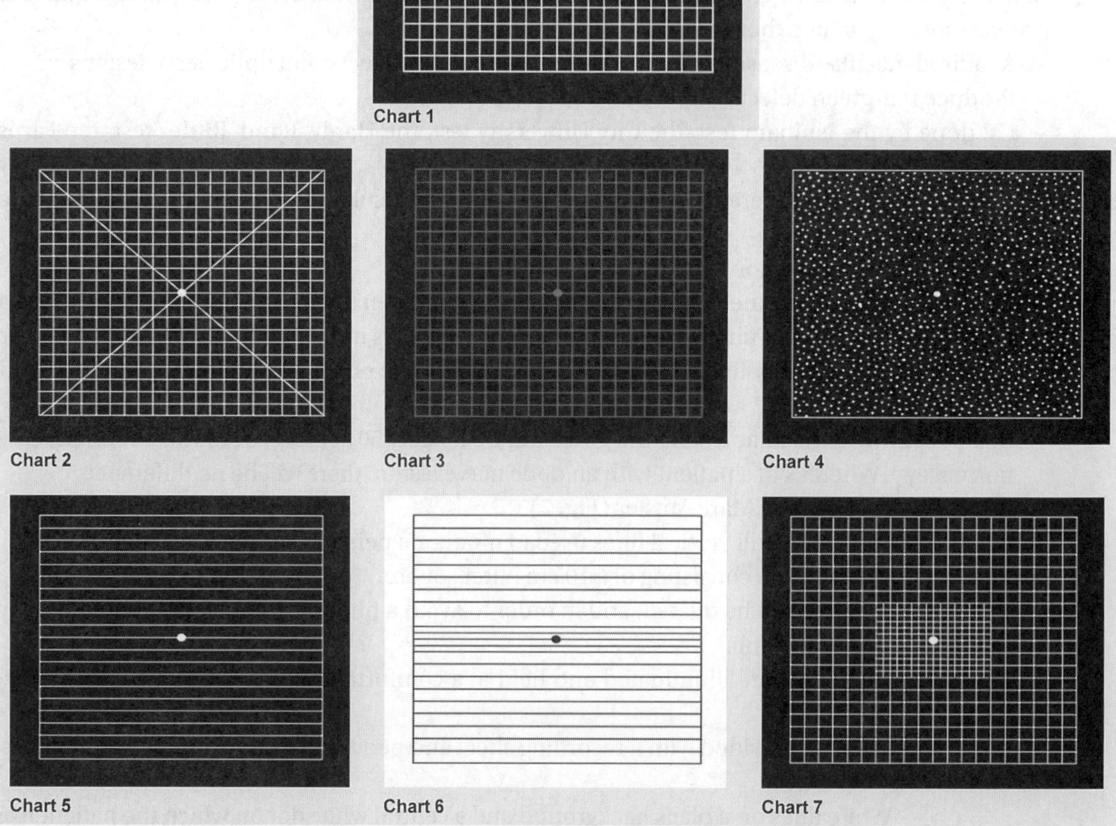

Fig. 7: Amsler grid. *(For Color version, See Color Plate 1)*

(E) *Contrast sensitivity:* Measure of minimum amount of contrast needed to distinguish a test object.
- Indirectly assesses the quality of vision
- Can detect early/subtle visual loss when VA is normal
- Spatial frequency is the number of dark light cycles per visual angle
- In macular disease, there is a marked impairment for intermediate and higher spatial frequencies.

(F) *Two-point discrimination test:* The ability to distinguish 2 illuminated point of light 2 mm diameter in size and 2 inches apart placed 2 feet away from patient's eye suggests good retinal function.
- Excellent method for testing macular functions in children and uncooperative adults in OPD clinic.

(G) *Entopic imaging:* Visual perceptions that are produced or influenced by native structures of one's own eye.
- If a focal source of light is pressed firmly against the exterior of eye through closed lids, the arborizing pattern of retinal blood vessels can be briefly made visible.
- Normal corpuscles are more than 15 corpuscles in one field
- Abnormal finding are failure to see any corpuscles or partial less of corpuscles in one part of the field, visibility of less number of corpuscles and slow corpuscular movement.

(H) Maddox rod test: When a patient sees a point source of light through the Maddox rod, a line perpendicular to axis of the parallel cylinders is perceived. Any break in this line in the center is indicative of a central/macular lesion.
- Very sensitive test that can be performed in outpatient clinic without requirement of any specific equipment.
- Maddox rod is used to assess the macular functions, the light source should be placed between 33 and 40 cm in front of eye and each should be tested uniocularly.

(I) *Laser interferometry:* Resolving power of macula is tested by using 2 coherent beams of light, which create a 3 D fringe pattern of retina
- Pupils are widely dilated and light beam is directed in to center of pupil
- Pupil is scanned until the fringe pattern is seen and patient indicates the orientation of bands of light
- Laser interferometry can thus be used in eyes with immature cataracts.

(J) *Microperimetry:* Also known as fundus perimetry
- Allows for exact topographic correlation between fundus details and its light sensitivity
- Microperimetry is a visual field test that incorporates perimetry and retinal imaging.

(K) *Potential visual acuity meter (PAM):* Main components of PAM are a bright light source miniature transilluminator Snellen chart and +12 D lens.

(L) *OCT:* Noninvasive noncontact imaging that produces high resolution cross-sectional image, useful in diagnosing macular disorders and to delineate retinal layers and detect subtle anatomical changes.

Test dependent on macular pigment: These tests require the presence of macular pigment for perception (outer plexiform layer).

1. *Haidinger's brushes:* Commonly used as a screening test for retinal pathology in strabismus patients with amblyopia.
   - Entopic phenomena
   - In this test diffusely illuminated source of plane polarized white or blue light is used
   - Brushes radiating from point of fixation to Maltese cross
   - Contrasting yellow or blue hues
   - Darker portion of Maltese pattern—yellow
   - Brighter pattern of Maltese pattern—blue,
   - Variation in absorption of plane polarized light by oriented molecules of xanthophylls in fovea
   - Yellow pigment disrupted -> Pathology in inner layer -> Brushes not seen
2. *Maxwell's spot:* A subject with normal macula will see a 3-degree dark ring surrounding fixation upon looking through a blue filter at a brightly illuminated white surface. Usually, a smaller dark spot is seen at a fixation point itself. The dark ring and spot will fade as the eye adapts to blue light.

- Some physiologists believe that perception of Maxwell's spot depends on the screening of photoreceptors by macular pigment.
- *Other tests:* Foveal flicker sensitivity, grating psychophysics, dark adaptometry, visual cycle, electrophysiological test

8. What are the theories of color vision? Describe the methods of evaluation of color vision. (10) (WBUHS MS 2022)

Color vision is the ability of eye to discriminate between color excited by the light of different wavelengths.

Theories of Color Vision

1. *Trichromatic theory:*
    - Given by Young and Helmholtz.
    - It postulated existence of three types of cones, each with a different photopigment maximally sensitive to either red, green, or blue.
    - The sensation of any given color is determined by relative frequency in pulse from each of the cone systems.

    Absorption Spectrum
    - Red sensitive cone pigments/Erythrolab: 570–590 nm
    - Green sensitive cone/Chlorolab: 535–550 nm
    - Red sensitive cone pigments/Cyanolab: 440–450 nm
2. *Opponent color theory by Hering:*
    - It states that some colors are mutually exclusive.
    - Cone photoreceptor linked together to form three opposing pair color.
    - Activation of one member of pair inhibit activity in other.
    - *Example:* Red-green and blue-yellow

Methods of Color Vision Evaluation

Ishihara Test

- Based on the principle of confusion in the pigment colors in red, green color defective for quick and accurate assessment of color vision deficiency of congenital origin
- Easy and rapid
- Used most commonly for screening
- It consists of total 25 plates

Function of pseudoisochromatic plates are:

	Subtype	Plate number	Intended origin
1	Introductory	1	Seen correctly by all subjects, identify malingering
2	Transformation	2–9	A number seen by a subject with normal color vision appear different to color deficient subjects
3	Vanishing	10–17	A number seen by a subject with normal color vision but cannot be seen by color deficient subject
4	Hidden digits	18–21	A number cannot be seen by a normal but seen by a color deficient subject
5	Classification	22–25	Types of deficiency (red/green) is obtained from comparing the relative contrast of the paired number

Interpretation:

- Out of initial 21 plates, if 17 or more plate are read correctly by an individual, his color sense should be regarded as normal.
- If 13 or less plates are correctly read, then patient has red-green color defect.

Hurdy-Rand-Rittler Test

- Test of choice for quantitative diagnosis of color blindness.
- It is a pseudoisochromatic test.
- Useful to identify protan, deutan, tritan defects.
- It consists of 24 plates with vanishing design containing geometric shape.
- 4 plates are introductory.
- 6 plates are for screening (4 for protan and deutan and 2 for tritan).
- 10 plates are for grading severity of protan-deutan defects.
- Last 4 plates for grading severity of tritan defects.

Lantern Test

The subject has to name the various colors shown to him using a lantern

He is rejected if he calls:

- Red as green and vice versa
- White light as green and vice versa
- White light as black

Farnsworth-Munsell 100 hue Test

- Very reliable and effective method for determining color vision defect
- Comprises 85 movable colored discs, arranged in four boxes of 22 colors in the first box and 21 colored discs in the rest, numbered in sequence undersurface.

The colors differ only in hue, and have equivalent brightness and saturation.

- Each group must be present in a row with the reference color at each end and the intervening disc in order of closest color match.
- The order of placement indicates the nature of the color defect

City University Color Vision Test

It is spectrographic test

- It is also a spectrographic test
- Central colored plate is matched to its closest hue from four surrounding color plates

Nagel's Anomaloscope Test

- The observer is asked to mix red and green color in a proportion to match the given yellow color hue
- It detects red-green deficiency

Holmgren's Wool Test

The subject is asked to make a series of color, matched from a selection of colored wool.

9. Write a short note on Contrast Sensitivity test. (5) (BHU MS 2015, WBUHS MS 2023)

Contrast Sensitivity Test

Contrast sensitivity is the ability to perceive slight changes in luminance between regions which are not separated by definite borders. In many diseases, loss of contrast sensitivity is more important and disturbing to the patient than the loss of visual acuity.

Types of Contrast Sensitivity

1. *Spatial Contrast Sensitivity:* It refers to detection of striped pattern at various levels of contrast and spatial frequencies. Patient is presented with sine wave grating and parallel light and dark bends and is asked to tell the minimum contrast at which the bars can be seen at each frequency. The width of the bars is the spatial frequency, which expresses the number of pairs of dark and light bars subtending an angle of 1 degree at the eye.

2. *Temporal Contrast Sensitivity:* Here the function is generated for time-related processing in the visual system by presenting a uniform target field modulated sinusoidal in time rather than as a function of spatial position.

   Recording of contrast sensitivity:
   1. *Arden gratings:* Booklet containing seven plates—one screening plate and six diagnostic plates. The contrast changes from top to bottom and covers a range of approximately 1.76 log units. The plates are studied at 57 cm, with spatial frequency increasing from 0.2 cycles/degree to 6.4 cycles/degree, each being double the frequency of the previous one. A score of 1–20 is assigned to each plate, depending upon the amount of plate uncovered. Sum of six plates with upper limit of 82 was established for normal subjects, with interocular difference of 12.
   2. *Cambridge low contrast gratings:* Consists of set of 10 plates containing gratings in a spiral bound booklet. Booklet is hung 6 m away on a wall. The pages are presented in pairs contain gratings and the other is blank, having same mean reflectance. The subject is simply required to choose which page top or bottom contains the gratings. The pages are shown in order of descending contrast and to stop when first error is made. When no error is made at plate 10, then a score of 11 is given.
   3. *Pelli-Robson chart:* This chart consists of letters which subtend an angle of 3 degrees at a distance of 1 m. Chart is printed on both sides. Letter sequence is different but otherwise identical. The letters are organized in triplets, two triplets in each line. The contrast decreases with each triplet. Log contrast sensitivity varies from 0.00 to 2.25.

      Chart is hung on the wall, middle of chart at subject's eye level. The subject is asked to spell or outline each letter on the chart starting from the upper left corner and reading horizontally across the line test is stopped when the subject guesses two of the three letters. The sensitivity is indicated by the finest triplet from which two of the three letters are named correctly.
   4. *The Visitech chart:* Contains sine wave gratings uses at a distance of 3 m from subject. Contrast is rested at several spatial frequencies and the subject has to identify the orientation of the gratings.
   5. Vector vision chart
   6. Fact CS chart

Diagnostic Application
- Before LASIK surgery
- ARMD
- Glaucoma
- Cataract
- Diabetic retinopathy

10. Write a note on Measurement of visual acuity in infants. (10) (TN MGRMU MS 2019)

Measurement of Visual Acuity in Infants

Indicators of Good Visual Acuity in Infants
- Normal pupillary response
- Elicitable optokinetic nystagmus

In an infant, fixation behavior develops at around 3 months of age. Development of adequate refixation reflex, permitting corer test, develops by 3–6 months of age.

The vergence response to interposition of base in/out prisms can be seen in children of 6 months of age.

The different between an infant with vision and a blind infant can be made early on, with the vestibule-ocular reflex induced nystagmus.

Infants greater than 4 months of age can be tested by optokinetic nystagmus.

Visual evoked response (VER) can assess pathologies of the optical pathway and cortical blindness.

The normal visual acuity in various age groups in infants are
- At birth—6/120 (20/400)
- 4 months—6/60 (20/200)

- 6 months—6/36 (20/120)
- 1 year—6/18 (20/60)

  Normal distant Snellen's visual acuity of 6/6 is achieved at around 2 years of age.

Tests for Visual Acuity in Infants

1. *Fixation behavior:* A normal fixation behavior of an infant can be described as CSM (central, steady, and maintained). "Central" and "steady" are terms used to describe monocular fixing behavior, while "maintained" is a term used to describe binocular fixing behavior when one of the eyes is covered.
2. *Menace reflex:* A reflex blinking of the child in response to a rapidly moving object perceived as a visual threat. It develops at 5 months of age. Afferent pathway is carried by the optic nerve and efferent is through the facial nerve.
3. *Optokinetic nystagmus test:* Passing a succession of black and white stripes in front of the eyes, elicits a nystagmus in the infant. This test is performed with an optokinetic drum having alternate black and white stripes, that is rotated.

   It gives a rough estimate of visual acuity in the infant. OKN-induced visual acuity is 6/120 in newborn that improves to 6/60 by 2 months, 6/36 by 6 months, and 6/6 by 20–30 months of age.
4. *Preferential looking test:* Based on the principle that an infant prefers to look at a pattern rather than a homogenous screen. Here, the child is presented 2 images, where one of them has a pattern and the examiner observes which image the child prefers to look at.
5. *Teller's acuity cards:* These cards contain different gratings of spatial frequencies. It is done in children up to 4 months of age and is based on the principle that children preferentially look at gratings rather than homogenous surfaces. Visual acuity is calculated on the basis of the gratings preferred by the child.
6. *Visually evoked response (VER):* It is used to assess the functional state of the visual system beyond the retinal ganglion cells.

   Flash VER assesses the integrity of macular and visual pathway.

   Pattern reversal VER gives a rough estimate of visual acuity. Visual acuity acquired by VER is 6/120 at the age of 1 month, 6/60 at 2 months of age, and 6/12 to 6/6 by 6 months to 1 year of age.
7. *Cardiff acuity cards test:* This test though commonly performed in children of 12–36 months of age, but can also be used in infants, as it is basically a pattern recognition test.
8. *Catford drum test:* Similar to optokinetic nystagmus test, except oscillating black dots of varying sizes are presented to the child, and the smallest dot that evokes pendular nystagmus denotes the level of visual acuity.

11. Write a short note on Sturm's conoid. (5) (TN MGRMU 2015)

Sturm's Conoid (Fig. 8)

It is optically defined as a geometrical configuration of light rays emanating from a single point source and refracted by the spherocylindrical lens. Also defined as a bundle of rays formed by an astigmatic optical system consisting of a primary focal line (stermi's) line, a circle of least confusion and a secondary focal line perpendicular circle of least confusion to the primary.

Sturm conoid is an optical condition in which refractive power of cornea and lens is not the same in all meridians, therefore instead of single focal point there are two focal points separated by focal interval.

1. *The focal interval of Sturm:* The distance between sagittal and tangential focal lines is called the focal interval of Sturm.
2. *Circle of least confusion/diffusion:* The smallest cross-section of a blur circle between the two focal lines formed by the astigmatic lens.

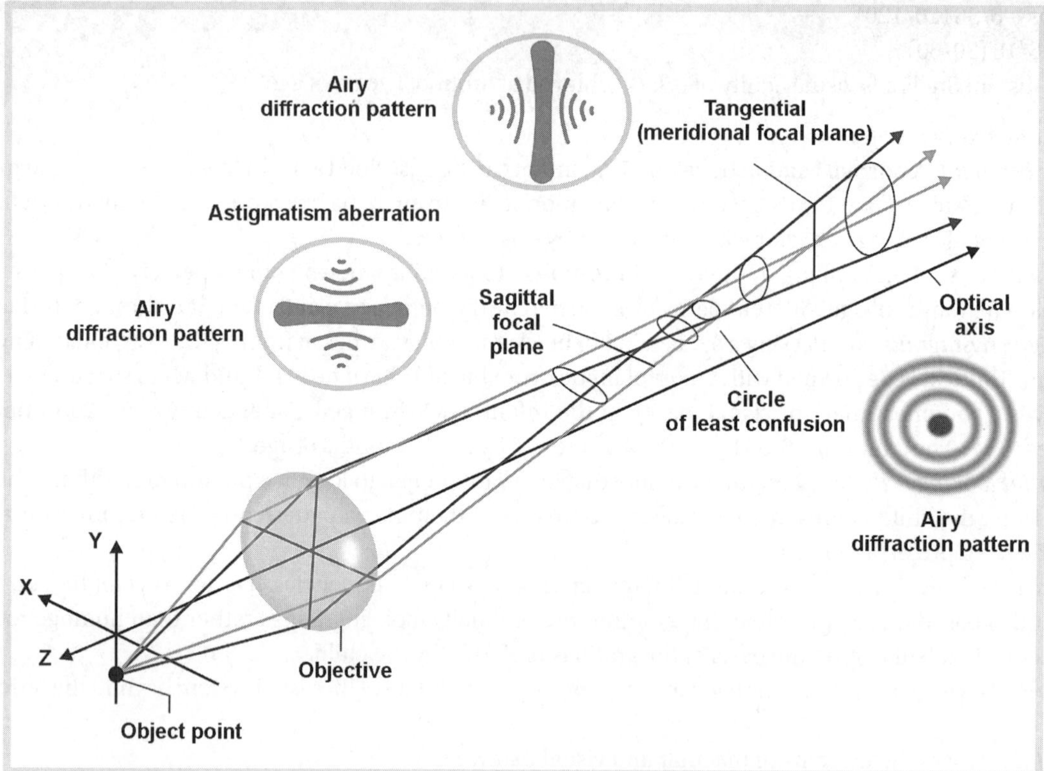

Fig. 8: Sturm's conoid. *(For Color version, See Color Plate 2)*

At point A, the vertical rays [V], the vertical rays are converging more than the horizontal rays [H]; so the section here is horizontal oval or an oblate ellipse.

At point B (first focus), the vertical rays have come to a focus while the horizontal rays are still converging and so they form a horizontal line (horizontal line).

At point C, the vertical rays are diverging and their divergence is less than the convergence of the horizontal rays; so a horizontal oval is formed here (horizontal oval).

At point D, the divergence of vertical rays is exactly equal to the convergence of the horizontal rays from the axis.

At point E, the section is a circle which is called the circle of least diffusion (circle of least diffusion). At point E, the divergence of vertical rays is more than the convergence of horizontal rays; so the section here is a vertical oval (divergence of vertical rays >> convergence of horizontal rays).

At point F (second focus), the horizontal rays have come to a focus while the vertical rays are divergent. So, a vertical line is formed here (vertical line at second focus).

Beyond f (as at point G), both horizontal and vertical rays are diverging and so the section will always be a vertical oval or prolate ellipse **(Fig. 9)**.

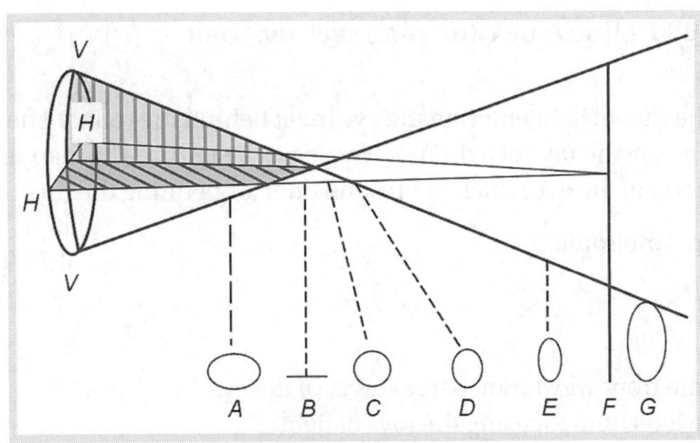

Fig 9: Sturm's conoid.

Source: Khurana AK. Optics and Refraction of Eye, 3rd edition. Amsterdam: Elsevier; 2013. Chapter 1, p. 27.

Etiology of Sturm's Conoid

Corneal Causes

It occurs due to abnormality of curvature of cornea (most common cause of astigmatism).

E.g., eyelid pressure, pterygium, corneal scars, corneal degeneration, keratoconus, mild corneal opacities.

Lenticular Causes

- It is comparatively rare.
  It may be—curvatural—lenticonus
- Positional—congenital tilting and traumatic subluxation of lens
  Index—developing cataract/nuclear sclerosis/index astigmatism. Focus of Sturm's conoid as per according to types of astigmatism:
  With the rule astigmatism:
  Vertical meridian of cornea is more curved. Myopic power is more in vertical meridian. E.g.: 3.0 D cyl × 180°

Against the Rule Astigmatism

Horizontal meridian of cornea is more curved. Myopic power is more in horizontal meridian. E.g., –3.0D cyl × 90°

Oblique astigmatism: Axis is not on or near 90° or 180°. Range of axis lies in-between 120°-150° and 60°-30°

E.g.: –3.0D cyl × 45°

Bi-oblique astigmatism: The meridians are not perpendicular

E.g.: –3.0D cyl × 90% –2.0 D cyl × 110°

Simple astigmatism:

- One focal point on retina and the other front or behind
  > Of 2 types simple myopic and simple hyperopic Compound astigmatism:
  Both the 2 focal points are in front or behind the retina
  Of 2 types compound myopic and hyperopic

Mixed Astigmatism:

> One focal point in front and other behind the retina

12. What is hypermetropia? Define types and management of it. (10) (WBUHS MS 2016)

Hyperopia

Hypermetropia occurs when the rays of light entering the eye meet behind the retina. The image of what the person sees is thus blurred. To see a clear image, the rays of light must focus on the retina. This happens when the eyeball is shorter than what it should be or the parts of the eye which are responsible for bending the rays of light are not able to do so.

Following are the causes of hypermetropia:
1. Hereditary
2. Prematurity
3. Hereditary
4. Flat cornea: The cornea is the front-most transparent layer of the eye
5. Lens defects which stop the lens from focusing the rays of light
6. Nanophthalmos: Here there is abnormal development of the eye

Types of hypermetropia **(Fig. 10)**:
Hyperopia can be classified in various ways:
1. Significant hyperopia—is defined as any degree of hyperopia sufficient to cause symptoms prompting clinical attention.
2. Simple hyperopia—is due to decreased axial length or decreased converging power of cornea, lens, and/or media (flattened cornea/decreased curvature, increased thickness of lens, etc.).
3. Pathologic hyperopia is due to atypical development, trauma, or disease of the eye (i.e., cataract, microphthalmia, nanophthalmos, aniridia, etc.).
4. Functional hyperopia is due to paralysis of accommodation. If affected, functional hyperopia is usually present at birth. Drugs, such as cycloplegics, can also cause transient hyperopia. Hyperopia may also be categorized by the degree of refractive error:
    1. Low hyperopia is +2.00D or less
    2. Moderate hyperopia ranges from +2.25 to +5.00D
    3. High hyperopia is +5.25D or more. High hyperopia may be associated with blurring of the optic disk margin, known as pseudopapilledema. It can be differentiated from true papilledema by the presence of normal caliber vasculature and normal-appearing juxtaposed retina.

Hyperopia may also be classified by the role of accommodation to visual functioning.
1. Facultative hyperopia is hyperopia that can be overcome by accommodation.
2. Absolute hyperopia cannot be overcome by accommodation.
3. Total hyperopia is the sum of facultative and absolute hyperopia.

Hyperopia may also be categorized based upon the outcome of noncycloplegic and cycloplegic refractions.
1. Manifest hyperopia is determined with noncycloplegic refraction, whereas
2. Latent hyperopia is determined with cycloplegic refraction. The magnitude of hyperopia is the sum of manifest and latent hyperopia.

Treatment

Contact lenses and prescription glasses

Surgical methods:
1. Conductive keratoplasty
2. Thermal laser keratoplasty
3. Hyperopic LASIK
4. Lens extraction

Complications of not treating hypermetropia:

1. Headaches
2. Eye strain
3. Blurry vision
4. *Squints or strabismus:* The type of strabismus is called accommodative esotropia and is usually associated with severe hyperopia.
5. *Lazy eye or amblyopia:* This is a serious condition and may need amblyopia exercises to correct loss of vision.

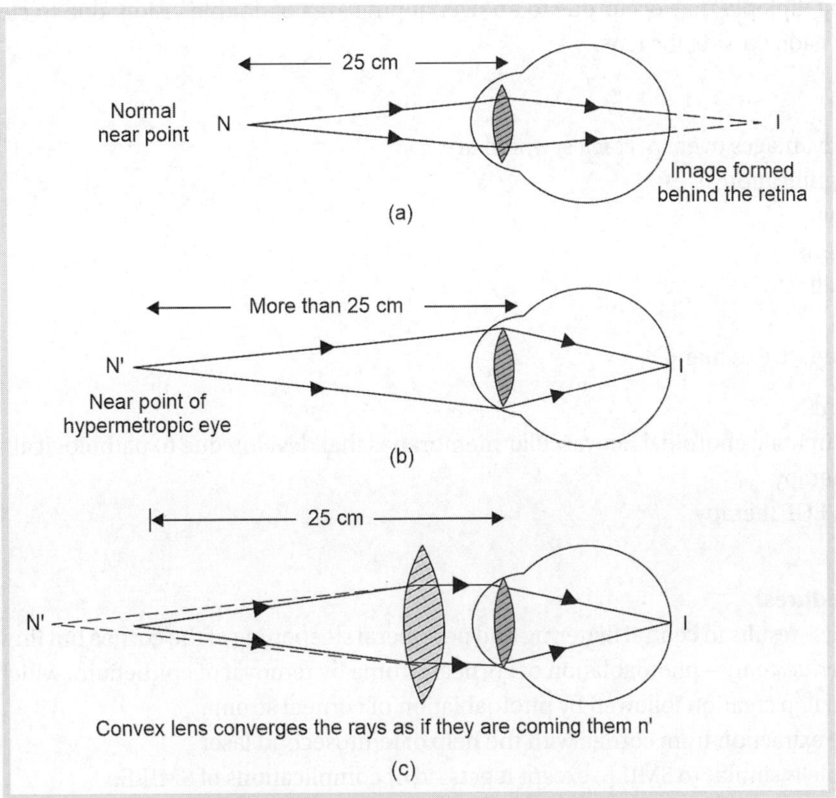

Fig. 10: Schematic diagram showing hypermetropia.

13. High Myopia—discuss the different types of optical correction. (10) (WBUHS MS 2018)

The different types of correction for high myopia include:

- Spectacles
- Contact lenses
- Medical management
- Refractive surgery

Spectacles

A minus correcting lens whose secondary focal point coincides with the far point of the eye is placed at the spectacle plane

Traditional myopia correction: Traditional eyeglasses correct myopia at the center of the retina, but not the relative hyperopia that exists in the peripheral retina. This might worsen peripheral hyperopia defocus and may result in myopia progression.

Optimal myopia correction: By contact lens having modified power in the Leu's periphery, replacing peripheral hyperopic defocus with myopic refocus, that might reduce risk of increasing myopia.

Problems caused by high minus lenses:

- *Lens weight and thickness:* Thick edges of a high minus lens are much more obvious to the observer than the thick centers. Edge thickness can be minimized by small lens size, high index materials, lenticular lenses and aspheric lens use. Lens weight can be minimized by use of plastic lenses.
- *Minification of image:* This can be addressed by fitting the lenses closer to the wearer's eye and use of contact lens.
- *Field of view:* Ring diplopia may occur due to an overlapping area of double vision, due to clear vision through the lens but blurred vision outside the lens.

Contact Lenses

These have a lot of advantages over spectacles, which are:

- Lesser image magnification
- Wider field of view
- Minimal aberrations
- Lesser prismatic effect
- Better cosmesis
- Greater accommodative demand

Medical Management

It is mainly aimed at treating choroidal neovascular membranes that develop due to pathological myopia.

- Photodynamic therapy
- Intravitreal anti-VEGF therapy

Refractive Surgery

Cornea-based procedures:

- *Radial keratotomy*—results in central flattering and peripheral steepening of the cornea but limited to –3D correction
- *Photorefractive keratectomy*—photoablation of corneal stroma by removal of epithelium, which later grows back
- *LASIK*—epithelial flap creation followed by photoablation of corneal stroma
- *SMILE*—lenticule extraction from cornea with the help of femtosecond laser
- *SILK*—the principle is similar to SMILE, except it gets rid of complications of SMILE.

Lens-based procedures:

- *Phakic IOL:* Implantation of angle fixated, iris clip or posterior chamber phakic IOL in front of the crystalline lens, in cases where a single cornea-based procedure is inadequate or corneal thickness do not permit any such procedures
- *Clear lens extraction*

14. Discuss about pathological myopia and its refractive challenges. (10) (DNB 2018)

Pathological myopia is rapidly progressive error which starts in childhood at 5–10 years of age and results in high myopia (6–8D) within early adulthood which is associated with degenerative changes in the eye.

It is unequivocal that in pathologic myopia is due to rapid axial growth of the eyeball which is outside the normal biological variations of development. It is definitely linked with hereditary factors and general growth process.
Clinical picture:

Symptoms

1. There is considerable visual defect due to higher degree of refractive error. Uncorrectable visual loss may occur due to degenerative changes.
2. Muscae volitantes and floaters
3. Night blindness in cases of marked chorioretinal degenerative changes

Signs

1. Prominent eyeballs
2. Corneal diameter appears large
3. Deep anterior chamber
4. Rapid change in refractive error with even increase by 4D yearly
5. Fundus changes:
   - Optic disc appears larger, pale and with myopic crescent at temporal edge. Peripapillary crescent encircling the disc may be present. A supertraction crescent is seen at the nasal edge.
   - Degenerative changes in the retina and choroid namely Foster–Fuch's spot
   - Acquired optic disc pit
   - Lattice degenerations
   - Lacquer cracks
   - Posterior staphyloma
   - Peripapillary intrachoroidal cavitation
   - Rhegmatogenous retinal detachment
   - Choroidal neovascularization
   - Macular retinoschisis
   - Macular hole
   - Peripapillary detachment
   - POAG
   - Complicated cataract
   - Dislocation of lens
   - Amblyopia

The prognosis of myopia depends largely on the age of the patient. Due to rapid alteration in refractive power, conservative treatment has to be revised periodically. The degenerative changes in the retina lead to irreversible damage to visual function which are not satisfactorily corrected completely, with residual visual defect.

Treatment

a. *Optical correction:* Meticulous use of optical correction with glasses or contact lenses for relieving visual strain and providing continuous clarity of distant vision. In cases of high myopes or pathologic myopia, full refractive correction can be rarely be tolerated. A compromise must therefore be adopted, where the refraction is reduced as little and possible with comfortable binocular vision, lens with greatest visual acuity is obtained without distress. The amount which has to be deducted usually varies from 1 to 3 D but in the highest grades lenses even weaker than these will be necessary. In such cases, glasses with high refractive index lens or lenticular forms are useful. In higher myopes, contact lenses provide better optical quality and benefits. They are free from the aberrations which are the unavoidable optical defects of thick spectacle lenses.
b. *Refractive surgery:*
   i. Corneal interventions:
      - Radial keratotomy—making deep radial incision sin the peripheral cornea leaving 4 mm of the central optical zone. On healing the incisions flatten the cornea, thereby reducing the refractive power
      - Photorefractive keratotomy: Surface ablation procedures can be helpful in myopia up to 6D, so early decision in cases of pathologic myopia is essential. Preferred procedure when the cornea is flat, thin corneas, deep set eyes, epithelial basement membrane dystrophy.
      - Epi-LASEK: Epithelial flap created with the help of blunt epikeratome and is reposited at the end of the surgery.
      - LASIK: It is the most practiced method where the anterior flap of the cornea is lifted with a microkeratome and excimer laser ablation to sculpt stromal bed to change the refractive error of the eye. Can be used in a patient with up to 12D of refractive error.
      - LASEK: The method is used to treat myopia in up to –15D of refractive error.

- Refractive lenticule extraction: Removal of an intrastromal lenticule from the cornea altering the thickness and curvature. Latest method is small incision lenticule extraction.

ii. Lens-based procedures:
- Refractive lens exchange—extraction of clear crystalline lens with suitable IOL placement
- Phakic refractive lenses

15. Astigmatism—discuss the types, signs and symptoms, investigations, and management.

(10) (TN MGRMU MS 2014, DNB)

Astigmatism is a type of refractive error wherein the refraction varies along different meridians. Consequently, the rays of the light entering the eye cannot converge to a point focus but form focal lines.

Broad Classification

Regular Astigmatism

The refractive power changes uniformly from one meridian to another, i.e., two principle meridian
Among this first group of classification is based on the etiology as follows:

Corneal astigmatism: It is the result of abnormal corneal curvatures. It is the most common cause of astigmatism.

Lenticular astigmatism: It is comparatively rare.

Curvatural: Small amount of curvatural astigmatism due to congenital abnormalities of curvature of lens is frequently seen. Marked curvatural cause is seen in lenticonus.

Positional: Small amount of astigmatism due to tilting of the lens is not uncommon. Congenital or traumatic subluxation is the reasons.

Index: Occur due to variable refractive index of the lens in different meridian in patients suffering from the diabetes and those developing cataract or nuclear sclerosis.

Retinal: Due to oblique placement of macula rarely.

Types of regular astigmatism:

1. With-the rule: The two principle meridian are placed at right angles to one another but the vertical meridian is steeper than the horizontal meridian.
2. Against-the-rule: In this type the two principle meridian are horizontal and vertical but the horizontal is steeper or more curved.
3. Oblique: The two principle meridian are not the vertical and horizontal but those are still at perpendicular to each other. Oblique type is usually found to be symmetrical or complementary.
4. Bi-oblique: Two principle meridian are not at right angles to each other.

In regular astigmatism, the parallel rays are not focused at a point rather as two focal lines. The refractive surface follows Sturm's conoid. The distance between the two focal lines is called focal interval of Sturm.

Refractive types of regular astigmatism:

1. Simple astigmatism: The rays of one meridian are focused on the retina and the other principle meridian are focused either in front (simple myopic) or back (simple hypermetropic) of the retina.
2. Compound astigmatism: In this type, the rays of light from both meridians are either focused in front (compound myopic) or at the back (compound hypermetropic) of the retina.
3. Mixed: In this condition rays of light refracted in one meridian are focused in front, while of the other meridian are focused at the back of the retina.

Irregular Astigmatism

It is characterized by the irregular change of refractive power in different meridian. There are multiple meridian which allow no geometrical analysis.

Etiological Types

i. *Corneal—found in patients with extensive corneal scars or corneal ectatic disorders.*
ii. *Lenticular*—It is due to variable refractive index of the lens substance.
iii. *Retinal*—seen due to distortion of the macular area due to scarring or tumors of retina and the choroid pushing the macular area.

Clinical Features

i. Blurring of vision while working at viewing precise distance relieved by rubbing of eyes. Circles appear elongated, point of light appears tailed off, a line appears like succession of strokes fused into blurred image.
ii. Asthenopic symptoms like headache, browache, eye strain, itching and heaviness of eyes.
iii. Tilting of the head in high degrees of astigmatism to reduce image distortion.
iv. Half closure of lids in order to make a stenopic slit and cutting out rays in one meridian.
v. Reading material maybe held close to eye.

Investigations

a. Retinoscopy will reveal difference in refractive power in the different meridians
b. Keratometry and corneal topography will reveal different corneal curvatures.
c. Astigmatic fan test
d. Jackson cross cylinder test
e. Slit lamp examination may reveal irregular corneal surface or ectasia
f. Placido's disc test

Treatment

Optical

For regular astigmatism, proper cycloplegic refraction to be done with appropriate spectacles prescription for regular use. Contact lenses can be used for lower degrees of astigmatic defect.

In cases of irregular astigmatism, usually contact lenses are better in relieving the symptoms.

Surgical

Regular astigmatism:

- Astigmatic keratotomy
- Limbal relaxing incision
- Photoastigmatic refractive keratotomy
- Astigmatic epi-LASIK
- Astigmatic LASIK
- Astigmatic C-LASIK

Irregular astigmatism:

- Corneal collagen cross linking
- Intracorneal ring segments
- Penetrating keratoplasty

16. Discuss anisometropia. (10) (TNMGRMU MS 2018)

Anisometropia

A condition of unequal refractive state between the eyes of an individual. A difference of 0.25D between the two eyes is technically termed anisometropia but not clinically significant. However, a difference of 1D results in a 2% change in retinal size of image, resulting in clinically significant anisometropia.

Causes

- Trauma to the eye
- Keratoplasty in one eye

- Asymmetric age changes
- Uniocular aphakia, post surgery

Types

- *Absolute:* The refraction of 2 eyes differs so much, that it becomes a problem. It can feather be subdivided.
  - *Simple*: One eye is emmetrope and the other eye is myope/hypermetrope.
  - *Compound*: Both eyes are myopic/hypermetropic
  - *Mixed*: One eye is myope and other eye is hypermetrope
  - *Compound astigmatic*: Both eyes are astigmatic but to an unusual degree
  - *Simple astigmatic:* One eye is myope/hypermetrope and the other eye is astigmatic
- *Relative:* Total refraction of the 2 eyes is same, but with different axial length, which results in formation of clear retinal images of unequal sizes.

Symptoms

- Eye strain
- Headache
- Nausea
- Tiredness
- Diplopia

Diagnosis

- Retinoscopy
- Testing for binocular single vision (BSV) status:
  - FRIEND test
  - Worth four dot test

Management

- Optical correction:
  - Spectacle correction (up to 4D difference)
  - Contact lenses
- Surgical management:
  - Corneal refractive surgery
  - Removal of crystalline lens
  - IOL implantation
  - Phakic IOL

17. Write a short note on Aniseikonia. (5) (BHU MS 2021)

Aniseikonia

Aniseikonia is a condition where the size and shape of the images formed in the two eyes are unequal. It is a common occurrence and a distressing symptom.

The inequality of the images may depend on two distinct factors: it may be an optical phenomenon depending on the difference of the size of the dioptric images formed on the retinae, or, it may be an anatomically determined difference in the distribution of the retinal elements.

Optical difference may be due to anisometropia, especially if the anisometropia is astigmatic. Although correction of the refractive error may increase aniseikonia.

Anatomical factor usually points that though the images formed on the retinae are similar, but the distribution on rods and cones may not be identical, so the image perceived by the brain would appear dissimilar.

Slight changes in size and shape of the images are normal and due to stereoscopic interpretation, normally not exceeding 5%.

In cases of squint, difference of 5–15% has been found, in which case the aniseikonia has an important bearing on the treatment and prognosis of the condition.

The difference in the images may be classified as follows:

i. *Symmetrical:* One image being larger either in all dimensions or in one meridian. Meridional change may be oblique.
ii. *Asymmetrical:* Image being distorted to some degree, like being progressively larger in one meridian, and smaller in another, the effect resembling that of a prism.

Symptoms: They include visual disturbance like blurred image, difficulty in fixation, tendency to diplopia, or even squinting.

Sometimes complaint of photophobia, headaches, general ocular discomfort and eye-strain common.

Clinical Investigation

The most accurate method depends upon the anomalous localization in space which results from the disparity in size of the images.

Treatment: The treatment of aniseikonia is the correction of the disparity in size of the image with iseikonic lenses, that lenses which cause magnification of the image size without introducing any refractive power by changing the direction of the pencil of rays of light.

18. Describe briefly Worth Four dot test. (5) (TN MGRMU MS 2018)

It is a dissociation test that can be used with both distance and near fixation and is a test for sensory anomalies in a patient with strabismus. This test helps in differentiation of binocular single vision (BSV), anomalous retinal correspondence (ARC), and suppression **(Fig. 11)**.

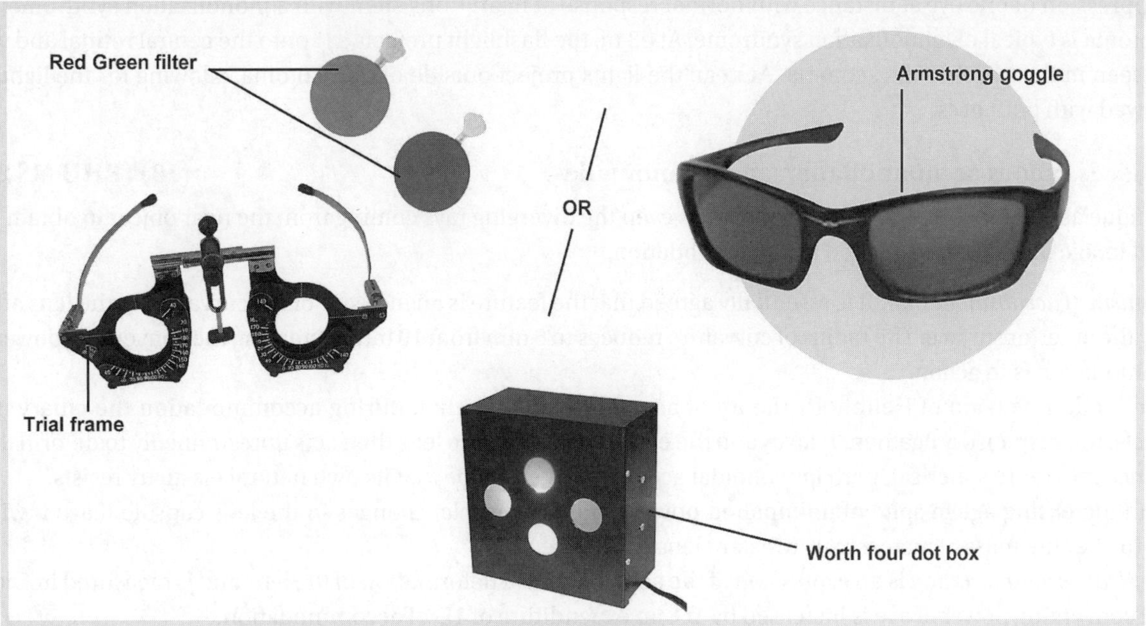

Fig. 11: Worth Four dot test. *(For Color version, See Color Plate 2)*

Procedure

- The patient wears red-green glasses (with red tinted lens before right eye and green tinted lens before left eye) or a trial frame with red and green filters placed in it.
- The patient is made to observe a box with 4 lights—one red, two green and one white, both for distant and near vision **(Fig. 12)**.

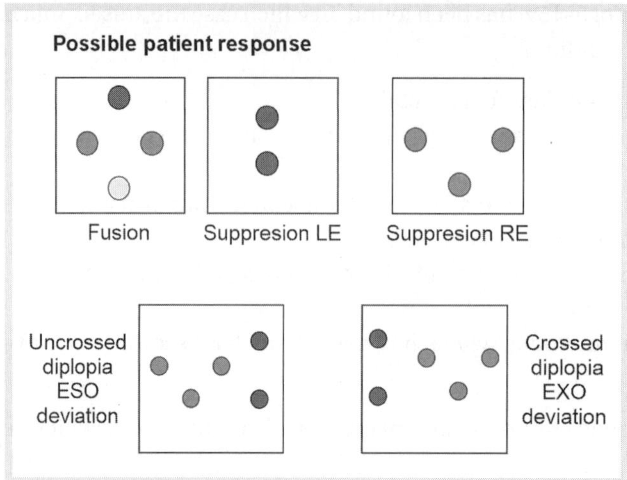

Fig. 12: Equipment Fort Worth 4-dot test.

Results

- If BSV is present, all four lights are seen.
- If all four lights are seen in the presence of a manifest squint, then harmonious ARC exists.
- If two red lights are seen, it indicates suppression in left eye.
- If three green lights are seen, there is suppression in right eye.
- If two red and three green lights are seen, it indicates the presence of diplopia.
- If red and green lights alternate, alternating suppression is present.
- Suppression of one eye at distance with normal response at near: Consistent with a monofixation syndrome. A 1–4° scotoma is typical of monofixation syndrome. At ≥3 m, the flashlight projects ≤1° onto the central retinal and will not be seen in the eye with the scotoma. At near, the lights project outside of the scotoma, allowing for the lights to be viewed with both eyes.

19. Discuss about accommodation and its anomalies. (10) (BHU MS 2015)

The unique ability of the eye by which it can focus even the diverging rays coming from the near object to obtain a clear defined image on the retina is called as accommodation.

Mechanism of accommodation: It is essentially agreed that the feature is an increase of the curvature of the lens affecting mainly the anterior surface. The radius of curvature reduces to 6 mm from 10 mm increasing the converging power while accommodation is in action.

The modern version of Helmholtz theory of accommodation is that, during accommodation the ciliary muscle contracts, the suspensory ligament relaxes and the elastic capsule of the lens then acts unrestrainedly to deform the lens substance into more spherical, perhaps conoidal accommodated shape that its own natural elasticity resists.

With increasing age in spite of unimpaired power of ciliary muscle, changes in the lens capsule leave it with less ability to alter the mass of increasingly resistant lens substance.

Physical accommodation is an expression of the actual physical deformation of the lens and is measured in Diopters. Thus if converging power of eye is increased by 1D, an expenditure of 1D of accommodation.

Physiological accommodation has unit of *myodiopter* which is taken as the contractile power of the ciliary muscle required to raise the refractive power of the lens by 1D.

Anomalies of accommodation:

Increased accommodation:

1. Excessive accommodation: The condition involves the production of an artificial myopia which varies from time to time. Both the far point and the near point are brought nearer to the eye and distance vision becomes blurred. Vision

is therefore improved by concave lenses. In the more marked degrees near vision also suffers, and after reading for some time the printed page becomes confused, which clears up after temporary rest. The prognosis of such a condition is food and treatment effective. Refraction should be done under full cycloplegia. Correction to be ordered after deducting 1D. In the worst cases the eye maybe kept mildly under the effect of atropine for a week or two in order to ensure absolute rest and allow the overexcited ciliary muscle to recover from its condition of irritability.

2. Spasm of accommodation: True spasm of ciliary muscle a condition similar to that brought by miotics is rare. The spasm is usually out of the control of the patient, amount may reach to 10D or more. The most effective treatment is the production complete ciliary paralysis with atropine and the cycloplegia to be kept for long time—4 weeks or more. Correcting spectacles are to be used.

Diminished accommodation:

1. Presbyopia: It is a condition of physiological insufficiency of accommodation due to reduced amplitude leading to progressive fall in near vision starting after 40–45 years of age. Age-related changes in the lens which includes decrease in elasticity of lens capsule and progressive increase in size and sclerosis of lens substance is the primary mechanism. Age-related decline in ciliary muscle tone due to uncorrected hypermetropia, general debility or pathology of eye. Optical correction is usually satisfactory and accepted.
2. Insufficiency of accommodation: The accommodative power of the eye is constantly below the lower limit of accepted normal variation of range. The failure may be lenticular in origin, arising from an undue sclerosis of the lens. Premature presbyopia affects physical accommodation only. This is a stable condition and gives rise to no symptoms except those of presbyopia which sets in an early age. The failure may be due to weakness of ciliary muscle and thus involve the physiological accommodation. This condition is usually labile. The symptoms are usually of asthenopia, eye-strain, fatigue, irritability. Near work is blurred and impossible. There is accompanying disturbance of convergence.
3. Ill-sustained accommodation: It is aggravated insufficiency. The range of accommodation is normal, but on any attempt to do near work for a prolonged period of time the accommodative power weakens, the near point recedes and near vision is blurred. Such a condition in mild form is relatively common in those who read in the evening when they are tired.
4. Inertia of accommodation: In this state the patient experiences the failure to alter the range of accommodation. It takes some time and effort on part of the patient to focus a near object after looking at the distance. For its correction refractive error to be corrected and accommodation exercises to be done.
5. Paralysis of accommodation: This may occur from local or general causes, the most important local cause is the exposure of the eye to parasympatholytic drugs. CNS causes like vascular disorders, cerebral syphilis.

   Failure of accommodation and convergence occasionally results from head injury. In paralysis of accommodation, the near point recedes and approximates the far point so as near objects appear blurred. The phenomenon of micropsia is seen. Pupils are slightly dilated. Seeing a near object needs extreme effort. The treatment of this condition is essentially the treatment of the primary cause.

20. Write a note on Convergence insufficiency. (10) (TNH MGRMU MS 2017)

Convergence Insufficiency

It is the inability to obtain and/or maintain adequate binocular convergence for any length of time without undue effort.

It is the most common cause of ocular asthenopia.

Etiology

- Primary or idiopathic
- Refractive errors (high hypermetropes, myopes)
- Presbyopia
- Muscle imbalance
- *Others:* Wide interpupillary distance, inadequate functional development

Clinical Features

- Asthenopia
- Unsatisfied with glasses
- Blurred near vision
- Intermittent crossed diplopia
- More common in people with a desk job

Diagnosis

- Near point convergence >10 cm
- Difficulty in attaining 30 degrees of convergence on synaptophore
- Prism convergence is low but prism divergence is normal

Differential Diagnosis

a. *Convergence paralysis:* Total lack of ability to overcome any amount of base out prism
b. *Accommodation effort syndrome:* Esophoria in near vision. Convex lenses help in this case, but not in convergence insufficiency.

Management

It has excellent prognosis. Children are to be treated when fusional vergence is poor and adults are treated when they become symptomatic.

i. *Optical treatment:*
    - Full correction for myopes
    - Under correction for hyperopes
ii. *Orthoptic treatment:*
    - To improve near point of convergence
    - To increase amplitude of fusion convergence
iii. *Prism therapy:* Using base-in prisms
iv. *Surgical treatment:* Medial rectus resection

21. Discuss about the management of Presbyopia. (10) (WBUHS MS 2023)

Presbyopia is the irreversible loss of accommodative ability of the eye that occurs due to aging. The pathophysiology of presbyopia can be explained by two theories: Lenticular and Extralenticular.

Lenticular theory: Sclerosis of nuclear lens tissue; senile changes in lens capsule leading to thicker, less extensible, brittle capsule; decreased distance between ciliary muscle and Leu's equator.

Extralenticular theory: Age-related hyalinization of ciliary processes and muscles; loss of elasticity in the zones; decreasing resistance of vitreous against accommodating lens capsule.

Management of Presbyopia

- *Optical correction by spectacles:*
    - Trial method: +0.25 D SPH increasingly added to the eye to be corrected and patient made to read at 40 cm, until the script is clearly visualized
    - Age method: Empirical method based on clinical experience obtained by prescribing a variety of patients

The glasses to be used by the patient can be:

- Monofocal lenses (reading glasses)
- Bifocal lenses
- Progressive lenses
- Optical correction by contact lenses:
    - Bifocal correction

- Multifocal correction
- Monovision correction

All of these are available as rigid gas permeable lenses and soft contact lenses.

- *Medical management:* The US-FDA has permitted the use of topical pilocarpine (1.25%) as a management of presbyopia.
- *Surgical correction:*
    - Lens-based procedures: Use of accommodative IOL or multifocal IOL following clear lens removal could be one of the options for correction of presbyopia
    - Cornea-based procedures:
        1. *Corneal inlays:* These improve vision by pinhole effect and increased depth of focus. They also reshape the surface of the cornea thus leading to correction of presbyopia.
        2. *Laser refractive surgery:*
            - PresbyLASIK
            - Monovision LASIK
            - Photorefractive keratectomy
            - Conductive keratoplasty
- Sclera-based procedures:
    1. Scleral implants
    2. Scleral laser micro-excision

22. Write short note on Jackson Cross Cylinder. (5) (TN MGRMU MS 2019)

Jackson Cross Cylinder (Fig. 13)

It is a spherocylindrical lens having a spherical power component combined with a cylindrical power component of twice the power of the sphere, and of opposite sign.

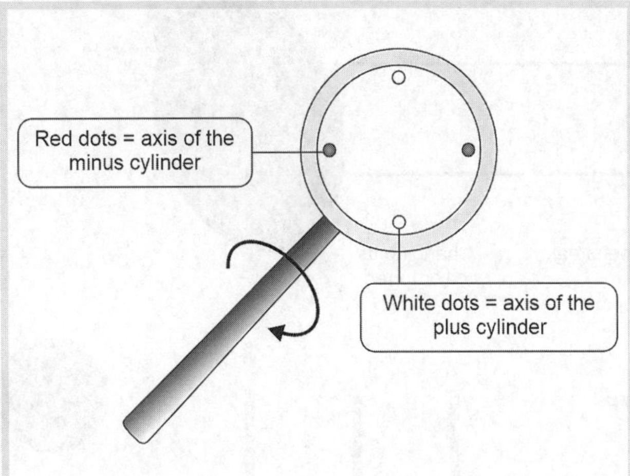

Fig. 13: The principal meridians are marked in the periphery. A handle is attached between the two marked axes. *(For Color version, See Color Plate 3)*

This instrument can be used to refine the power and the axis of a prescription with a cylindrical power.

After finding the spherical power of the patient by subjective refraction, the cylinder axis and then the cylindrical power can be determined by a JCC (Jackson Cross Cylinder).

If astigmatism is present, then first refinement of the axis is done, followed by refinement of the power, as correct axis can be found in the presence of incorrect power, but the full cylindrical power will not be found in the presence of an incorrect axis.

For refinement of axis:

- Cylindrical axis determined by retinoscopy is placed on the trial frame
- JCC held with handle parallel to the axis of the cylinder in the trial frame and the patient asked about which of the flip positions is perceived better
- In case, both the positions of JCC are seen with equal clarity, it is presumed that the axis of the cylinder is correct
- A minus cylinder is rotated by 10 degrees towards the negative axis of JCC and a plus cylinder rotated by the same extent towards its corresponding positive axis
- This is continued until both the flip positions are seen with same clarity by the patient; this gives the correct axis of the cylinder.

For refinement of power:

- After cylindrical power is placed in trial frame after
- retinoscopy, JCC is placed with any of the axis parallel to the axis of the cylinder in the trial frame
- If both the flip positions are perceived equally, no adjustments in power are required
- If any of the flip positions are seen to improve the visual acuity then, the corresponding correction is placed in the trial frame, and the process is continued until neutral point is achieved.

23. Write a short note on Maddox rod. (5) (TN MGRMU MS 2022)

Maddox Rod

The Maddox rod consists of several red cylinders of glass placed parallel to each other in a frame. This converts the appearance of a white spot of light into a red streak. The optical properties of the rods cause the streak of light to be perpendicular to the axis of the glass rods. When the glass rods are horizontal the streak will be vertical and vice versa.

When a single Maddox rod is used, and placed in front of right eye, the right eye sees a red streak which cannot be fused with unaltered white spot of light seen by the left eye **(Fig. 14)**.

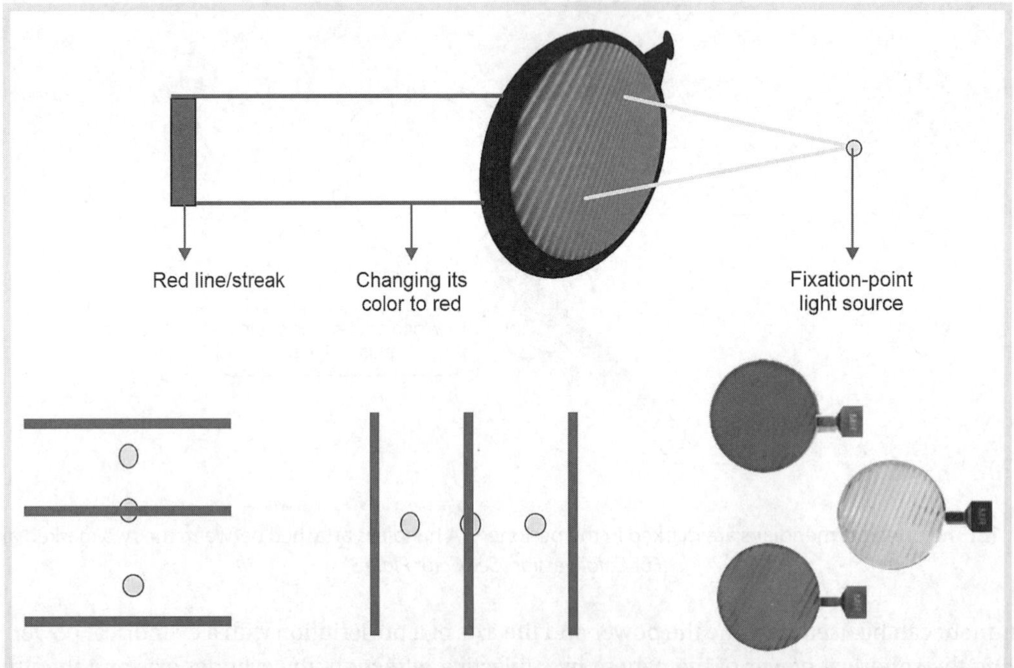

Fig. 14: The working of Maddox rod. *(For Color version, See Color Plate 3)*

The double Maddox rod test is used to test cyclodeviation. A Maddox rod is placed in front of each eye in a trial frame with the lines vertically so that the patient sees a horizontal image. The patient or the examiner rotates the axes if the rods until the lines are perceived to be parallel. The degree of cyclodeviation and direction can be determined by the angle of rotation that causes the line images to appear horizontal and parallel. Traditionally a red Maddox rod is placed before right eye and a white Maddox rod in front of left eye.

The amount of dissociation is measured by the superimposition of the two images using the prisms. The base of the prism is placed in the position opposite to the direction of the deviation.

Both vertical and horizontal deviations can be measured but difference between phoria and tropia cannot be identified.

24. Discuss Maddox Wing test. (10) (TNMGRMU MS 2022)

Maddox Wing Test (Fig. 15)

It is an instrument by which the amount of phoria for near (at 33 cm) can be measured.

Principle

To dissociate two dissimilar images of near phoria.

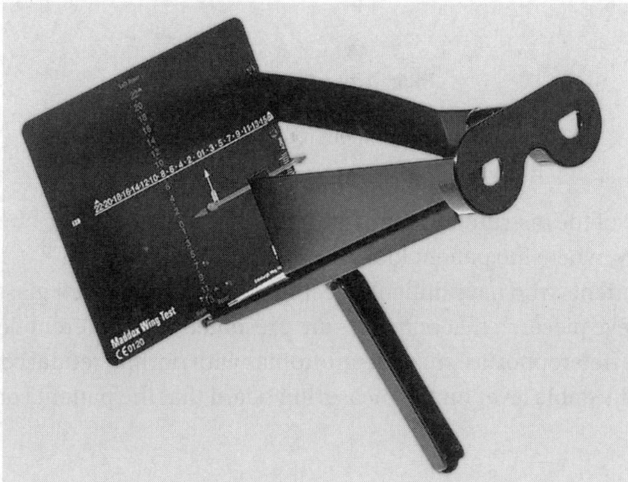

Fig. 15: Maddox wing. *(For Color version, See Color Plate 4)*

Procedure

- It is a quantitative and subjective method.
- The right eye sees a white vertically placed arrow and a red horizontally placed arrow.
- The left eye sees two series of numbers, one oriented vertically and the other placed horizontally.
- The arrows are observed to point towards these numbers, when seen with both the eyes.
- The room should be brightly lit and patient should wear full optical correction.
- The examiner asks the patient to hold the instrument and identify the number that the white vertical arrow and red horizontal arrow point to.

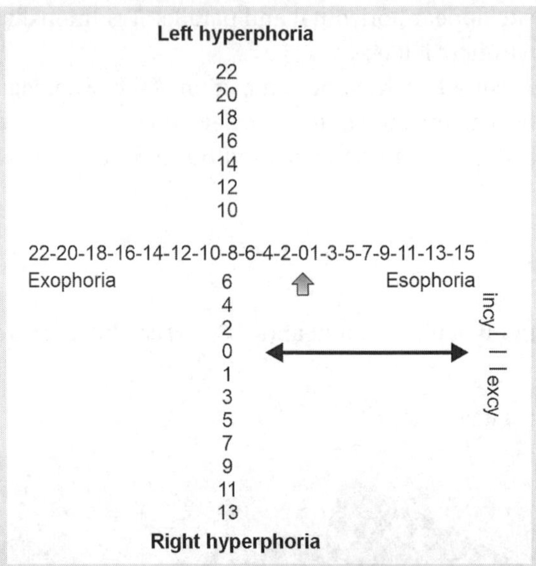

Fig. 16: Measurement for Maddox Wing test.

Components

- *Handle:* Located at the base of the instrument; retractable
- *Eye piece:* Located anteriorly, where the patient looks into
- *Eye piece lens holder:* For patients who have difficulty seeing the board with their glasses
- *Septa:* 2 septa separate the eye piece, so that both eyes are presented with different field of view
- *Scale card:* Used to measure heterophorias, small heterotropias with normal retinal correspondence and also torsion
- *Torsion lever:* There is an adjustable lever on the measuring board that the patient can subjectively align to measure torsion.

Advantages (Fig. 16)

- Test is reliable as patient uses accommodation
- Horizontal, vertical and cyclophorias can be simultaneously measured
- Can be used in children
- Handheld instrument

Disadvantages

- Interpupillary distance is not adjustable
- Purely subjective test
- Cannot be performed in patients with accommodation insufficiency
- Contraindicated in patients with suppression and abnormal retinal correspondence

25. Write briefly regarding the principles of retinoscopy and the correct procedure of performing retinoscopy. (10) (WBUHS MS 2014)

Retinoscopy is the most valuable method of estimating the optical state of the eye. It is an objective method of finding out the error of refraction by utilizing the technique of neutralization.

Optics

In retinoscopy an illuminated area of the retina serves as an object, and the rays emanated from this area illuminate the pupillary area and form its image at the far point of the eye. When the immediate source of light is moved across the eye, the behavior of the luminous reflex in the pupil will be dependent on the refractive status of the eye. If the image is formed between the observer and the patient, the movements of the reflex and the external light are in opposite directions; if it falls outside this region, either behind the patient's eye or behind the observer's eye, the image and light move in the same direction.

When the far point of the patient's eye corresponds to the nodal point of the observer's eye, a *neutral point* occurs.

The detailed optics is most easily considered in three stages: first, the *illumination stage,* second *the reflex imagery stage,* third *the projection stage.*

Retinoscopy optics in emmetrope:
In emmetropia, the light rays emanating from the illuminated area of the fundus are parallel to each other and the examiner projects the image of F_1 to f_1 and that of F_2 to f_2. The light source when move upwards, the image also moves along the plane mirror.

Retinoscopy in hypermetrope:
In hypermetropia, the rays emerging from the illuminated area of the fundus are divergent, so the examiner projects the image of F_1 to f_1 and of F_2 to f_2. In this case the image moves along the movement of the plane mirror **(Fig. 17).**

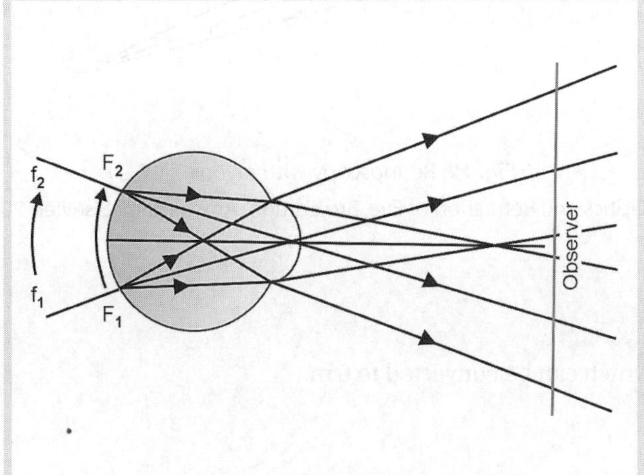

Fig. 17: Retinoscopy of hypermetrope.
Source: Khurana AK. Optics and Refraction of Eye, 3rd edition. Amsterdam: Elsevier; 2013. chapter 5, p. 129.

Retinoscopy in myope **(Fig. 18):**

A. *Myopia with <1D:* In myopia of less than 1D, the emergent rays from the illuminated area of the fundus are convergent and meet at a point behind the observer sitting at 1 m from the patient. The movement of the final image remains along the movement of retinoscope.

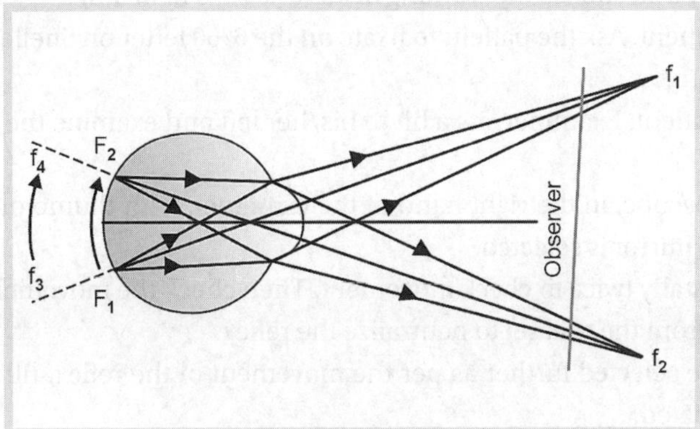

Fig. 18: Retinoscopy for myopia <1 D.
Source: Khurana AK. Optics and Refraction of Eye, 3rd edition. Amsterdam: Elsevier; 2013. chapter 5, p. 130.

B. *Myopia equal to 1D:* In such patients, the nature of the emergent rays remains same. The final image is formed at the pupillary plane, so the examiner does not appreciate any movement of the pupillary shadow.

C. *Myopia with >1D:* In these patients, the emergent light rays from the illuminated fundus are convergent at a point between the patient and examiner. The final image here moves opposite to the direction of the retinoscope or plane mirror **(Fig. 19)**.

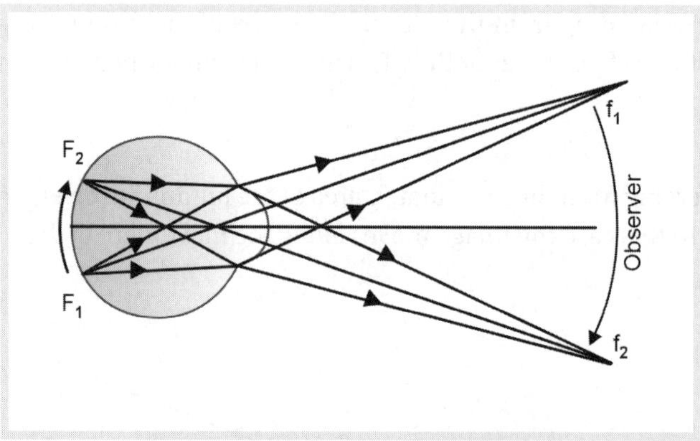

Fig. 19: Retinoscopy with myopia >1D.

Source: Khurana AK. Optics and Refraction of Eye, 3rd edition. Amsterdam: Elsevier; 2013. chapter 5, p. 130.

Procedure of Retinoscopy

Prerequisites of Retinoscopy:

i. A dark room, 6 m long or which can be converted to 6 m
ii. A trial lens set
iii. A trial frame
iv. Distance vision chart
v. Near vision chart
vi. Retinoscope: Priestly Smith retinoscope/streak retinoscope

Method

- Greet the patient and explain the procedure
- Check for dilatation of pupil and cycloplegia
- Make the patient sit properly and choose the working distance as 2/3 m or 1 m
- Put the trial frame on the patient. Ask the patient to fixate on the 6/60 letter on Snellen's chart.
- Turn off the lights of the room.
- Start with right eye of the patient. Examiner sits a bit to his/her left and examine the patient's right eye with his/her right eye.
- Ideally using a streak retinoscope, in the right hand of the examiner, with thumb on the sleeve to make the streak horizontal or vertical. Plane mirror is selected.
- The streak is moved horizontally twice to check movement. Then check the movement vertically.
- Select the appropriate lens from the trial set to neutralize the reflex.
- The higher power lenses are selected further as per the movement of the reflex, till it is neutralized and the entire pupillary aperture is illuminated.
- Record the vertical and horizontal readings as the power cross.
- Repeated for the other eye, with the examiner observing the left eye of the patient with his or her left eye.

26. Discuss the different principles of automated refraction (10) (WBUHS MS 2020)

Automated refraction is conducted by automated refractometers, those are devices incorporating banks of lenses for measuring the refractive state of the eye.

The basic principles of refractometers are described as under:

- *Scheiner double pinhole principle:* Double pinhole apertures are placed before pupil to isolate 2 small bundles of light from a distant source of light.

  If the eye is emmetropic, the rays of the 2 bundles form a single focus on the retina. But if the eye is myopic (2 bundles cross each other before reaching retina) or hyperopia (2 bundles are visualized before they cross each other), 2 separate bundles are visualized. By adjusting the position of the object (mechanically or optically) until one focus of light is seen by the patient, the far point of the patient's eye and refractive error can be determined.
- *Optometer principle:* A convex lens and a movable target are placed in front of the eye to be examined, such that focal point of the lens, lies at the level of spectacle plane of the eye.

  It target lies at first principle focus of the lens, rays will be parallel at the spectacle plane and focus on the retina of an emmetropic eye. As this is a movable target, light from target on par side of lens enters eye with vergence depending on the position of target. Vergence of light in the focal plane of optometer lens is linearly related to displacement of target, this can be used to assess the refractive status of the eye.
- *Meridional refractometry:* In the presence of astigmatism, the spherical refraction measured in 3 axes, the position of the principle axes and their refractive power can be found by mathematical calculation.
- *Grating focus principle:* A moving grating of light is projected into the eye, the focus of the grating on the retina is then analyzed by a photodetector.
- *Automated retinoscopy principle:* Neutralization of retinoscopic reflex is not performed but the speed of reflex in each meridian is determined.
- *Continuously variable spherocylinder power:* Any refractive correction can be simulated by the sum of—a variable sphere or two variable cross cylinders.

27. Discuss about the merits and demerits of each of subjective and objective refraction—short note. (5) (WBUHS DO)

Subjective Refraction

The process to determine by subjective means the combination of spherical and cylindrical lenses necessary to provide best visual acuity with accommodation relaxed.

Principles of Subjective Refraction

- Accommodation in relaxed state
- Maximum plus; minimum minus
- Back vertex distance to be considered for high prescription individuals

Advantages of Subjective Refraction

- Can be done in the absence of special instruments and good pupillary reflex
- Can be used for verifying values obtained by objective refraction
- Glasses can be prescribed at first visit

Disadvantages of Objective Refraction

- May give variable results due to accommodation
- Requires patient cooperation

- Not possible in small children
- Not possible in senile and mentally retarded patients

Objective Refraction

The refractive error of an eye is determined without any significant input from the patient.

Components of Objective Refraction

- Retinoscopy
- Autorefractometry
- Keratometry

Advantages

- Can be used in patients who are senile or uncooperative
- Can be used in children
- There is a specific end point, such as neutralization in retinoscopy
- Accommodation can be relaxed by use of cycloplegics

Disadvantages

- May not be possible to prescribe glasses in first visit
- A good fundal glow or pupillary reflex is required
- Corneal ectasias make it difficult to determine the refractive state of the eye

28. Write a short note on Back Vertex distance. (5) (TNMGRMU 2016)

Back Vertex Distance (Fig. 20)

It is the distance from the back surface of a corrective lens, i.e., spectacle or contact lens to front of the cornea. It is important while converting glass prescriptions to contact lenses, especially in prescriptions >±4.00 D.

The standard vertex distance is about 12 mm.

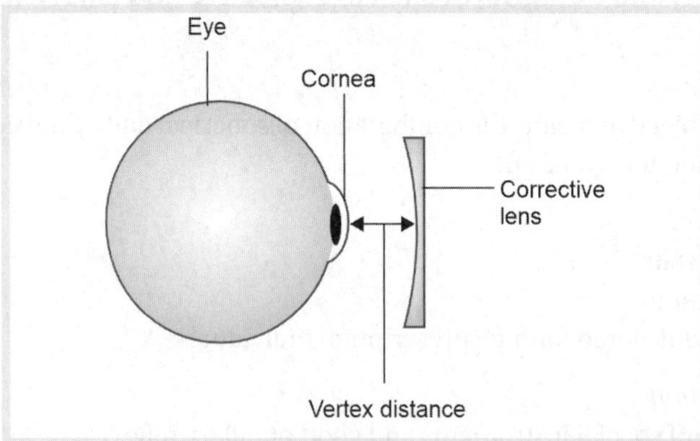

Fig. 20: Back vertex distance.

The optical effect of a lens varies with the back vertex distance. Increasing back vertex distance leads to:

- Convex lens becoming stronger
- Concave lens becoming weaker

Shorter vertex distances increase the field of view, through the viewing zone of the lens **(Fig. 21)**.

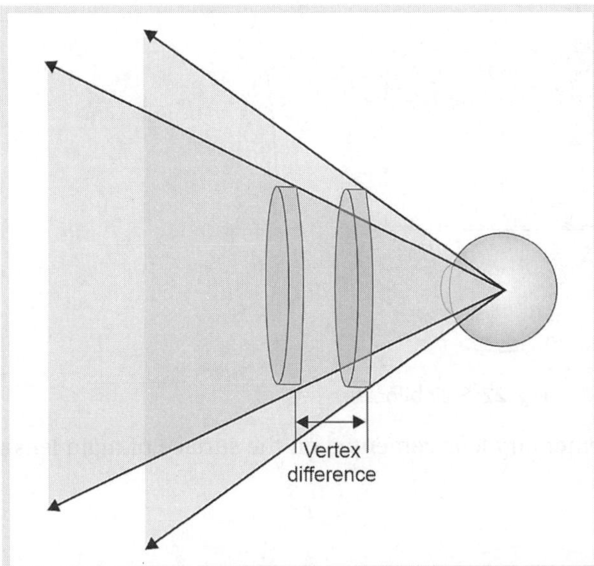

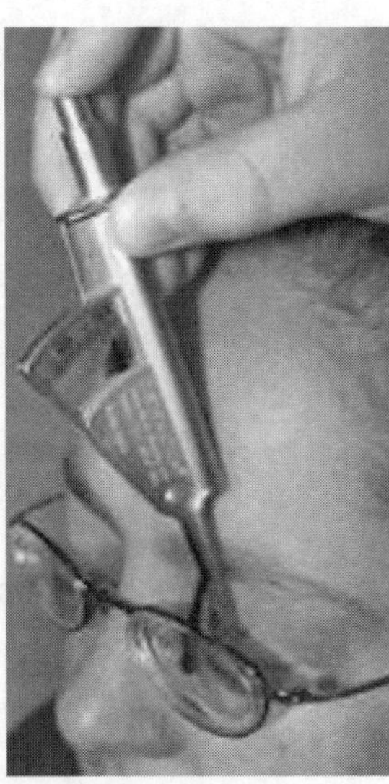

Fig. 21: Short vertex distance. *(For Color version, See Color Plate 4)*

The measurement of back vertex distance is carried out with the help of a *Distometer*.

Retinal image size is influenced by the back vertex distance of a corrective lens. Contact lenses have shorter vertex distances than spectacles, hence image sizes are changed less.

The effective power of a corrective lens varies with the back vertex distance. The effective power of a contact lens can be calculated from its spectacle power with the help of a formula

$$Fc = Fs/1\text{-}dFs$$

Where Fc = power of contact lens, Fs = power of spectacle and d = back vertex distance in meters.

29. Bifocals—short note. (5) (TNMGRMU MS 2018)

Bifocals

These are lenses with two focal powers, one for distant vision and the other for near vision.

Indications

- Presbyopes
- Myopes with esophoria for near; with poor accommodation
- Aphakia
- Hypermetropia with esotropia for near

Contraindications

- Intolerant or unstable patients
- Marked astigmatism and anisometropia
- Certain occupations—such as, golf, where full field of—distance vision is required.

Types

- *Split bifocals* ***(Fig. 22)****:* 2 separate lenses in the same frame. It has become obsolete at present.

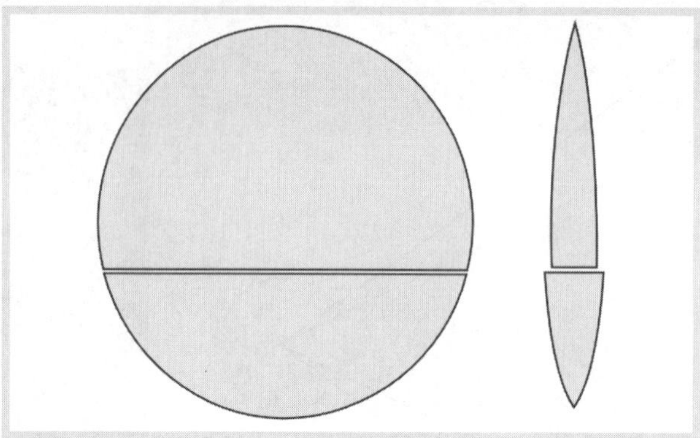

Fig. 22: Split bifocals.

- *Cemented water bifocals* ***(Fig. 23)****:* Supplementary lens cemented on the surface of main lens with glass of same refractive index.

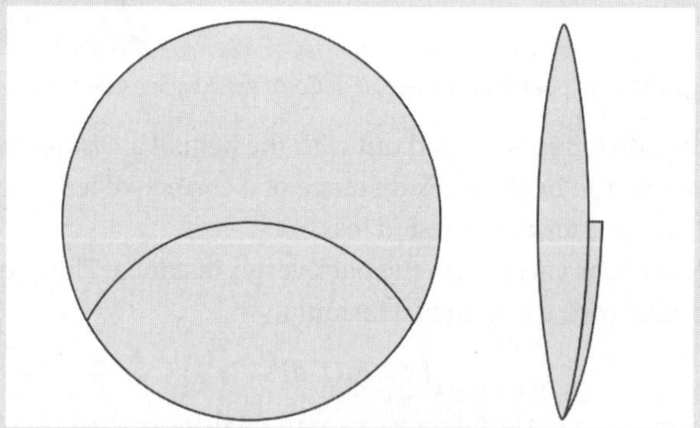

Fig. 23: Cemented bifocals.

- *Fused bifocals* ***(Fig. 24)****:* Made by combining a lens of crown glass with a segment of flint glass of higher refractive power cemented on the hollow of crown glass lens.
    - Round segment
    - Flat topped "D segment"
    - Flat topped "rectangular segment"
    - Curve topped

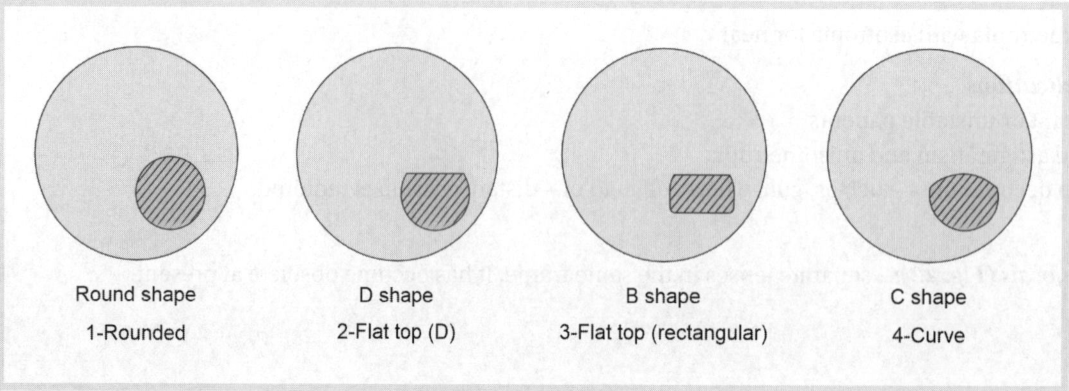

Fig. 24: Fused bifocals.

- *Solid bifocals (Fig. 25):* It is made up of a single piece of glass where two curves are ground upon one spherical surface.

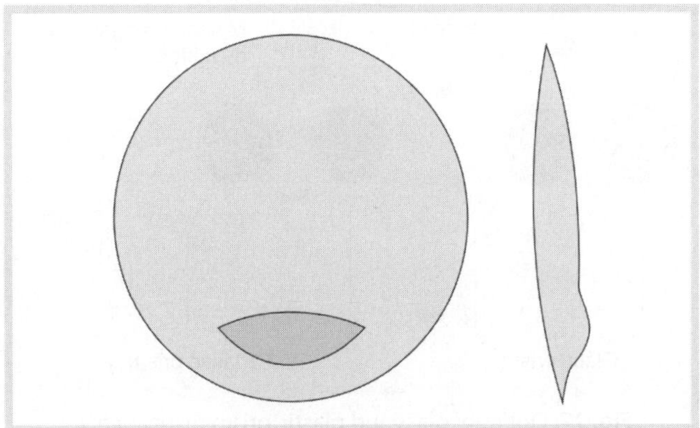

Fig. 25: Solid bifocals.

30. Write a short note on Optics of prisms and its clinical use. (10) (BHU MS 2014)

Optics of Prisms (Figs. 26 and 27)

Prisms are refracting media bounded by two plane surfaces inclined at a finite angle. They have a **base** and an **apex**.

As a ray of light traverses the prism, it is deviated towards the base of the prism, which is perceived as if coming from the apex.

Prism power is the amount of deviation produced as a ray of light traverses a prism. This is measured in Prism Diopter (Δ), which is the number of centimeters of linear deviation undergone by a ray of light when measured at 100 cm from the prism.

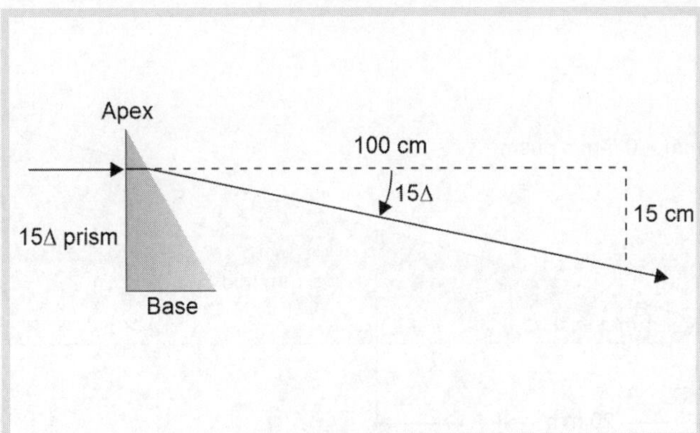

Fig. 26: Optics of prism.

There are 2 main positions that prisms can be used in, these are—*Prentice position* and *Minimum Angle of Deviation (MAD)*.

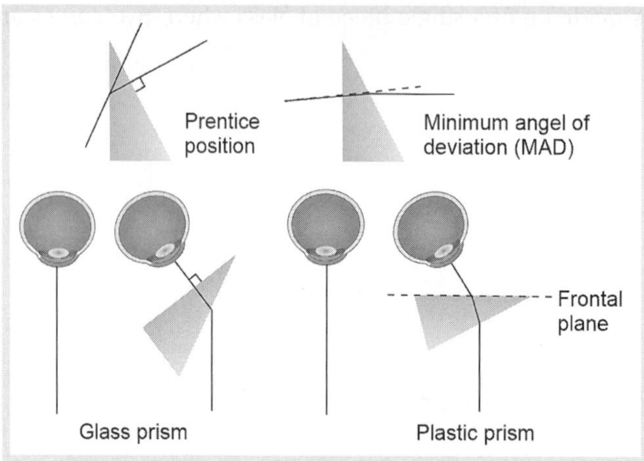

Fig. 27: Optics of glass and plastic prism respectively.

Glass prisms are used in prentice position, while plastic prisms are used in minimum angle of deviation.

In case of prentice position, light enters or leaves the prism, perpendicular to one face of the prism. The MAD position is achieved by holding the prism with its back surface perpendicular to the direction of the fixation object, which for distant objects corresponds to the frontal plane position.

Fresnel prism (Fig. 28): The power of a prism is related to the angle formed by its sides. But when ground into spectacle lens, this can make one edge of the spectacle very thick. Hence, the alternative is pressed prism, in which the angled surface is broken up into a series of much smaller prismatic surfaces at the same angle.

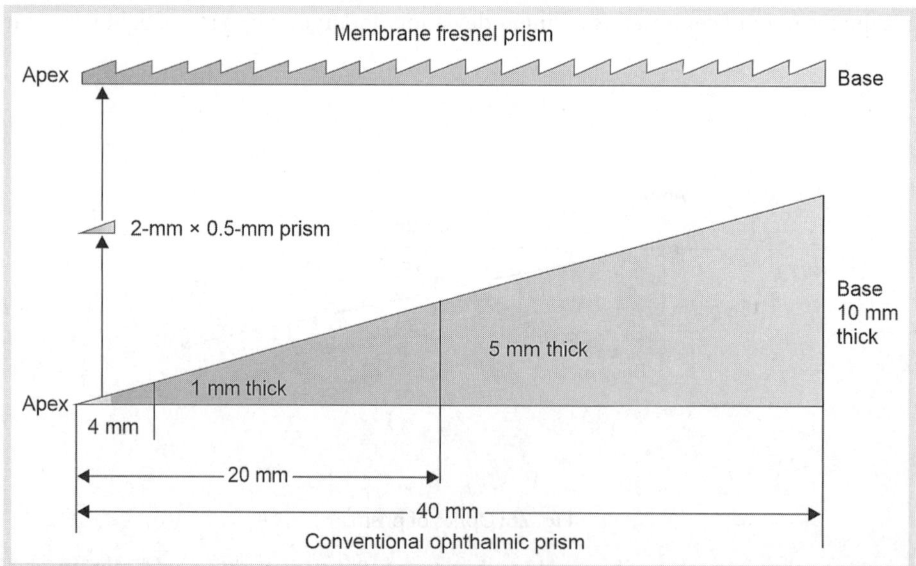

Fig. 28: Fresnel prism optics.

Clinical uses of Prisms

1. *Prism adaptation test:* In case of partially accommodative esotropia, base out prisms are used to determine the maximum adapted angle, to reduce under-correction rate following surgery.
2. *Vertical prism test:* To assess fixation preference in children with straight eyes. No movement is observed induced by vertical strabismus in an amblyopic eye.

3. *Prism alternate cover test:* Estimates the amount in prism diopters required to neutralize the full deviation including any latent phoria.
4. *Detection of anomalous retinal correspondence (ARC):* Occurrence of diplopia in a patient of manifest strabismus after prism neutralization is suggestive of ARC.
5. *To relieve diplopia:* Prisms are used to neutralize diplopia in primary gaze, in case of paralytic or restrictive strabismus.
6. *Convergence insufficiency:* Base-out prisms are used to exercise eyes with convergence insufficiency.
7. *Nystagmus:* Prisms can be used to bring the eyes to null point, in order to relieve anomalous head posture.
8. *Ophthalmic instruments:* Instruments such as—slit lamp biomicroscope, Koeppe's goniolens, applanation tonometer, indirect ophthalmoscope, keratometer, synaptophore, operating microscope, etc.—require prisms for their construction.

31. Discuss the uses of contact lenses in ophthalmology. (10) (TN MGRMU MS)

Contact lenses are optical correction worn in apposition with the cornea which has some practical advantages over spectacles. The lens moves very largely with the eye, and vision through it is therefore much less prone to peripheral distortion which occurs on eccentric viewing through a powerful spectacle lens. The size of the retinal image is also more physiological, thus facilitating binocularity in anisometropia or uniocular aphakia.

Indications

1. Optical indications:
   - Anisometropia
   - Unilateral
   - High myopia
   - Keratoconus
   - Irregular astigmatism
2. Therapeutic indications:
   - Corneal diseases—nonhealing corneal ulcer, bullous keratopathy, filamentary keratitis and recurrent corneal erosion syndrome.
   - Diseases of iris—aniridia, coloboma, albinism to avoid glare
   - Glaucoma for drug delivery
   - Amblyopia opaque contact lenses
   - Bandage soft contact lenses after keratoplasty.
3. Preventive indications:
   - Prevention of symblepharon and restoration of fornices in chemical burns
   - Exposure keratitis
   - Trichiasis
4. Diagnostic indications:
   - Gonioscopy
   - ERG
   - Examination of fundus in the presence of irregular corneal astigmatism
   - Fundus photography
   - Goldmann's three-mirror examination
5. Operative:
   - Goniotomy operation for congenital glaucoma
   - Vitrectomy
   - Endocular photocoagulation
6. Cosmetic indications:
   - Corneal scars
   - Cosmetic scleral lenses in phthisis bulbi

Contraindications

- Mental incompetence or irresponsibility
- Diseases of lacrimal apparatus
- Diseases of ocular surface and adnexa
- Episcleritis and scleritis
- Iridocyclitis
- Seventh nerve palsy
- Upper limb disability
- Poor personal hygiene
- Dry eyes

Clinical uses of Various Contact Lenses in Special Situations

Scleral Rigid Gas Permeable Lenses

1. *Patients with irregular or abnormal corneal topography:*
    - High astigmatism due to keratoconus or other causes of corneal ectasia
    - Traumatized eye with mechanical trauma or chemical burn
    - Postrefractive surgery ectasia and corneal irregularity
    - Aniridia and microphthalmos
    - PMD
    - Neurotrophic keratitis
2. *Patients with high refractive error:*
    - Centration difficulty
    - Intolerance to corneal RGP or hydrogel lenses
3. *Therapeutic applications:*
    - Severe dry eye conditions like cicatrizing pemphigoid, Sjogren syndrome and SJS
    - Lagophthalmos due to poor lid closure or absent lid closure
    - Intractable trichiasis and lid margin keratinization

Hybrid Contact Lens

These lenses consist of RGP center and silicone hydrogel skirt

Uses

- In astigmatism
- Patients with unstable vision with soft toric contact lenses
- Patients wearing RGPs with comfort issues
- Presbyopic patients with astigmatism
- Soft multifocal wearers looking for better visual acuity
- Irregular cornea patients looking for new options

Extended Wear Hydrogel Soft Lenses

Uses

- Elderly aphakic patients having handling problems
- Younger patients to avoid frequent handling problems
- Patients in profession with irregular working hours
- Patients habitual of falling asleep with the lenses on

Extended Wear RGP Lenses

Uses

- Metabolic problems with hydrophilic extended wear
- Visual problems

- Allergic reactions like giant papillary conjunctivitis
- Superior limbic keratoconjunctivitis due to soft lenses
- All patients who have high grade refractive errors needing thicker lenses

Therapeutic Contact Lenses

- *High water content:* Descematocele for support, aphakic and pseudophakic bullous keratopathy, coexistent corneal or anterior segment inflammation.
- *Moderate water content*
- *Low water content:* Epithelial defect in relatively dry eye, when minimal lens movement is required.

Cosmetic Lenses

Uses

- Disfigured corneas
- Vision disturbing conditions like albinism, iris colobomas, aniridia, diplopia, polycoria
- Occlusion therapy in small children

Drug Delivery Systems

The incorporation of the drug into lens material favors a prolonged release of the active medication toward the post lens tear film in contact with corneas where the drug has to penetrate.

Achieving a sustained and prolonged release of ophthalmic drugs allows to reduce the frequency of application and also the required dose to achieve healing.

32. Write a short note on Optical biometry. (5) (TN MGRMU MS 2020)

Optical Biometry

- Ocular biometry involves the measurement of anatomical dimensions of the eye including axial length, corneal curvature and anterior chamber depth.
- These measurements are primarily required for calculation of intraocular lens implant after cataract surgery.
- Optical and ultrasound biometry are the two different modalities which are used, and they have their sets of advantages and disadvantages.
- Optical biometry is a non-contact automated modality used for measuring optical biometric parameters. Two models are widely available that employ two different techniques:
- Laser partial coherence interferometry (PCI) and optical low-coherence reflectometry (OLCR). Both techniques carry the advantage of performing keratometry in addition to measuring the axial length.
- The introduction of this method has significantly improved the accuracy of axial length measurement. This method takes the retinal pigment epithelium as end point of optical measurement.
- Commercially available optical biometers include: (i) IOL Master (ii) Lens Star

Working principle of IOL Master: It works on the PCI method which relies on laser Doppler technique for AL measurement. Corneal curvature is measured by conventional keratometry. AC depth is determined as the distance between the optical sections of lens and cornea. IOL power calculated by the software incorporating the internationally accepted formulae.

Working principle of Lens Star: Lens star LS900 provides highly accurate laser optic measurements for every section of the eye and is the first to measure thickness of the crystalline lens.

Central corneal thickness is measured by optical coherence biometry. It employs a unique dual zone keratometry method for corneal curvature. Pupillometry is done in ambient light conditions. Measurement of lens thickness is key to optimal IOL power prediction.

Formulae for calculating IOL Power

- *First generation:*
  Theoretical: Binkhorst formula

Colenbrander–Hoffer formula
Gill's formula
Regression—SRK-I formula

P = A-2.5L-0.9K, where P = power of IOL; A is constant specific for each lens; L is axial length in mm and K is average keratometry in diopters.

- *Second generation:*
  Theoretical: Modified Binkhorst formula
  Regression—SRK-II formula

The formula remains as SRK-I, the A constant is modified on basis of axial length.
If L is <20 mm – A + 3.0D
L is 20-20.99-A + 2.0D
L is 21-21.99-A + 1.0D
L is 22-24.5 mm-A
L is > 24.5 mm-A-0.5D
Modified SRK-II formula:

If L is <20mm – A + 1.5D
L is 20-21 mm - A +1.0D
L is 21-22mm - A+ 0.5D
L is 22-24.5 mm - A
L is 24.5-26 mm - A- 1.0D
L is >26mm - A - 1.5D

- *Third generation:*
  Holladay I formula
  Hoffer's Q formula
  SRK-T Formula
- *Fourth generation:*
  Holladay II formula
  Haigis formula
- *Fifth generation:*
  Hoffer H-5 formula
  Barrett Universal II formula
  Olsen formula
  Hill-RBF formula

Ultimately the choice of formula is up to the surgeon for selecting the appropriate IOL, and effort should be made to reach the best possible accuracy.

33. Discuss the various intraocular lens power calculations, its merits and demerits.
(5) (TN MGRMU 2020)

Formulae for calculation of IOL power can be of two major types:
- Regression formulae
- Theoretical formulae

Regression Formulae
- These are empiric formulae generated by retrospective analysis of postoperative refraction of large numbers of IOL implantations, in an attempt to predict IOL power.
- Most common: SRK and SRK II formulae.

Theoretical Formulae

- Based on theoretical model of the eye (Gullstrand eye). The eye is considered as a two Leu's system, i.e., cornea and IOL.
- On the basis of calculation of effective lens position (ELP), the IOL calculation formulae can be subdivided into various generations.

1st Generation Formula

A constant value was considered in all cases for IOL power calculation. ELP of 4 mm was considered in all patients. *A constant* was used in IOL power calculation in the SRK formula. The Binkhorst formula considers a postoperative constant anterior chamber depth for IOL power calculation. However, abnormally high or low values were obtained for very short or very long eyes.

2nd Generation Formula

Better results were obtained by polynomial regression formulae. Theoretical formulae considered AC depth in relation to axial length of the eye.

3rd Generation Formulae

Third generation theoretical formulae use axial length along with K readings of the corned for IOL power calculation. These formulae were found to be significantly more accurate compared to previous formulae.

4th Generation Formulae

A wide variety of variables were considered for IOL power calculation. Even though these formulae are more accurate in general, but third generation formulae are more for eyes with extremely high axial length. Personalizing the A constant for different eyes leads to a better refractive outcome.

5th Generation Formulae

Variables required for calculation of IOL are—K reading, axial length, anterior chamber depth.

34. Write a short note on Trifocals lens. (5) (TN MGRMU MS 2015)

Trifocal Lens

These lenses were introduced to achieve spectacle independence after cataract surgery, particularly for intermediate vision, such as computer work, car driving, music playing, etc. These glasses may be required despite satisfactory near and distance vision by dividing light into three focal points. They are of following designs:

Fine Vision Iol (PhysIOL)

It is the first diffractive trifocal lens made up of 25% hydrophilic acrylic IOL in addition to a near foci (+ 3.5D) with four closed haptics. An asymmetric distribution of energy among the three foci (near, intermediate and far) for improved vision. This IOL is based on a fully diffractive optic with gradual attenuation of step height. When pupil is dilated, the peripheral steps are exposed, more light passes to distant vision than near and intermediate focal points and approximately 15% energy is lost.

Micro Fine Vision (Micro f) is its toric version.

AT LISA Trifocal IOL:

It is a diffractive IOL (+3.33D near and +1.66D intermediate)

Reduces 14.3% light loss. The portion of light energy sent to intermediate focal point is same at all pupil size (30%). It has plate haptic design.

Both IOLs are injectable. But, AT LISA trifocal IOL are prefolded and preloaded, whereas fine vision IOL (PhysIOL) must be manually folded and then inserted into cartridge.

PanOptix Trifocal IOL:

One of the most popular trifocal IOL that warrants mention in this regard is PanOptix (by Alcon). It has a smaller central diffractive region, better light utilization and also corrects for spherical aberrations of the cornea.

Trials comparing trifocal lenses (PanOptix) with EDOF IOL showed better visual acuity at distance, near and especially intermediate ranges, better contrast sensitivity and lesser complaints of halos and glare in the former.

35. Write short note on low vision aids. (5) (BHU MS 2021)

Vision rehabilitation begins with a low vision evaluation and is followed by training and referral to resources and specialized services.

Visual rehabilitation aims to assess and address the whole person by considering five areas:

1. Reading and access to text
2. Valued daily life activities
3. Patient safety
4. Continued participation in activities despite vision loss
5. Psychosocial well-being

Types of Low Vision Aids

a. *Technology and electronic devices:* Smartphones and tablets are now increasingly helping in visual rehabilitation by magnifying images, use of audio options to send texts, send emails, read books and newspapers, read bar codes, navigate unfamiliar areas. Smart speakers and virtual assistant also can be very useful for individuals with vision impairment. Audio books available as Digital Accessible Information System (DAISY) format is being used now by patients with low vision. A variety of video magnifier devices combine cameras and screens to allow not only magnification, but also modification of contrast and color. The major disadvantages with electronic devices are cost and training requirements. E.g., Soundscape app, VoiceOver screen reader in operating system, iVision app, Be my Eyes app, TapTap See app, etc.

b. *Optical devices:* Most commonly used method can be use of *High Adds,* i.e., +4.00D adds or simple over the counter readers, as long as patients can maintain the closer focal distance and use supplemental lighting if beneficial. Patients often use readers in power ranges +6.00D–+12.00D, with appropriate base-in prism and focal distance. The Kestenbaum rule would estimate that a patient with 20/200 acuity would require 200/20 or 10.00 D add. Alternatively, computer glasses with the intermediate powers in the upper segment of the bifocal can be useful.

c. *Magnifiers:* Wide range of optical magnifiers are available with and without illumination. There are two methods of calculating the magnification of magnifiers. *Simple or nominal* magnification is the dioptric power divided by 4, assuming the object is held at the anterior focal point of the magnifier. *Commercial* magnifiers are often labeled with a "trade magnification" power calculated as (dioptric power of magnifier)/4+1.

d. *Telescopes:* Bioptic telescopes are spectacle mounted set to focus at distance, they are mounted in the upper portion of spectacle lens. Patients with good contrast sensitivity and intact central field are optimal candidates for bioptic telescopes.

e. *Nonoptical aids:* An armamentarium of tools are available to assist patients with impaired vision. Simple and practical devices like large-format watches, remote controls, bold letter computer keyboards, needle threaders, talking clocks, timers.

36. Explain the working principle of synoptophore and its clinical role. (10) (TN MGRMU 2015)

A synaptophore is an instrument which presents separate images to the eye. It compensates for the angle of squint and allows stimuli to be presented to both the eyes simultaneously. An instrument for diagnosing imbalance of eye muscles and treating them by orthoptic methods.

Working Principle

Haploscopic principle **(Fig. 29)**: It is based on the principle of division of physical space into two separate areas of visual space each of which is visible to only one eye.

The object and its image are "conjugate" being join by the optical system so that if test object pictures are placed in a chosen position relative to each other it follows that the image will be directed into similar relative positions.

By altering the position of the test objects in an instrument that their image can be made to stimulate selected retinal areas as required.

Optics

The instrument consists of two cylindrical tubes with mirrored right-angled bend and a +6.50D lens in each eyepiece. This optically sets the distance as equivalent to about 6 meters. The image of the test object slide is situated at the principle focus of the lens.

Rays of light emanating from the principal focus will after refraction through the lens in eye piece emerge as parallel rays, this means that the eye when viewing the image is relaxed or focused for distance, no accommodation is required.

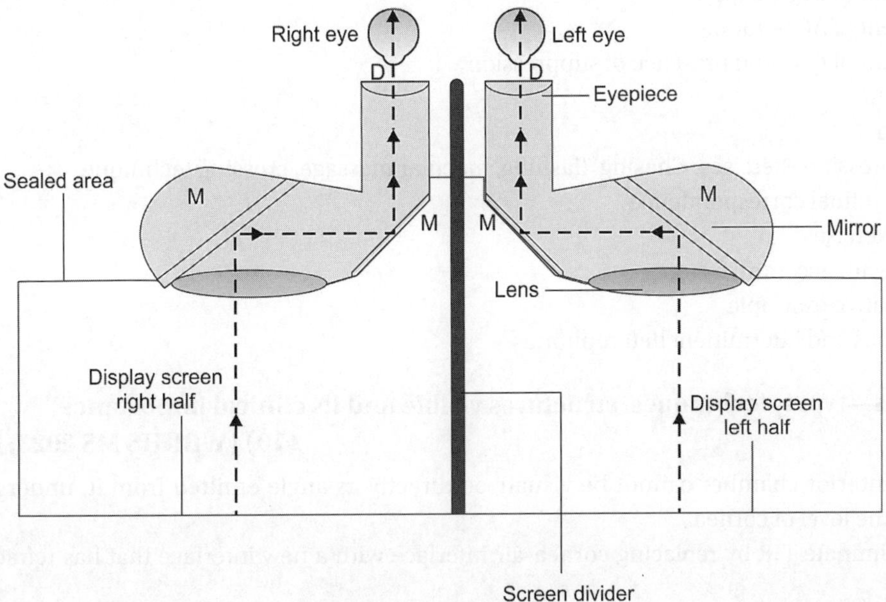

Fig. 29: Haploscopic principle.

Slides used for the various grades of Binocular vision:

1. Simultaneous perception slides—foveal, macular, paramacular, peripheral
2. Fusion
3. Stereopsis
4. Special purpose slides:
   a. After image slides
   b. Haidinger brushes
   c. Slide with number or letters

Clinical uses of Synaptophore

1. *Diagnostic uses:*
   a. Measurement of deviation:
      - With each eye fixing (paralytic squint)
      - Objective angle and subjective angle (to measure ARC)
      - In different gaze positions (incomitant squints)
      - Horizontal, vertical and torsional deviations can be measured
   b. Special functions like adaptability to function in aniseikonia with the help of special slides
   c. "After image" testing
   d. Assessment of binocular status:
      - Simultaneous macular perception
      - Fusion
      - Stereopsis—for foveal, macular and paramacular retinal areas

e. Measurement of range of fusion
f. Cases with incomplete suppression can also be tested by using differential illumination and by using flashing devices
g. Appreciation of entoptic phenomenon, Haidinger brushes
h. Measurement of inter pupillary distance
i. Measurement of fusional vergence
j. Measurement of angle kappa
k. Measurement of AC/A ratio
l. Measurement of type and presence of suppression

2. *Therapeutic uses:*
   a. Suppression
      - Antisuppression exercises: Chasing, flashing, macular massage, crossing technique
   b. Anomalous retinal correspondence
      - Fusion exercises
   c. Amblyopia with eccentric fusion
   d. Accommodative esotropia
   e. Heterophorias and intermittent heterophorias

37. Gonioscopes—types, techniques, structures visible and its clinical importance. (10) (WBUHS MS 2023, DO 2016, 2017)

The angle of the anterior chamber cannot be visualized directly as angle emitted from it, undergoes total internal reflection (TIR) at the level of cornea.

Goniolenses eliminate TIR by replacing cornea-air interface with a new interface that has refractive index greater than cornea.

Types of Gonioscopy

- Direct gonioscopy
- Indirect gonioscopy
  - Indentation
  - Nonindentation
  - Manipulative

Direct Gonioscopy (Fig. 30)

Anterior curve of goniolens is such that critical angle is not reached and light rays refracted at contact lens-air interface.

Examples: Koeppe's lens, Richardson-Shaffer lens, Hoskins-Barkan lens, Swan Jacob lens

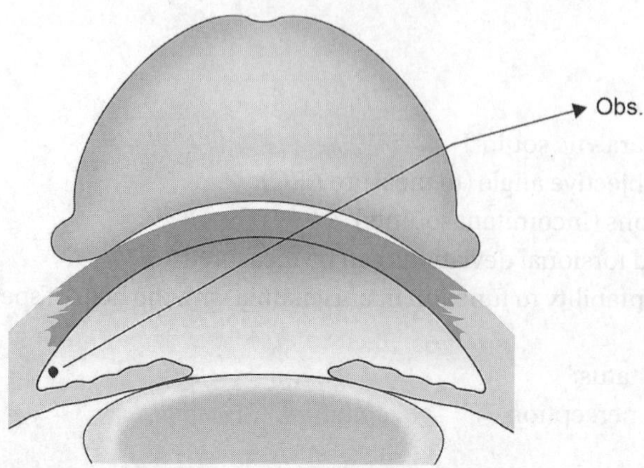

Fig. 30: Optics of direct gonioscopy.

Technique:

- The patient lies in supine position, with eye to be examined, under topical anesthesia.
- Goniolens is placed on the cornea using balanced salt solution or methyl cellulose.
- Examiner holds goniolens in one hand and the light source in another, and observes the whole 360° of the angle, by moving their position.
- Panoramic view of the angle can be achieved.
- Provides a straight view rather than an inverted view.
- Angle is deep in supine position, so it is difficult to view the angle.

Indirect Gonioscopy

The light rays emitting from the angle are reflected by the mirror inside the goniolens, hence the image obtained is inverted.

Examples: Indentation—Goldman single mirror, Goldman 3 mirror, Allen Thorpe

Nonindentation—Zeiss four mirror, Sussman four mirror

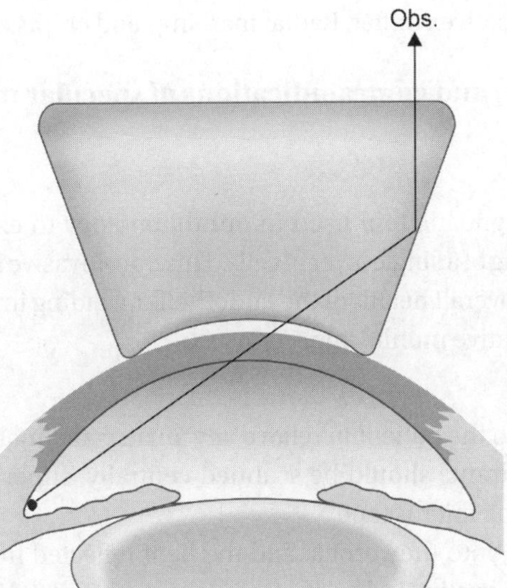

Fig. 31: Optic of indentation gonioscopy.

Technique of nonindentation gonioscopy:

- After anesthetizing the cornea, coupling gel is inserted into the cup of the goniolens.
- Goniolens is placed and tipped on the cornea.
- Slit lamp beam is focused which shows the inverted angle image.
- The surface of the gonioprisms is larger than the cornea, hence coupling gel is required.

*Technique of indentation gonioscopy **(Fig. 31)**:*

- Similar to indentation gonioscopy except, no coupling gel is required as the curvature of the goniolens is at par with the curvature of the cornea.
- Varying amounts of pressure is applied and the examiner observes its effect on the width of angle of anterior chamber.
- Increased pressure over central cornea displaces aqueous towards the angle, hence widely opening the angle.

Manipulative gonioscopy:

It is a variant of indirect gonioscopy when the patient is asked to look into the mirror being looked at by the examiner, hence bring into better view the angle structures of the opposite angle.

Structures Seen on Gonioscopy

- *Schwalbe' line*
  - It is the anterior most structure observed on gonioscopy.
  - It represents the peripheral termination of the Descemet's membrane.
  - It is seen as a faint white to translucent line, located by identifying the meeting point of the corneal wedge.
- *Trabecular meshwork*
  - It lies between the Schwalbe's line (anteriorly) and scleral spur (posteriorly).
  - It is smooth in infants and becomes coarse and pigmented with age. The anterior part is non-functional and non-pigmented, while the posterior portion is functional and pigmented.
    Posterior portion overlies the canal of Schlemm, where the aqueous escapes into, from the anterior chamber.
- *Scleral spur:* Anterior most projection of the scleral; situated posterior to trabecular meshwork; appears as a dense, white, shiny band. Identification of scleral spur indicates gonioscopically open angle.
- *Ciliary body band*
  - Appears as a pink to brown or slate gray band, just behind the scleral spur.
  - It is visible due to the insertion of iris into the ciliary body.
- *Root of iris:* Iris contour is slightly convex or flat. Radial markings and crypts are present.

38. Describe the technique, uses, and contraindications of specular microscopy. (10) (WBUHS MS 2017)

Specular Microscopy

Specular microscopy is a pivotal diagnostic tool used in ophthalmology to examine the corneal endothelium, the innermost layer of the cornea consisting of a single layer of cells. This non-invasive technique provides critical information on cell density, morphology, and the overall health of the endothelium, aiding in the diagnosis of endothelial disorders, pre-surgical evaluation, and postoperative monitoring.

Technique

The procedure is first fully explained to the patient to relieve any anxiety and make the patient comfortable. The cornea is systemically scanned, and all quadrants should be scanned centrally, superior, inferior, temporal, and nasal. The specular microscope is a light-reflecting microscope.

The slit beam of light is projected onto the cornea, and the light reflected from the tissue interface helps form the image. The difference between the refractive index of aqueous humor and endothelial cells gives rise to specular or mirror-like reflection on the posterior surface.

The reflected light is approximately 0.02% of the incident beam of light. If a broad beam of light is used, the reflected beam from the stroma and epithelium obscures a clear view of the endothelium. Liang described 4 distinct zones on specular microscopy using a slit beam of evaluation:

- *Zone 1:* Epithelium/coupling fluid of lens
- *Zone 2:* Corneal stroma
- *Zone 3:* Endothelium
- *Zone 4:* Aqueous humor

Uses

- Endothelial changes after surgery
- Contact lens endotheliopathy
- Pseudoexfoliation-induced endotheliopathy
- Endotheliopathy after ocular inflammation (e.g., uveitis, endotheliitis)
- Endotheliopathy after forceps injury
- Endotheliopathy in corneal dystrophy
- Drug-induced endotheliopathy

- Corneal guttata
- Fuchs endothelial corneal dystrophy
- Posterior polymorphous endothelial dystrophy
- Congenital hereditary endothelial dystrophy
- Iridocorneal endothelial syndrome
- Senile endothelial degeneration

Contraindications of Specular Microscopy

Absolute

a. Severe corneal opacification
b. Active ocular infection
c. Acute ocular trauma

Relative

a. Shallow anterior chamber
b. Severe photophobia
c. Uncooperative patient

39. Explain confocal laser microscopy with diagram. (5) (TN MGRMU MS 2022)

Confocal Optics (Fig. 32)

- When an imaging system and illumination system focus on the same small point, the system is described as confocal.
- The contrast and resolution of the image are increased by minimizing the amount of scattered light.

This is achieved by:

- Using a laser source of illumination
- Observer viewing through a pinhole or slit.

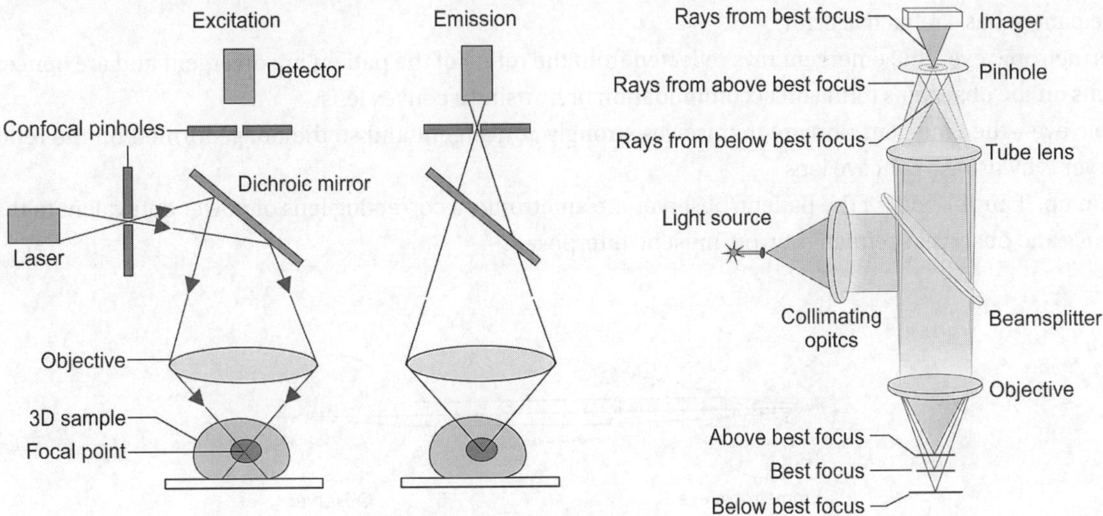

Fig. 32: Optic of confocal laser microscopy.

Components

Pinholes

- Objective lenses
- Low-noise detectors
- Fast scanning mirrors
- Filters for wavelength selection

- Laser illumination

This principle of confocal optics is used in various instruments to view various parts of the eye in great detail, some of which have been described below.

Confocal Microscopy of Cornea

Microscopic examination of the various layers of living cornea. It helps to study changes in cornea in contact lens wearers. Limbal microstructures can be observed.

- *Scanning laser polarimetry:* It measures the thickness of RNFL to detect early glaucomatous damage.
- *Confocal laser scanning ophthalmoscope (CSLO):* This technology is used by Heidelberg retinal tomograph.

A laser light (670 nm) enters through one pinhole and focuses on a plane of retina or optic disc. The reflected light passes through a confocal pupil that allows only reflected light from that specific plane to enter the photodetector. A reference plane has to be defined in this case.

40. Discuss optical principle and working of direct ophthalmoscope. (10). (WBUHS MS 2014)

Ophthalmoscopy is the method of examination of the internal structures of the eye by an ophthalmoscope. It is primarily done to assess the fundus oculi and the media opacities. The ophthalmoscope was first invented by Babbage in 1848 but the usage was not wide until it was modified by von Helmholtz in 1850.

Direct Ophthalmoscopy is the most widely used examination method for routine fundus examination.

Optical principle (Fig. 33)

The modern day direct ophthalmoscope is basically based on the basic principle of von Helmholtz's glass plate ophthalmoscope. A convergent beam of light from the ophthalmoscope is shined onto the patient's pupil. The rays which are emergent from the fundus of the eye being examined reaches the observer's retina through the viewing apparatus of the ophthalmoscope. The emergent rays are parallel which are coming from the retina of the patient's eye are then brought to focus on the retina of the observer (emmetropic) once accommodation is relaxed.

When the patient has a refractive error:

- Hypermetropic eye—the emergent rays reflected from the retina of the patient are divergent and are hence brought to focus on the observer's retina on accommodation or by using a convex lens.
- Myopic eye—the emergent rays are themselves strongly convergent and so the image formed on the retina of the observer is by using a concave lens

To sum up, if any or both of the patient/observer are ametropic, a correcting lens of power equivalent to the sum of the patient's and observer's refractive errors must be interposed.

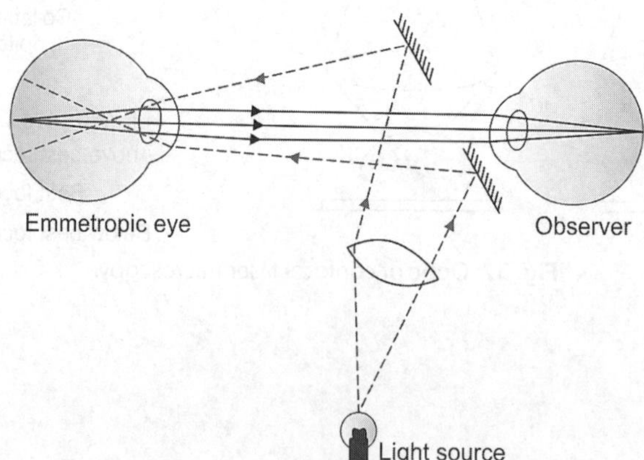

Fig. 33: Schematic diagram of optical principle of direct ophthalmoscope.

Source: Khurana AK. Optics and Refraction of Eye, 3rd edition. Amsterdam: Elsevier; 2013. Chapter 12, p. 457.

Characteristics of the Image Formed (Fig. 34)

When in direct ophthalmoscopy, the image formed is erect, virtual and magnified to about 14 times in emmetropes.

The emergent rays from the illuminated area of retina AB are parallel. These parallel rays intercepted by the observer is projected behind the patient's eye A_2B_2. These points theoretically are situated at the observer's minimal distance of distinct vision. The image of the patient's fundus A_1B_1 is equal to the size of the fundus AB examined.

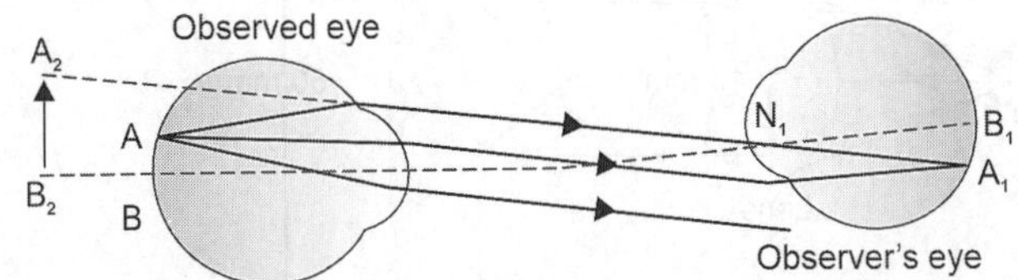

Fig. 34: Characteristics of the image formed in direct ophthalmoscopy.

Field of Vision in Direct Ophthalmoscopy

The field of vision in direct ophthalmoscopy is always less than the field of illumination. It is affected by the following factors:

- It is directly proportional to the size of the pupil of the examined eye
- Also it is directly proportional to the axial length of the observed eye
- It is inversely proportional to the distance between the observer's and the examined eye.

Technique

- The procedure to be done in dark room with the patient seated and looking straight ahead
- The patient's right eye to be examined by the observer's right eye and the left eye with left.
- Light is reflected into patient's pupil.
- Once the red reflex is seen, observer to move to the eye as close as possible.
- The fundus view should be focused by dialing the Reskoss disc which has several plus and minus powered lenses.
- Once focus is set, the disc, macula, vessels should be examined.

41. Describe with diagram the optical principle of indirect ophthalmoscope. (10) (WBUHS MS 2016)

Binocular indirect ophthalmoscopy, introduced by Nagel in 1864, is most commonly used method for examination of posterior segment. Indirect ophthalmoscopy is of great application and requires much skill and practice by the anterior and posterior segment surgeons.

Optical Principle

The principle is based on making the eye highly myopic by placing a strong convex lens in front of patient's eye so the emergent rays from an area of the fundus are brought to focus as a real inverted image between the lens and the examiner's eye.

Optical System of Binocular Indirect Ophthalmoscope ***(Fig. 35)****:* Binocularity is achieved by reducing the interpupillary distance of the examiner from about 60 mm average to 15 mm using prisms or mirrors. This artificial reduction in the IPD requires larger pupillary dilation of the patient for proper binocular viewing.

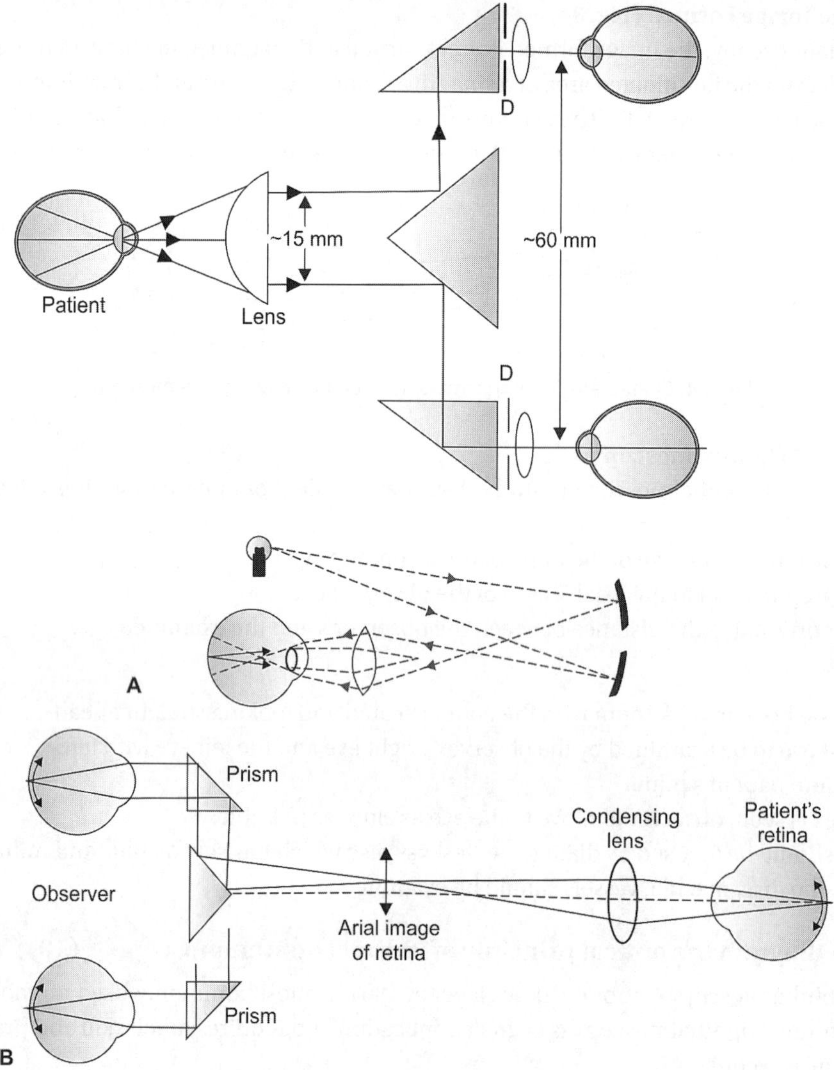

Fig. 35: Optics of indirect ophthalmoscope.
Source: Khurana AK. Optics and Refraction of Eye, 3rd edition. Amsterdam: Elsevier; 2013. Chapter 12, p. 461.

Field of illumination: The field in myopia is more, less in hypermetropia when compared to emmetropia.

Image formation:

a. *In emmetropia* ***(Fig. 37)****:* The emergent rays from the illuminated area of the retina in an emmetropic are parallel and hence brought to focus by the condensing lens at its principle focus. An inverted real image of retina is formed in between the examiner's eye and the lens
b. *In hypermetropes* ***(Fig. 38)***: The rays emergent from illuminated retina are themselves of diverging character, appearing to come from an imaginary point behind the retina (erect, virtual). This imaginary object is used by the condensing lens, forming an inverted, real image, located in front of principle focus.
c. *In myopes* ***(Fig. 36)***: The illuminated area of retina lets emergent rays which are convergent, forming and inverted image in front of the eye. The condensing lens then helps to form the final image located within its own focal length.

Characteristics of the image formed: The image formed by indirect ophthalmoscopy is real, inverted and magnified. Magnification depends upon the dioptric power of the condensing lens, position of the lens in relation to patient's eye and its refractive status. With stronger power of lens image will be smaller but brighter and with more field of vision.

Relative positions of the image formed **(Figs. 36 to 38)**:
- In emmetropia, the emergent rays are parallel and focused at the principle focus of the condensing lens.
- In hypermetropia, the emergent rays are divergent, hence focused farther away from the principle focus.
- In myopia, emergent rays are convergent and are therefore focused near the principle focus of lens.

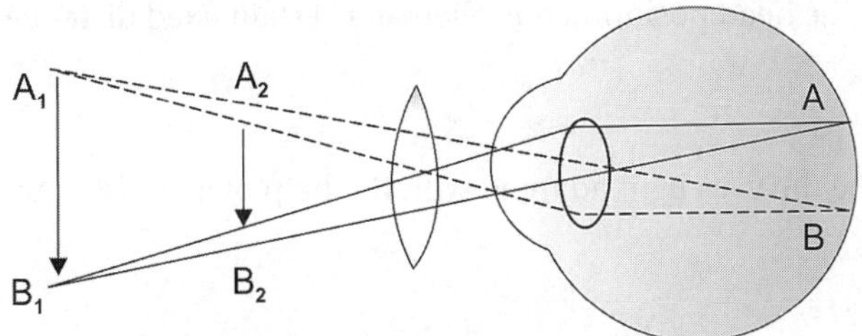

Fig. 36: Image formation in myopia.
Source: Khurana AK. Optics and Refraction of Eye, 3rd edition. Amsterdam: Elsevier; 2013. Chapter 12, p. 462

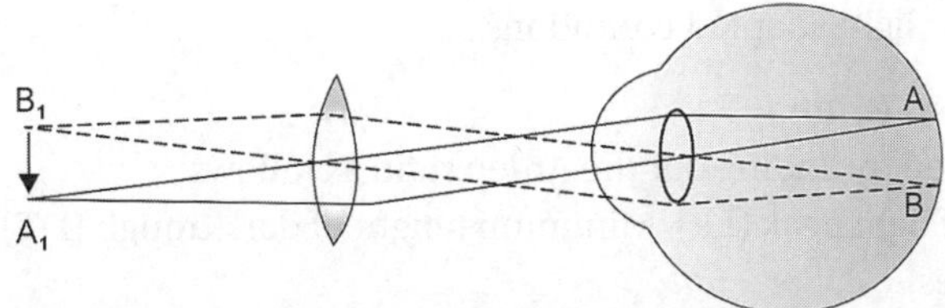

Fig. 37: Image formation in emmetropia.
Source: Khurana AK. Optics and Refraction of Eye, 3rd edition. Amsterdam: Elsevier; 2013. Chapter 12, p. 462.

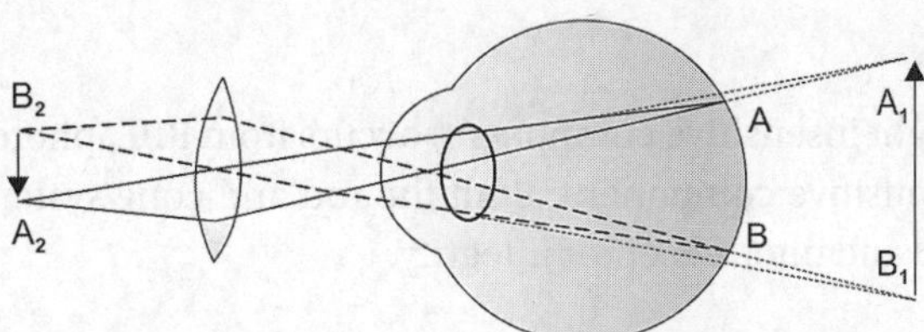

Fig. 38: Image formation in hypermetropia.
Source: Khurana AK. Optics and Refraction of Eye, 3rd edition. Amsterdam: Elsevier; 2013. Chapter 12, p. 461.

Image magnification: Lateral magnification in an indirect ophthalmoscope is a function of power of patient's eye. A 20D lens will produce a magnification of 3 times, a 30D lens forming 2 times.

The field of observation is always greater than the field of illumination in indirect ophthalmoscopy. The size of the pupil does not affect the size of the field of observation as long as it is larger than the examiner's pupil.

42. Write a short note on EOG. (5) (TN MGRMU 2015)

Electrooculography (EOG) is based on the measurement of resting potential of the eye exists between cornea(positive) and back of retina (negative) during fully dark adapted and fully light adapted conditions.

Electrophysiological basis of EOG:
The outer retinal layers are electronegative and inner retinal layers are electropositive. The internal electropositivity is transmitted to the cornea while the outer electronegativity is transmitted to periocular tissues. A potential difference of 2–19 mV is recorded by millivoltmeter connected to 2 electrodes.

Technique of Recording

Prerequisites
Good fixation, normal extraocular motility, visual field of at least 60 degree.

Electrodes

Placed over the orbital margins near the medial and lateral canthi serve as active electrodes. A forehead electrode serves as a ground electrode

Patient's Position and Fixation

Patient sits erect in a room with the head position controlled at a certain fixed distance from 3 fixation lights which are places in patient's line of vision.

Stimulus Light

An arrangement is made to make the eyes light adapted with the help of a bright, long duration stimulus. The pupil is dilated with mydriatics.

Recording

The patient is asked to move the eye sideways (medially and laterally) by fixating right and left fixation lights alternately and keep there for few seconds, during which recording is done. After standardized period of light adaptation, responses are recorded for 15 minutes under dark adapted condition. The stimulus lights are then turned on again and responses are recorded for 15 minutes under light adapted conditions.

Measurement and Interpretation of Results

Results of EOG are then interpreted by finding out the Arden ratio as follows:
Arden ratio = Maximum height of light peak (LP)/Minimum height of dark trough (DT)
[DT-8–12 minutes, LP-6–9 minutes]
Normal value 1.85 or above
Subnormal value 1.65–1.85
Abnormal value—below 1.65

Components of EOG

- *Dark trough (DT):* This is the light insensitive component, occurs from RPE, photoreceptors, inner nuclear layer.
- *Light peak (LP):* This is light sensitive component. Both the rod and cone systems contribute to EOG light rise. It appears to be a measure of RPE and photoreceptor integrity.

Clinical Applications

EOG reflects the presynaptic functions of the retina, any disease that interferes with functional interplay between the RPE and the photoreceptors will produce an abnormal or absent light rise.

EOG is Affected in

Retinitis pigmentosa, vitamin A deficiency, retinal detachment, toxic retinopathies, retinal vascular occlusions

Patients with vitelliform macular degeneration often show a striking reduction of EOG in the presence of a normal ERG.

43. Write a short note on electroretinogram. (5) (TN MGRMU MS 2022)

Electroretinogram is a corneal measure of an action potential produced by retina when it is stimulated by light of adequate intensity.

Principle: Sudden illumination of retina will cause simultaneous activation of all retinal cells to generate current that passes through vitreous and extracellular space. High RPE resistant prevent summated current from passing posteriorly, small portion of summated current which escape through cornea is recorded as ERG.

Electrophysiological basis of ERG (Fig. 39)

1. A wave:
   - Corneal negative wave
   - Arises from photoreceptors

- Origin—light fall on photoreceptor producing hyperpolarization (outer portion of photoreceptor becomes positive and inner becomes negative, hence cornea becomes negative).
- Both rods and cones contribute to A wave.

2. B wave:
   - Corneal positive wave.
   - Arises from Muller cells, represent activity of bipolar cells.
   - Origin—light fall on photoreceptor causing hyperpolarization. K+ leakage and absorption by Muller cells causes depolarization of Muller cells.
3. C wave:
   - Corneal prolonged negative wave with low amplitude.
   - Represent metabolic activity of pigment epithelium.
   - Origin: Negative wave generated by RPE in response to rod signal only because rods cells are in direct contact with apical end of RPE.

Types of ERG

According to Stimulus Zone

1. Full field
2. Focal
3. Multifocal

According to Type of Stimulus

1. Single flash
2. Flicker fusion
3. Red flash
4. Blue filter
5. Pattern ERG

According to Retinal Adaptation

1. Scotopic
2. Photopic
3. Mesopic

Role of ERG

- Child with poor vision—to rule out any dystrophy

To Diagnosis

- Labor congenital amaurosis
- Juvenile X-linked recessive disorders
- Congenital stationary night blindness in myopia

In Prognosis of

- Retinitis pigmentosa
- Cone rod dystrophy

Evaluate Toxicity

- Metallic intraocular foreign body
- Vitamin A deficiency
- HCQ toxicity

Other Uses

- Retinal detachment

- Vascular occlusion
- Diabetic retinopathy

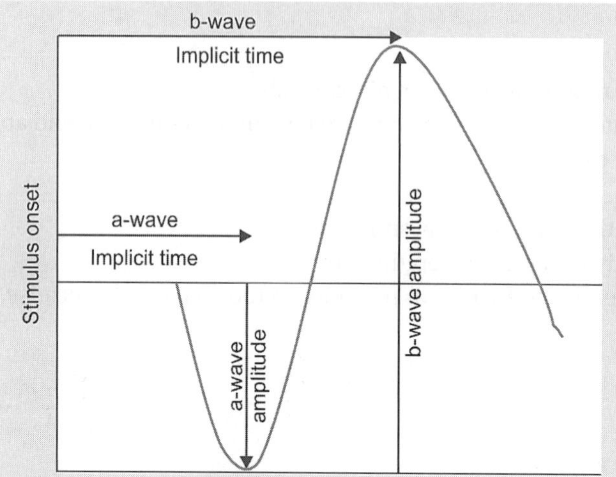

Fig. 39: VEP waveforms.

44. Write a short note on visual evoked potential (VEP). (5) (TN MGRMU MS 2018)

VEP is an electrophysiological test to record the electrical activity of the visual cortex in response to visual stimulation. VEP depends on the integrity of the visual pathway starting from the eye to the occipital cortex. Currently for VEP, the Standard International society for clinical electrophysiology of vision (ISCEV) protocols are followed to assess the anterior visual pathway from the eye to the optic nerve anterior to the optic chiasma.

Patient Preparation

a. Refractive correction
b. Uniocular recording
c. Pupil undilated
d. The other eye patched

The electrodes are placed in the occipital lobe, forehead and either in earlobe/mastoid/vertex. Types of VEP with its waveform:

a. *Pattern reversal VEP:* With the luminance same, the checkerboard blocks reverse 2 times per second.
   Waveform—the waves appear 75 ms, 100 ms, 135 ms after the stimulus hence named—N75, N100, N135. There are 2 negative and 1 positive wave.
b. *Pattern onset/offset VEP:* The blocks of checkerboard go on & off with time, keeping the luminance same. It is on for 200 ms and off for 400 ms. This type is specially used for malingering patients and those with nystagmus.
   Waveform—positive wave C1 at 75 ms, C3 at 150 ms and negative wave C2 at 125 ms.
c. *Flash VEPs:* This type uses a flash which subtends 20 degrees of the visual field. Flash rate is 1 per second.
   Waveform—multiple positive and negative waves.

Uses of VEP

i. To assess the prognosis of poor vision before planning for surgery
ii. To assess and monitor visual function in children and infants.
iii. Evaluation of optic nerve
iv. Rule out malingering.

45. Write a short note on Cover Test. (5) (BHU MS 2020)

Cover Tests

The cover tests are helpful in detecting heterotrophia and heterophoria.

Prerequisites:

- Patient should have foveal fixation in each eye.
- Patient should be able to pay attention and cooperate with the examiner
- Patient should have preserved ocular movements.

There are three main types of cover tests, which are—*cover-uncover, alternate cover and simultaneous prism and cover.*

Cover-uncover Test

This test is again subdivided into 2 components. (I) Cover test and (II) Uncover test, which is tested for both distant and near fixation with an accommodative target **(Flowchart 1)**.

Cover test (Fig. 40)

- This is a qualitative test, which is used to detect heterotrophia.
- After assessment of corneal light reflex, fixating eye is covered and the deviating eye is observed for movements to take up fixation.
- No movement indicates orthotropia. Adduction in deviating eye indicates exotropia, whereas abduction suggests esotropia. Downward movement is suggestive of hypertropia and upward movement points to hypotropia.

Uncover test

- A qualitative test useful in detection of heterophoria.
- Either of the eyes are covered and kept under cover for 2–3 seconds. The cover is then removed to observe any movement in the covered eye. If the covered eye had deviated under cover, a refixation movement would be observed when the cover is removed.
- Movements are indicative of latent strabismus of respective direction, as observed in cover test.
- Here, the smoothness and speed of recovery is the evidence of the strength of motor fusion.

Alternate Cover Test

- It is a test used to detect both latent and manifest strabismus.
- As the patient fixates, occluder is moved from one eye to the other, where movement of each eye is observed when it is uncovered. However, it does not distinguish between latent and manifest strabismus.

Flowchart 1: Cover–uncover test.

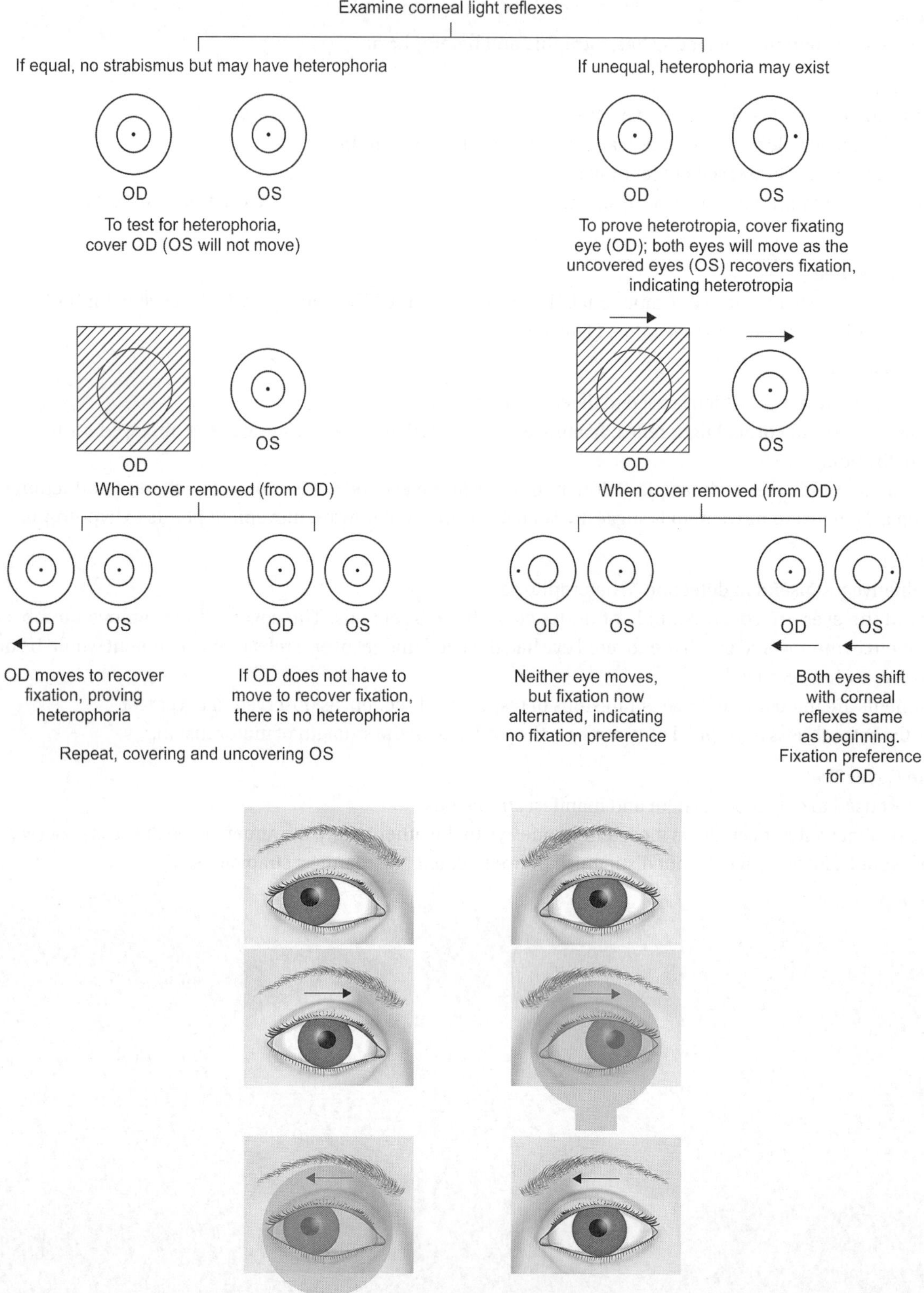

Fig. 40: Cover test.

Simultaneous Prism and Cover Test (Fig. 41)

- It measures the manifest deviation during binocular viewing. It provides the best indication of size of deviation.
- A prism is placed in front of deviating eye with the fixation eye kept covered. Movement is observed in the deviated eye with increasing power of prisms until no movement can be observed.

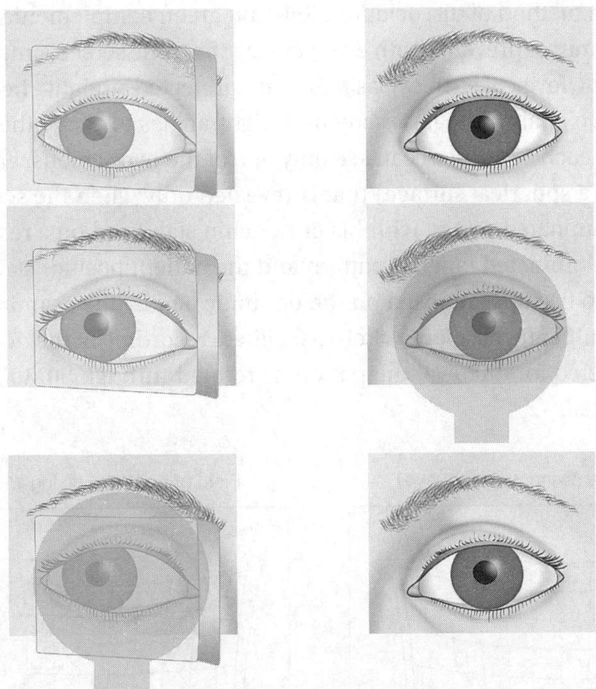

Fig. 41: Prism and cover test.

46. Write a short note on Hess Chart. (5) (TN MGRMU MS 2021)

A Hess chart is plotted to aid in the diagnosis and monitoring of a patient with incomitant strabismus such as an extraocular muscle palsy or a mechanical or a myopathic limitation. The chart is commonly prepared using either the Hess Screen or Lees Screen which facilitate plotting of the dissociated ocular position as a measure of extraocular muscle action.

Principle

The principle is the foveal projection. The chart is plotted based on the Hering's and Sherington laws of ocular motility.

Hess Screen (Fig. 42)

The original test used a black screen on which was marked a square-meter tangent scale. The tangent nature of the coordinate lines converts equidistant points, seen in a virtual sphere like a perimeter, into a two-dimensional chart. The test relies on color dissociation using red/green complementary filters. This maximizes the ocular deviation. A red target is illuminated or projected at the juncture where each tangent line crosses. A green light is projected by the patient and each plot is recorded. The test is repeated for the opposite eye resulting in a chart showing an inner and outer range of ocular rotation for each eye. The Hess screen contains a tangent pattern displayed on a dark grey background. Red lights that can be individually illuminated by a control panel indicate the cardinal positions of gaze within a central field (15° from primary position) and a peripheral field (30°); each square represents 5° of ocular rotation. The eyes are dissociated by the use of reversible goggles incorporating a red and a green lens, the red lens in front of the fixating eye and the green lens the non-fixating eye. Red points of lights are illuminated at selected positions on the screen. The patient holds a green pointer and is asked to superimpose a green light over each red light in turn. In orthophoria the two lights should be more or less super-imposed in all positions of gaze. The goggles are then reversed and the procedure repeated. Software is available that facilitates the plotting of a Hess chart using a standard desktop computer screen.

Lees Screen

The Lees screen is a modification of the Hess screen. It is used to obtain the same information about incomitant strabismus, but using a different method of dissociation. Red and green complementary color dissociation is replaced with a double-sided mirror. The mirror prevents both eyes viewing the same screen simultaneously, although the patient perceives both images seen by the fovea of each eye as if they are projected straight ahead.

This apparatus consists of two opalescent glass screens at right-angles to each other, bisected by a two-sided plane mirror that dissociates the eyes; each of the eyes can see only one of the two screens. Each screen has a tangent pattern (two-dimensional projection of a spherical surface) that is revealed only when the screen is illuminated. The patient is positioned facing the non-illuminated screen with his or her chin stabilized on a rest. Using a pointer, the examiner indicates a target point on the illuminated tangent pattern and the patient positions a pointer on the non-illuminated screen, at a position perceived to be superimposed on the dot indicated by the examiner. The non-illuminated screen is briefly illuminated by the examiner using a footswitch to facilitate recording of the dot indicated by the patient. When the procedure has been completed for one eye, the patient is rotated through 90° to face the previously illuminated screen and the procedure repeated.

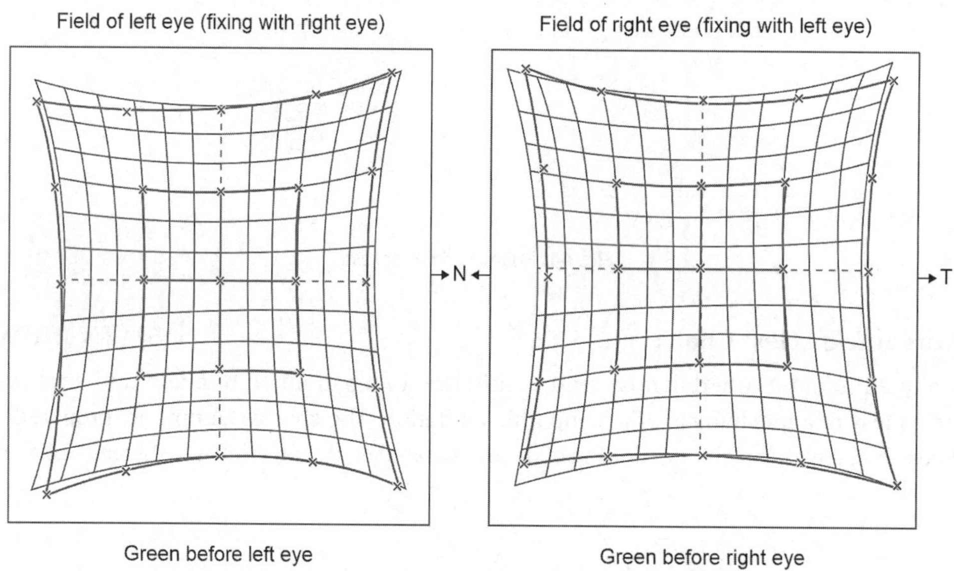

Fig. 42: Hess chart. *(For Color version, See Color Plate 4)*

47. Discuss about Amsler Grid in brief. (10) (BHU MS 2015)

The Amsler grid evaluates the 20 degrees of the visual field centered on fixation. It is principlely useful in screening for and monitoring macular disease, but will also demonstrate central visual field defects originating elsewhere. Patient with chronic macular diseases like CNVM, CSCR, should be provided with Amsler grid at home for regular monitoring.

There are seven charts available, each consisting of a 10 cm outer square.

Chart 1: It consists of a white grid on black background, the outer grid enclosing 400 smaller 5 mm squares. When viewed at about 1/3rd of a meter, each small square subtends an angle of 1 degree.

Chart 2: It is also white grid on black background with has two diagonal lines that aid fixation for patients with a central scotoma.

Chart 3: Instead of white squares, it has red squares. The red-on-black design aims to stimulate long wavelength foveal cones. It is used to detect subtle color scotomas and desaturation in toxic maculopathy, optic neuropathy and chiasmal lesions.

Chart 4: It consists of only random dots and is used mainly to distinguish scotomas from metamorphopsia as there is no form to be distorted.

Chart 5: It consists of horizontal lines and is designed to detect metamorphopsia along specific meridian. It is of particular importance in the evaluation of patients describing difficulty reading.

Chart 6: Similar to chart 5 but has a white background and the central lines are closer together, enabling more detailed evaluation.

Chart 7: This chart includes a fine central grid, each square subtending an angle of a half degree, and is more sensitive.

Technique of Amsler grid test:

The pupils should not be dilated and in order to avoid a photostress effect, the eyes should not have been ideally examined on slit-lamp. A presbyopic refraction correction should be used if appropriate. The chart should be well illuminated and held at a comfortable reading distance, optimally around 33 cm.

- One eye is covered
- The patient is asked to directly look at the central dot with uncovered eye, to keep looking at it, and to report any distortion or waviness of the lines on the grid.
- Reminding the patient to maintain focus on the central dot, is asked then if there is any blurring areas or blank spots anywhere on the grid. Patients with macular diseases often report there is wavy lines, whereas those with optic nerve involvement tend to remark that some lines are missing or faint but not distorted.
- The patient is asked whether he/she can see all the four corners and all four sides of the square- a missing corner or border should raise the possibility of causes other than macular disease, such as glaucomatous field defects or Retinitis pigmentosa.
- The patient maybe provided a pen and sheet to record and draw the anomalies **(Fig. 43)**.

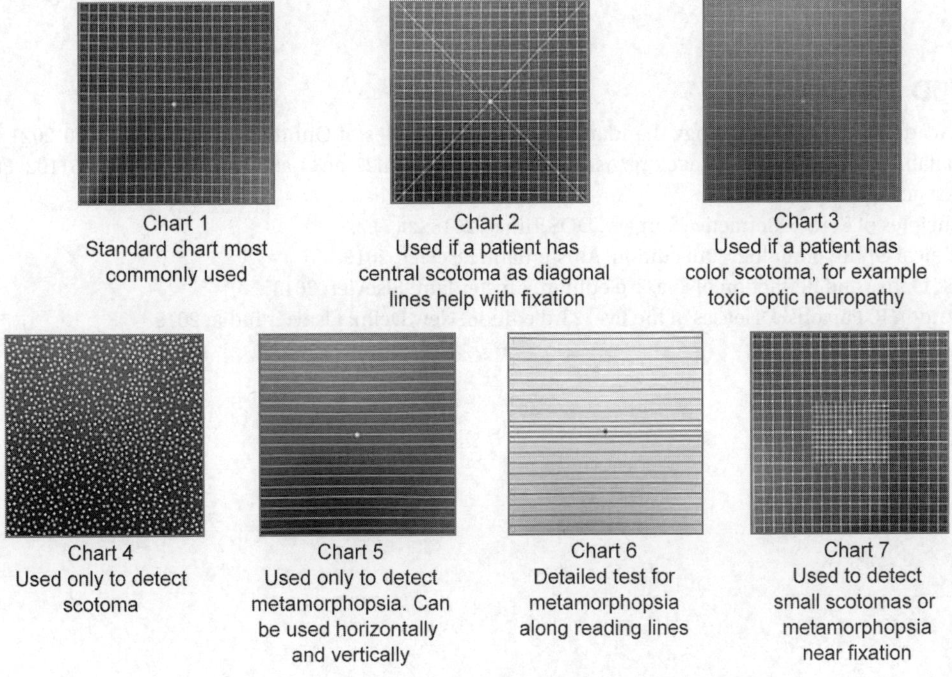

Fig. 43: Types of Amsler grid test. *(For Color version, See Color Plate 5)*

48. Write a short note on Titmus fly test. (5) (TN MGRMU MS 2017)

Titmus Fly Test

It is a contour stereotest. It is performed at a distance of 40 cm. The Titmus test consists of 3D polaroid vectograph consists of two plates in the form of booklet viewed through polaroid spectacles they are present right angle to each other they have pictures like fly, circles, animals. This test uses crossed Polaroid filters to present slightly different aspects of the same object to each eye. The test comprises three sections:

The Housefly: Which shows large disparities and should be seen in depth by most subjects.

Stereoacuity range of random dot butterfly is:

Bottom of lower wing: 1150 sec of arc

Tip of abdomen: 700 sec of arc

Top of upper wing: 2000 sec of arc

The right side of the test booklet contains a large housefly to test gross stereopsis (3000 seconds).

It is especially useful in young children.

The child is asked to pick up one of the wings of fly between finger and thumb. If patient sees stereoscopically he will reach out to above plates.

Animals: There are 3 rows of 5 animals, one animal in each row having a crossed disparity which ranges from 100, 200, 400 secs of arc. It is performed if gross stereopsis is present.

The subject is asked which animal stands out.

One disadvantage of this test is that it contains monocular cues.

Circle patterns: This section consists of 9 patterns containing four circles.

One of the circles in the pattern contains a graded disparity (crossed), so that when it is viewed binocularly it is seen to float in front of the others.

The disparities of the circles range from 800 to 40 secs of arc. It consists of nine squares each containing four circles.

Only one of the circles in the pattern in each square contains a graded disparity (crossed), so that when it is viewed binocularly it is seen to float in front of the others. The disparities of the circles range from 800 to 40 secs of arc.

If the subject has passed other two tests, he is asked to push-down the circle that stands out, beginning with the first set.

SUGGESTED READING

1. American Academy of Ophthalmology. Fundamentals and Principles of Ophthalmology, AAO 2020-2021 BCSC Section 3. [online] Available from https://www.aao.org/Assets/b415860a-b6ec-4f22-ac33-a6fb8e668065/636312511027800000/bcsc1718-s02-pdf. [Last accessed March, 2025]
2. Dave A. Principles of Kerato-Refractive Surgery. DOS Times. 2015;20(7):2.
3. Kanski J. Clinical Ophthalomology, 9th edition. Amsterdam: Elsevier; 2019.
4. Khurana AK. Optics and Refraction of Eye, 3rd edition. Amsterdam: Elsevier; 2013.
5. Sihota R, Tandon R. Parsons' Diseases of the Eye, 23rd edition. New Delhi: Elsevier India; 2019.

3

CHAPTER

Eyelid

Prabrisha Banerjee, Koustav Bhunia

QUESTIONS

1. **Describe the anatomy and development of eyelids with a labelled diagram.** **(10) (DNB 2024)**
2. **Discuss meibomian gland dysfunction.** **(10) (DNB 2018)**
3. **Trichiasis—Short Note** **(5) (BHU MS 2018)**
4. **Lagophthalmos—Short Note** **(5) (BHU MS 2017)**
5. **Mention principles of ptosis surgery. How will you manage a case of congenital ptosis with Marcus Gunn Jaw-Winking Phenomenon?** **(5+5) (DNB 2020)**
6. **Discuss the management of congenital ptosis with Marcus Gunn Jaw-Winking Phenomenon.** **(5) (DNB 2020)**
7. **Describe sling surgery for ptosis.** **(10) (TNMGRMU MS 2021)**
8. **Discuss entropion.** **(10) (RGUHS MS 2018)**
9. **Describe surgical management of entropion.** **(10) (BHU MS 2020)**
10. **Cicatricial entropion—Short Note** **(5) (TNMGRMU MS 2019)**
11. **Describe the classification and surgical management of ectropion.** **(10) (TNMGRMU 2022/BHU 2018)**
12. **A 75-year-old female presented with an ulcerated lesion in the medial side of the left lower eyelid for 2 years, size 15 mm × 10 mm. Discuss its differential diagnosis and management.** **(10) (DNB 2019)**
13. **Lid tumor excision.** **(10) (BHU MS 2021)**
14. **Write briefly on eyelid coloboma.** **(10) (DNB 2019)**

1. Describe the anatomy and development of eyelids with a labelled diagram. (10) (DNB 2024)

In a young adult:

- The interpalpebral fissure height is approximately 10-11 mm
- The horizontal fissure length is 30-32 mm
- The upper and the lower lid meet at the medial canthus and the lateral canthus at an angle of 60°.
- Lateral canthus rests against the globe, but the medial canthus is displaced away by the lacus lacrimalis comprising the caruncle and the plica semilunaris.
- The lateral canthal angle lies 2 mm higher than the medial canthal angle.
- The upper eyelid covers 2 mm of the cornea in primary gaze, and the lower lid rests on the inferior limbus.
- The eyelid consists of the following structural planes
  - The skin and subcutaneous fascia
  - The orbicularis oculi muscle
  - The orbital septum

- The eyelid retractors
- The tarsal plates and conjunctiva

- The attachment of superficial fibers of the levator palpebral superioris muscle to the orbicularis muscle and the subcutaneous tissue gives rise to the skin crease (6-7 mm in males, 7-8 mm in females).
- The eyelid skin is very thin and devoid of any subcutaneous fat.
- The orbicularis muscle consists of three parts, namely, orbital, pre-septal, and pre-tarsal
  - Orbital part - originates from the frontal process of the maxilla, orbital process of the frontal bone and the medial canthal ligament, passes around the orbital margins and inserts just below the points of origin. It helps in the forced closure of the eyelids.
  - Pre-septal part - lies over the orbital septum. The upper eyelid has a superficial and deep head originating from the medial palpebral ligament and the posterior lacrimal crest. The fibers pass over the septum superiorly and inferiorly and insert at the lateral palpebral raphe.
  - Pre-tarsal part - lies over the tarsal plate. The upper and lower lid muscles originate from a superficial head (from the medial palpebral ligament) and a deep head (from the lacrimal fascia and posterior lacrimal crest). The fibers pass laterally and are inserted into Whitnall's tubercle. The muscle fibers arising from the posterior lacrimal crest (Horner's muscle) help in the drainage of tears.
  - The palpebral part helps in the gentle closing of the eyelids.
- Orbital Septum - multi-layered fibrous membrane which inserts superiorly into the periosteum over the superior orbital rim. It merges with the fibers of levator aponeurosis above the superior tarsal border.
- Orbital Fat - there are 2 pockets of fat; nasal and central in the upper lid posterior to the orbital septum and 3 pockets of fat in the lower lid.
- Retractors - levator palpebral superioris originates from the lesser wing of sphenoid. The muscular part is 40 mm, runs horizontally, the aponeurotic part is 20 mm in length becomes vertical after crossing Whitnall's ligament. It inserts onto the tarsal plate, the medial horn into the posterior lacrimal crest and the lateral horn at Whitnall's tubercle. Few fibers insert into the skin and form the skin crease, and in the superior fornix. It is supplied by the Oculomotor nerve. Capsulopalpebral fascia acts as lower lid retractor. The other lid retractors are Muller muscle for the upper lid and inferior tarsal muscle for the lower lid.
- Tarsal plates - the upper tarsal plate measures 11 mm, while the lower tarsal plate is 3-4 mm. The tarsal plate contains meibomian glands.
- Conjunctiva - lines the posterior surface of the lid, composed of non-keratinizing squamous epithelium. Harbors the accessory lacrimal glands.
- Blood supply - The eyelid is mainly supplied by the supraorbital and lacrimal arteries.
- Lymphatics - Medial side drains into the submandibular glands, lateral part drains into the superficial preauricular glands and deep cervical nodes.
- The structures of upper and lower eyelid are given in **Figures 1 and 2**, respectively.

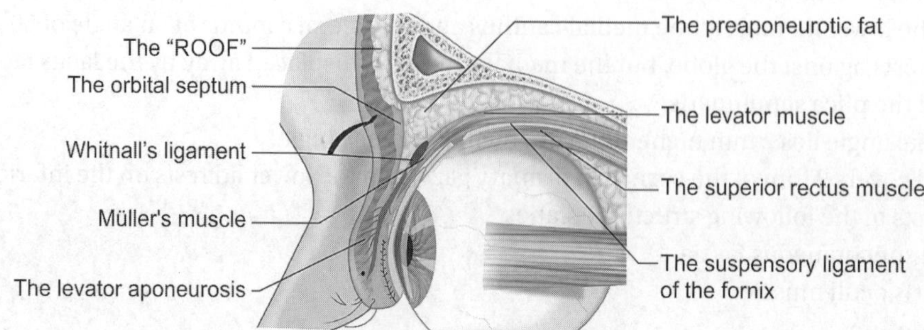

Fig. 1: Anatomy of upper eyelid.

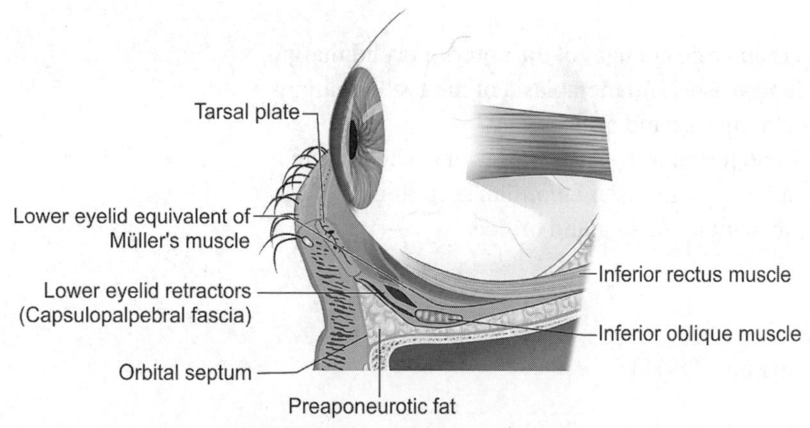

Fig. 2: Anatomy of the lower eyelid.

2. Discuss meibomian gland dysfunction. (10) (DNB 2018)

Definition- It is the chronic, diffuse abnormality of the meibomian glands, commonly characterized by terminal duct obstructions and/or qualitative/quantitative alterations of its secretions leading to a spectrum of ocular surface diseases.

- According to the International Workshop on Meibomian Gland Dysfunction, MGD can be an obstructive disease or it can be caused by a hyposecretory state.
- Obstructive MGD can be cicatricial secondary to trachoma, mucous membrane pemphigoid, or atopy) and non-cicatricial secondary to seborrheic dermatitis, rosacea, or atopy.
- Pathophysiology—Obstruction is the most common cause of MGD. The underlying pathophysiology is epithelial hyperkeratinization, which causes duct obstruction, leading to meibum stasis, cystic dilation, and eventually acinar atrophy due to disuse, and gland dropout.
  - *Aging:* Meibomian gland acinar epithelial cell atrophy and decreased lipid production occurs with aging.
  - *Microbiome: Staphylococcus epidermidis*, *Staphylococcus aureus*, and *Propionibacterium acnes* are most commonly involved. These bacteria produce lipolytic enzymes and release inflammatory mediators, leading to lipolysis in the tear film.
  - *Environmental stress:* Low-humidity environments cause increased meibum production. This leads to ductal dilation and a decrease in the number of functioning meibocytes, causing gland atrophy and hyposecretion.
  - *Hormonal effects:* Androgens stimulate meibum secretion and suppress inflammation, while estrogens tend to increase inflammation.
  - *Contact lens use:* Contact lenses result in irreversible meibomian gland dropout in the long run.
  - *Medications:* Medications like β-blockers and carbonic anhydrase inhibitors, and retinoic acid leads to hyposecretion.
  - *Congenital:* Reduced number of or absent meibomian glands is seen in patients with Turner syndrome, ectrodactyly with ectodermal dysplasia and cleft lip and palate (ECC syndrome), and anhidrotic ectodermal dysplastic syndrome, and in distichiasis.
- High delivery state of MGD occurs due to release of a large lipid volume at the lid margin. Seborrheic dermatitis and acne rosacea are 2 common causes of high-delivery MGD.
- Symptoms:
  - Burning
  - Foreign-body sensation
  - Redness of the eyelids
  - Conjunctival injection
  - Filmy vision

- Clinical signs:
  - Seborrheic and eczematoid changes of the anterior eyelid margin
  - Telangiectatic blood vessels and metaplasia of the eyelid margins
  - Pouting of the meibomian gland orifices
  - Foamy discharge and irregularity at the posterior eyelid margin
  - Turbid, cheesy, or toothpaste-like meibomian secretions
  - Posteriorly displaced meibomian gland orifices
- Evaluation

  Tear film volume
  - Tear osmolarity
  - Tear film break-up time (TBUT)
  - Schirmer test
  - Corneal and conjunctival staining
  - *Slit lamp assisted grading recommendations:* Photographic assessment for comparison with healthy controls and other set of patients used for developing grading scales
  - *Lipid layer thickness (LLT):* Lipiview interferometer used, LLT cutoff < 60nm used
  - *In vivo confocal microscopy (IVCM):* gland dilatation, acinar diameters calculated; high sensitivity and specificity
  - *Noncontact infrared meibography:* Infrared light used; objective and repeatable; drug and age-related gland loss identified.

  Staging of MGD are mentioned in **Table 1**.

TABLE 1: Staging of MGD.

Stage	MGD Grade	Symptoms	Corneal Staining
1	+ (minimally altered expressibility and secretion quality)	None	None
2	++ (mildly altered expressibility and secretion quality)	Minimal to mild	None to limited
3	+++ (moderately altered expressibility and secretion quality)	Mild-to-moderate	Mainly peripheral
4	++++ (severely altered expressibility and secretion quality)	Marked	Peripheral and Central

- Management
  - Optimization of working environment, reduction in screen time, regular warm compress.
  - Expression of accumulated secretions.
  - Topical azithromycin – broad spectrum macrolide antibiotic with anti-inflammatory property.
  - Artificial lubricants for use.
  - Topical emollients help stabilize tear film
  - Topical Cyclosporine A 0.05%, or topical steroid in severe stages, helps reduce inflammation.
  - Increase in dietary omega 3-fatty acid intake (1.5 gm daily).
  - Oral tetracyclines in severe MGD.
  - Intraductal probing – aids in mechanical opening and dilatation of the blocked meibomian gland orifices and ducts. Initially, 1 to 2 mm Maskin probes aid in dilating the ducts, followed by 4 to 6 mm probes to achieve ductal patency.
  - Electronic Heating Device - This delivers heat simultaneously to the palpebral conjunctiva of both upper and lower lids. Concurrently, it also helps express meibomian gland content by providing pressure to the outer eyelid surfaces in a pulsatile manner. Example: LipiFlow (Johnson and Johnson), Systane iLux and Systane iLux MGD Thermal Pulsation Systems (Alcon) are handheld devices.

3. Trichiasis—Short Note (5) (BHU MS 2018)

- Trichiasis is defined as inward growth of normal lashes.
- In trichiasis, the lash follicle is normal, but the direction of lash growth is abnormal.
- There may be misdirection of the follicles in associated inflammation.
- Trichiasis may be classified as major (> 5 cilia), or minor (< 5 cilia)
- Causes—Chronic blepharitis, chemical injury, thermal burns, Herpes Zoster, eyelid trauma, eyelid surgery, atopic disease, vernal keratoconjunctivitis, cicatricial conjunctival diseases, meibomitis, eyelid tumors, trachoma
- Eyelids should be looked for scarring, symblepharon, margin keratinization and the cornea should be stained to detect keratopathy.
- Complications—Ocular irritation, lacrimation, punctate epithelial erosion, corneal abrasion, corneal ulcer, pannus formation
- Management:
  - Manual epilation of trichiatic lashes and bandage contact lens offer short-term relief.
  - Electrolysis with radiofrequency needle causes permanent destruction of the roots of the trichiatic lashes. (Contraindicated in patients with pacemaker). However, there are chances of recurrence and patients may require multiple sittings.
  - Argon laser ablation is useful for a few darkly pigmented trichiatic lashes.
  - Cryotherapy—Reduction of the temperature to -25 degrees destroys the lash bulb without inducing tissue necrosis. A double freeze-thaw technique is used. It leads to hypopigmentation of the skin. Risk of recurrence is present.
  - Trephination/Eyelash bulb extirpation - less commonly used.
  - Surgical excision—Localized area of trichiatic lashes with eyelid laxity can be managed with wedge excision and direct closure.

4. Lagophthalmos—Short Note (5) (BHU MS 2017)

- Lagophthalmos is defined as incomplete closure of the eyes.
- The underlying pathophysiology includes facial nerve palsy, proptosis, eyelid retraction, and anterior lamellar shortening due to scarring.
- Facial nerve palsy is the most common etiology of lagophthalmos.
- Facial nerve palsy can be idiopathic (Bell's palsy) or secondary to infection (viral, bacterial, mastoiditis), trauma, tumor (cerebropontine tumors, parotid tumor), iatrogenic (parotid surgery, mastoid surgery, excision of cerebropontine tumors).
- Evaluation comprises
  - Detailed history—onset, duration, past surgery, trauma, pain and discharge in ear, hearing loss, neurosensory deficits, past medical history like diabetes mellitus, myasthenia gravis, sarcoidosis, past history of Botulinum toxin injection.
  - Upper motor neuron disease—will spare the frontalis muscle
  - Lower motor neuron disease—will lead to loss of forehead furrows, brow ptosis, upper lid retraction, lagophthalmos, reduced blink rate, lower lid ectropion, loss of nasolabial fold, oral droop, and difficulty in speech.
  - Lagophthalmos is measured as the vertical height at the greatest distance of the palpebral fissure.
  - Bell's phenomenon should be documented.
  - Nocturnal exposure of cornea should be enquired.
  - Corneal sensation.
  - Corneal staining to detect exposure keratopathy.
  - Tear film assessment.
  - Other facial muscles should be assessed.
  - Examination of other cranial nerves.
  - To look for signs of aberrant regeneration, hemifacial spasm

- Investigation—Computed tomography (CT) of brain with contrast helps to detect space-occupying lesions, magnetic resonance imaging (MRI) brain with contrast aids in detecting neurovascular conflict.
- Management
  - Initially, in the acute phase, artificial tears are prescribed to maintain the tear film. Taping of the eyelids with ointment at night is advocated. Patient is advised physiotherapy.
  - Severe lagophthalmos, poor Bell's phenomenon, reduced corneal sensation, and dry eyes are indications for surgical intervention in the form of lateral tarsorrhaphy.
  - If there is nil or mild improvement in the eyelid closure after six months, gold weight/platinum weight implant is applied.
  - In mild-to-moderate lid retraction cases, Muller muscle and levator palpebral superioris recession is the treatment of choice.
  - Lower lid ectropion can be corrected by lateral tarsal strip with or without a spacer graft depending on the severity.
- In lagophthalmos secondary to proptosis, the underlying cause should be diagnosed and treated.
- In anterior lamellar scarring, hyaluronic acid gel filler can be useful. In anterior lamellar shortening, a full-thickness skin graft is needed.

5. Mention principles of ptosis surgery. How will you manage a case of congenital ptosis with Marcus Gunn Jaw-Winking Phenomenon? (5+5) (DNB 2020)

6. Discuss the management of congenital ptosis with Marcus Gunn Jaw-Winking Phenomenon. (5) (DNB 2020)

- Ptosis or blepharoptosis is defined as drooping of the upper eyelid in the primary gaze.
- There are mainly two components of ptosis surgery:
  1. Functional— improvement in superior visual field prevention of amblyopia
  2. Cosmetic—achieving a good eyelid contour symmetrical palpebral fissure height in both eyes
- Congenital ptosis with Marcus Gunn Jaw-Winking Phenomenon
- Margus Gunn Jaw Winking Syndrome (MGJWS) is associated with 2%-13% cases of congenital ptosis.
- It is mostly unilateral but can be bilateral rarely.
- It manifests as a coordinated synkinetic movement of the upper eyelid and the jaw due to an abnormal connection between the motor branches of the trigeminal nerve and the superior division of oculomotor nerve.
- There are 2 types of trigemino-oculomotor synkinesis as follows:
  - External pterygoid-levator synkinesis: Lid elevates when the mouth is widely open.
  - Internal pterygoid-levator synkinesis: Lid elevates on teeth clenching
- It is often associated with strabismus, monocular elevation deficiency.
- Detailed history and reviewing past photographs are highly recommended.
- Ocular examination:
  - Visual acuity and refraction.
  - Cover test for unveiling hypotropia and rule out any component of pseudoptosis.
  - Extraocular motility.
  - Pupillary examination.
  - Examination to look for any giant papillary conjunctivitis or symblepharon.
  - Corneal sensation and dry eye evaluation.
  - Fundus examination.
- Ptosis evaluation:
  - *Palpebral fissure height (PFH):* Vertical aperture height between upper and lower lid in the pupillary plane with eyes in primary gaze. Normal value is 9-10 mm.
  - *Margin-reflex distance 1 (MRD1):* The distance between upper eyelid margin and corneal light reflex. Normal value is 4 mm.

- The difference of 2 mm in MRD 1 between the 2 eyes = mild ptosis, difference of 3 mm = moderate ptosis and 4 mm = severe ptosis respectively.
  - Levator action—amount of excursion measured after negating frontalis action when the eyelid moves from extreme downgaze to extreme upgaze. It is graded as:-
    Less than 4 mm - Poor
    5 to 9 mm - Fair
    9 to 11 mm - Good
    Greater than 12 mm - Excellent
    Iliff test: If the upper lid returns to its original position immediately after eversion of the upper lid, then the LPS action is considered to be good.
  - Margin crease distance (MCD): Distance between the lid margin and skin crease in downgaze. Normal MCD is 7 to 8 mm in men and 8 to 10 mm in women. In congenital ptosis, MCD is usually absent or faint.
  - Lagophthalmos
  - Bell's phenomenon
  - The lid excursion should be measured and graded as mild = 2 mm, moderate = 2 mm to 5 mm, and severe = higher than 5 mm
- The indications for ptosis correction in a pre-school child are
  - Anisometropia
  - Amblyopia
- In cases with strabismus, first strabismus surgery is done, followed by ptosis correction.
- It is important to ascertain if the ptosis or the wink is the main concern of the patient and the parents.
- In MGJWS with mild-to-moderate excursions, frontalis sling surgery is preferred.
- In MGJWS with severe excursions, or in case the patient and parents are more concerned about the wink, levator extirpation with frontalis sling surgery is performed.
- In amblyopic children, the patching should be continued after the ptosis correction.

7. Describe sling surgery for ptosis. (10) (TNMGRMU MS 2021)

- The tarsofrontalis sling surgery is aimed to harness the action of the frontalis muscle to elevate the eyelids.
- Normally, the frontalis muscle contributes 10 mm to 15 mm of elevation.
- Indications for sling surgery:
  - Poor Levator function
  - Marcus Gunn Jaw-Winking Syndrome
  - Blepharophimosis
  - Ptosis in Third Nerve Palsy
  - Myasthenia Gravis
  - Chronic Progressive External Ophthalmoplegia
- The various materials used for the sling can be classified as mentioned in **Table 2**:

TABLE 2: Classification of various materials used for the sling.

Autogenous	*Allogenic*	*Synthetic*
Fascia lata	Banked fascia lata	Silicon rod
Palmaris longus tendon		Prolene
Temporalis fascia		Mersilene Mesh
		Gortex

- Techniques:
  - Fox pentagon technique:
    - General anesthesia is used for children, local anesthesia for adults.

- Two eyelid markings are made 2 mm from the lid margin at the medial and lateral limbus.
- Two eyebrow markings are made just above the eyebrows corresponding to the medial and lateral canthus. A central forehead marking is made in the pupillary plane 1cm above the eyebrow.
- Stab incisions are made on the markings.
- The silicon rod is passed through the forehead, medial eyebrow, medial pre tarsal orbicularis, lateral pretarsal orbicularis, lateral eyebrow, and both the ends are placed inside a sleeve and buried at the forehead wound **(Fig. 3)**

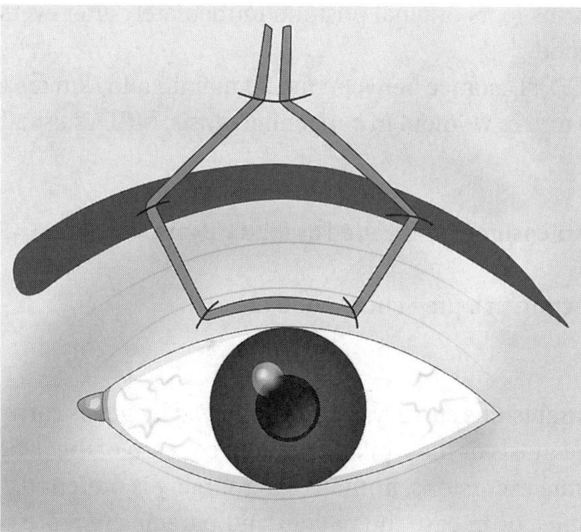

Fig. 3: Fox pentagon frontalis sling surgery.

- Crawford technique-
  - Double triangle technique **(Fig. 4)**
  - Usually done with autogenous fascia lata.
  - The child must be more than 3 years of age for the legs to develop completely for harvesting fascia lata.

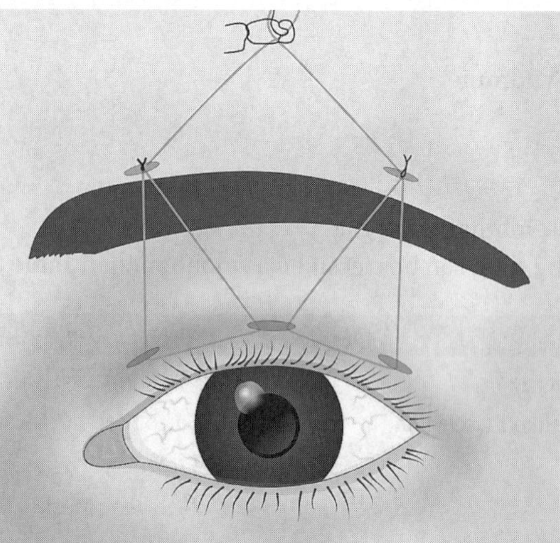

Fig. 4: Crawford technique.

- Complications—undercorrection, overcorrection, lagophthalmos, exposure keratopathy, eyelid contour defects, granuloma, silicone rod exposure, and extrusion.

8. Discuss entropion. **(10) (RGUHS MS 2018)**

9. Describe surgical management of entropion. **(10) (BHU MS 2020)**

10. Cicatricial entropion—Short Note **(5) (TNMGRMU MS 2019)**

- Entropion is defined as inward turning of the eyelid margin.
- It can be unilateral or bilateral.
- There are 4 types of entropion:
  - Involutional
  - Cicatricial
  - Acute spastic
  - Congenital
- Involutional entropion
  - Caused by horizontal laxity of the eyelid, attenuation or disinsertion of eyelid retractors, and overriding by the preseptal orbicularis oculi muscle over the pretarsal muscle fibers.
  - Enophthalmos due to orbital fat atrophy is a contributing factor.
- Cicatricial entropion
  - Transconjunctival scarring leads to the cicatricial entropion.
  - It is caused by chemical injury, burn injury, trauma, eyelid surgery, topical glaucoma medications, Stevens Johnson syndrome, ocular pemphigoid, Herpes zoster infection, and trachoma.
- Acute spastic entropion
  - This is seen in patients with reflex blepharospasm.
  - Initially this is reversible once the underlying cause of ocular irritation is treated.
  - Untreated cases may become permanent and need surgical correction.
- Congenital entropion
  - This is the rarest form.
  - The underlying pathogenesis includes abnormal insertion of the lower lid retractors, posterior lamella insufficiency, and kinking of the tarsal plate.
  - This needs surgical correction.
- Symptoms - watering, ocular irritation due to the rubbing of the eyelashes and the lid margin against the ocular surface, photophobia
- Evaluation -
  - The eyelid should be assessed for horizontal lid laxity
  - *Snap back test:* The middle portion of the lower eyelid is fully displaced by pulling it down. After releasing the lid, it should immediately return to its original position in a healthy lower eyelid.
  - The grading scale depends on how long the lower lid takes to spring back into the globe.
  - *Grade 0:* Takes less than 2 seconds
  - *Grade I:* Takes 2 or 3 seconds
  - *Grade II:* Takes 4 or 5 seconds
  - *Grade III:* Takes more than 5 seconds but returns to its normal position with blinking
  - *Grade IV:* Never returns back to the normal position
  - *Pinch test:* The patient is asked to look up with an open mouth. The skin of the lower eyelid below the lashes is grasped and the distance the lid can be distracted from the globe is measured.
  - A healthy lid will not distract more than 6 mm from the globe.
  - Punctum is assessed to look for punctal entropion.
  - Eyelid distraction test - to assess the medial and lateral canthal laxity. Distraction of the lateral canthal more than 2 mm shows canthal laxity. Medial canthal laxity is examined by the displacement of the lower punctum from its resting position and graded as grade 0 (at plica semilunaris), grade 2 (medial limbus), and grade 4 (mid pupil).

- The signs for lower lid retractor disinsertion should be examined. The eyelid margin rolls over the inferior limbus in such cases and poor movement of the eyelid when the patient looks down.
- Ocular surface examination for associated trichiasis, posterior lamellar scarring, lid margin keratinization, punctate keratopathy, epithelial defect and corneal abrasion.

- Grade of entropion:
  - *Grade 1:* Inward turning of the posterior lamella
  - *Grade 2:* Inward turning of the grey line
  - *Grade 3:* Inward turning of the anterior lamella
- Management
  - The stimulus inducing acute spastic entropion should be addressed.
  - Acute spastic entropion due to blepharospasm can be managed with botulinum toxin injection at the initial stages.
  - Elderly patients with involutional entropion can get temporary relief with botulinum toxin injection and taping of lower lid.
- Surgical management
- Involutional entropion –
  - Everting suture – prevents upward movement of preseptal orbicularis fibers, tightens lower lid retractors **(Fig. 5)**.

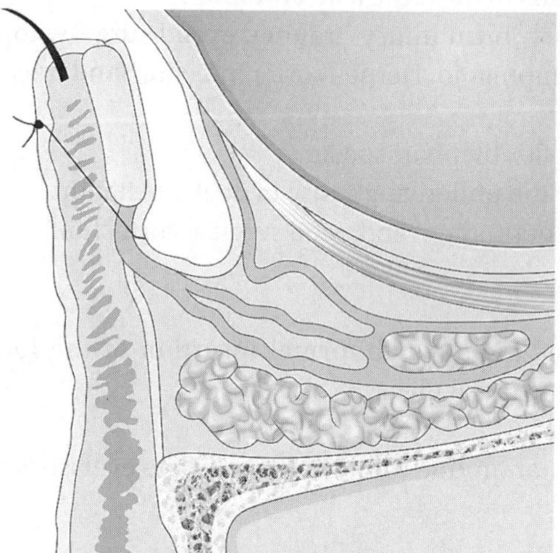

Fig. 5: Everting suture.

  - Weis procedure—the full thickness eyelid split below tarsal plate creates a scar that prevents overriding of the preseptal fibers of the orbicularis and the everting sutures tighten the lower lid retractors **(Fig. 6)**

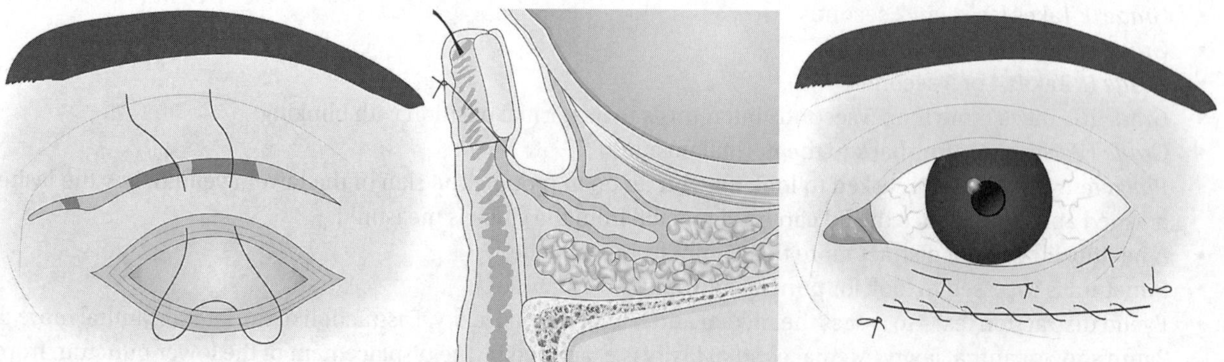

Fig. 6: Weiss procedure.

- Lateral tarsal strip—for significant horizontal eyelid laxity, canthal laxity, lateral tarsal strip is performed with everting sutures.
- Quickert procedure—comprises traverse lid splitting, horizontal lid shortening and everting sutures. It provides long-term cure for entropion.
- Jones procedure—lower lid retractor plication. It is indicated in lower lid retractor disinsertion and recurrent entropion **(Fig. 7)**.

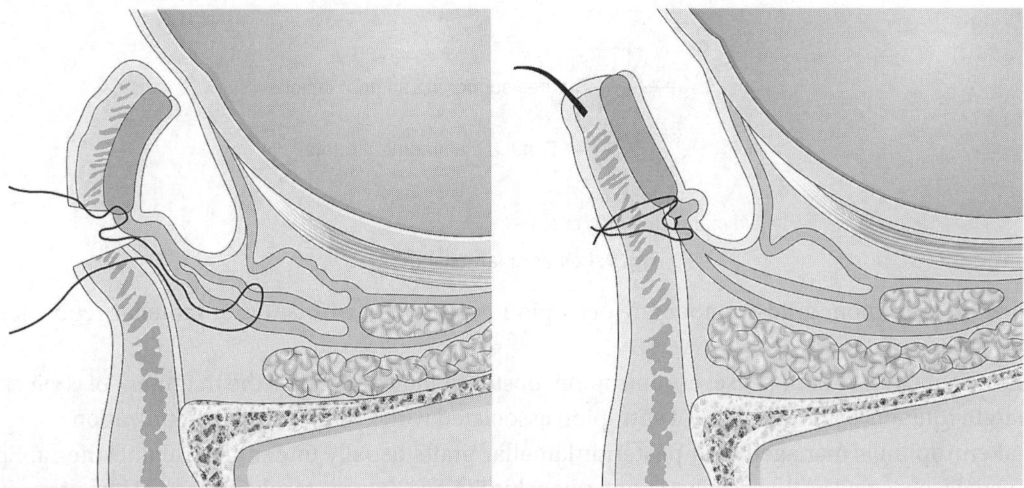

Fig. 7: Jones procedure.

- Cicatricial entropion—
  - Mild lower lid cicatricial entropion can be treated with tarsal fracture and everting sutures. Lower lid should not be retracted more than 1.5mm below limbus **(Fig. 8)**.

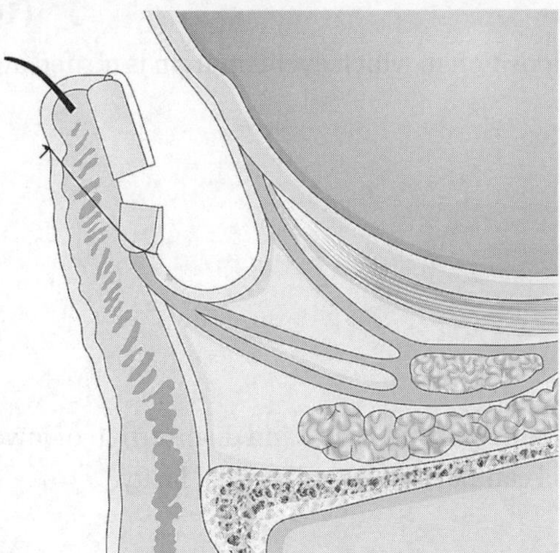

Fig. 8: Tarsal fracture.

  - For moderate to severe cases where lower lid retraction is more than 1.5 mm below - posterior lamellar graft is needed.
  - Oral mucus membrane or hard palate graft are usually used **(Fig. 9)**.

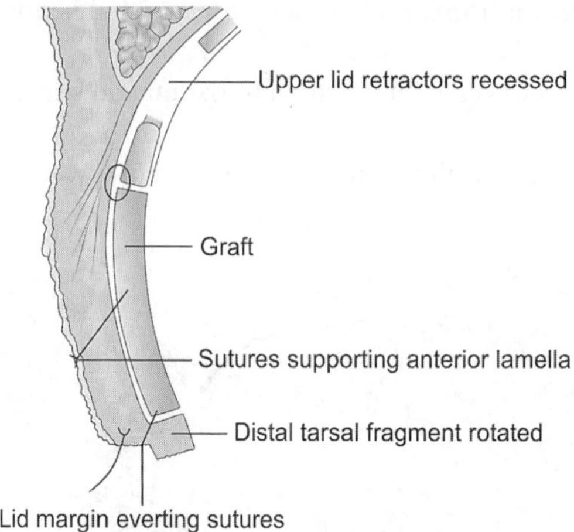

Fig. 9: Posterior lamellar graft.

- In upper lid entropion, mild-to-moderate entropion is corrected with anterior lamellar repositioning with or without eyelid split.
- In presence of tarsal scarring or severe entropion, posterior lamellar graft is the treatment of choice.
- Lid margin rotation is done in cases of entropion associated with eyelid margin keratinization.

- Congenital entropion is managed with posterior lamellar grafts usually under general anesthesia. Epiblepharon cases are usually observed as they resolve spontaneously with age. In non-resolving cases, Hotz procedure is done.
- *Complications:* Wound dehiscence, infection, hematoma, overcorrection, undercorrection, recurrence, scarring, lateral canthal deformity.

11. Describe the classification and surgical management of ectropion.

(10) (TNMGRMU 2022/BHU 2018)

- Ectropion is defined as eyelid malposition in which eyelid margin is turned away from the globe.
- Lower lid is commonly involved.
- The types of ectropion are:
  - Involutional ectropion
  - Paralytic ectropion
  - Cicatricial ectropion
  - Mechanical ectropion
  - Congenital ectropion
- Involutional ectropion:
  - Occurs due to senile changes, horizontal lid laxity, and disinsertion of lower lid retractor.
  - There can be associated medial canthal and lateral canthal laxity.
- Paralytic ectropion:
  - Seen in facial nerve palsy
  - Poor tone of orbicularis muscle
  - Associated with lagophthalmos
  - Punctal eversion is commonly seen
- Cicatricial ectropion:
  - Occurs secondary to scarring and shortening of anterior lamella.
  - Mainly seen in trauma, chemical injury, burn, atopic dermatitis, and post blepharoplasty, eyelid reconstruction, or orbital surgery.
  - Lamellar ichthyosis also presents with cicatricial ectropion.

- Mechanical ectropion:
  - Commonly caused by eyelid tumor pulling down the eyelid margin with its weight.
- The eyelid should be assessed for horizontal lid laxity
- Snap back test - should be performed
- The grading scale depends on how long the lower lid takes to spring back into the globe.
- *Grade 0:* Takes less than 2 seconds
- *Grade I:* Takes 2 or 3 seconds
- *Grade II:* Takes 4 or 5 seconds
- *Grade III:* Takes more than 5 seconds but returns to its normal position with blinking
- *Grade IV:* Never returns back to the normal position
- Pinch test—A healthy lid will not distract more than 6 mm from the globe.
- Punctum is assessed to look for punctal ectropion, erosion.
- Eyelid distraction test—to assess the medial and lateral canthal laxity. Rounded lateral canthal tendon, and distraction of the lateral canthus more than 2mm shows canthal laxity.
- Medial canthal laxity is examined by the displacement of the lower punctum from its resting position and graded as grade 0 (at plica semilunaris), grade 2 (medial limbus), and grade 4 (mid pupil).
- The signs for lower lid retractor disinsertion should be examined. A distinct white band is seen under the tarsal plate in cases of disinsertion of retractors when the patient looks down.
- Ocular surface examination for associated exposure keratopathy, epithelial defect and corneal abrasion.
- Bell's phenomenon and the tone of orbicularis muscle should be documented.
- Anterior lamella should be measured from the supraorbital rim (just below the eyebrow) to the eyelid margin at the central part joining the center of the pupil aperture, medially parallel to the medial limbus and laterally along the line joining the lateral limbus.
- Grading of ectropion:
  - *Grade 1:* Punctal eversion
  - *Grade 2:* Punctal eversion + visible palpebral conjunctiva
  - *Grade 3:* Fornix is visible
- Management:
- Involutional ectropion:
  - Simple ectropion without much lid laxity can be treated with inverting sutures.
  - Horizontal eyelid laxity can be addressed with eyelid shortening procedure like wedge excision.
  - Lateral tarsal strip takes care of the horizontal lid laxity as well as lateral canthal laxity.
  - Medial canthal laxity can be corrected by medial canthal plication.
  - In case of marked excess of skin, horizontal lid shortening should be combined with blepharoplasty.
- Paralytic ectropion:
  - Monitoring in the initial phase, patients should be encouraged to participate in physiotherapy to promote spontaneous resolution. Artificial tears and taping at night for lagophthalmos.
  - Mild punctal ectropion can be corrected by medial spindle procedure.
  - Punctal ectropion with medial canthal tendon laxity needs medial spindle as well as medial canthal plication **(Fig. 10)**. If the orbicularis tone is poor, then medial canthoplasty is recommended.
  - Horizontal lid laxity should be simultaneously corrected with eyelid shortening procedures (wedge resection or lateral tarsal strip)

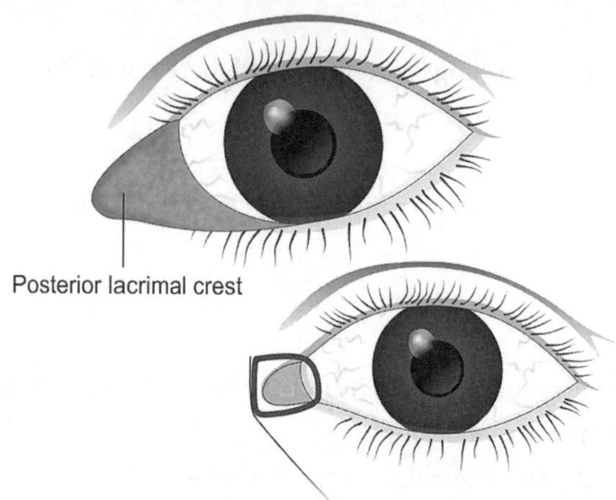

Fig. 10: Medial canthal plication.

- Cicatricial ectropion:
  - Cicatricial ectropion secondary to glaucoma medications, dermatitis can be managed by stopping the offending medication, short term use of steroid ointment.
  - Ectropion secondary to anterior lamellar shortening needs full thickness skin graft. The most common donor sites are contralateral upper eyelid skin, post auricular, pre auricular, supraclavicular region, and volar surface of the arm.
  - In cases of linear scar due to trauma, Z-plasty is the treatment of choice **(Fig. 11)**.

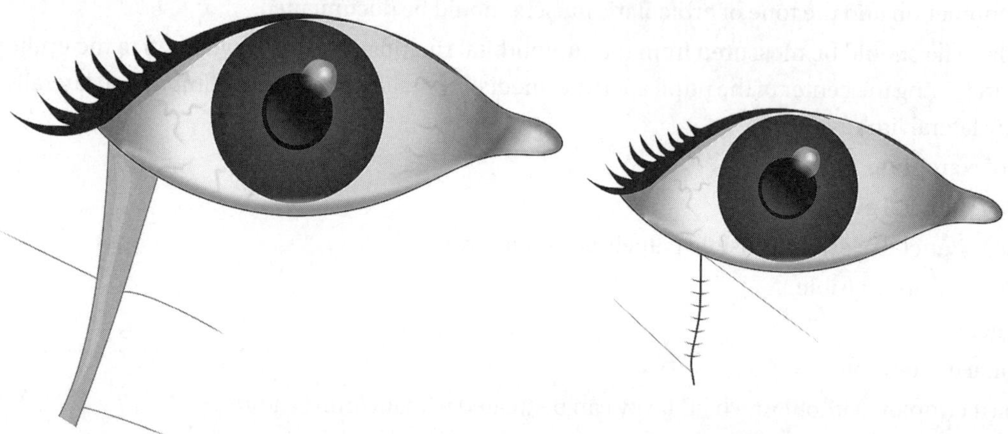

Fig. 11: Z-plasty for linear scar causing cicatricial ectropion.

- Mechanical ectropion is corrected by treating the underlying cause.
- Congenital ectropion occurs mainly because of anterior lamellar shortening. Hence, full thickness skin graft is required in those cases.
- Complications—wound dehiscence, hematoma, infection, overcorrection, undercorrection, scarring, entropion, recurrence, graft necrosis, graft failure.

12. A 75-year-old female presented with an ulcerated lesion in the medial side of the left lower eyelid for 2 years, size 15mm*10 mm. Discuss its differential diagnosis and management. (10) (DNB 2019)

- The ulcerated lesion can have the following differentials:
  - Basal cell carcinoma (BCC)—can be the noduloulcerative variant with rolled edges and telangiectasias over the lesion.

  - Squamous cell carcinoma (SCC)—ulcerating squamous cell carcinoma has a similar appearance but lacks telangiectasia.
  - Melanoma—superficial spreading melanoma manifests as a plaque with irregular boundaries and variable pigmentation.
  - Merkel cell carcinoma
  - Trichoepithelioma
  - Sebaceous gland carcinoma (SGC)
- Management
- Detailed history about the onset, progression, change in color, bleeding, other swelling or lump in the body, weight loss, systemic illness or already diagnosed associated syndromes, family history, immunodeficiency, immune disorder, fair skin, inability to tan, exposure to the predisposing factors like PUVA, past surgical history, genetic predisposition.
- Examination
  - Eyelid should be thoroughly examined for—size, location of the lesion, borders, induration, presence of pigmentation, ulceration, telangiectatic vessels, loss of eyelashes, regional lymphadenopathy.
  - Ocular surface should be minutely evaluated for pagetoid spread in case of sebaceous gland carcinoma.
  - Globe invasion—Invasion into the globe should be ruled out.
  - Orbital invasion—The extent of spread should be determined especially in medial canthal BCC.
  - The whole body should be examined for similar mass lesion.
- Investigation
  - In suspected cases of orbital involvement, MRI is indicated.
- BCC is a locally invasive tumor, hence the primary aim is local control.
- The management comprises both surgical and non-surgical modalities.
- Small lesions— curettage, electrodessication, vaporization with CO_2 are the treatment modalities available.
- Lesions <10 mm - cryotherapy can be used.
- Lesions <2 cm, superficial lesions—Topical imiquimod 5% which induces interferon alpha apoptosis has shown good results.
- Mohs micrographic surgery with frozen section is the treatment of choice **(Fig. 12)**.
  In absence of Mohs micrographic surgery, around 3 mm margin clearance is obtained under frozen section.
- Vismodegib—is a hedgehog pathway inhibitor which is helpful in recurrent, invasive BCC.
- In orbital involvement—exenteration is needed.
- Radiotherapy—is used as an adjuvant following exenteration, excision of ill-defined lesion, perineural spread. 40-70 Gy. 3Gy/session, over 5weeks.
- Immune checkpoint targets like cytotoxic T lymphocyte antigen 4 Ipilimumab and Programmed Cell Death I inhibitor Pembrolizumab has shown promising results.
- Here, the mass involves around 50% of the lower lid at the medial side.
- Imaging in the form of CT or MRI is needed to ascertain the depth of the lesion and rule out orbital involvement.
- Punctum and canaliculus involvement should be assessed and the patient should be counseled about epiphora following surgery.
- Tumor should be excised with an average clear margin of 3 to 3.5 mm.
- The eyelid reconstruction can be done by Tenzel's semicircular rotational flap, or tarsoconjunctival advancement flap (Hughes).
- For medial canthal lesions, excision followed by full thickness skin graft, rhomboid flap, glabellar flap are the few available options.

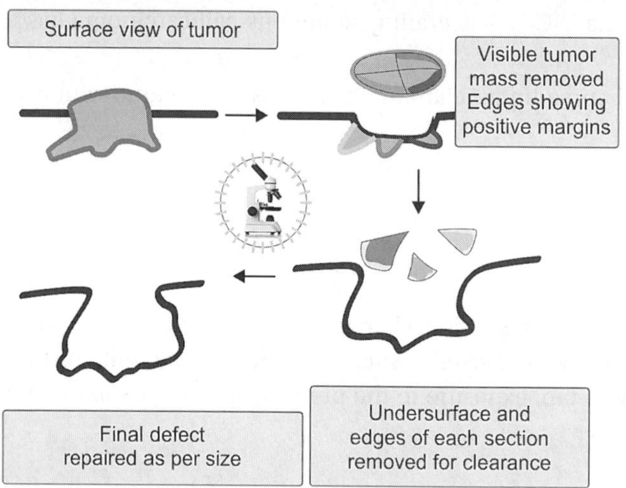

Fig. 12: Pictorial representation of Mohs micrographic surgery.

- There is 5%-15% chances of recurrence. The risk factors are medial canthus lesion, infiltrating histopathological type, perineural invasion, associated with xeroderma pigmentosum.

13. Lid tumor excision. (10) (BHU MS 2021)

- Principle of eyelid tumor excision:
  - Complete removal with sufficient margin clearance to minimize recurrence and metastasis.
  - For small lesions, excision biopsy can be done.
  - For large lesions, excision can be done with frozen section.
  - In view of unavailability of frozen section facility, initially incision biopsy can be taken to confirm the diagnosis and proceed for wide excision or excision biopsy can be done with adequate margins and the reconstruction can be planned after obtaining margin clearance from histopathology.
  - Conjunctival map biopsy should be performed in suspected cases of pagetoid disease.
  - In case of regional lymphadenopathy, sentinel lymph node biopsy should be done.
  - Efforts should be made to preserve the vital structures like the lacrimal drainage apparatus.
  - "No touch" technique should be implemented while removing the mass lesion.
  - The margin of resection for BCC is 3mm, SCC is 4mm, SGC is 5mm, and melanoma 5mm respectively
- Eyelid reconstruction aids in achieving anatomical integrity, restoring function and cosmesis.
- Eyelid reconstruction needs an anterior lamella and a posterior lamella.
- The various eyelid reconstruction techniques are mentioned **Table 3:**

TABLE 3: Various eyelid reconstruction techniques.

Defect	*Technique*
<25%	• Laissez-Faire • Direct closure • Direct closure with lateral cantholysis
25%-50%	• Lateral semicircular rotation flap (Tenzel's)**(Fig. 13)** • Tarsoconjunctival flap—Horizontal tarsoconjunctival transposition flap (Hewes)
50%-75%	Bridged advancement flap (Cutler–Beard)
75%-100%	• Rhomboid cheek flap • Free tarsoconjunctival graft and myocutaneous advancement flap • Tarsoconjunctival advancement flap • Lid switch flap (Mustarde) • Temporal forehead transposition flap (Fricke)

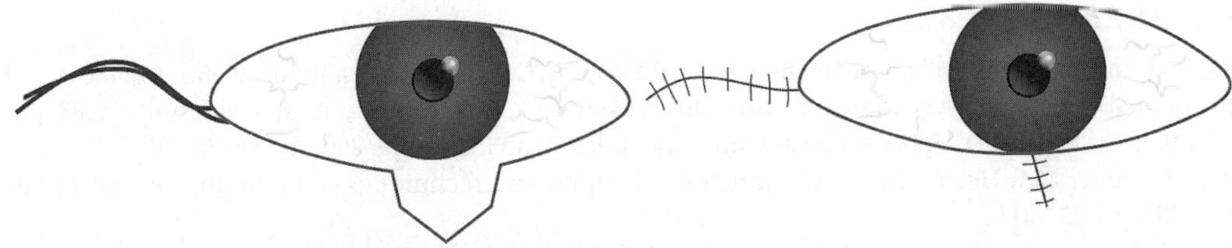

Fig. 13: Lateral semicircular rotational flap (Tenzel's)

14. Write briefly on eyelid coloboma. (10) (DNB 2019)

- Eyelid coloboma can be congenital or acquired.
- Congenital eyelid coloboma can be unilateral or bilateral.
- Upper eyelid is most commonly involved, and the most frequent site is the junction of the medial and middle-third of the eyelid **(Fig. 14)**.
- It is postulated to be a part of the facial cleft.
- Eyelid coloboma is often associated with several syndromes like Fraser syndrome, Goldenhar syndrome, Treacher Collins syndrome, CHARGE Syndrome, frontonasal dysplasia.
- The underlying pathophysiology remains unclear, it can be due to the defect in the apoptosis of the mesenchymal cells.
- It is important to look for microphthalmia, lipo-dermoids, keratoconus, iris coloboma, exposure keratopathy.
- Nouby has devised a classification of eyelid coloboma as follows in **Table 4**:

TABLE 4: Classification of eyelid coloboma.

Grade	*Finding*
Coloboma without cryptophthalmos	
Coloboma with abortive cryptophthalmos	
Coloboma with complete cryptophthalmos	
Classic cryptophthalmos	Absence of normal structure and eye covered with skin
Severe cryptophthalmos	Severe deformity of nose and ectropion of the upper lip

- Management is focused on corneal protection and amblyopia treatment.
- Indications for early surgical intervention in these cases include corneal exposure due to lid defect.
- Surgical correction:
- For small upper lid defects—direct closure, direct closure with cantholysis, Tenzel's semicircular flap
- For moderate to severe upper lid defects—Tenzel's semicircular flap, Mustarde's lid switch flap, Cutler Beard method
- For small lower lid defects - direct closure with or without cantholysis
- For moderate lower lid defects—posterior lamella can be reconstructed with Hughes flap, anterior lamella requires full thickness skin graft, advancement of cheek skin
- For larger lower lid defects—hard palate graft or mucoperiosteal graft is used for posterior lamella, Mustarde's cheek rotation flap, nasolabial flap are used for anterior lamella.

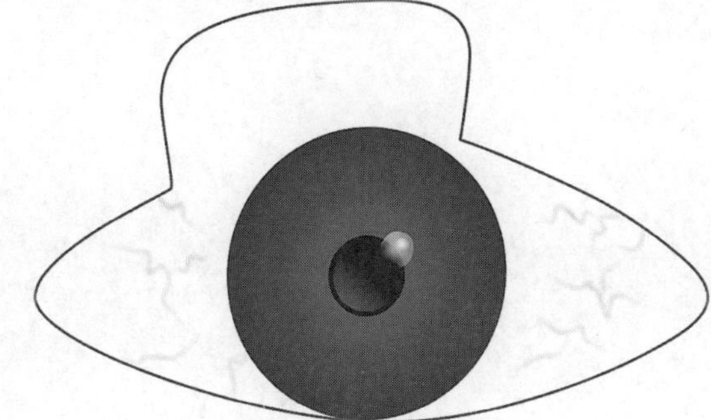

Fig. 14: Congenital upper eyelid coloboma.

SUGGESTED READING

1. Bernardini FP. Management of malignant and benign eyelid lesions. Curr Opin Ophthalmol. 2006;17(5):480-4.
2. Collin JRO. Manual of systematic eyelid surgery, 3rd edition. New York, Edinburgh: hurchill Livingstone; 1983. pp. 76-95.
3. Kakizaki H, Malhotra R, Selva D. Upper eyelid anatomy: an update. Ann Plast Surg. 2009;63(3):336-43.
4. McCord CD, Codener MA, Hester TR. Eyelid surgery. Principles and techniques, 1st edition. New York: Lipincott-Raven publishers; 1995. pp. 252-311.
5. Subramanian N. Reconstructions of eyelid defects. Indian J Plast Surg. 2011;44:5-13.
6. Takahashi Y, Leibovitch I, Kakizaki H. Frontalis suspension surgery in upper eyelid blepharoptosis. Open Ophthalmol J. 2010;4:91-7.

4

CHAPTER

Orbit

Prabrisha Banerjee, Puja Chowdhury, Koustav Bhunia

QUESTIONS

1. **A 60-year-old woman came to OPD with unilateral proptosis. Discuss the differential diagnosis, evaluation, and management of the case. (3+3+4) (DNB 2018)**
2. **A 3-year-old child presented in OPD with unilateral proptosis. Discuss the differential diagnoses, evaluation, and management of the case. (3+3+4) (BHU MS 2017)**
3. **Describe the clinical features and management in a case of orbital cellulitis. (5) (MS WBUHS 2014, DO 2015)**
4. **Clinical features, investigations, and treatment of thyroid ophthalmopathy. (10) (MS WBUHS 2021)**
5. **Orbital apex syndrome—short note. (5) (MS WBUHS 2015)**
6. **Write briefly on lateral orbitotomy. (10) (MS BHU 2020)**
7. **Write briefly on enophthalmos. (10) (MS RGUHS)**
8. **Write briefly on orbital implants and their clinical importance. (10) (WBUHS MS 2018)**
9. **Briefly discuss the indications, advantages and disadvantages of various types of orbital exenteration. (5) (BHU MS 2019)**
10. **Give the morphological classification of contracted socket. Discuss the strategies for managing a contracted socket. (10) (DNB 2017 WBUHS)**

1. A 60-year-old woman came to OPD with unilateral proptosis. Discuss the differential diagnosis, evaluation, and management of the case. (3+3+4) (DNB 2018)

2. A 3-year-old child presented in OPD with unilateral proptosis. Discuss the differential diagnoses, evaluation, and management of the case. (3+3+4) (BHU MS 2017)

- Proptosis is defined as the protrusion of the eyeball out of the orbit by 2 mm or more.
- It can have a unilateral or bilateral presentation.
- The differential diagnosis for unilateral proptosis in different age groups in descending order of frequency are as follows in **Table 1**:

TABLE 1: differential diagnosis for unilateral proptosis in different age groups.

Children	*Adult*	*Senile*
• Orbital cellulitis • Capillary hemangioma • Dermoid cyst • Venolymphatic malformation • Rhabdomyosarcoma • Granulocytic sarcoma • Optic nerve glioma	• Thyroid eye disease • Orbital inflammatory disease • Cavernous hemangioma • Schwannoma • Meningioma	• Lymphoma • Thyroid eye disease • Metastasis in orbit

- Evaluation of a case of proptosis comprises:
  - Detailed history
  - Ocular examination and evaluation of proptosis
  - Systemic examination
  - Imaging and investigation
- Detailed history that helps to formulate differential diagnosis must include:
  - Age of onset
  - Nature of onset—sudden or gradual
  - Progression—slow, rapid, or intermittent
  - Pain
  - Postural variation
  - Associated diminution of vision
  - Associated diplopia
  - Associated history of fever, headache, weight gain/loss, tremors, change in appetite, cold or heat intolerance, bowel disturbances
  - History of respiratory tract infection, blood dyscrasia
  - History of trauma
  - History of any systemic illness
  - Drug history
  - History of smoking
  - Past surgical history
- Clinical examination:
  - Visual acuity
  - Color vision
  - Pupillary reaction
  - Hirschberg reflex
  - Ocular motility
- Examination of proptosis:
  - Inspection of face—for facial asymmetry seen in neurofibromatosis, fullness in temporal fossa seen in sphenoid wing meningioma
  - Unilateral/bilateral involvement
  - Dystopia or direction of displacement
  - Eyelid signs—to look for eyelid retraction, lateral flare, eyelid lag, lagophthalmos
  - Signs of inflammation—congestion, eyelid edema, chemosis
  - Palpation of the orbital rim—to detect any discontinuity in the orbital rim, to feel the palpable mass, to check if finger insinuation can be achieved.
  - Palpation of the mass/lesion—the following characteristics of the mass/lesion should be observed during palpation: Size, consistency (firm/soft), margins (well-defined/ill-defined), shape, temperature, tenderness, reducibility, mobility, skin over the mass.
  - Retrobulbar resistance (RBR)
  - Feel for any thrill—present in vascular tumors, or vascular malformation
  - Asymmetry between the two eyeballs can be assessed by Nafziger's view, or Worm's eye view.
  - *Exophthalmometry:* Hertel is used most commonly. Naugle's exophthalmometer is used in lateral orbital wall defects.
  - *Globe displacement:* Horizontal and vertical (2 Ruler test)—to measure dystopia.
  - Measurement of superior, and inferior scleral show, lagophthalmos, and levator palpebral superioris action in cases of thyroid eye disease.
  - Regional lymph node palpation—pre- and postauricular, submandibular, and cervical.

- Cranial nerve examination (II, III, IV, V, and VI)
- Valsalva maneuver
- Auscultation—to hear bruit with the bell of the stethoscope in arteriovenous malformation and fistula.
- Slit lamp examination to look for conjunctival congestion, chemosis, corkscrew vessels, Salmon patch, exposure keratopathy, superior limbic keratopathy, Lisch nodules.
- Intraocular pressure—a rise in intraocular pressure is noted in proptosis due to altered scleral rigidity.
- Gonioscopy—to look for blood in Schlemm's canal.
- Fundoscopy may reveal optic disc edema, optociliary shunt, optic atrophy, choroidal folds, venous engorgement.

- Systemic examination should include the nasopharynx, oral cavity, thyroid gland, respiratory system, and gastrointestinal system.
- MRI is preferred for soft tissue lesions and vascular lesions. Contrast enhancement is recommended in certain cases like neoplastic lesions, vascular lesions, and suspected optic nerve perineuritis.
- CT scan is required to detect bony lesions like osteoma, bone erosion, or remodeling due to orbital mass as observed in pleomorphic adenoma, in suspected cases of dumb-bell dermoid.
- Ultrasound B scan (USG B scan) is less commonly used these days.
- Management **(Flowchart 1)**:

Flowchart 1: Management.

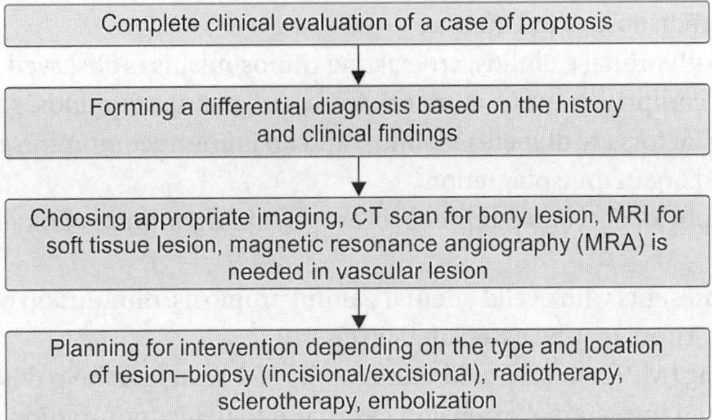

- In the 60-year-old patient the likely cause will be neoplastic lesion like lymphoma or thyroid eye disease. Imaging will aid in the diagnosis **(Flowchart 2)**.

Flowchart 2: Diagnosis of MRI orbit with contrast.

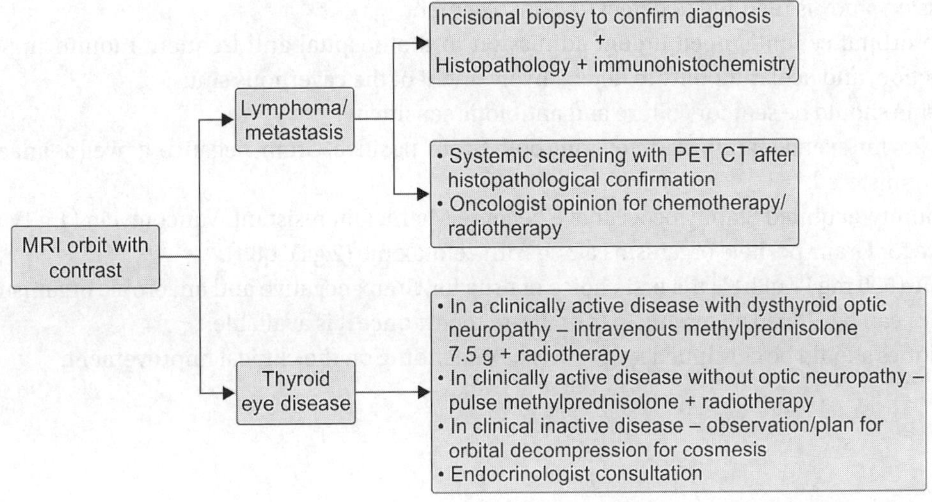

- In a 3-year-old child, the likely differential and their management are as follows in **Table 2**:

TABLE 2: Differential diagnosis and management.

Diagnosis	*Management*
Orbital cellulitis	Hospital admission + blood and urine culture + IV antibiotics + ENT consultation for pansinusitis
Capillary hemangioma	Usually self-limiting, resolves with age. In case of optic nerve compression, risk of amblyopia, treatment with beta blockers based on body weight
Dermoid cyst	Excision biopsy
Venolymphatic malformation	Sclerotherapy with bleomycin injection
Rhabdomyosarcoma	Incisional biopsy for histopathological confirmation, oncologist consultation for chemotherapy
Granulocytic sarcoma	Peripheral blood smear examination
Optic nerve glioma	Observation, treatment needs to be started in case of diminished vision at presentation or progression

3. Describe the clinical features and management in a case of orbital cellulitis.

(5) (MS WBUHS 2014, DO 2015)

- The most common cause of orbital cellulitis is sinusitis. Orbit's location adjacent to the paranasal sinus, and the thin wall of lamina papyracea predispose to infections.
- In about 86–98% patients with orbital cellulitis, co-existing rhinosinusitis is observed.
- The other common causes comprise trauma, dental abscess, and panophthalmitis.
- The common predisposing factors are diabetes mellitus, and an immunocompromised state like immunodeficiency disease, chemotherapy, and organ transplantation.
- Gram-positive bacteria Staphylococci and Streptococci are the most common etiological agents in the adult and the pediatric population.
- Clinically orbital cellulitis presents with eyelid edema, painful proptosis, diminution of vision, ophthalmoplegia, and chemosis **(Figs. 1A and B)**. There may be associated fever.
- Magnetic resonance imaging (MRI) or computed tomography (CT scan) can help detect orbital infections.
- MRI is preferred in suspected intracranial extension cases and to detect non-radiopaque foreign bodies like wood, bamboo, etc.
- CT scan (thin cuts) is a better modality for detecting bone involvement, and radiopaque foreign bodies.
- In orbital cellulitis, CT scan and MRI orbit display inflammatory edema of the orbital soft tissue in T2WI with orbital fat stranding along with proptosis.
- A fat suppression study is required to detect CNS involvement.
- Patients with orbital cellulitis need urgent admission to the hospital and frequent monitoring of visual acuity, pupillary reaction, and ocular motility to detect involvement of the cavernous sinus.
- Blood and urine should be sent for culture and antibiotic sensitivity.
- Broad-spectrum intravenous antibiotics covering both Gram-positive, Gram-negative, as well as anaerobic organisms should be administered.
- As the community-acquired Staphylococci have become Methicillin resistant, Vancomycin (1 g IV q12h) is the first drug of choice for Gram-positive organisms along with cefotaxime (2 g IV q8h).
- Metronidazole (500 mg IV q8h) is the first choice of drug for Gram-negative and anaerobic organisms.
- The antibiotics can be altered according to the culture report once it is available.
- The IV antibiotics should be continued for 1–2 weeks depending on the clinical improvement.

- The role of systemic steroids remains controversial. However, it should be started only after a good response to the IV antibiotics. Systemic steroids should be avoided in immunocompromised and diabetic patients.
- A nasal decongestant should be started and an ENT consultation is needed for associated sinusitis. These patients may need functional endoscopic sinus surgery.
- Orbital cellulitis is an emergency. It can lead to the following complications if it is not managed timely **(Table 3)**.

TABLE 3: Complications of orbital cellulitis.

Compressive optic neuropathy	Cavernous sinus thrombosis (CST)
Central retinal artery occlusion (CRAO)	Septic emboli
Exposure keratopathy	Brain abscess
Exudative retinal detachment	Meningitis

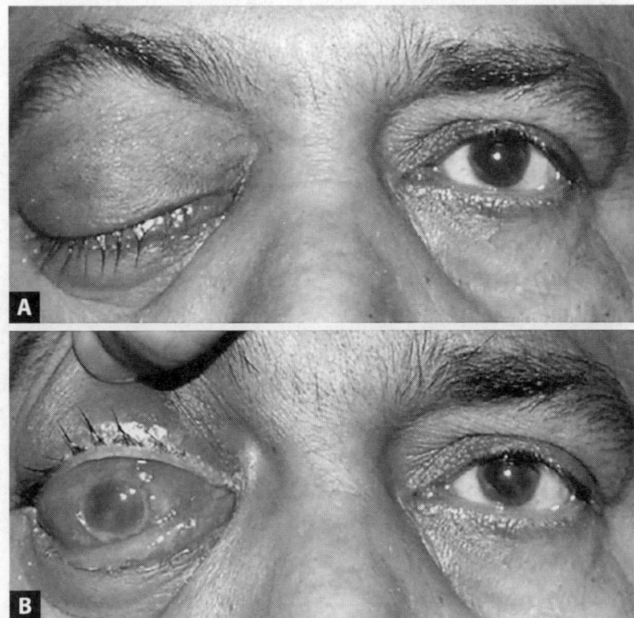

Figs. 1A and B: A 50-year-old male presenting with right eye orbital cellulitis. *(For Color version, See Color Plate 5)*

4. Clinical features, investigations, and treatment of thyroid ophthalmopathy. (10) (MS WBUHS 2021)

- Thyroid eye disease, also known as Grave's disease, is an autoimmune disorder mostly associated with hyperthyroidism.
- It is the most common cause of unilateral and bilateral proptosis in adults.
- However, it can manifest in primary hypothyroidism or euthyroid state as well.
- The risk factors are: age, females are more predisposed, smoking, tobacco chewing, radioactive iodine therapy, post-ablative hypothyroidism, and stress.
- The auto antibodies to thyroid stimulating hormone receptor activate the orbital fibroblasts to produce glycosaminoglycans leading to tissue edema and adipogenesis.
- Thyroid eye disease has an active and a quiescent stage **(Fig. 2)**.

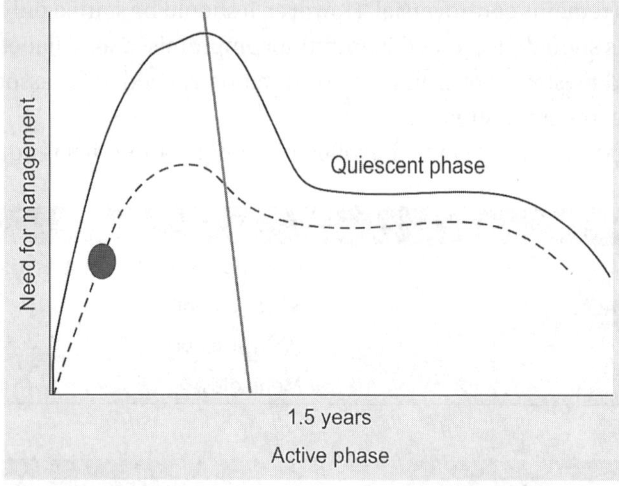

Fig. 2: Rundle's curve describing the phases.

- Clinical signs:
  - Lid signs: Kocher's sign—Staring appearance
  - Vigouroux sign—Eyelid fullness or puffiness
  - Rosenbach's sign—Tremors of eyelids (when closed)
  - Riesman's sign—Bruit over the eyelids
  - Von Graefe's sign—Upper lid lag on downgaze
  - Dalrymple's sign—Upper eyelid retraction
  - Stellwag's sign—Incomplete and infrequent blinking
  - Grove sign—Resistance to pulling the retracted upper lid
  - Boston sign—Uneven, jerky movements of the upper lid on inferior gaze
  - Jellinek's sign—Abnormal pigmentation of the upper lid
  - Gifford's sign—Difficulty in everting the upper lid
  - Means sign—Increase superior scleral show on upgaze
  - Enroth's sign—Edema of the lower lid
  - Griffith's sign—Lower lid lag on upward gaze
  - *Restrictive myopathy:* The GAG deposition in the muscles leads to swelling and motility disorder, presents as diplopia and strabismus. Inferior rectus is the most commonly involved muscle followed by medial, superior, and lateral rectus. After the active phase is over, fibrosis sets in leading to permanent restrictive myopathy.
  - *Proptosis:* Swelling of the extraocular muscles, adipogenesis leads to axial proptosis in the majority of the cases.
  - *Soft tissue involvement:* Manifests as grittiness, redness, watering due to dry eyes, superior limbic keratopathy, eyelid edema, conjunctival congestion, and chemosis.
  - *Dysthyroid optic neuropathy (DON):* Occurs secondary to apical compression by the enlarged extraocular muscles, increased orbital contents. The other mechanisms are ischemia due to compromised vascular supply, and mechanical stretching of the optic nerve.
- A detailed history comprising onset, progression, presence of diurnal variation in swelling, cold or heat intolerance, loss or gain of appetite, weight loss or weight gain, thyroid status, history of smoking, chewing, radioactive iodine, thyroidectomy should be taken.
- A thorough ophthalmic evaluation comprises visual acuity, pupil reaction, Hirschberg reflex, ocular motility, slit lamp examination, intraocular pressure (often raised due to elevated episcleral venous pressure), and fundoscopy. Proptosis should be assessed with Hertel's exophthalmometer
- Clinical activity is assessed with the clinical activity score (CAS)

- Clinical activity score gives each point to the following clinical features: orbital pain at rest, orbital pain with movement, chemosis, caruncular edema, conjunctival injection, and eyelid injection.
- CAS score >3 out of 7 signifies clinically active TED.
- VISA classification/International Thyroid Eye Disease Study (ITEDS) grades clinical activity based on certain subjective and objective examination of Vision, Inflammation, Strabismus, and Appearance. VISA grading helps to assess clinical response to the treatment.
- VISA score >4 indicates clinical activity.
- Investigations:
  - Thyroid function tests, Anti-TSH R antibody, anti-thyroglobulin antibody, antithyroid peroxidase (TPO) antibody.
  - *Imaging:* MRI/CT is indicated in unilateral proptosis, in suspected dysthyroid optic neuropathy, in VISA score > 4, for planning orbital decompression.
  - The common findings on imaging include tendon sparing enlargement of the extraocular muscles, increased orbital fat, apical compression of the optic nerve, and lacrimal gland enlargement **(Fig. 3)**.
  - Barret's index and fat effacement give an estimation of apical compression of optic nerve.
  - Color vision, contrast sensitivity, visual field test
  - Visually evoked potential (VEP)

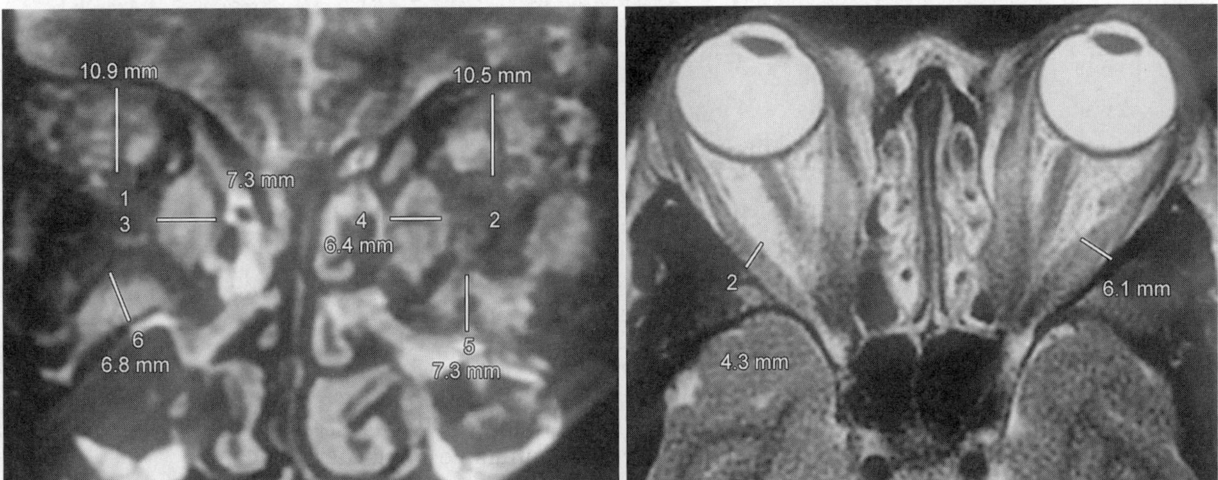

Fig. 3: MRI orbit showing enlarged recti muscles, hyperintense signal on T2WI indicating edema, and apical compression.

- Management **(Flowchart 3)**:
  - To act on modifiable risk factors—to stop smoking, to maintain euthyroid state.

Flowchart 3: Management.

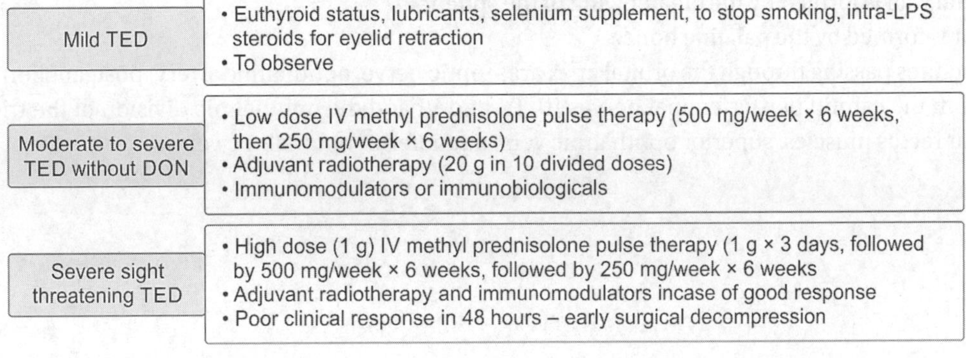

- Immunomodulators:
  - Azathioprine 50 mg BD or mycophenolate 500 mg BD for 6 months or more
- Newer drugs in the management of TED **(Table 4)**:

TABLE 4: Newer drugs in the management of TED.	
Teprotumumab	Inhibits insulin-like growth factor 1 signaling
Tocilizumab	Humanized monoclonal antibody against IL-6 receptor

- Orbital decompression **(Table 5)**:
  - Indications in active phase
    - DON not responding to medical management
    - Severe TED with gross proptosis and exposure keratopathy
    - Globe subluxation

    Indications in quiescent phase—cosmesis

TABLE 5: Orbital decompression.	
Fat removal orbital decompression	2–3 mm
Bone removal orbital decompression	
1 wall	2–3 mm
2 wall	4–5 mm
3 wall	6–7 mm

  - Order of surgery for cosmesis in quiescent phase
  - Orbital decompression → Squint surgery → Lid surgery
  - For upper eyelid retraction—blepharotomy, Muller muscle and LPS recession can be done
  - For lower lid retraction—spacer graft, lower lid retractor recession is done.

5. Orbital apex syndrome—short note. (5) (MS WBUHS 2015)

- Orbital apex syndrome (OAS) is a complex neurological disorder characterized by proptosis, ptosis, ophthalmoplegia with diplopia or diminution of vision due to the involvement of multiple cranial nerves.
- It is also known as Jacod syndrome.
- The common etiological factors are neoplastic, vascular, infectious, or inflammatory conditions.
- The spread from the adjacent paranasal sinus and hematogenous spread are responsible for the orbital involvement.
- Anatomy of the orbital apex **(Fig. 4)**:
  - Orbital apex is a connection between the orbit and the central nervous system.
  - The roof is formed by the lesser wing of the sphenoid.
  - The medial wall is formed by the ethmoid bone.
  - The lateral wall is formed by the greater wing of the sphenoid.
  - The floor is formed by the palatine bone.
  - The structures passing through the orbital apex are—optic nerve, ophthalmic artery, postganglionic sympathetic fibers from the carotid plexus, cranial nerves III, IV, and VI and the ophthalmic division of the trigeminal nerve (V1), four rectus muscles, superior ophthalmic vein, and inferior ophthalmic vein.

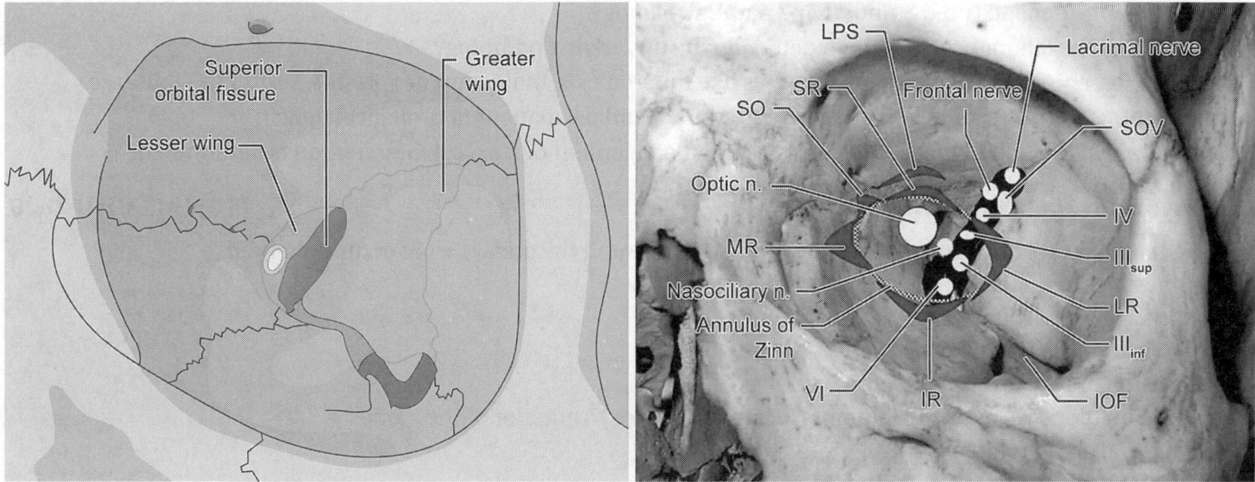

Fig. 4: Anatomy of the orbital apex. *(For Color version, See Color Plate 6)*

- The causes of orbital apex syndrome are mentioned in **Table 6**:

TABLE 6: Causes of orbital apex syndrome.

Etiological condition	*Entities*
Infections	• Orbital cellulitis, sinusitis can involve the orbital apex. *Staphylococcus, Streptococcus,* and *Pseudomonas* are the most common causal agents. The toxins produced by the bacteria cause disseminated infection. Another important and frequent etiological agent is Mycobacterium tuberculosis • Fungi like Mucor and Aspergillosis can involve the orbital apex
Inflammatory	Orbital inflammatory diseases like sarcoidosis, IgG4 disease, sclerosing idiopathic orbital inflammatory disease, granulomatosis polyangiitis can lead to orbital apex syndrome
Neoplastic	Mass lesions at the orbital apex like cavernous hemangioma, schwannoma, or metastatic lesions from breast carcinoma, lungs, or lymphoma may involve the orbital apex
Vascular	Carotid cavernous fistula, cavernous sinus thrombosis
Traumatic	Penetrating injury, intraorbital foreign body

- Patient may present with ptosis, ophthalmoplegia, pain, proptosis, diplopia and diminution of vision. Pain over the trigeminal sensory distribution is noted in Tolosa–Hunt syndrome.
- *Investigation:* Imaging guides in delineating the extent of the disease. MRI with contrast is the imaging modality of choice. CT is needed when suspecting bony lesions or when MRI is contraindicated.
- *Laboratory tests:* The imaging guides in deciding the ancillary tests required for the further management. The range of the test comprises:
  - Complete blood count with peripheral blood smear
  - Erythrocyte sedimentation rate and C-reactive protein
  - Blood culture
  - Venereal Disease Research Laboratory (VDRL) test, treponema pallidum hemagglutination assay (TPHA), rapid plasma reagin (RPR)
  - Mantoux test, high-resolution computed tomography (HRCT) chest, interferon-gamma release assay (IGRA) for tuberculosis
  - Blood sugars, glycosylated hemoglobin
  - Angiotensin-converting enzyme, serum calcium for sarcoidosis
  - Perinuclear and cytoplasmic anti-neutrophil cytoplasmic antibodies (pANCA and cANCA) and anti-nuclear antibody (ANA)
  - Serum IgG4

- Management—depends on the underlying pathophysiology
- Imaging and the laboratory tests aid in detecting the underlying pathology.
- Systemic screening is also mandatory in cases like tuberculosis, malignant neoplasms, serum IgG4 disease.
- Intervention within 48 hours help to reduce morbidity and permanent neurological deficit.
- Depending on the underlying pathology, medical management or surgical intervention is determined.

6. Write briefly on lateral orbitotomy. (10) (MS BHU 2020)

- Lateral wall of the orbit is formed by the zygomatic bone and the greater wing of the sphenoid.
- It lies next to the middle cranial fossa.
- It is the strongest orbital wall.
- The indications for lateral orbitotomy
  - Excision biopsy of intraconal tumors
  - Excision biopsy of extraconal tumors located posterior to equator of the globe
  - Lacrimal gland tumors
  - Orbital decompression in thyroid orbitopathy
  - Removal of intraorbital foreign body
  - Drainage of orbital abscess or hematoma
- Lateral orbitotomy approaches **(Fig. 5)**:
  A. Sub-brow incision (Stallard-Wright incision)
  B. Extended upper lid crease incision
  C. Lateral canthotomy-cantholysis incision (Berke's incision)

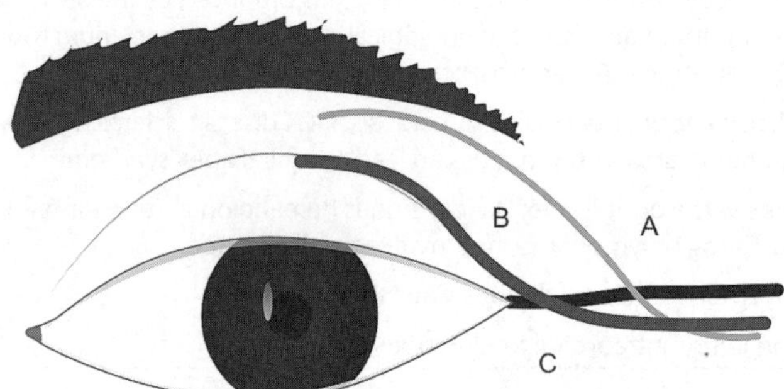

Fig. 5: Surgical approach for lateral orbitotomy.

Steps of Lateral Orbitotomy

- The surgery is done under general anesthesia.
- Extended upper lid crease incision is given.
- Soft tissue dissection done to expose the periosteum.
- Periosteum is elevated to expose the lateral orbital rim (frontozygomatic suture).
- Periorbita is lifted and pushed medially.
- If osteotomy is needed, incision is given below the frontozygomatic suture and at the lower part of the lateral orbital rim.
- Bone is removed either will the help of oscillating saw or osteotome and mallet.
- The periorbita is opened with a T-shaped incision **(Fig. 6)**.
- Lateral rectus has to be disinserted if needed.
- Incision or excision biopsy is accomplished **(Fig. 7)**.
- The bone fragment is replaced in position with the help of cyanoacrylate glue or wire/prolene suture **(Fig. 8)**.
- Periosteum is sutured with 6-0 Vicryl sutures.
- Skin and orbicularis are closed in layers.
- Complications of lateral orbitotomy—vision loss, orbital hemorrhage, ptosis, diplopia, strabismus, injury to lacrimal gland leading to dryness, rounding of lateral canthus, infraorbital hypoesthesia, CSF leakage, pupillary dysfunction (damage to ciliary ganglion)

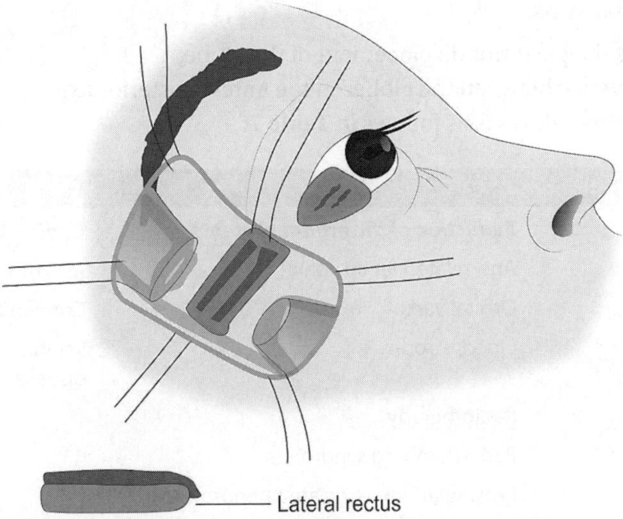

Fig. 6: Periorbita incised and orbital fats and LR muscle exposed.

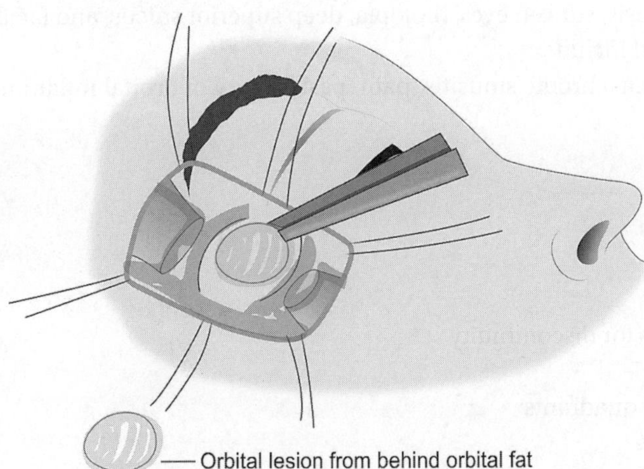

Fig. 7: Excision of the orbital mass.

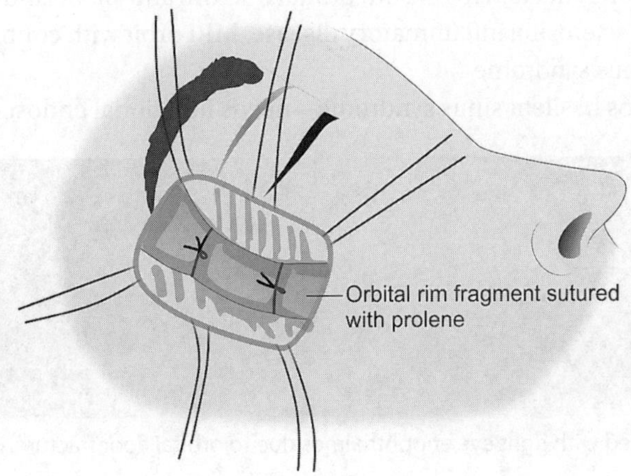

Fig. 8: Bone placed back and sutured with prolene suture.

7. Write briefly on enophthalmos. (10) (MS RGUHS)

- Enophthalmos is defined as the posterior displacement of the globe.
- There should be 2 mm difference between the globes in the anteroposterior axis.
- The pathophysiology of enophthalmos is as follows in **Table 7**:

TABLE 7: Pathophysiology of enophthalmos.

Enlargement of orbit	*Reduction of the orbital contents*	*Contracture of orbital contents*
Blow out fracture of orbital floor	Age-related fat atrophy	Metastatic scirrhous breast cancer
Silent sinus syndrome	Orbital varix	Congenital fibrosis syndrome
Deficient sphenoid wing	Lipodystrophy	Sclerosing idiopathic orbital inflammatory disease
Bony remodeling by orbital tumor	Radiotherapy	
	Parry-Romberg syndrome	
	Prostaglandin-associated periorbitopathy	
	Orbital decompression surgery	

- Patient can present with ptosis, sunken eyes, diplopia, deep superior sulcus, and facial asymmetry
- Clinical examination should include:
  - Detailed history—trauma, chronic sinusitis, pain, past history of orbital inflammation, family history, previous drug history
  - Vision
  - Hirshberg
  - Presence of Hypoglobus
  - Pupil reaction
  - Ocular motility
  - Palpation of orbital rims for discontinuity
  - Retrobulbar resistance
  - Finger insinuation in all quadrants
  - To look for hypoesthesia
  - Valsalva maneuver for orbital varix
  - To look for pulsation in absent sphenoid wing
  - Hertel exophthalmometry **(Fig. 9)**
- *Imaging:* Non-contrast CT orbit is needed to rule out orbital fracture and silent sinus syndrome. For detecting orbital varix, orbital metastasis, and sclerosing inflammatory disease, MRI orbit with contrast is required.
- ENT consultation in silent sinus syndrome
- Management of enophthalmos in silent sinus syndrome—needs functional endoscopic sinus surgery.

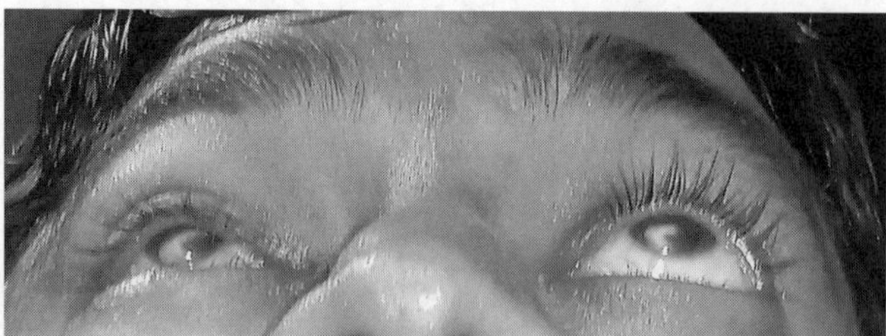

Fig. 9: A 35-year-old male presented with right eye enophthalmos due to orbital floor fracture. *(For Color version, See Color Plate 6)*

- Indications for repair of isolated orbital floor fractures (**Table 8**):

TABLE 8: Indications for repair of isolated orbital floor fractures.

Immediate	• Trapdoor fracture in children • Oculocardiac reflex without any spontaneous regression • Early hypo- or enophthalmos suggesting a large floor fracture
Within 2 weeks	• Diplopia in the functionally important gaze directions • Fracture >50% of the area of the orbital floor • Enophthalmos >2 mm
Observation	• No significant enophthalmos or hypo-ophthalmos • Minimal diplopia (not in primary or down gaze)

Surgical management of enophthalmos with isolated orbital floor fracture:

Freeing all entrapped herniated tissue

↓

Sufficient subperiosteal exposure and identification of fixed base posterior to the globe

↓

Positioning of graft (titanium/polymer plate) behind the globe axis
Reconstruction of defect with graft or plate fixed to base with screws

↓

Assessing FDT before closure (in layers)

- Orbital varix can be treated with sclerotherapy depending upon its location and the supplying vessel after MR angiography or digital subtraction angiography.
- For the deep superior sulcus, dermal fillers can be used for better cosmesis.

8. Write briefly on orbital implants and their clinical importance. (10) (WBUHS MS 2018)

- The ideal characteristic features of orbital implants are:
  - Mimics normal globe as closely as possible.
  - Biologically inert.
  - Replaces the needed volume and allows space for a prosthesis of adequate thickness
  - Has minimal rate of infection, exposure, and extrusion.
  - Provides socket motility transmitted to prosthesis
  - Lightweight, centered within muscle cone, anchored to orbital tissues
  - Able to get integrated with prosthesis for transfer of motility
  - Affordable and easily available
- The types of the orbital implants are as follows in **Table 9**:

TABLE 9: Types of orbital implants.

Biogenic	***Non-integrated***	***Semi-integrated***	***Fully integrated***	***Expandable Implants***
Dermis fat graft is indicated in children, patients having reduced surface along with loss of volume	Non-porous	Have attachments for extraocular muscles on anterior surface	• Porous implant • Allows fibrovascular ingrowth	Expands in vivo and promotes orbital growth
	No integration with orbital tissue	Allows good motility	Minimal chances of migration and extrusion	Used in congenital microphthalmos and anophthalmos

Contd...

Contd...

Biogenic	Non-integrated	Semi-integrated	Fully integrated	Expandable Implants
	Do not allow attachment to muscles unless wrapped	Readily available	Transmits movement through a motility peg on the anterior surface	Self-expanding tissue expanders—made of osmotically active hydrogel, becomes 8 times of their original size by absorbing body fluids
	E.g.: PMMA sphere, silicon spheres	• Erosion on conjunctiva can cause discomfort • Extrusion rate is higher • Prosthesis needs to be customized according to these implants	Expensive	E.g.: • Hemispherical socket expanders—used to stretch fornix for putting prosthesis • Orbital expanders—used in anophthalmos • Pin SETEs—used in sockets appearing enophthalmic with an implant inside
		E.g.: Allen, Iowa Universal, Castroviejo	E.g.: Natural hydroxyapatite, synthetic hydroxyapatite, porous polyethylene (Medpor)	

Orbital implant after evisceration is depicted in **Figure 10**.

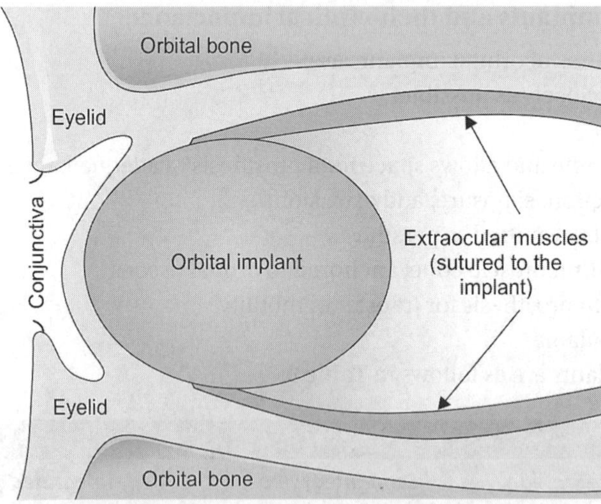

Fig. 10: Orbital implants after evisceration.

- Implants in orbital wall fracture **(Table 10)**:

TABLE 10: Implants in orbital wall fracture.

Metallic	Non-metallic		Composite
Titanium	Porous	Non-porous	Porous polypropylene + Titanium (Synpor/Titan)

Contd...

Contd...

Metallic	*Non-metallic*		*Composite*
Cobalt alloy	Polyethylene (Medpor)	Silicon	
	Polycaprolactone (Osteomesh)	Polydioxanone	
	Polytetrafluoroethylene (Gore-tex)	Polyetheretherketone (PEEK)	
	Hydroxyapatite		

9. Briefly discuss the indications, advantages and disadvantages of various types of orbital exenteration. (5) (BHU MS 2019)

- *Definition:* Exenteration is the radical surgical procedure involving removal of the soft tissues of the orbit, including muscles, nerves, vessels, fat, orbital contents, and periorbital lining of the cavity.
- Modern exenteration was introduced by Arlt.
- *Indications of exenteration are:*
  - Primary orbital malignancies of adnexa. Example: Squamous cell carcinoma, basal cell carcinoma, sebaceous carcinoma, uveal melanoma as primary mode of surgery; also those not responding to chemotherapy or radiotherapy.
  - Aggressive life-threatening fungal infections: Orbital zygomycoses (mucormycoses) not responding to treatment or involving 3 or more orbital quadrants
  - Malignant epithelial tumors of lacrimal gland (adenoid cystic carcinoma)
  - Destructive/painful/progressive tumors of sinuses, eyelids, conjunctiva (malignant melanoma), face encroaching into orbital anatomy.
  - Grossly deformed orbital cavity post trauma or in neurofibromatosis for better cosmesis.
- Types of exenteration **(Table 11)**:

TABLE 11: Types of exenteration.

Stage	*Type*	*Surgical technique*	
Subtotal exenteration	I	Eyelids and bulbar/palpebral conjunctiva spared	*Advantages*: Few complications, fast wound healing, allow use of prosthesis, better cosmesis *Disadvantages:* Difficulty in detecting local tumor recurrence
	II	Eyelids and palpebral conjunctiva spared	
	III	Eyelid skin and deeper muscle spared	
Total exenteration	IV	Eyelid excision	*Advantages:* Facilitates tumor free/disease free condition *Disadvantages:* More complications, delayed wound healing, fistula formation, needs customized prosthesis, poor cosmesis, chances of CSF leak, intracranial infection
Radical exenteration	V	Orbital cavity bones resection	
	VI	Adjacent structures like the sinus removal	

10. Give the morphological classification of contracted socket. Discuss the strategies for managing a contracted socket. (10) (DNB '2017, WBUHS)

- Contracted socket is the shrinkage of all or part of orbital tissue causing shallowing of the fornices and decrease in the orbital volume and thus causing the inability to retain prosthesis.
- Factors leading to contracted socket are mentioned in **Table 12**:

TABLE 12: Factors leading to contracted socket

Intrinsic	***Extrinsic***
Radiation given to anophthalmic sockets in children with retinoblastoma	Poor surgical technique—excessive orbital tissue dissection leading to poor healing and fibrosis
Chemical burn specially alkali burn	Non-placement of implant or small size of implant in the primary surgery
Trauma leading to excessive tissue loss, conjunctival scarring	Absence of conformer which keeps the conjunctiva stretched
	Use of ill-fitting, sharp edged prosthesis

- Morphological classification of contracted socket **(Table 13)**:

TABLE 13: Morphological classification of contracted socket.

• Anophthalmic contracted socket	• Most common-seen after enucleation or evisceration
• Ophthalmic contracted socket	• Following chemical or radiation injuries
• Microphthalmic contracted socket	• Seen in microphthalmos
• Hypoplastic contracted socket	• In congenital underdeveloped bony socket

- Gopal Krishna classification of contracted socket **(Table 14)**
  Grade 1: The socket is characterized by a shallow lower fornix or shelving of the lower fornix.
  Grade 2: Loss of the upper and lower fornices
  Grade 3: Loss of the upper, lower, medial, and lateral fornices
  Grade 4: Loss of all fornices and reduction of the palpebral aperture in horizontal and vertical dimensions
  Grade 5: In some cases, there is recurrence of contraction of the socket after repeated trials of reconstruction
- Management of contracted socket:
  - Prevention is the best mode of management. Careful orbital tissue dissection during primary surgery. Placement of an orbital implant of adequate size during primary surgery. Applying a conformer in the postoperative period and using a well-fitting prosthesis with smooth edges.

TABLE 14: Gopal Krishna classification of contracted socket.

Grade 1	Inferior fornix formation suture (FFS) ± Mucus membrane graft (MMG)
Grade 2	Both eyelids MMG + Superior + Inferior FFS
Grade 3	• If implant present, then MMG + FFS or Amniotic membrane transplant (AMT) or Dermis Fat Graft (DFG) • In absence of implant, adequate surface, secondary ball implant is done • Socket without implant and inadequate surface—DFG can be done
Grade 4	To be treated as Grade 3 with lateral cantholysis
Grade 5	Temporalis muscle transfer or microvascular graft is recommended

SUGGESTED READING

1. Honavar SG. Medical management of thyroid eye disease - A paradigm shift. Indian J Ophthalmol. 2020;68:1515-18.
2. Krishna G. Contracted sockets - I (Aetiology and types). Indian J Ophthalmol. 1980;28:117-20.
3. Nesi FA, Lisman RD, Levine MR. Evaluation and current concepts in the management of anophthalmic socket. In: Nesi FA, Lisman RD, Levine MR (Eds). Smith's ophthalmic plastic and reconstructive surgery, 2nd edition. Maryland Heights: Mosby; 1998. pp. 1079-124.
4. Sokoya M, Cohn JE, Kohlert S, Lee T, Kadakia S, Ducic Y. Considerations in Orbital Exenteration. Semin Plast Surg. 2019;33(2):103-5.
5. Topilow NJ, Tran AQ, Koo EB, Alabiad CR. Etiologies of Proptosis: A review. Intern Med Rev (Wash D C). 2020;6:10.
6. Yadalla D, Jayagayathri R, Padmanaban K, Ramasamy R, Rammohan R, Nisar SP, et al. Bacterial orbital cellulitis – review. Indian J Ophthalmol. 2023;71:2687-93.

CHAPTER

Lacrimal Apparatus

Shashwat Bhattacharyya, Puja Chowdhury

QUESTIONS

1. **Epiphora—short note** **(5) (BHU MS 2019)**
2. **A 14 months child presents with watering in eyes from birth and regurgitation present on pressure over lacrimal sac region. Discuss the management of this case** **(10) (BHU MS 2019)**
3. **Describe causes and management of congenital nasolacrimal duct obstruction: causes and management.** **(3+7) (WBUHS MS 2019)**
4. **Conjunctiva-DCR, indications, contraindications and complications. what RE the types of tube available.** **(10) (DNB 2018)**
5. **Describe the techniques of repair of canalicular injury. (5) DNB 2018**
6. **What are the contraindications of DCR. What are causes of failed DCR and what steps can be taken to prevent it. What is Sump syndrome. How can it be prevented** **(10) (DNB 2020)**
7. **Balloon dacryoplasty—short note** **(5) (DNB 2019)**

1. Epiphora—short note (5) (BHU MS 2019)

Definition: It is the condition of inadequate drainage of tears, leading to overflow at eyelid margin

Causes:

- *Physiological:* Most commonly presents due to lacrimal pump failure, as a result of lower lid laxity or weakness of the orbicularis oculi muscle
- *Mechanical obstruction:*
    - *Punctal causes:*
        i. Eversion of lower punctum commonly in old age due to lower lid laxity, chronic ectropion , chronic blepharitis
        ii. Punctal obstruction due to congenital absence of puncta; cicatricial closure following trauma, chemical injury, burns; eye drops like pilocarpine; by foreign body or concretions
    - *Canalicular cause:* Congenital or acquired (foreign body, stricture, infection)
    - *Lacrimal sac causes:* Trauma, infections like TB or syphilis, stones, atony of sac, congenital mucosal folds
    - *Nasolacrimal duct causes:* Congenital non-canalization, imperforated membrane valves, trauma, infections , tumors or strictures

2. A 14 months child presents with watering in eyes from birth and regurgitation present on pressure over lacrimal sac region. Discuss the management of this case (10) (BHU MS 2019)

The probable diagnosis of the above mentioned case is Congenital Nasolacrimal duct obstruction. It occurs due to failure in canalization of the last portion of lacrimal drainage system, i.e., region of valve of Hasner. If spontaneous resolution of epiphora fails to occur even after first year of birth, it indicates Congenital Nasolacrimal duct obstruction.

Signs of the disease:

- *Epiphora:* Chronic or intermittent watering of eye on affected side, overlapping with any URTI or viral conjunctivitis
- Matting of lashes
- Mucopurulent reflex or discharge by gentle pressure over lacrimal sac area
- Normal anterior segment findings
- *Fluorescence Dye Disappearance test (FDDT):* Highly specific test showing only a fine line of dye should remain 5–10 Minutes under inspection with a blue light

Differential diagnosis:

- Punctal atresia
- Congenital glaucoma
- Chronic conjunctivitis (chlamydial)
- Keratitis
- Uveitis
- Congenital dacryocystocele

Treatment:

- Conservative:
  - *Massage over lacrimal area suggested by rupturing of membranous obstruction by hydrostatic pressure:* Index finger placed over common canaliculi to block reflux, thumb rolled over sac massaging downwards
  - *Probing and irrigation:* Diagnostic and therapeutic—if symptoms are mild-to-moderate, can be delayed until 12–24 months of age, under general anesthesia—punctal dilatation by 00 Bowman lacrimal probe coated with antibiotic ointment inserted into punctum perpendicular to lid margin then turned medially parallel to lid margin.
    A single lacrimal probing successfully resolves congenital NLDO in 90% patients below 13 months age
    Presence of fluorescein dye injected through punctum, in inferior meatus of the nose indicates good patency.
    Results of probing: Hard stop-medial wall of lacrimal sac
    + lacrimal bone cause obstruction
    Soft stop-canalicular or common canalicular block
- *Surgical intervention:* If probing fails–
  - Intubation with silastic tubing with or without balloon dilatation of NLD (balloon dacryoplasty)
  - Endoscopic DCR
  - Conventional DCR
    Intubation: with the help of a lacrimal stent, indicated in children with:
    - Recurrent epiphora despite repeated NLD probing
    - Indicated in canalicular stenosis, punctal agenesis

  Nasolacrimal intubation after failed probing has reported success rate greater than 70%.

  Commonly used stents is the Crawford stent (olive tip) and hook.

The lacrimal stent can be secured with a square knot near punctum; or endoscopically directly sutured to lateral wall of nose, or limbs of stent secured by passing through a silicon band or sponge in inferior meatus of nose.

Self-retaining bicanalicular lacrimal stent comes preloaded with rigid inserter or monocanalicular stent in children with one patient canaliculus.

The proximal end of stent has a punctal plug to self- secure it at punctum.

Balloon dacryoplasty: Balloon catheter dilatation of nasolacrimal canal with introduction of a collapsed balloon catheter inside duct followed by inflation. Expensive, and not of much use due to high success rate of probing.

DCR is reserved for children with persistent epiphora following intubation or/and balloon dacryoplasty, extensive developmental anomalies, older children with epiphora having NLDO.

3. Describe causes and management of congenital nasolacrimal duct obstruction: causes and management. (3+7) (WBUHS MS 2019)

In children the majority of nasolacrimal duct obstruction (NLDO) is Congenital, which presents as persistent tearing up.

- *Site of obstruction:* The blockage occurs most commonly at the distal end of the duct, by a membrane obstructing the Valve of Hasner at nasal end of NLD.
- *Epidemiology:* Congenital NLDO affects around 11% of all normal newborns; no gender or genetic predisposition is present. Maybe unilateral or bilateral (one-third cases).
- Common causes of CNLDO:
    - Membrane obstructing Valve of Hasner at distal nasal end of the nasolacrimal duct, having delayed involution.
    - Generalized stenosis of the duct/inferior meatus
    - Narrow inferior nasolacrimal canal, usually in cases of midfacial abnormalities (Goldenhar syndrome, craniosynostosis, hemifacial microsomia)
    - Maldevelopment of punctum and canaliculi (congenital proximal lacrimal outflow dysgenesis)
    - Associated dacryocele (distended lacrimal sac)
    - Premature births, association with Down's syndrome
- *Clinical presentation:* Usually mentioned by the caregiver of child and seen on examination as follows:
    - Persistent epiphora, increased tear lake in undisturbed eyes
    - Occasional discharge and stickiness of eyelids
    - Pus/mucopurulent discharge (reflux) released on pressure over the lacrimal sac area through the puncta; occasional matting of eyelids.
    - Periocular skin may be chapped from recurrent wetting
    - The symptoms worsens with attacks of URTI
- *Evaluation:* Diagnostic tools:
    - *Fluorescein dye disappearance test:* Retention of dye in thickened tear film strip meniscus 5 minutes after instillation indicates poor outflow.
      In unilateral cases, comparison to healthy side may be done.
    - Primary Probing started with 00 Bowman's probe as early as 6 months may be done in persistent watering without improvement. Probing is diagnostic as well as therapeutic.
      Under local or general anesthesia.
    - *Cycloplegic refraction:* To rule out anisometropic amblyopia in cases where obstruction persists beyond first year of life
- Differential diagnoses:
    - *Nasolacrimal sac obstruction:* More watery discharge than mucopurulent; obstruction at valve of Rosenmuller.
    - *Congenital glaucoma:* Raised intraocular pressure with corneal edema
    - *Foreign body conjunctiva and eyelids:* Congested, hyperemic conjunctiva; retained material seen on eversion of lids.
    - *Corneal abrasion/ulceration:* Positive staining of cornea
    - Acute conjunctivitis
    - Dacryocele, Mucocele
    - Trichiasis, epiblepharon
- *Treatment*: Early diagnosis helps in better recovery.
    - *Conservative management:* Below one year of age, observation is usually advised. Spontaneous resolution by 13 months age of child is seen in upto 93% cases, and upto 44% resolution between 1 to 2 years age.
      Topical antibiotic eyedrops in cases of acute infection, discharge and lacrimal sac massage to be given by caregiver. Crigler maneuver is adopted as the first line of management during the observation period up to 12 months age **(Fig. 1)**.

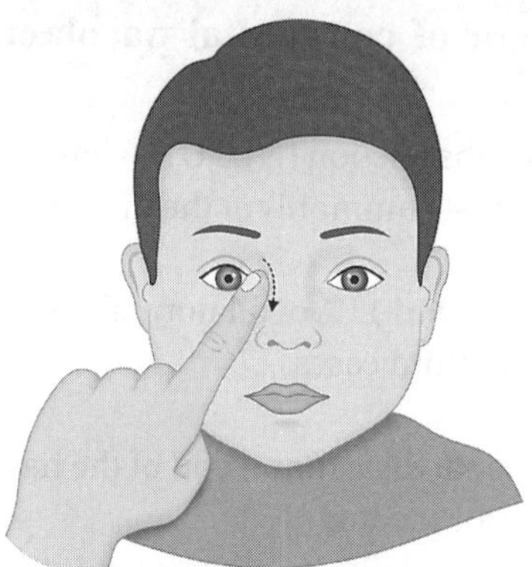

Fig. 1: Crigler massage.

- Invasive therapy:
  - Probing and irrigation **(Figs. 2A and B)**:

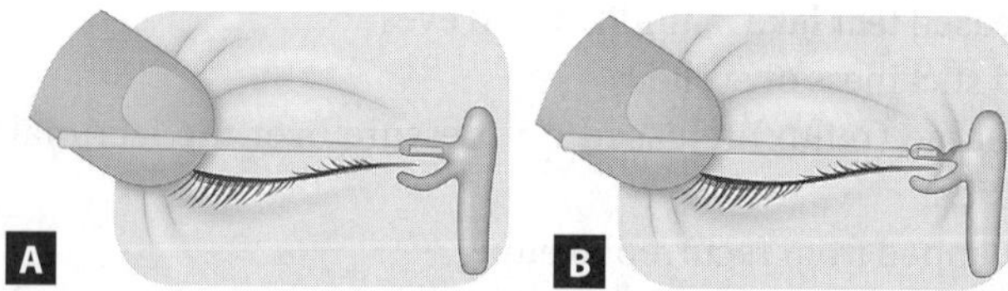

Figs. 2A and B: (A) After punctal dilatation, Bowman's probe in right upper horizontal canaliculus with lateral traction on the eyelid; (B) "Soft stop" encountered when probe tip blocked by canalicular obstruction (soft issue) with medial movement of eyelid skin. "Hard stop" is felt when probe crosses common canalicular system and pushed against lacrimal sac wall and lacrimal bone

- The High pressure irrigation creates positive pressure inside the lacrimal pump system and breaks membranous obstruction if any.
- Probing is an invasive blind procedure, which can be done under general anesthesia, is generally considered after the age of 1 year with success rate potentially decreasing with age.

4. Conjunctiva-DCR, indications, contraindications and complications. What RE the types of tube available. (10) (DNB 2018)

Conjunctiva-DCR is the surgical procedure when the medial canthus is dissected and utilized as the entry point of drainage apparatus (Teflon catheter with Pyrex tube or Jones glass tube) for entry into the lacrimal sac space as alternative to conventional DCR. It can be done by external approach or endoscopically **(Fig. 3)**.

- Indications:
  - Single or both canalicular blockage: Chemical
    Blockage (drugs like Fluorouracil, Docetaxel, Pilocarpine, Timolol, Idoxuridine), trauma, burn injury
  - Chronic NLDO with canalicular blockage
  - Canalicular fibrosis/failed previous stenting surgery due to trauma (laceration), radiation, cicatricial states
  - Lacrimal pump failure, Bell's palsy with hyperlacrimation
- Contraindications:
  - Carunculitis
  - Symblepharon (Steven Johnson syndrome)
  - Medial entropion, history of medial tarsorrhaphy
  - Nasal pathologies: Severe Deviated nasal septum, hypertrophic middle turbinates, nasal polyps
  - Ocular surface lesions, malignancies

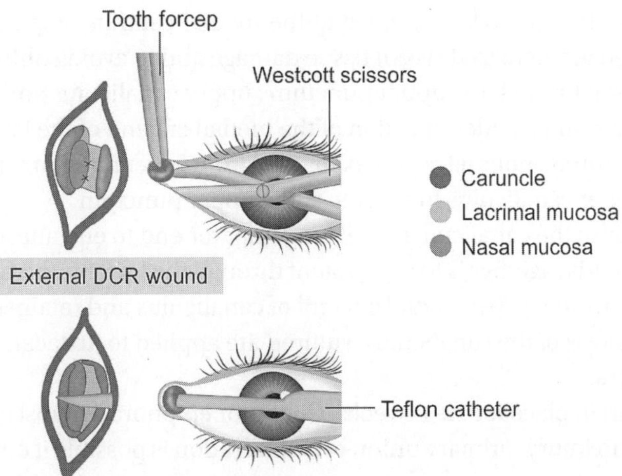

Fig. 3: Conjunctiva-DCR. *(For Color version, See Color Plate 7)*

- Complications:
  - *Failure of tube to drain:* Placement of too long a tube, which touches the nasal septum usually in cases of deviated nasal septum and large middle turbinates.
  - *Lateral migration of the tube:* Seen with loose tube, in contact with the septum. Replaced with a shorter tube, with a modified neck collar named Putterman-Gladstone tube.
  - *Medial migration of tube:* Loss of tube end in medial canthal tissues due to laxity of tissues and poor support to tube; replaced with tube with larger collar.
  - *Granuloma formation:* Conjunctival granuloma around Pyrex tubes commonly formed, prevented with steroid drops.
  - *Closure of the soft tissue opening:* A lost tube must be replaced within one week; if not possible to find tube, new opening is created with Teflon sheathed IV cannula.
  - *Spontaneous expulsion of tube:* Rare due to flanged tubes used presently.
- Tubes commonly used as stents in DCR are:
  - *Jones tube:* Prototype glass rod
  - *Putterman-Gladstone tube:* frosted
  - *StopLoss Jones tube:* Flanged **(Fig. 4)**
  - *Metaireau tube (M-tube):* Silicon tube coated with PVP

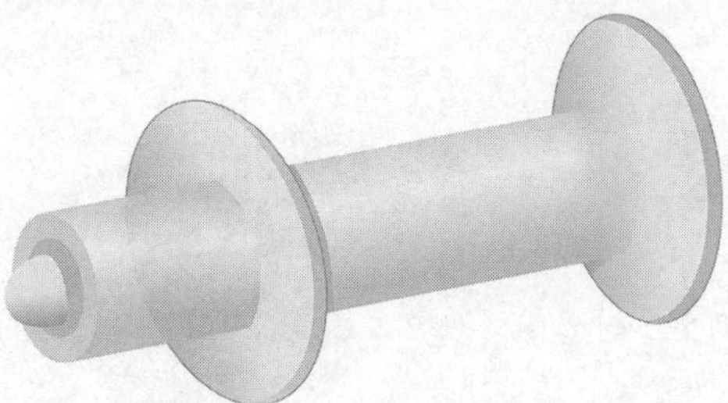

Fig. 4: StopLoss Jones tube.

5. Describe the techniques of repair of canalicular injury. (5) (DNB 2018)

Avulsions of the medial canthus necessarily involve damage to the lacrimal canaliculi or sac which should be simultaneously dealt with. Steps of the repair are stated **(Fig. 5)**:

- The repair should be ideally operated under a microscope
- The cut medial end of the canaliculus is identified preferably by intubating the upper canaliculus and injecting air while keeping thumb pressure over sac

- Bubbles coming out through the saline lake created at the medial canthus help identifying the medial end of the canaliculus. Dyes are avoided for increased risk of tissue damage and to avoid confusion.
- The Worst pigtail probe passed through the upper punctum , upper canaliculus and manipulated into the sac end of lower canaliculus gives good results in identification of the medial cut end of the lower canaliculus.
- A silicon thread/stent (of an intravenous jelco) is next passed from lower punctum and lateral cut end of canaliculus through the sac and then upper canaliculus to emerge at the upper punctum
  - This way the two cut ends of the canaliculi are held together for end to end anastomosis using 9-0 nylon
  - Another way to hold the ends together is to pass a stent through the lower punctum, lateral cut part of canaliculus and engage into the already identified medial cut end of canaliculus and retained there.
  - After end to end anastomosis of the canaliculus, sutured are applied to juxtacanalicular tissue.
  - Lid repair is done in layers.
  - Stent is allowed to remain in place for 12-14weeks. Check for epiphora in subsequent visits.
  - In rest of the eyelid margin injury, primary union of lid laceration is possible if one-fourth or less of the lid margin is lost.

Causes of canalicular injury involve traumatic damage or surgical excision of tumors.

Postoperative care:
Application of antibiotic ointment over surgical site 3–4 times daily, oral analgesics, oral antibiotics. Removal of stent after 3 months of surgery.

Potential complications:
- Canalicular stenosis at laceration site
- Punctal erosion and canalicular slitting
- Injury to opposite canaliculus

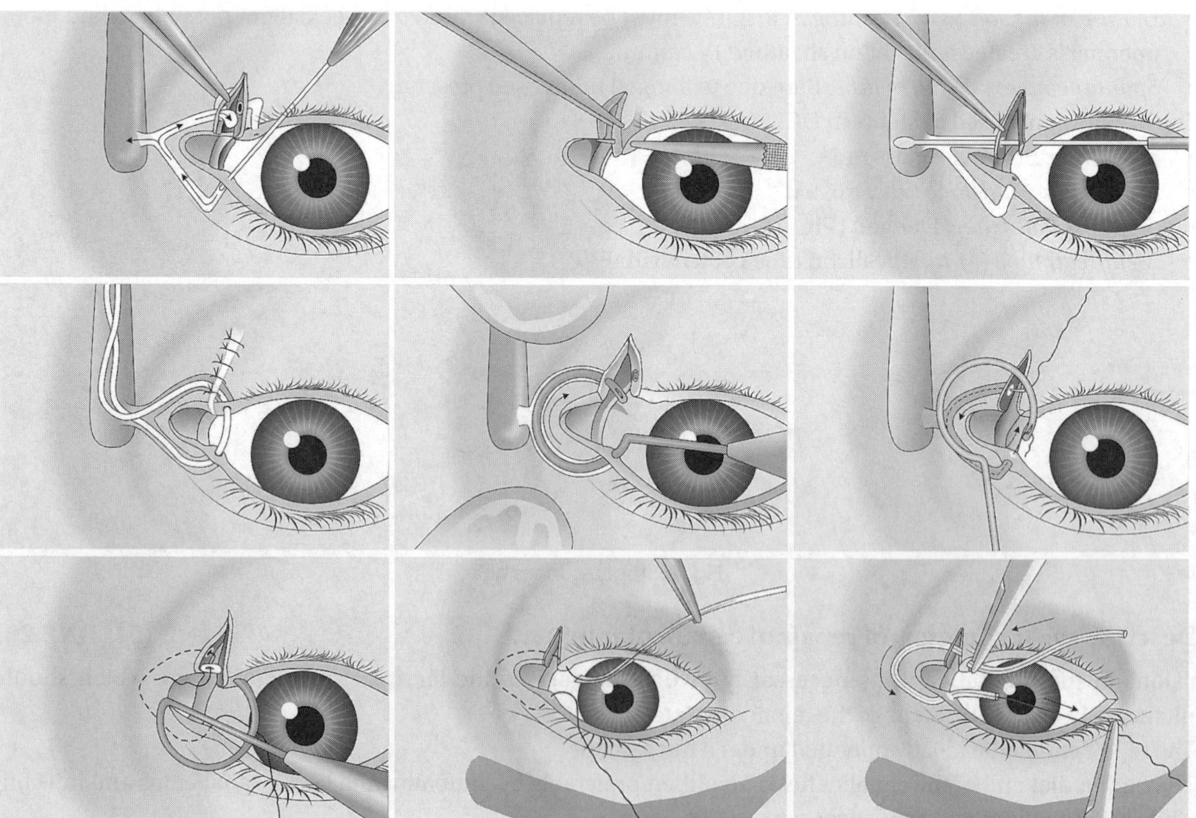

Contd...

Contd...

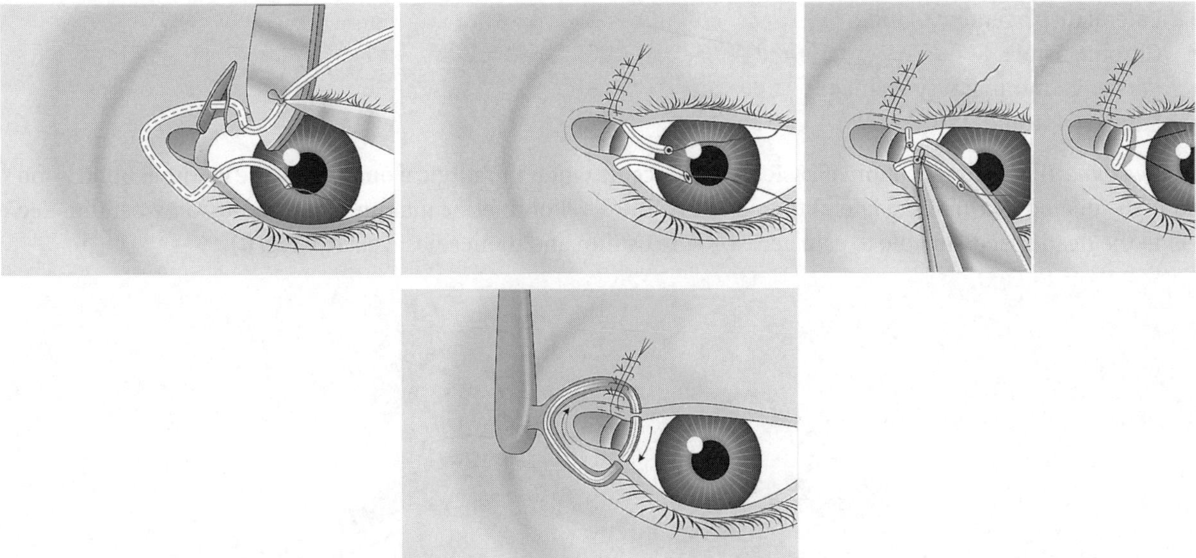

Fig. 5: Repair of canalicular injury.

Source: Modified from-Dutton J, Waldrop TG. Ch. 74. Atlas of Oculoplastic and Orbital surgery, 1st edition. pp. 225, 227.

6. What are the contraindications of DCR. What are causes of failed DCR and what steps can be taken to prevent it. What is Sump syndrome. How can it be prevented (10) (DNB 2020)

Dacryocystorhinostomy is the surgical procedure for treatment of chronic dacroscystitis in elderly as well as young population.

Contraindications of DCR:

- External DCR:
  - TB of lacrimal sac
  - Malignancy of lacrimal sac
  - Immunocompromised individuals, uncontrolled diabetes
  - Atrophic rhinitis
  - Presence of canalicular/common canalicular block
- Endonasal DCR:
  - History of midfacial trauma
  - Lacrimal sac neoplasm
  - *Septal anomalies:* Large middle turbinate/nasal polyp/tight nostrils
  - Granular inflamed nasal mucosa

Causes of failed DCR:

- *Functional failure:* Persistent epiphora after DCR surgery with absence of anomaly/pathology in eyelids and ocular surface despite anatomical patency of lacrimal drainage system; occurs due to:
  - Canalicular obstruction
  - Small lacrimal sac (in primary Nasolacrimal duct obstruction mostly): disturbs transmission of hydrostatic pressure
  - Thick maxilla
  - Anteriorization of ethmoid sinus
  - Absence of mucous dacryocystitis
- *Pathological failure:* Postoperative complications
  - Delayed wound healing, bleeding, granuloma, infection

- Rhinostomy fibrosis
- Lateral displacement of tube
- Chronic fistula
- Persistent intranasal synechiae
- Sump syndrome

Sump syndrome: It is a complication of DCR surgery, occurs when the surgical opening in the lacrimal bone is too small or too high- dilated lacrimal sac lateral to and below the level of inferior margin of the rhinostomy ostium- secretion collect in the dead space - unable to gain access to the ostium and thence nasal cavity **(Fig. 6)**.

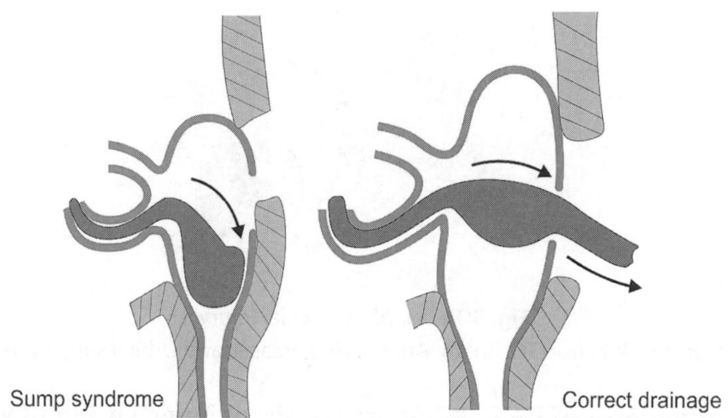

Fig. 6: Sump syndrome.

Prevention of sump syndrome:
- Make large mucosal flap of sac and larger rhinostomy ostium
- Nasal mucosal flap should be slightly lower vertically than lacrimal sac flap- facilitate easy passage of hydrostatic flow
- Avoiding overriding of flaps of both sides (lacrimal sac and nasal mucosa)—only close proximation to maintain patency of passage

Steps for prevention of failed DCR:
- *Nasal bleeding:* Can be controlled by adequate pressure or packing by cellulose hemostatic agent intraoperatively and post-operatively. Head elevation for 20 minutes and nasal packing can suffice well.
- Persistent epiphore managed by leaving the silicon tube in canalicular system for longer (~3 months), which helps dilate the canaliculi and maintain drainage.
- Wound infections though rare can be dealt with preoperative as well postoperative antibiotics coverage, warm compresses, maintaining local hygiene.
- Recurrent obstruction of surgical fistula/ostium may be cleared with radiosurgery cutting tip to clear any membranes, or by pushing small muscle hooks through it. Silicon tubes if need to be removed before stipulated time, are replaced to maintain patency.
- Persistent intranasal synechiae can be prevented with Oxymetazoline nasal anticongestants, avoiding nose blowing postoperatively; in extreme cases endoscopically release may be needed.
- In cases of small, fibrotic sac or ducts, with partial NLD obstructions Balloon dacryoplasty is indicated.
- To prevent false passage and fistula, repeated syringing and probing postoperatively is avoided.
- Preoperative evaluation of nasal pathologies like nasal polyps, deviated nasal septum, thickened/inflamed sinus and its walls to estimate chances of surgical failure, and better decision on choice of surgery

7. Balloon dacryoplasty—Short note (5) (DNB 2019)

Balloon catheter dilatation is a commonly recommended minimally invasive modality of surgery in Congenital Nasolacrimal duct obstruction **(Fig. 7)**.

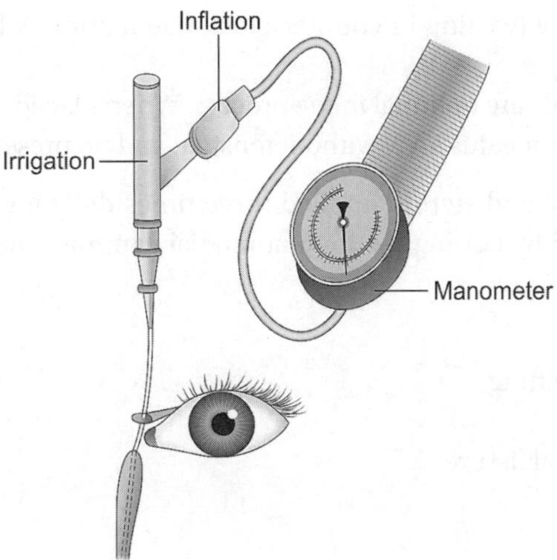

Fig. 7: Punctal dilatation.

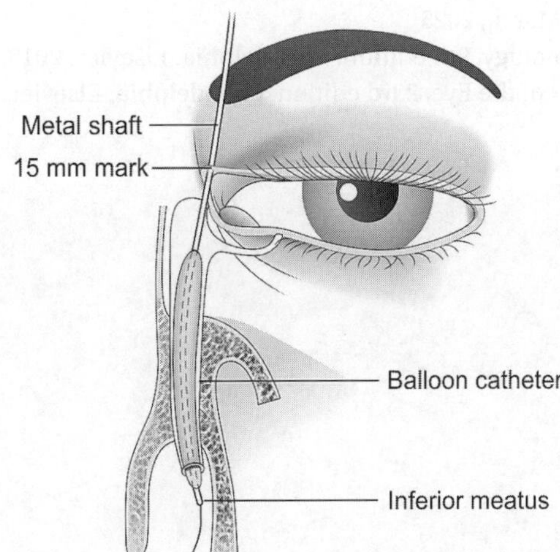

Fig. 8: The metal shaft of catheter going inside the upper punctum through superior canaliculus, the balloon catheter lying inside the lacrimal sac and nasolacrimal duct.

Indications:
- Congenital nasolacrimal duct obstruction, with failed probing and irrigation
- Partial NLD obstruction with fibrotic narrowing/restenosis of lacrimal duct/sac, specially following silicon tube implants

Surgical steps: Performed under general anesthesia **(Fig. 8)**.
Following punctal dilatation and probing with
- Bowman's probe, The deflated balloon catheter
(LacriCath pump and catheter) is passed through inferior canaliculi to the lacrimal sac—then vertically into the lacrimal duct. Size 3 mm is indicated for children 2 years or older; 2 mm for younger group.
- Advancement of catheter down the duct till the highest black mark is at the punctum (15 mm mark). This positions the balloon at the Valve of Hasner.
- The water pressure (manometer) is pushed up to 8 atm, maintained for 90 sec then balloon is deflated. Again balloon is reinflated for 60 sec.
- The balloon is now deflated and the catheter is retracted 5 mm, till 10 mm mark such that second highest black mark is at the punctum—this repositions the balloon at the lacrimal sac and upper duct. The step of inflation with water to 8atm pressure, maintaining for 90 sec then deflating. Repeating the process for another 60 sec is done.

- The catheter is gently removed by twisting in counter-clockwise manner while retracting and outflow system is irrigated with BSS.
- Placing the silicon intubation stents are optional in the process. When placed, silicon button is introduced such that the knotted loop is placed at lower meatus level without tension, and no pressure is exerted at puncta.

Postoperative care: Topical antibiotic and steroid applied three times daily for a week into the eye. After 3 months postoperatively, the tube is removed by cutting the loop at medial canthus, and pulling the tubing out of nose with Bayonet forceps.

Complications

- Punctal erosion and canalicular slitting
- Corneal abrasion and discomfort
- Dislocation of tubing into palpebral fissure

SUGGESTED READING

1. AAO 2023-2024 BCSC section 7 part 3: Oculofacial Plastic and Orbital surgery. [online] Available from https://www.aao.org/Assets/9b6632e1-2ef2-4d0b-9152-689786ffd9cc/638343096464930000/oculofacial-plastic-surgery-subspecialty-day-2023-syllabus-pdf?inline=1 [Last accessed March, 2025].
2. Salmon JF. Kanski's Clinical Ophthalmology, 9th edition. Philadelphia: Elsevier; 2019. pp. 100-10.
3. Sihota R. Tandon R. Parsons' Diseases of the Eye, 23rd edition. Philadelphia: Elsevier; 2019.

6

CHAPTER

Conjunctiva

Smiti Rani Srivastava, Rituparna Ghosh

QUESTIONS

1. **Write in brief symptoms, signs and management of adenovirus keratoconjunctivitis. (10) (WBUHS MS 2021)**
2. **Enumerate two immunosuppressive agents used in allergic eye diseases. Elaborate their mechanism of action and side effects. (10) (DNB 2020)**
3. **Ophthalmia neonatorum. (10) (WBUHS MS 2019)**
4. **Write briefly surgical treatment of pterygium and advanced strategies to decrease pterygium recurrence. (10) (WBUHS MS 2023)**
5. **Describe the clinical features, evaluation and management of ocular manifestations of Steven Johnson Syndrome. (3+3+4) (DNB 2020)**
6. **Describe vernal keratoconjunctivitis. What is medical and surgical management? (3+4+3) (DNB 2022)**
7. **Clinical features, histopathology and management of ocular surface squamous neoplasia (OSSN). (3+4+3) (WBUHS DO 2019)**
8. **Describe the etiopathogenesis and histopathology of OSSN. Write briefly on the use of antimetabolites in the management of OSSN. (2+3+5) (DNB 2018)**

1. Write in brief symptoms, signs and management of adenovirus keratoconjunctivitis. (10) (WBUHS MS 2021)

- Adenovirus keratoconjunctivitis is known as epidemic keratoconjunctivitis. It is highly contagious disease form of viral conjunctivitis. It can be sporadic or epidemic which is transmitted by contact with respiratory or ocular secretions or by fomites such as contaminated towels. It may occur in epidemics in workplace, schools and swimming pools.
- The serotypes involved are EKC 8, 4, 19, and 37. Serotypes 53 and 54 are found as causative organisms for recent outbreak.

Clinical presentation—they present with three classical syndromes.
- Simple follicular conjunctivitis (multiple serotypes)
- Pharyngoconjunctival fever (Serotype 3, 4,7)
- Epidemic keratoconjunctivitis (Serotypes 8, 9, 37, subgroup D)

Symptoms
- *Systemic:* Fever, malaise, fatigue, headache, UTI, respiratory tract infections and GIT symptoms.
- *Ocular:*
  - Watering
  - Burning sensation
  - Foreign body sensation
  - Photophobia
  - Blurring of vision

Signs (Fig. 1)

- *Systemic:* Tender preauricular lymphadenopathy
- *Eyelid:* Eyelid edema
- *Conjunctiva:*
  - Hyperemia, chemosis, follicular reaction prominent.
  - Papillae may be seen.
  - Membrane or pseudomembrane – can cause scarring after resolution.
  - Pinpoint sub-conjunctival hemorrhage (petechial)
- *Cornea:*
  - Epithelial microcysts nonstaining – early stages
  - Punctate epithelial keratitis – after 1 week.
  - Subepithelial anterior stromal infiltrates – immune response to the virus. It may persists or recur over months or year.
  - Mild anterior uveitis
- *Complication:* Can lead to scaring of conjunctiva, symblepharon formation, dacryocystitis and irregular astigmatism.

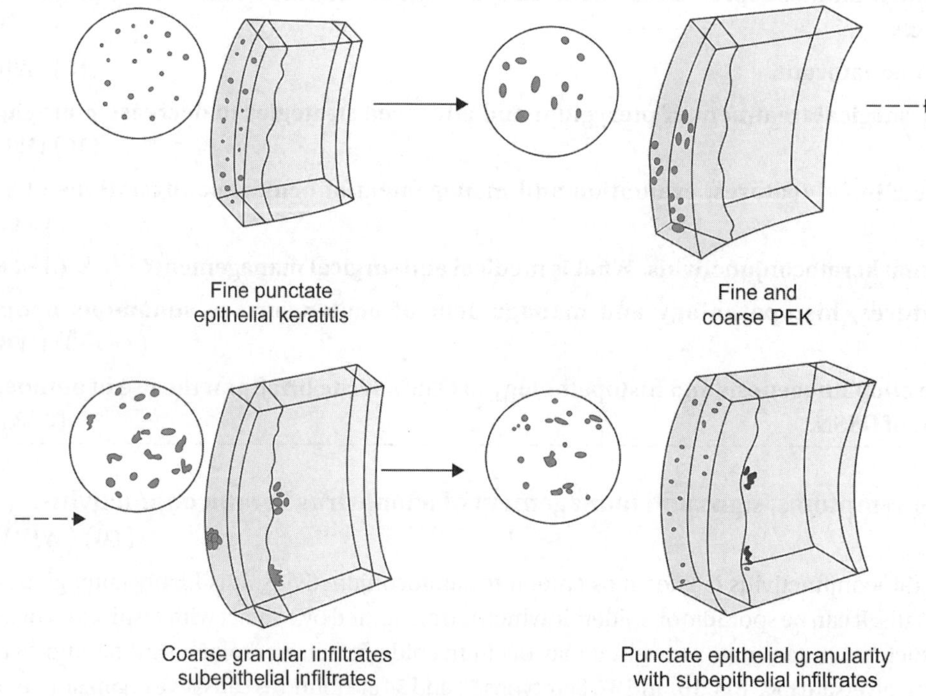

Fig. 1: Schematic diagram showing the progression of epithelial keratoconjunctivitis.

Management

Diagnosis

- Investigations are not required usually. Diagnosis is based on ocular and systemic examination and history. EKC is suspected in patients with bilateral follicular conjunctivitis associated with petechial conjunctival hemorrhage, conjunctival membrane or bilateral subepithelial infiltrates.
- Signs and symptoms of cases are noted. Watery discharge of viral conjunctivitis is a differentiation from bacterial conjunctivitis where the discharge is thick purulent.
- Investigation is required when its nonresolving and when diagnosis is doubtful.
- Giemsa stain shows mononuclear cells in adenoviral conjunctivitis.

Nucleic acid amplification techniques like PCR is sensitive and specific for adenoviral conjunctivitis for detection of viral DNA.

Viral culture with isolation is standard. It has specificity about 100% but sensitivity is variable.

Cell culture and immunoassay can be done.

Polymerase Chain Reaction

RPS adeno detector (Rapid pathogen screening, AD1)—The AdenoPlus is done by collecting tear samples and microfiltration technology. It uses enhanced second-generation device by RPS which is approved by FDA. It had sensitivity 90% and specificity 96%.

Treatment

- Spontaneously recovery occurs usually.
- Cold compression is required to reduce the symptoms.
- Proper hand hygiene maintenance and avoidance of sharing of fomites is very important.
- Artificial tear (preservative free) 4–8 times/day for 1–3 weeks.
- Antihistamine (epinastine 0.05% b.i.d) and vasoconstrictor drops if itching is severe.
- Weaker topical steroid (loteprednol 0.2% b.i.d or 0.5% q.i.d, fluorometholone 0.1% ointment q.i.d) can also be tried with caution with slow taper. Topical corticosteroids prolong the adenoviral shedding, so there use should be reserved for patients with severe symptoms and signs like conjunctival membrane and bilateral subepithelial infiltrates.
- Topical antibiotics are considered if secondary infection is suspected.
- Topical cyclosporine 1% may be used when other therapies fail.
- Anti-viral ganciclovir gel can be prescribed for early resolution. Antiviral like acyclovir, ganciclovir, cidofovir (1 mg/kg/day) 3 times a week, IDU may be helpful.
- Povidone-iodine with topical steroid (Dexamethasone 0.1%) can reduce subepithelial infiltrates.

  As the disease is highly contagious, following precautions are very important, like:
  - NSAIDs drops may be used when steroid weaning circumstances occur.
  - Topical antibiotics can be used to control secondary bacterial infection.
  - In severe cases, topical corticosteroids are prescribed. Its resolute scar and symblepharon formation. Topical steroid (Prednisolone 0.5% q.i.d or dexamethasone 0.1% ointment q.i.d) may be needed for severe form of the disease with acute membrane/pseudo membrane or subepithelial infiltrations.
  - Discontinuation of contact lens is must until resolution occurs.
  - Removal of symptomatic pseudo membrane or membrane by peeling.

  Follow up is must in 2-3 weeks, but frequent follow up is needed if condition worsens significantly.

2. Enumerate two immunosuppressive agents used in allergic eye diseases. Elaborate their mechanism of action and side effects. (10) (DNB 2020)

Ocular allergic diseases are most common disease nowadays, as air pollution, atopy, pollen, genetics, inflammatory agents are main causes.

Allergic conjunctivitis can be sub-classified as:

- Acute,
- Perennial,
- Seasonal.

These are vernal keratoconjunctivitis (VKC), seasonal allergic conjunctivitis (SAC), atopic keratoconjunctivitis (AKC), and perennial allergic conjunctivitis (PAC).

Pathophysiology: Acute, seasonal and perennial forms are IgE or type I mediated hypersensitivity due to contact with allergen which releases inflammatory markers and causes mast cell degranulation. Giant papillary conjunctivitis leads to direct mechanical injury causes type I and IV hypersensitivity reactions.

Immunosuppressive agents are any drug or substance which suppresses immune response. The immunosuppressive are recommended for in cases of refractory allergic conjunctivitis.

Indications of immunosuppressants:

- To control long standing inflammation.
- *Corticosteroid sparing agents:* When corticosteroid related toxicity like glaucoma precipitates during treatment regimen.
- As adjuvant to corticosteroid.

Corticosteroids

Mechanism of action

- It has a dose dependent mechanism of action. Lower doses acts on intracellular receptors and in higher doses it acts on transcellular receptors.
- It inactivates nuclear factor-κB that prevents the transcription of pro-inflammatory factors i.e., IL-1, IL-2, TNF which activates anti-inflammatory mediators like IL-10 and lipocortin – 1.
- This results prevention of vasodilatation, migration and activation of inflammatory cells.
- It also acts as an immunosuppressant by decreasing humoral B-cell immunity and reduces the T-cell activation by inhibition of IL-2.

Side effects

Side effects of topical corticosteroids

- Ocular hypertension
- Secondary glaucoma
- Reactivation of corneal herpetic infections
- Posterior subcapsular cataract
- Central serous chorioretinopathy

Side effects of systemic steroids

- Gastritis
- Fluid retention and hypertension
- Dose dependent increase in blood sugar level
- Steroid induced myopathy
- Cushingoid features and weight gain
- Induced osteoporosis
- Impaired wound healing and susceptible to infection
- Dyslipidemia

Monitoring

- Intraocular pressure monitoring regularly and optic disc assessment are necessary.
- Before prescribing systemic steroids, a baseline bodyweight, blood pressure measurement, glycemic monitoring are required.
- If a maintenance dose is given baseline bone mineral density scan are required.
- For introduction of systemic steroid, infections like tuberculosis, syphilis and viral serology should be checked.
- Oral calcium (500 mg/day) and vitamin D (500-1,000 IU/day) are prescribed along with systemic steroid.

T-cell inhibitors

Mechanism of action:

- These are the calcineurin inhibitors which causes prevention of the T- cell activation by IL-2.
- In the T-cell cytoplasm, the drug binds with immunophilins.
- Cyclosporine bind with cyclophilins, but tacrolimus bind with FK binding protein.
- These complexes inhibit calcineurin activity competitively so the transcription of cytokine genes is prevented.
- IL-2 gene is essential for T-cell activation and proliferation.
- These effects on T-helper, T-suppressor and T cytotoxic cells.
- It causes immunosuppression by blocking T-cell activity.

Side effects of cyclosporine:

- Stinging, burning sensation in the eye
- Pain
- Redness
- Foreign body sensation
- Swollen eyelids

- Blurring of vision
- Tearing of eyes

Systemic side effects of cyclosporine:

- High blood pressure
- Increased hair growth
- Inflamed gums
- Tremors
- Nausea
- Diarrhea
- Headache

3. Ophthalmia neonatorum. (10) (WBUHS MS 2019)

- Ophthalmic neonatorum is also known as neonatal conjunctivitis. It is the conjunctival inflammation in first 28 days of life (neonatal period).
- Incidence - 12% of neonate.
- Mode of infection - vaginal delivery in an infected mother which is transmitted to infant.
- Causative agent - C. trachomatis, N. gonorrhoeae and herpes simplex virus (HSV-2).
  C. trachomatis is the most common organism to cause moderate to severe conjunctivitis.
  Staphylococcus causes mild conjunctivitis.
  Congenital nasolacrimal duct obstruction leads to mild watery eyes with bacterial conjunctivitis.
- *Latent period*
  - Chemical exposure - within the first 24 hours.
  - Gonococcal - first week
  - Staphylococcal and other bacteria - end of first week
  - Herpes simplex virus (HSV) - 1-2 weeks
  - Chlamydia - 1-3 weeks
- *Risk factors*
  - Infected mother's birth canal
  - Maternal HIV infection or other STDs exposure
  - Infant suffering from pneumonia, otitis media or any skin diseases
  - Premature rupture of membranes
  - Ocular trauma while delivery/ postdelivery infection
  - Preterm baby and poor prenatal care
- *Pathophysiology*
  Newborns are prone to have conjunctivitis due to poor development of immune system.
  - Decreased tear production
  - Decreased level of IgA in tear
  - Decreased immune function
  - Absence of lymphoid tissue in conjunctiva

Decreased lysozyme activity

- *Signs*
  - Mild sticky discharge
  - Mucopurulent discharge after pressing near the lacrimal sac region suggestive of NLD blockage.
  - Severe chemosed eyelids
  - Preseptal or orbital cellulitis
  - Periocular vesicles may occur due to HSV infections.
  - In severe cases, corneal ulceration may be there
  - Pseudomembranes are also seen in chlamydial conjunctivitis.
  - Congenital glaucoma can be present.

- *Investigations*
  - Prenatal testing of STI
  - Conjunctival scraping for nucleic acid amplification (PCR) of Chlamydia, HSV.
  - Gram and Giemsa staining of conjunctiva shows multinucleated giant cells in HSV infection.
  - Conjunctival swabs are taken with calcium alginate or sterile cottoned-tip applicator for bacterial culture in chocolate agar or Thayer-Martin medium to detect Chlamydia infection.
  - Papanicolaou smear detects epithelial cells with HSV infection.
- *Treatment*

a. Prophylaxis
   - Povidone iodine 2.5% application in eye causes prevention of conjunctivitis.

b. Chemical conjunctivitis is treated with artificial tears.

c. Mild conjunctivitis - broad spectrum antibiotic such as chloramphenical, erythromycin or fusidic acid ointment can be used for treatment.

d. Moderate - severe conjunctivitis - microscopy with Gram staining detects the organism. Oral erythromycin can treat this condition.

e. Severe conjunctivitis—Topical erythromycin treat the acute condition along with ceftriaxone.

f. Gonococcal infection—Third generation of cephalosporin is effective in these cases. First line of treatment of hospitalization and single dose of oral ceftriaxone 25–50 mg/kg/day with irrigation of eye with sterile isotonic solution.

g. Herpes simplex infection - high dose of oral acyclovir is effective including the severe cases like encephalitis.

Complications: Corneal ulceration /globe perforation

Differential diagnosis:

- Dacryocystocele
- Congenital glaucoma
- NLD obstruction
- Cellulitis
- Keratitis

Prognosis: The severity of disease can be prevented by early intervention.

4. Write briefly surgical treatment of pterygium and advanced strategies to decrease pterygium recurrence. (10) (WBUHS MS 2023)

- Pterygium is wing shaped fibrovascular subepithelial degenerative interpalpebral conjunctival tissue approaching towards limbus onto cornea.
- It is a common ocular surface lesion.
- Ultraviolet rays, hot n dry climate are responsible for its progression.
- Frequently asymptomatic
- Presents with Grittiness, irritation decreased vision due to visual axis obscured or induced astigmatism.
- Sunglasses or goggles advised to avoid ultraviolet ray, dust and wind. Artificial tear drops q.i.d used for lubrication.
- Low potency Topical steroid advised in tapering dose to reduce inflammation.

Indication of surgery:

- Progression of pterygium toward the visual axis.
- Interference of vision by astigmatism.
- Cosmetic purpose.

Surgical treatments are:

- Simple excision (bare sclera) technique (D' Ombrain) is associated with excising the head and body of pterygium which gives bare sclera area to re-epithelize. Recurrence rate is 80%.

- *Conjunctival autograft:* Superotemporal part of bulbar conjunctiva of the same or other eye is suitable for autograft. Autograft is sutured after removal of pterygium. Large graft and good dissection of tenon tissue from conjunctival graft n recipient bed is required to reduce recurrence
  - *Latest technique:* Air assisted dissection, here air is injected with 30 gauge needle into side of the cap of head which makes a plane between pterygium head n cornea.
    - No suture no glue auto blood graft fixation: Here after excision of pterygium a thin film of blood is left over bare area and conjunctival autograft is placed over it.

To avoid recurrence techniques are:

1. *Amniotic membrane grafting:* Has advantage of preservation of bulbar conjunctiva. AM is placed over bare sclera with BM facing up and stroma down. AM minimize fibroblast proliferation, help in epithelial development, suppress TGF-β and prevent recurrence. Fibrin glue can be added for good adherence.
2. Adjunctive therapy:
   - *MMC:* They inhibit fibroblastic proliferation and suppress vascular ingrowth and thereby reduce the recurrence but corneal edema and necrotizing scleritis can occur.
   - Beta irradiation.
   - Anti-VEGEF Ranibizumab in drops or sub conjunctival injection
   - Fluorouracil
3. Double-sliding conjunctival flap procedure.
4. Tissue tuck surgery – uses cryopreserve AMT.
5. P.E.R.F.EC.T – Pterygium extended removal followed by extended conjunctival transplant) Considered as best technique in recurrent cases. Disadvantage is long duration of surgery. It has Best outcome close to zero % recurrence. Surgery consists of removal of conjunctiva , tenon including semilunar fold nasally. Superiorly n inferiorly conjunctiva tenon is removed to the superior n inferior recti leaving bare sclera. Media recti inferior recti were bridled. Superotemporal conjunctival autograft dissected. Dissection of conjunctiva from tenon done by injecting BSS. This autograft is sutured at bare sclera with margin of conjunctiva host n sclera. paracaruncular area is repaired too.

   Ideal graft should be transparent, free from tenon and then transferred to the pterygium site so that it will heal with minimal scarring and recurrences.
6. P.E.R.F.A.M.T. (Pterygium extended removal followed by amniotic membrane transplantation)
7. Limbal stem cell transplantation: The procedure allows the epithelialization of peripheral cornea, limbus and denuded sclera by the corneal epithelium.
8. Primary closure – head and body of the pterygium are excised followed by tenonectomy which is extended beneath the conjunctiva to the adjacent rectus MS. Around the limbus superiorly and inferiorly relaxation incision is given in conjunctiva n closed .
9. Stocker method – it is conjunctival Z plasty for primary closure to prevent recurrence.
10. Rotational conjunctival autografting – CRA , It is mainly attempted to prevent recurrences. Here 90 degree rotation autograft of excised pterygium tissue is done and resutured by 10-0 nylon in its bed.

    Risk of recurrence:
    - Young in age.
    - Africo-American and Hispanic Patients
    - Double pterygia (both nasal and temporal).

    Careful surgery, proper follow up and aggressive topical steroid is very useful to prevent recurrences.

5. Describe the clinical features, evaluation and management of ocular manifestations of Steven Johnson Syndrome. (3+3+4) (DNB 2020)

Steven Johnson Syndrome – is an acute life threatening rare dermatological disorder which involves mucous membranes and epidermis with blisters formation which rapidly spreads and forms bullae and finally causing necrosis and sloughing of epidermal layer.

TEN and SJS are disease of same spectrum. TEN being more life-threatening. SJS is defined when less than 10% of total body surface area is affected. Through ophthalmic examination, early intervention, frequent follow-ups is required to avoid blindness

Presentation (Table 1)

TABLE 1: Severity of eye involvement.

	Severity of eye involvement			
Staining location and treatment recommendations	***Mild***	***Moderate***	***Severe***	***Extremely severe***
Lid margin	No stain	Stain <1/3 of lid margin length	Stain >1/3 of lid margin length on at least 1 lid	Stain >1/3 of lid margin length on more than 1 lid
Cornea	No stain	No stain	Any epithelial defect more than punctate staining	Any epithelial defect wider than punctate staining
Conjunctiva (bulbar and peripheral)	Hyperemia, without stain	(+) Stain, <1 cm in greatest diameter	(+) Stain >1 cm	Multiple areas of stain >1 cm
Treatment recommendation	Medical	Medical and close observation	Medical and urgent ANT	Medical and urgent ANT (may require repeat ANT)

Systemic

- Initial stages comprises of fever, malaise, cough, anorexia and rhinorrhea
- Mucosal – blister and hemorrhagic crusting of lips
- Blisters on tongue, oropharynx nasal mucosa and genitalia also common.
- *Skin:* Tender cutaneous eruptions on face, extremities and trunk which forms macules, papules, atypical target lesions and vesicles or bullae. The denuded area appears like severe burns which tends to get secondary infection.

Ocular

- *Symptoms:*
  Acute stage: More than 50% patients get affected in mild to severe eye disease.
  - Eyelid:
    - Mild lid edema with hemorrhagic crusting of lid margins.
    - Ocular irritation due sloughing of eyelid margin epithelium
  - Conjunctiva:
    - Hyperemia, chemosis n hemorrhagic blisters in bulbar conjunctiva
    - Conjunctival membrane and pseudo membrane formation in palpebral conjunctiva
    - Dry eyes
  - Cornea:
    - Pseudo membrane formation
    - Acute epithelial defect

Chronic stage:

Eyelid:

- Lagophthalmos
- Cicatricial ectropion, trichiasis, metaplastic lashes, ankyloblepharon
- Cicatricial entropion
- Severe meibomian gland disease

Cornea:

- Persistent epithelial defects
- Scarring vascularization and keratinization

- Corneal perforation
- Limbal stem cell deficiency

Conjunctiva

- Keratinization of conjunctiva
- Subconjunctival scarring

Dry eye – due to fibrosis of lacrimal gland ductulus and loss of goblet cells due to conjunctival metaplasia.
Anterior segment – anterior uveitis
Posterior segment – Pan Ophthalmitis

Management

Investigations:

1. Recent history of changes of dosage of drug or introduction of new medications.
2. Skin biopsy of affected areas shows full thickness keratinocyte necrosis with perivascular lymph histiocytic infiltrate.
3. Granulysin can be detected from fluid of bullae.

Systemic treatment:

- Discontinuation of culprit drug or source
- General supportive measures to maintain the hydration, electrolyte balance, protein replacement etc.
- Systemic steroids
- Intravenous immunoglobulin,
- Immunosuppressants like cyclosporine, azathioprine,
- Systemic antibiotic as a prophylaxis against the skin or other systemic infection.

Ocular treatment:

- Mild to moderate cases pseudomembrane debridement with cotton tipped applicator and daily saline flush.
  - Scleral ring with large haptic lens with central zone removed prevent symblepharon formation
  - Lysis of symblepharon with sterile glass rod.
  - Topical moxifloxacin 4 times
  - Topical steroid 6 times
  - Ciclosporin 4 times
  - Preservative free artificial tears
  - Soft CL/ scleral CL
- Severe cases with eye lid involvement with or without involvement bulbar conjunctiva:
  - Medical management
  - Amniotic membrane should be applied with glue or sutured covering superior and inferior fornixes and to be repeated if needed

Chronic disease:

- *DED ocular xerosis:* All the three components of tear film aqueous, mucin and lipid are involved. Topical cyclosporine improves goblet cell density. Frequent dose of preservative free artificial tears helps to replenish aqueous deficient DED. Punctal occlusion with cautery or plugs can improve the dry eye.
- Abnormalities of eyelid and lashes like ectropion entropion, trichiasis distichiasis can be treated surgically.
- Tarsorrhaphy is used to treat lagophthalmos.
- Mucous membrane grafting or scleral lenses like PROSE lenses are used in posterior eyelid margin scarring.
- conjunctival disease and corneal complication should be addressed after inflammation subsides i.e., 3 to 6 months post SJS
- Posterior eyelid margin keratinization causes corneal disease due to repetitive mechanical microtrauma inducing corneal epithelial defect, infection, perforation and stromal melting. Transretinoic acid ointment, scleral CL like PROSE therapy and MMG is the treatment. PROSE is prosthetic replacement of the ocular surface ecosystem.

- Eyes with limbal stem cell deficiency can be benefitted with SLET therapy.
- In end stage, ocular Steven Johnson Syndrome – keratoprosthesis is the mainstay.

6. Describe vernal keratoconjunctivitis. What is medical and surgical management? (3+4+3) (DNB 2022)

Vernal keratoconjunctivitis (VKC) or Spring catarrh is a sub classification of allergic conjunctivitis, which presents as recurrent bilateral asymmetric IgE and cell mediated hypersensitivity commonly found in boys.

It consists of papillary, limbal and mixed type.

Characteristics

- The most common symptom is itching.
- Males are affected than females. (2:1) ratio
- Children to young adults are mostly prone for this disease.
- The signs and symptoms are mostly seen in warm, dry climate with a peak incidence during late spring and summer.
- But chronic cases are found throughout the year.
- Family history of atopy should be excluded which includes allergic rhinitis, asthma and eczema.
- Frequently it becomes perennial form and recurrent in spring time.

Etiology

- It is due to IgE mediated reaction via mast cell reaction.
- Activated eosinophils are also responsible for inflammation.
- Type 4 hypersensitivity mediated CD4 T helper cells with immunomodulators i.e., IL-4, IL-5, FGF can cause VKV symptoms and can be perennial.

Pathophysiology

- Hyperplasia of conjunctival epithelium in upper tarsal conjunctiva presents as multiple papillae.
- Hyperplastic tissues projected downwards into subepithelial tissue.
- The adenoid layer consists inflammatory cells like eosinophils, plasma cells, lymphocytes and histiocytes.
- Fibroblast cells proliferate and cause hyaline changes resulting giant papillae.

Symptoms

- Intense itching,
- Lacrimation
- Foreign body sensation
- Photophobia
- Thick mucoid discharge
- Blepharospasm
- Blurring of vision.

Signs

- Ecchymosis of eyelids due to rubbing of eyelids,
- Conjunctival congestion
- Copious, ropy, mucoid discharge
- Giant papillae in upper tarsal conjunctiva
- Limbal swelling with Horner-Trantas spots which are degenerated epithelial cells and eosinophils.
- If cornea involves shield ulcer in severe cases as plaques containing fibrin and mucus accumulates in microerosions areas.
- It may be associated with keratoconus.

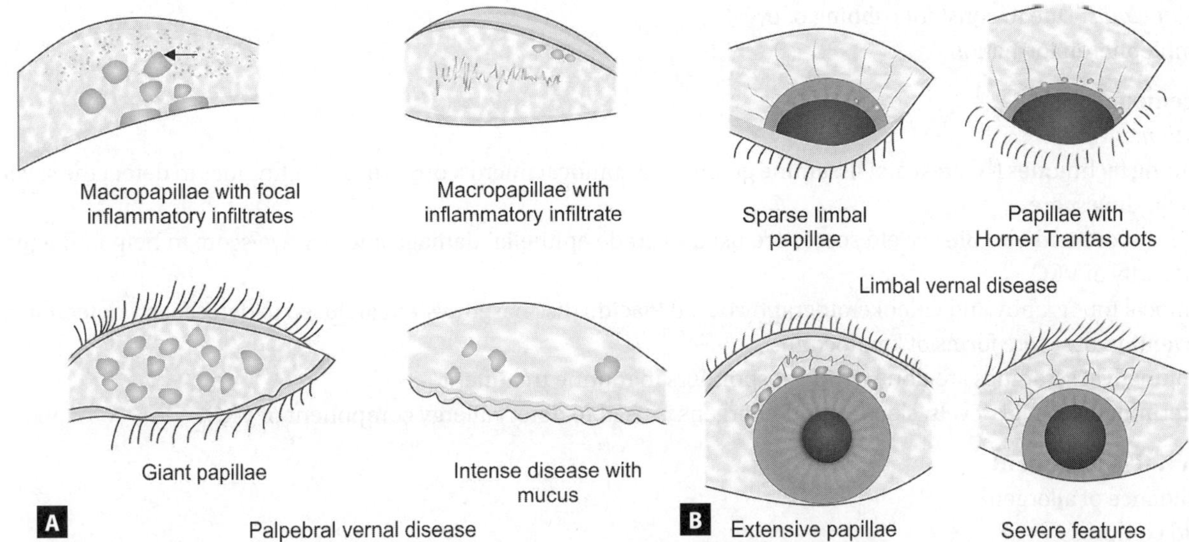

Figs. 2A and B: Different forms of vernal keratoconjunctivitis—palpebral vernal disease, limbal vernal disease, extensive papillae, and severe features.

Types (Figs. 2A and B)

1. *Palpebral type:*
   - It involves upper tarsal conjunctiva which causes hyperemic conjunctiva, diffuse papillary hypertrophy giving cobblestones appearance.
   - Macropapillae (<1 mm) have a flat-topped polygonal shaped.
   - Focal or diffuse inflammatory infiltrates is seen in severe cases.
   - In severe cases giant papillae (>1 mm in diameter in flattened tops) i.e., cobblestones forms as smaller lesions conjoins in upper tarsal plate.
   - Mucus deposition occurs in between of lesions.
   - Superficial punctate erosions, plaques, subepithelial scars are also seen in associated keratopathy in severe form.
   - Pseudogerontoxon is a sign of chronicity, is characterized by a paralimbal band of superficial scarring present in inflamed limbus.
2. *Limbal type:*
   - It can be associated with palpebral form of VKC or solely.
   - Due to aggregation of eosinophils and degenerated epithelial cells over limbal area got thickened, gelatinous white spots are known as Horner Trantas spots.
   - Triangular congestion of bulbar conjunctiva in palpebral area is noted.
   - Limbal disease is severe in topical areas.
3. *Mixed type:*
   - It is a combination of palpebral and bulbar forms.

Complications

- Conjunctival fibrosis
- Limbal stem cell deficiency
- Pannus formation
- Corneal neovascularization
- Macro-erosion of epithelium
- Shield ulcers
- Corneal scar formation
- *Pseudoxerontoxon:* A waxing and waning gray white lipid deposition in periphery and superficial stroma can occur.

- *Keratoconus:* Due to constant rubbing of eyes.
- Symblepheron formation

Management

Evaluation:

- Staining techniques (fluorescein, lissamine green) and confocal microscopy are few techniques to detect the severity and grading score.
- Oxford score and Van Bijsterveld scores are used to grade epithelial damage and dry eye score to help in diagnosis of severity of VKC.
- Confocal topography and videokeratography based Placido disc based system are used to detect early detection and prevention of severe forms of keratoconus.
- Conjunctival scrapings are done in non-responders in routine treatment.
- Determination of IgE levels, skin tests for allergens is used to detect allergy component of VKC.

Conservative treatment

- Avoidance of allergen
- Cold compress
- To prevent excessive glare and photophobia dark goggles are used.

Medical management

A. *Local treatment*
   - Mast cell stabilizer (sodium cromoglycate, nedocromil sodium 2% b.i.d, iodoxamide. 1% q.i.d) are useful to reduce the moderate forms of VKC and is required for long-term treatment to reduce inflammatory cells.
   - Antihistamines (emedastine, epinastine, levocabastine, bepotastine 1.5%) are used for acute attack.
   - Combined preparations of antihistamine and vasoconstrictor (antazoline with xylometazoline) are also used.
   - Dual action antihistamine and mast cell stabilizers (azelastine 0.05%, ketotifen 0.025%, olopatadine 0.1% b.i.d) are necessary to reduce the symptoms speedily.
   - Topical steroid (fluorometholone 0.1%, prednisolone 0.5%, rimexolone 1%, loteprednol 0.2% or 0.5%) are usually used for short period with tapering for severe acute exacerbations.
   - Stronger steroid like prednisolone 1%, dexamethasone 0.1% ointment can also be used in severe cases, but risk of steroid induced glaucoma has to be concerned.
   - Supratarsal steroid injection (0.5–1 mL) like dexamethasone (4 mg/mL) or triamcinolone (40 mg/mL) can also be introduced for severe palpebral type.
   - *Immune modulators:* Cyclosporine (*Dosage:* 0.05% to 2% b.i.d to q.i.d topically) indicated in allergic eye disease as a steroid sparing agent, if steroids are contraindicated, ineffective or not tolerated. It is a calcineurin inhibitor which selectively inhibits T lymphocyte proliferation. It decreases inflammatory cytokines as it blocks lymphocyte proliferation.
   - Tacrolimus (0.1%) is most commonly used in these cases. It can be used in severe allergic conjunctivitis and in refractory cases. It also decreases inflammation by selectively inhibiting T lymphocyte proliferation. It also reduces conjunctival fibroblast and interleukin 1b production. Used as an alternative to cyclosporine in non-responded cases.
   - Peeling and or wiping of corneal plaque followed by topical steroid and antibiotic drops is the standard treatment for nonhealing shield ulcers. Amniotic membranes graft is used in severe cases.

B. *Systemic treatment*:
   - Oral antihistamines and antileukotrines are used to improve the severity of VKC.
   - Antibiotics (doxycycline 50–100 mg daily for 6 weeks or azithromycin 500 mg daily for 3 days) to control VKC associated blepharitis.
   - Intranasal corticosteroids are advised on ocular symptoms of allergic rhinoconjunctivitis.
   - Systemic treatment with T-lymphocyte signal transduction inhibitors like cyclosporin or tacrolimus may improve severe and refractory cases.
   - Omalizumab is an anti-IgE recombinant, humanized, non-anaphylactic antibody, directed against the receptor binding domain of IgE may be administered in VKC patients, who are having high levels of IgE.

- Aspirin (0.5–1g/day) may be also useful in steroid sparing agent in VKC, but it should be avoided in children for the risk of Reye's syndrome.
- Allergic specific immunotherapy (SIT) is effective to improve IgE associated VKC.

Surgical management:

- Bandage contact lens for the relief in case of persistent epithelial defects.
- Superficial keratectomy to remove plaque and to promote re-epithelialization.
- Surface restoration surgery like amniotic membrane grafting with keratectomy is done in deep ulcers.
- Limbal stem cell transplantation is advised in severe and persistent limbal implantation.
- Oral mucosal grafting is done as invasive procedure **(Fig. 3)**.

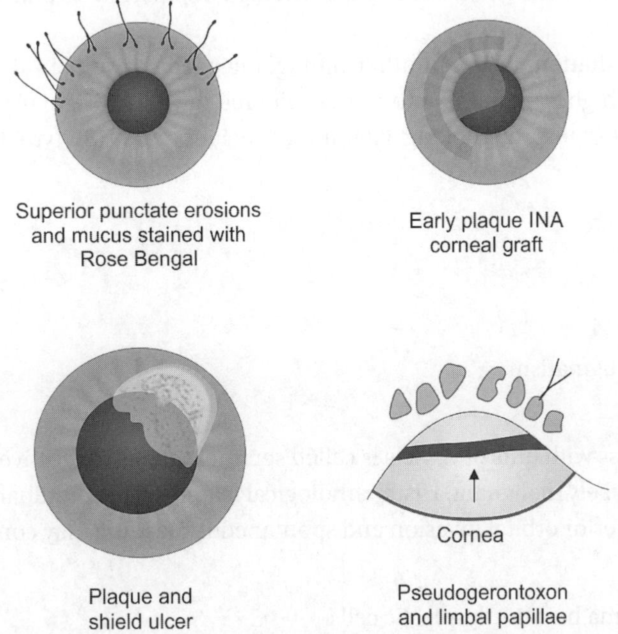

Fig. 3: Keratopathy in vernal disease, A-superior punctate erosions and mucus stained with Rose Bengal.

7. Clinical features, histopathology and management of ocular surface squamous neoplasia (OSSN). (3+4+3) (WBUHS DO 2019)

8. Describe the etiopathogenesis and histopathology of OSSN. Write briefly on the use of antimetabolites in the management of OSSN. (2+3+5) (DNB 2018)

Ocular surface squamous neoplasia or OSSN is a precancerous or cancerous lesion of conjunctival, cornea and limbal epithelium. It can present as squamous dysplasia, corneal intraepithelial neoplasia (CIN) and squamous cell carcinoma (SCC). Based on the ability of invasion in conjunctiva, it may be subdivided into mild, moderate, severe **(Table 2)**.

TABLE 2: Lee and Hirst Classification of OSSN.

Benign OSSN	• Papilloma • Pseudotheliomatous hyperplasia
Preinvasive OSSN	• Conjunctival /corneal carcinoma in situ
Invasive OSSN	• Squamous carcinoma • Mucoepidermoid carcinoma

Incidence—0.02-3.5/100000 in population.

- Male preponderance (older)
- Dark skinned
- Age (20-88 years); average age - 60 years
- Xeroderma pigmentosa and HIV infections are associated with early age.

Etiopathogenesis

1. UV-B light - role of sunlight and UV-B light exposure damages DNA repair mechanism. It also causes p53 gene mutation. Defective DNA repair mechanism also responsible for OSSN in xeroderma pigmentosa. Fair skinned with light colored iris are more prone.
2. Human papilloma virus (HPV): Genotypes 6, 8, 11 causes benign lesion. HPV 16 and 18 can also cause the malignant lesion.
3. Stem cell theory: UV-B irradiation HPV and other mutagenic agents results in dysfunctional limbal stem cells. Concentration of stem cells highest in nasal limbus is considered the likely origin of OSSN.
4. Other causes: HIV, chemical exposure, smoking, vitamin A deficiency and HSV type 1 virus.

Clinical features

Symptoms:

- Foreign body sensation
- Irritation
- Redness
- Diminished vision due to astigmatism.

Signs:

- Elevated pearly-grey mass with tufts of vessels is called sentinel vessels suggestive of malignancy.
- Larger lesions are most likely malignant. Histopathological features like epibulbar vasculature, corneo-scleral or intraocular invasion, anterior orbital invasion and spontaneous bleeding may confirm malignancy.

CIN has three clinical variants:

1. Papilliform - Sessile papilloma harbors dysplastic cells.
2. Gelatinous - It is a combination of Acanthosis and dysplasia.
3. Leukoplakic - Due to hyperkeratosis, parakeratosis and dyskeratosis this type of lesion occurs.

Invasive OSSN:

- Plaques like, gelatinous or papilliform growth appears in limbal and bulbar conjunctiva, most commonly appears in interpalpebral fissure zone. Broad base is often present in limbal area and spreads over cornea and conjunctiva. It has sharp borders and grows outward may be diagnosed as leukoplakia.
- It usually presents over epithelial basement membrane causes superficial lesions and neoplastic cells penetrate sclera along with engorged conjunctival vessels causes malignancy.

Histopathology:

- Preinvasive OSSN is classified as mild moderate and severe depending upon extent of dysplasia in epithelium.
- *Mild:* CIN grade 1—dysplasia in lower third of epithelium.
- *Moderate:* CIN grade 2—dysplasia in middle third of epithelium.
- *Severe:* CIN grade 3—also called carcinoma in situ—has full thickness epithelial involvement with intact basement membrane.
- Invasive carcinoma is when basement membrane is breached and cells infiltrate into stroma.
- Mucoepidermoid carcinoma is an aggressive variant of SCC.
- Dysplastic squamous cells and malignant goblet cells with mucin staining is a classical feature.

Management of OSSN

- *Investigations:*
  1. History taking - Frequent episodes of redness, degrees of ocular irritation secondary to inflammation can be noted in these patients.
  2. AS-OCT - Hyper reflective thickened epithelium and abrupt transition from normal to abnormal tissue are noted in ultra-high resolution OCT. It makes a differentiation between pterygium and abnormal conjunctival tissue.
  3. Impression cytology - It is a noninvasive method to detect and monitor OSSN. A cytobrush is used to collect the exfoliated cells from the conjunctival surface. Malignant cells have poor cell detachment and desquamate from mucosal surface. This cell to cell relationship is maintained by using cellulose acetate paper. Biopore membrane is the procedure of choice now a day. Keratinization is the key to monitor these patients.
  4. UBM - If malignancy suspicion is noted like scleral or corneal surface invasion, then UBM is a choice.
  5. Confocal microscopy - It is a simple and non-invasive diagnostic tool is used to identify recurrence and the after effect of chemotherapeutic agents.

Treatment

- *Medical:*
  Topical chemotherapeutic agents:
  - IFN-α2b - It is a cytokine which have antiproliferative, cytotoxic, antiviral and antigenic properties. A subconjunctival injection 3 million IU/0.5 mL at dosage is administered weekly till resolution occurs. Topical eye drop 1 million IU/mL is advised as four times for 1–2 months after resolution which may take around four months on average. The efficacy rate after topical is around 80–100%.
  - 5-FU - It acts as a pyrimidine analog which blocks DNA synthesis by incorporating with RNA. One to five cycles are given to patient where one month on treatment and three months are weaning period. The recurrence rate is 20%. The efficacy rate is 100%. The disadvantage of 5-FU are mild ocular irritation and conjunctivitis like appearance.
  - MMC - An antimetabolite which alkylates DNA and causes disruption of RNA production. The lower concentration medication can be applied for a month but higher concentration medication can be applied for one week followed by 2–3 weeks off. Ocular pain, limbal stem cell loss, punctal stenosis can be disadvantages. The efficacy is around 80-100%.
- *Surgical:*

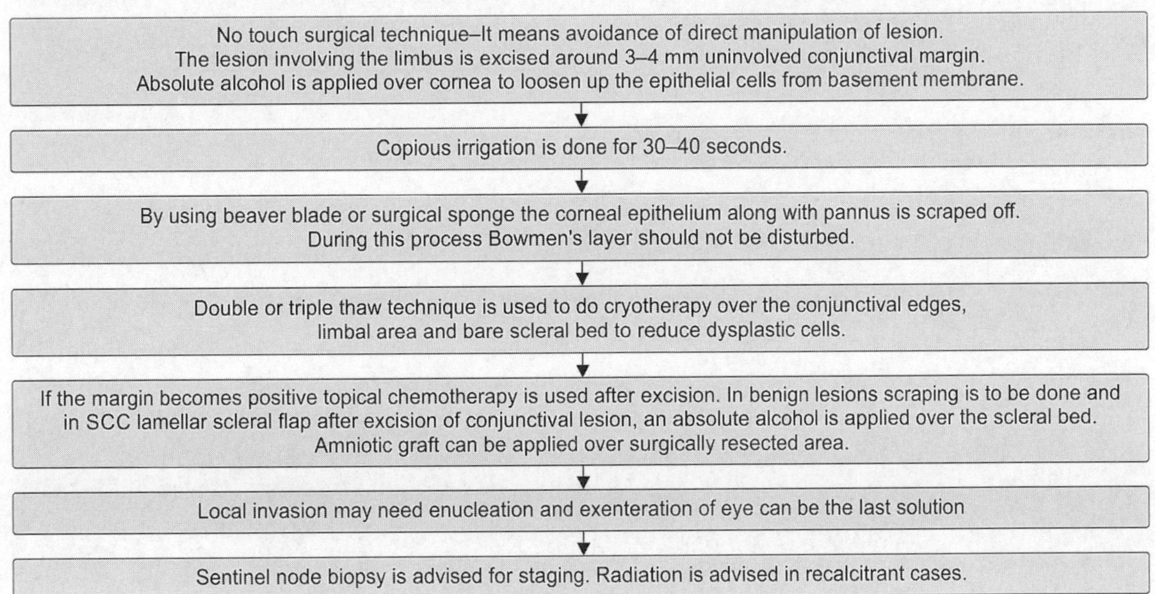

SUGGESTED READING

1. AAO 2020-2021 BCSC SECTION 8: External Diseases and Cornea. [online] Available from https://www.berri.es/libreria_medica/EXTERNAL-DISEASE-AND-CORNEA-(Basic-and-Clinical-Science-Course-2021-2022)/AAO%208%20Weisenthal/9781681044460/357349/cod=357349#:~:text=Section%208%20discusses%20the%20structure%20and%20function%20of,transplants%20from%20the%20eye%20bank%20Association%20of%20America [Last accessed March, 2025].
2. AAO. Eyewiki. [online] Available from https://eyewiki.org/Main_Page [Last accessed March, 2025].
3. Gerstenblith AT, Robinowitz MP. The Wills eye manual, 6th edition. Philadelphia: Lippincott Williams & Wilkins; 2012. p. 110.
4. Salmon JF. Chapter 6: Conjunctiva. In: Salmon JF (Ed). Kanski's Clinical Ophthalmology, 9th edition. Philadelphia: Elsevier; 2019.

7

CHAPTER

Dry Eye

Smiti Rani Srivastava, Rituparna Ghosh, Puja Chowdhury

QUESTIONS

1. **Describe the neural pathway for tear secretion by lacrimal gland. What are the tests for evaluating tear film. Describe etiopathogenesis of Sjogren's syndrome. (3+3+4) (WBUHS MS 2018, DNB)**
2. **Tests for evaluating tear film—short note. (5) (WBUHS MS 2016, DO 2015)**
3. **Define dry eyes as per DEWS 2 report. Role of anti-inflammatory in management of dry eye. (2+3) (DNB 2019)**
4. **Discuss the etiopathogenesis and management of dry eye. (10) WBUHS MS 2023**

1. Describe the neural pathway for tear secretion by lacrimal gland. What are the tests for evaluating tear film. Describe etiopathogenesis of Sjogren's syndrome. (3+3+4) (WBUHS MS 2018, DNB)

Lacrimal gland is a branched tubule-alveolar gland (serous acinus) with serous secretions called tears.

The main lacrimal gland is situated in the fossa for lacrimal gland, formed by the orbital plate of frontal bone, in the anterolateral part of roof of orbit.

Tears are continuously secreted throughout the day by main lacrimal gland (reflex) secretions and accessory lacrimal gland (basal) secretions.

- Reflex secretion occurs in response to sensations from the cornea and conjunctiva, probably produced by evaporation and breakup of tear film.
- Afferent pathway of this secretion is formed by the fifth cranial nerve and efferent by parasympathetic (secretomotor) supply of lacrimal gland.
- Normal rate of tear production is about 1.2 microlitres/min, tear volume in eye at any time is 7 microliters, turnover rate being 7 minutes.

The accessory lacrimal glands include:

- Glands of Krause
- Glands of Wolfring
- Intraorbital glands
- Glands of caruncle and plica semilunaris

Nerve supply of the main lacrimal gland: **(Fig. 1)**

1. *Sensory nerve supply:* Lacrimal nerve, a branch of ophthalmic division of the fifth cranial nerve
2. *Sympathetic nerve supply:* Arises from the superior cervical ganglion as postganglionic fibers which from the carotid plexus of the cervical sympathetics.

   From the sympathetic plexus around the internal carotid artery, some fibers join the deep petrosal nerve, then the nerve of pterygoid gland, then ultimately reach the lacrimal gland through the lacrimal nerve branch of V1.
3. *Secretomotor fibers:* Derived from superior salivary nucleus.

The lacrimatory nucleus receives afferent fibers from the hypothalamus for emotional response and from the sensory nuclei of trigeminal nerve for reflex lacrimation secondary to irritation of cornea and conjunctiva.

Preganglionic parasympathetic fibers from lacrimatory nucleus(pons)—Nervus intermedius (sensory root of facial nerves)- Geniculate ganglion of facial nerve—Greater superficial petrosal nerve + Deep petrosal nerve (sympathetic)- Nerve of pterygoid canal (Vidian nerve)—Sphenopalatine ganglion (preganglionic parasympathetic fibers relay here)- Zygomatic nerve (post ganglionic fibers)

- Zygomaticofacial branch—Lacrimal nerve-Lacrimal gland

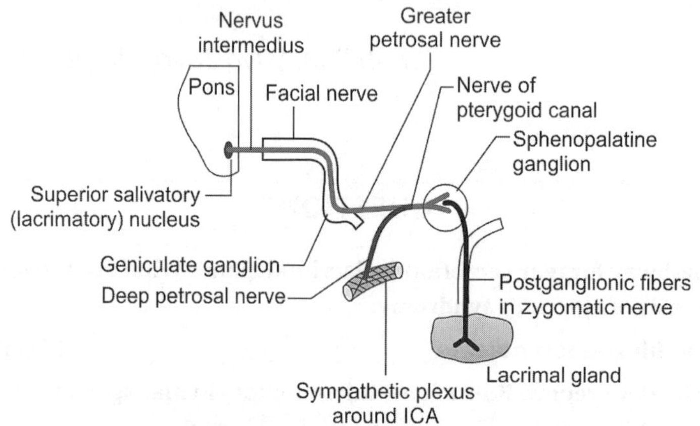

Fig. 1: Pathway from brain to lacrimal gland.

2. Tests for evaluating tear film—short note. (5) (WBUHS MS 2016, DO 2015)

Tear film adequacy can be assessed by the following tests **(Fig. 2)**

1. *Schirmer test:* Test for tear quantity by checking extent of wetting of a 5 × 35 mm Whatman filter paper number 41 over 5 minutes, placed in lower fornix at inner two- third and outer one-third junction.
   - Schirmer 1 test gives value of both basal and reflex tearing, using open eye technique.
   - Schirmer 2 test gives value of reflex secretion of tears, after rubbing an anesthetized nasal mucosa with cotton
   - 15 mm is the cut off value; less than that indicates diminished tear production
2. *Tear film breakup time (TBUT):* Interval between a complete blink and the appearance of the first randomly distributed dry spot on cornea, observed after instilling fluorescein drop in fornix and examining in cobalt-blue light of slit lamp.
   - 10 seconds is the cutoff; lesser values indicate mucin deficiency in tear film
3. *Vital staining:* Using dyes to histologically make transparent structures on ocular surface visible
   - *Fluorescein staining:* Water soluble chemical resorcinolphthalein stains areas of denuded corneal surface as the epithelial barrier is broken. Sensitive test for Keratoconjunctivitis sicca used in diagnosis of Sjogren's syndrome.
   - *Rose Bengal staining:* 1% aqueous solution used to stain mucus, debris, devitalized cells useful in diagnosis of KCS. Grading system of 0-3 used, where 3 indicates gross staining. Also counting stained dots on cornea by grading system of 1-5 are quantified system.
   - *Lissamine green staining:* Similar to Rose Bengal stain, dark green water-soluble stains dead degenerated cells and mucus.
4. *Marginal tear strip or tear meniscus:* Height of 0.5 mm on slit lamp examination is considered normal. Lesser value indicates dry eye with tear deficiency.
5. Tear film enzymes:
   - *Lysozyme levels:* Presents 20% of protein contents of tear; decreased levels in dry eye (early indicator).
   - *Tear lactoferrin levels:* Clinical tool in diagnosing dry eye syndrome
6. *Tear pH & osmolarity:* Normal 7.0, shows hypertonicity and alkaline shift in KCS - specific diagnostic test.*Conjunctival biopsy and impression cytology:* Cellulose acetate filter material used in non-invasive technique to diagnose squamous metaplasia/keratinization of epithelial cells. Staging system 0 to 5 used, where 0 is normal cellular structure and 5 indicates advanced keratinization.

Sjogren's etiopathogenesis (4): **(Flowchart 1)**

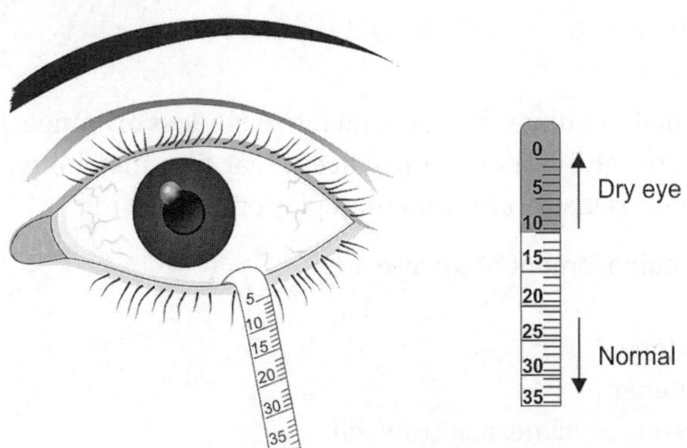

Fig. 2: Schirmer's strip test.

Flowchart 1: Pathogenesis of Sjogren's syndrome.

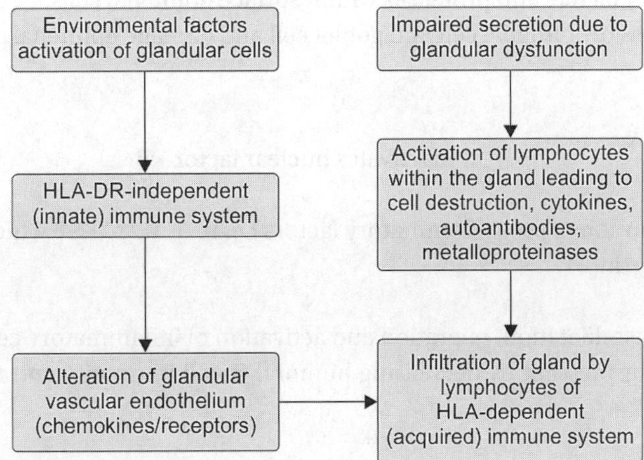

- Sjögren's syndrome (SS) is a chronic autoimmune disease associated with functional disorders of the exocrine glands (e.g., parotid and lacrimal glands) and extraglandular manifestations.
- Sjögren's syndrome (SS) is manifested by keratoconjunctivitis sicca (dry eye), xerostomia (dry mouth) and other extraglandular abnormalities.
  - Primary SS is defined as the presence of the above manifestations without additional connective tissue disease.
  - Secondary SS involves an association with RA, SLE or other connective tissue diseases. Patients with fibromyalgia and chronic fatigue syndrome frequently present with sicca symptoms but may fail to meet strict criteria for the diagnosis of SS.
- SS is primarily a disorder of women, occurring 9-10 times more commonly in women than men. This predominance of SS in women seems to be related to the immunoregulatory properties of the sex hormones. Most women with SS are afflicted in their perimenopausal years. SS is a disorder that may possess important clues to the etiology, pathogenesis and treatment of autoimmunity as well as malignancy.
- In a 2013 review by G Nocturne and X Mariette of the pathogenesis of SS (26), three key steps were identified based on the initial genome-wide association study (GWAS):
  1. Aberrant activation of the innate immune response, especially through the interferon (IFN) and NF-KB pathways
  2. Atypical recruitment to lymphoid follicles mediated by CXCR5
  3. T-cell activation with ascending HLA susceptibility along the IL-12-IFN-γ axis.
- BAFF was considered to be vital in coordinating the innate and adaptive immune responses to the disease. They also highlighted the pathophysiological role of natural killer (NK) and epithelial cells as well as the dysfunction of the neuroendocrine system.
- The development of primary SS is strongly associated with MHC class II genes, most specifically HLA-DR and DQ alleles.
- Importantly, classic clinical features of Sjögren syndrome may also be seen in infections with certain viruses. These include hepatitis C virus, human immunodeficiency virus (HIV), and human T-cell lymphotrophic virus (HTLV). (See DDx.)

  Most patients with primary Sjögren syndrome have two specific antibodies: against Ro (SS-A) and La (SSB) antigens.

3. Define dry eyes as per DEWS 2 report. Role of anti-inflammatory in management of dry eye. (2+3) (DNB 2019)

Definition

Dry eye is a multifactorial disease of the ocular surface characterized by loss of homeostasis of the tear film, accompanied by ocular symptoms like discomfort and visual disturbances. Tear film instability, hyperosmolarity, ocular surface inflammation and damage, and neurosensory abnormalities play etiological role

Anti-inflammatory drugs used in management of dry eye are:

1. Corticosteroids
2. Nonsteroidal immunomodulators
3. NSAIDs—e.g., ketorolac, nepafenac
4. Antibiotics—e.g., doxycycline, minocycline, azithromycin

Role of anti-inflammatory drugs in management of dry eye – **Table 1**.

- Tear osmolarity is an important factor to cause dry eye. Tear hyperosmolarity aggravates the cascade signaling events which releases inflammatory factors and proteases within surface epithelial cells.
- Inflammatory cells cause loss of epithelial cell and goblet cell and damage epithelial glycocalyx of ocular surface.

Corticosteroids

Mechanism of action

It inactivates nuclear factor-κB

Which prevents the transcription of pro-inflammatory factors i.e. IL-1, IL-2, TNF which activates anti-inflammatory mediators like IL-10 and lipocortin – 1.

This results prevention of vasodilatation, migration and activation of inflammatory cells.

It also acts as an immunosuppressant by decreasing humoral B-cell immunity and reduce the T-cell activation by inhibition of IL-2.

T- cell Inhibitors

Mechanism of Action

- These are the calcineurin inhibitors which causes prevention of the T- cell activation by IL-2. IL-2 gene is essential for T-cell activation and proliferation which effects T-helper, T-suppressor, and T cytotoxic cells.
- In the T-cell cytoplasm, the drug binds with immunophilins.
- Cyclosporine binds with cyclophilins, but tacrolimus binds with FK binding protein.

↓

- The complex inhibits calcineurin activity competitively so the transcription of cytokine genes is prevented.

- It causes immunosuppression by blocking T-cell activity.

TABLE 1: Treatment of dry eye disease.

Drug	*Loading dose*	*Maintenance dose*
Corticosteroids Prednisolone	1-1.5 mg/kg/day Pulse dose – 500 mg stat (IV)	5-7.5 mg/day
T-cell inhibitors – Cyclosporine	2.5-5 mg/kg/day in two divided doses	0.5 mg/kg/day
Tacrolimus	0.05-0.1 mg/kg/day	
Antimetabolites–Methotrexate	7.5-10 mg/once a week which is increased 2.5 mg + Folic acid 1 mg * 5 days or 5 mg *1 day	Reduced by 0.5 mg/kg every month

Contd...

Contd...

Drug	*Loading dose*	*Maintenance dose*
Mycophenolate mofetil	2 g/day (2 divided doses) for 6 months.	0.5-3 mg/dL
Alkylating agents – cyclophosphamide	10-15 mg/kg (500-750 mg) (IV)	
Azathioprine	2-3 mg/kg/day in two divided doses Increased by 0.5 mg/kg/day	Reduced by 0.5 mg/kg every month
Alkylating agents – Cyclophosphamide	Pulse dose 10-15 mg/kg	1-3 mg/kg/day

4. Discuss the etiopathogenesis and management of dry eye (10) (WBUHS MS 2023)

Etiopathogenesis—**Flowcharts 2 and 3.**

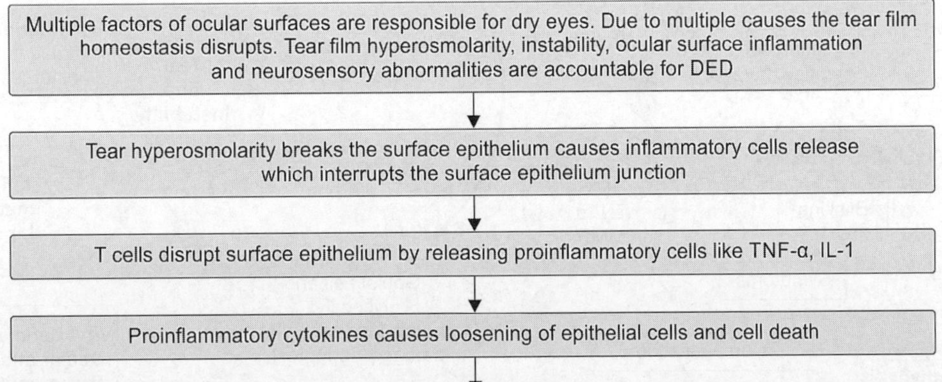

Flowchart 2: Pathogenesis of dry eye disease.

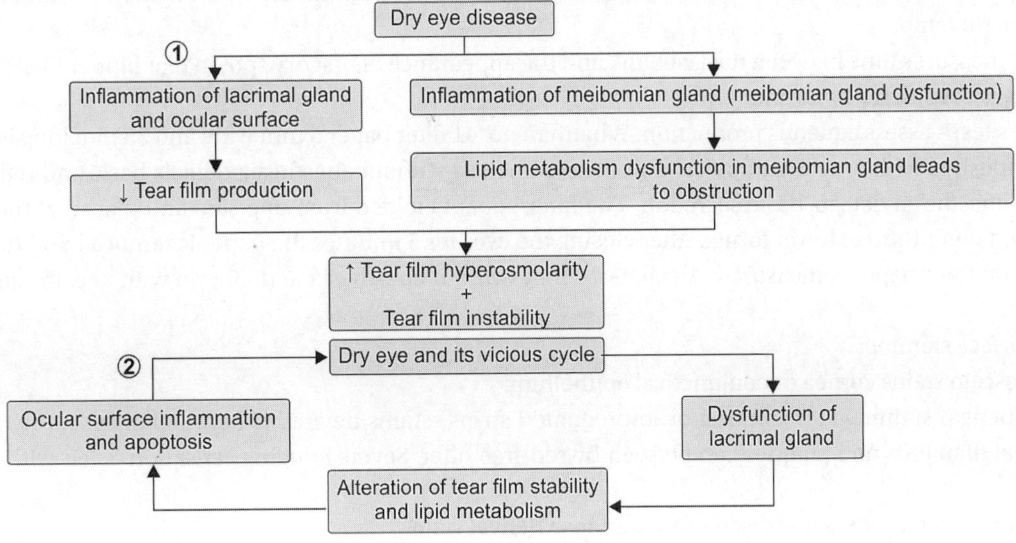

Flowchart 3: Pathophysiology of DED.

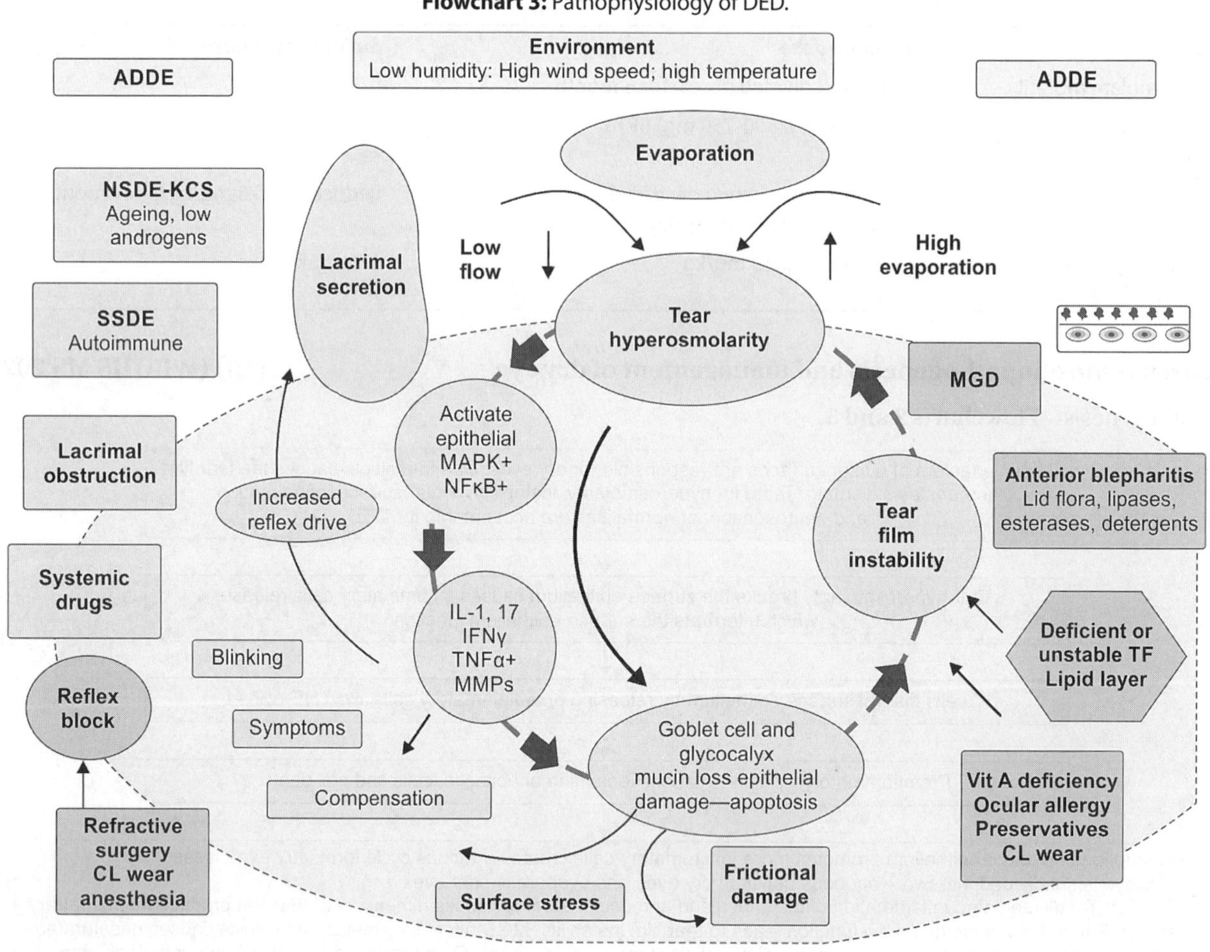

Courtesy: The ocular surface—TFOS DEWS II Report Executive Summary.

Diagnosis

- Tear break-up time - assess evaporative dry eye
  - Fluorescein is instilled in lower fornix and patient is asked not to blink and tear film is observed under cobalt blue filter of slit lamp.
  - TBUT measures time between the last blink and the appearance of first dry spot in tear film. A TBUT of Less than 10 sec, is considered abnormal.
- Schirmer's test - assess aqueous production. Whatman no. 41 filter paper 5 mm wide and 35 mm long is used. It can be accomplished with or without topical anesthesia. The test without anesthesia detects basic and reflex secretion and with anesthesia detects basic secretion. The filter paper is folded from one side and placed at the junction of middle and outer third of lower fornix. After closing the eyes for 5 minutes the paper is removed and the amount of moisture on filter paper is measured. A value <10 mm without anesthesia and <6 mm with anesthesia considered abnormal.
- Ocular surface staining:
  - Fluorescein stains cornea or conjunctival epithelium.
  - Rose Bengal staining (1% solution or impregnated strips) stains devitalized epithelial cells. Any pre-existing corneal filaments and plaques can be seen by red-free filter. Severe stinging sensation is felt with rose Bengal stain.
  - Lissamine green causes less discomfort than rose Bengal stain.

Other investigations are:
- Fluorescein clearance test
- Tear film osmolarity test
- Tear constituent measurement
- Phenol red thread test
- Tear meniscometry
- Impression cytology

TABLE 2: Dry eye severity scale.

Dry eye severity scale	*Level 1*	*Level 2*	*Level 3*	*Level 4*
Discomfort, severity and frequency	Mild and/or episodic; occurs under environmental stress	Moderate episodic or chronic, stress or no stress	Severe frequent or constant without stress	Severe and/or disabling and constant
Visual symptoms	None or episodic mild fatigue	Annoying and/or activity limiting, episodic	Annoying, chronic and/or constant, limiting activity	Constant and/or possibly disabling
Conjunctival congestion	None to mild	None to mild	+/-	+/++
Conjunctival staining	None to mild	Variable	Moderate to marked	Marked
Corneal staining (severity/ location	None to mild	Variable	Marked central	Severe punctate erosions
Corneal/tear sign	None to mild	Mild debris, reduced meniscus height	Filamentary keratitis, mucus clumping, increased tear debris	Filamentary keratitis, mucus clumping, increased tear debris, ulceration
Lid/meibomian glands	MGD variably present	MGD variably present	Frequent	Trichiasis, keratinization, symblepharon
TFBUT (Second)	Variable	<= 10	<= 5	Immediate
Schirmer test(mm/5 min)	Variable	<= 10	<= 5	<= 2

Treatment (Table 2)

Level 1: *Lifestyle modification*
- Frequent blinking while reading, reducing the screen time, and limited use of contact lens.
- Artificial tear substitutes including gels and ointments frequently.
- Preservative free topical medication preferred.
- Warm compresses, lid hygiene for blepharitis.
- If lagophthalmos is present taping and lateral tarsorrhaphy in extreme cases.

Level 2
- Preservative free tear substitutes advised in DED.
- Anti-inflammatory agents like topical steroids, T-cell inhibitors like cyclosporine (0.05%).
- Tetracyclines
- Punctual plugs - Long lasting collagen plugs or silicone plugs can be used.
- Moist chamber spectacle and spectacle side shields are used.

Level 3
- Serum eye drop from autologous or umbilical cord serum (20-100%).
- Contact lenses - Silicone hydrogel retain moisture for 12-16 hours.
- Permanent punctal occlusion
- Punctual cautery is done by laser cautery or surgical thermal coagulation in moderate to severe keratoconjunctivitis sicca.

Level 4

- Systemic anti-inflammatory agents.
- Surgery – tarsorrhaphy in severe cases.
- Salivary gland auto-transplantation
- Mucous membrane or amniotic membrane transplantation.

SUGGESTED READING

1. Craig JP, Nelson JD, Azar DT, Belmonte C, Bron AJ, Chauhan SK, et al. TFOS DEWS II Report Executive Summary page 4-6. Ocul Surf. 2017;15(4):802-12.
2. Eyewiki. Dry eye disease. [online] Available from https://en.wikipedia.org/wiki/Dry_eye_syndrome#:~:text=Dry%20eye%20syndrome%2C%20also%20known%20as%20keratoconjunctivitis%20sicca%2C,mild%20and%20occasional%20to%20severe%20and%20continuous.%20%5B3%5D [Last accessed March, 2025].
3. Salmon JF. Chapter 8. Kanski's Clinical Ophthalmology, 9th edition. Philadelphia: Elsevier; 2019.

8

CHAPTER

Episclera and Sclera

Smiti Rani Srivastava, Rituparna Ghosh

QUESTIONS

1. **Classify scleritis. Describe the clinical features, investigations, diagnosis and management of posterior scleritis. (2+2+2+2+2) (DNB 2021)**
2. **Short note on necrotizing scleritis. (5) (WBUHS MS 2018)**
3. **Short note on systemic association of scleritis. (5) (WBUHS DO 2018)**

1. Classify scleritis. Describe the clinical features, investigations, diagnosis and management of posterior scleritis. (2+2+2+2+2) (DNB 2021)

Scleritis is a severe ocular inflammatory condition which affects the sclera i.e., the outer coat of the eye. It may be idiopathic or caused by infectious or noninfectious condition. Viruses, bacteria, fundi and parasites can cause infectious scleritis. 50% of the patients of scleritis are associated with autoimmune diseases in which rheumatoid arthritis and systemic vasculitis are most common. It affects middle aged females more commonly.

Classification of Scleritis (Flowchart 1):

Flowchart 1: Classification of scleritis.

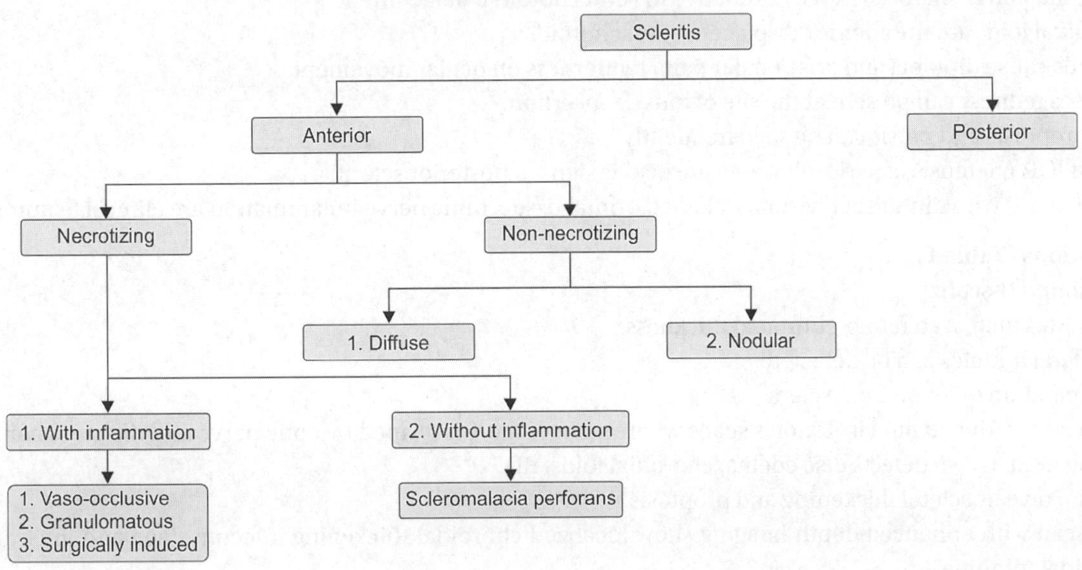

- Anterior non-necrotizing—most common form
  - *Diffuse:* It features with anterior sclera edema with dilation of deep episcleral vessels.
  - *Nodular:* This occurs in a large number of patients who is having past history of herpes zoster ophthalmicus.

- Anterior necrotizing with inflammation—It is extremely grave and aggressive form of scleritis which needs systemic immunotherapy to reduce inflammation and diminished vision.
  - *Vaso-occlusive:* In rheumatoid arthritis, it is commonly found. Non-perfused episclera with underlying single area of sclera edema and conjunctiva can be seen.
  - *Granulomatous:* It is associated with granulomatosis with polyangiitis or PAN.
  - Surgically induced
- Scleromalacia perforans (necrotizing scleritis without inflammation)—It is characterized with progressive scleral thinning without vascular congestion.
- Posterior (with or without anterior scleritis)

Posterior Scleritis

It is a vision threatening condition seen mostly under the age of 40 years. It occurs bilaterally in 35% cases. 33% of cases over the age of 55 years have associated systemic diseases. It may or may not be associated with anterior scleritis.

It is seen commonly behind the insertion of rectus of muscle.

Clinical features

- It usually presents with varied symptoms which may range from discomfort to boring pain and tenderness to palpation (very common), may radiate to forehead, brow, and jaw.
- Diminished vision
- Pain associated with ocular movement
- Protrusion of eyeball
- Lid swelling
- Diplopia due to restrictive ocular movement

Pain does not correlate with severity of the diseases.

Signs:

a. Slit lamp biomicroscopy—It shows corneal edema, shallow anterior chamber with anterior bowing of iris, mild to moderate AC cells.
b. Exudative retinal detachment appears like yellowish brown subretinal exudative material.
c. Uveal effusion is characterized by exudative RD and choroidal detachment.
d. Choroidal folds are the anterior displacement of choroid.
e. Myositis cause diplopia and arise ocular pain, tenderness on ocular movement.
f. It causes redness can present at the site of muscle insertion.
g. Mild proptosis and ptosis can be seen frequently.
h. Raised IOP, chemosis of periorbital area are ocular signs of posterior scleritis.
i. Disc edemas with diminished vision, inflamed orbital tissue, optic nerve inflammation are clinical features.

Investigations (Table 1)

- Ultrasound B-scan:
  - It notes increased retino-choroidal thickness.
  - Scleral nodules can be detected.
  - Separation of tenon from sclera

T-sign is seen due to fluid in Tenon's space where stem of the T is formed by optic nerve and the cross bar is the gap containing fluid. It also detects disc edema, choroidal folds, RD.

- CT scan reveals scleral thickening and proptosis.
- OCT scan with enhanced depth imaging show localized choroidal thickening in acute stage and in chronic stage choroidal thinning.
- FA can detect early pinpoint leaks with late pooling with SRF.
- ICGA - It shows choroidal vasculitis, zonal hyperfluorescence, choroidal perfusion delay, enlargement of draining choroidal veins and hypo fluorescent dark spots.

- Mantoux test, Quantiferon Gold is done to rule out TB.
- RPR and FTA-Abs test is done for syphilis.
- Rheumatoid factor and anti-citrullinated protein antibodies, ANA, ACE, lysozyme, ANCA, HLA-B 27, CBC, CMP can be done.
- X-ray chest and sacroiliac joints.

TABLE 1: Diagnostic tests.

Test	*Associated disease*
PPD or Quantiferon Gold	Tuberculosis
• RPR • FTA-Abs	Syphilis
• Rheumatoid factor • Anti-CCP	Rheumatoid arthritis
ANA	Systemic lupus erythematous
• ACE • Lysozyme • Chest X-ray	Sarcoidosis
ANCA	Granulomatous polyangiitis; polyarteritis nodosa
HLA-B27	Ankylosing spondylitis; psoriasis

Management

- It needs urgent and aggressive treatment.
  - First line treatment:
    - Oral NSAIDs used for 2 weeks and then review, e.g., Tablets Indomethacin 25 mg tds, Ibuprofen 600–800 mg qds.
  - Second line treatments:
    - Oral corticosteroids—given when oral NSAIDs is not responding. Dose is (1 mg/kg/day or 60–80 mg of prednisolone daily). It tapered slowly within few weeks.
  - Third line treatments:
    - Immunosuppressive/anti-metabolites agents—it is used after 1 month of failure of oral steroid treatment. Commonly used agents are i.e., methotrexate (max 25 mg/week) and mycophenolate mofetil (1,500 mg BID) and azathioprine are advised.
  - Fourth line treatment:
    - Biologics such as infliximab, rituximab are also helpful in systemic associated scleritis. Cyclophosphamide can be used primarily in patients with associated systemic vasculitis like GPA.

2. Short note on necrotizing scleritis. (5) (WBUHS MS 2018)

This form of scleritis occurs around the age of 60 years, bilateral in 60% cases and if not treated at initial stage, it may result in vision threatening condition.

It may range from trivial to severe self-limiting recurrent attacks.

It is associated with connective tissue disorders in 50% cases like rheumatoid arthritis, SLE, PAN, Wegener's granulomatosis, IBD, HZO and also with other miscellaneous systemic conditions such as TB, sarcoidosis, syphilis, leprosy, lyme disease, etc.

Types:

1. Necrotizing scleritis with inflammation.
2. Necrotizing scleritis without inflammation

Clinical features

Necrotizing scleritis with inflammation: intense congestion of vessels and pain are the key features.

1. Vaso-occlusive
2. Granulomatous
3. Surgically induced

Symptoms: Persistent, severe boring pain, which is gradual in onset and radiates to the temple, brow or jaw. Sleep is disturbed with pain.

Signs:

a. *Vaso-occlusive:* Scleral edema with nonperfused episcleral and conjunctiva mainly associated with rheumatoid arthritis.
b. *Granulomatous:* Starts with injection near limbus and extends very rapidly to sclera, episclera, conjunctiva and adjacent cornea. It is associated with Wegener granulomatosis and Polyarteritis nodosa
c. *Surgically-induced:* Starts within 3 weeks or more after a patient with RA followed by ECCE, squint correction, trabeculectomy, scleral buckling, pterygium excision, etc. They remain localized to one segment unlike other types.

Complications

- Acute infiltrative stromal keratitis
- Sclerosing keratitis
- Peripheral ulcerative keratitis
- Uveitis (in aggressive scleritis)
- Glaucoma (leading to vision loss)
- Hypotony (due to ciliary body detachment and ischemia)
- Perforation of sclera (very rare)

Necrotizing scleritis without inflammation (Scleromalacia Perforans) absence of vessel congestion and pain.

Elderly women with long term rheumatoid arthritis get affected commonly

- *Symptoms:* Irritation in eyes with no pain and vision loss
- *Signs:* Necrotic scleral plaques starting near limbus then slowly progressing with no vascular congestion. Scleral thinning and exposure of underlying uvea seen in due course of time but globe perforation is extremely rare.

Investigations

- Total hemogram, serum uric acid, ESR, FBS, ACE, CH 50.
- X-ray chest and sacroiliac joints,
- Mantoux test,
- VDRL, FTA-ABS for syphilis, RPR
- USG B-scan
  - Serum for RF, ANA, ANCA (p-ANCA, c-ANCA), Antiphospholipid antibodies.
  - FA can help to diagnose necrotizing scleritis by identifying vascular nonperfusion.

Treatment

Necrotizing scleritis with inflammation

1. Systemic corticosteroids in high dose and sometimes with topical prednisolone
2. IVMP as pulse may be given
3. Immunomodulatory and biologic agents—for refractory cases
4. Surgery—for progressive disease even after treatment, Scleral patch graft and tectonic lamellar keratoplasty can be done.

Scleromalacia Perforans

**Medical therapy*

1. Oral NSAID first line of treatment
2. Topical NSAID

3. Topical tear substitute
4. Topical ciclosporin

**Systemic immunosuppressive therapy*

- Corticosteroid oral 1 mg/kg/day then tapered
- Cyclophosphamide oral 2–3 mg/kg/day

**Surgery:* Scleral patch graft etc., if uvea is exposed

**Protection from trauma*

3. Short note on systemic association of scleritis. (5) (WBUHS DO 2018)

Various diseases may be associated with scleritis, which are mainly autoimmune in nature such as rheumatoid arthritis, Wegener granulomatosis, Polyarteritis nodosa, relapsing polychondritis, etc.

1. *Rheumatoid arthritis:* It is most common systemic association of scleritis, particularly necrotizing type. It is more commonly seen in females around the age of 3rd decade. It is symmetrical, destructive, inflammatory polyarthropathy with extra articular manifestations like pulmonary nodules, multifocal neuropathy, septic arthritis, secondary amyloidosis, carpal tunnel syndrome etc.

   Bilateral swelling of small joints of hands involving proximal interphalangeal joints with joint instability, subluxation, subcutaneous nodules and vasculitis, sparing distal interphalangeal joints are seen most commonly.
2. *Wegener granulomatosis:* It is idiopathic, multisystem granulomatous disease with generalized small vessel vasculitis affecting respiratory tract and kidneys in around 5th decade of life with progressive, granulomatous and necrotizing scleritis associated with c-ANCA in over 90% cases. Occlusive retinal vasculitis, orbital inflammatory disease, peripheral ulcerative keratitis, nasolacrimal obstruction, dacryocystitis and rarely tarsoconjunctival diseases also seen.

   Upper respiratory tract involvement by necrotizing granulomatous inflammation results in saddle shaped nasal deformity, nasal septal perforation and fistulae. Lower respiratory tract involvement may result in lung infiltration, cavitation and nodules. Necrotizing granulo nephritis, vasculitis involving skin, spleen, heart and adrenals are also seen.
3. *Polyarteritis nodosa:* It is a collagen vascular disease affecting medium sized or small arteries, more commonly in 3rd to 6th decades of life in males with aggressive necrotizing scleritis, peripheral ulcerative keratitis, orbital pseudotumor, occlusive retinal periarteritis with fever, arthralgia, myalgia, purpura, renal involvement with hypertension, coronary arteritis , heart failure, myocardial infarction, GI bleeding, stroke, multifocal neuropathy associated with eosinophilia and hypergammaglobulinemia.
4. *Relapsing polychondritis:* It is rare idiopathic small vessel vasculitis involving cartilage of various organs resulting in recurrent, progressive inflammation in 5th decade of life with non-erosive polyarthritis, necrotizing and non-necrotizing scleritis, acute anterior uveitis, cardiac valve dysfunction, cochlear or vestibular damage leading to hearing loss, tinnitus, vertigo, saddle shaped nose due to collapsing of nasal cartilage, recurrent swelling of pinnae and cough, stridor, hoarse voice due to involvement of tracheobronchial cartilage.

SUGGESTED READING

1. AAO 2020-2021, BCSC Section 9: Uveitis and Ocular Inflammation. [online] Available from https://store.aao.org/basic-and-clinical-science-course-section-09-uveitis-and-ocular-inflammation.html [Last accessed March, 2025].
2. Eyewiki. Scleritis. [online] Available from https://eyewiki.org/Scleritis [Last accessed March, 2025].
3. Gerstenblith AT. The Wills Eye Manual, 6th edition. Philadelphia: Wolters Kluwer; 2012. p. 124.
4. Robertson R, Ansari FA, Gafoor S, Idolor ON, Amakye D. Review of Ophthalmology—Posterior scleritis: a diagnostic challenge. Cureus. 2024;16(6):e61537.
5. Salmon JF. Chapter 9 Episclera and Sclera. Kanski's Clinical Ophthalmology, 9th edition. Philadelphia: Elsevier; 2019.

9

CHAPTER

Cornea

Sony Sinha, Smiti Rani Srivastava

QUESTIONS

1. **Discuss corneal collagen cross linking.** **(10) (WBUHS DO 2018)**
2. **Discuss corneal Topography.** **(10) (RGUHS MS 2021)**
3. **Write briefly on Corneal vascularization.** **(5) (TN MGRMU MS)**
4. **Write briefly on Fuchs' endothelial dystrophy.** **(10) (WBUHS DO)**
5. **Briefly describe herpes simplex epithelial keratitis. Outline the management.** **(5+5) (WBUHS DO 2018)**
6. **Discuss interstitial keratitis.** **(10) (WBUHS MS 2023)**
7. **What is keratoconus? Describe its clinical signs and recent management.** **(1+4+5) (WBUHS MS 2023, DO 2018)**
8. **Write briefly on peripheral ulcerative keratitis (PUK).** **(10) (TN MGRMU MS 2019)**
9. **Stains in fungal corneal ulcer—write short note.** **(5) (WBUHS MS)**

1. Discuss corneal collagen cross linking. (10) (WBUHS DO 2018)

Key pathogenetic mechanism in corneal ectatic disorders is progressive degradation of stromal collagen interlamellar covalent bonds (cross-links) leading to loss of stromal integrity and tensile strength.

CXL = C3R aims to generate the interlamellar covalent bonds by photoactivation of adjacent collagen fibrils aided by riboflavin.

Progression of keratoconus can be halted by cross-linking corneal stromal collagen using the classical Dresden protocol where de-epithelialized cornea is exposed to 0.1% riboflavin phosphate eye drops @ once every 3 minutes for 30 minutes for photosensitization. De-epithelization is assisted by application of a drop of alcohol every 5 minutes for 30 minutes followed by debridement of the central 2-9 mm. This is followed by photo-oxidation with 3 mW/cm^2 ultraviolet A light after which a bandage contact lens or soft contact lens is put till the epithelium heals. This technique requires a corneal thickness of 380-400 microns after epithelial removal.

Latest modifications in this regard include:

Defining progression as increased K max with corresponding 1 D change in subjective refraction or a greater or equal to 5% decrease in thinnest pachymetry in the preceding 6 months.

Accelerated/high-fluence CXL takes into account the fact that the total energy required for effective CXL is 5.4 mN/cm^2. As per the Bunsen-Roscoe law of reciprocity, this can be achieved by new protocols of 9 mW/cm^2 over 10 minutes or 18 mW/cm^2 over 5 minutes. Any further acceleration would be ineffective due to depletion of oxygen within the corneal stroma. Prior enrichment with oxygen can lead to better outcomes.

Pulsed accelerated CXL uses pulses of 1 second at 1 second intervals with 8 minutes photo-oxidation 230 mW. Use of pulsed fluence enables improvement in oxygen content of the stroma which can get depleted rapidly within 10-15 seconds of continuous exposure.

Stromal lenticule assisted CXL or contact lens assisted CXL where the lenticule or CL is soaked in riboflavin solution for 20 minutes, used in a corneal thickness of 350 microns. This is laid on the epithelium of cornea.

A corneal thickness less than 330 microns is liable to cause endothelial toxicity on ultraviolet light exposure. Some ways to temporarily improve corneal thickness include the following:
- Isotonic riboflavin combined with 10% hydroxypropyl methylcellulose over the cornea.
- Hypoosmolar riboflavin combined with 0.9% phosphate buffered saline or 0.9% sodium chloride causes 10% increase in pachymetry.
- Hyperosmolar concentrations of riboflavin 0.15%/0.25% or 0.5% using BAK/tetracaine/EDTA to increase its penetration into the corneal stroma can be used with Epithelium-on CXL. Transepithelial CXL without such enhancement leads to a shallower demarcation line with variable results.

In *TREK + CXL,* asymmetrical CXL is customized to target areas of ectasia for stabilization in corneal thickness up to 330 microns. There is topography guided epithelial removal by photorefractive keratectomy. It is centered on the steepest cone with ablation of tissue 20 microns.

Topography guided cross-linking is centered on the posterior float with administration of variable fluence of 10 J/cm^2 in the center and 3 mJ/cm^2 at the periphery with eye tracking.

Time is customized to pachymetry at the end of riboflavin soak while the irradiation intensity is constant at 3 mW/cm^2. An online CXL calculator has been developed to assist in such decisions based on the Lambert-Beer equation.

Combined modalities of treatment like *SMILE with CXL* or femtosecond laser assisted INTACS with CXL are also being used.

There is now a tendency to perform early CXL in 18-19 years old patients with pachymetry less than 450 microns without waiting for actual progression to be demonstrated.

PACK-CXL is photoactivation of chromophore with CXL used as an adjuvant for treatment of infectious keratitis to prevent perforation while the chromophore like Rose Bengal inhibits matrix metalloproteinases and cytokines.

CXL after phototherapeutic keratectomy (PTK) leads to faster and better epithelial regeneration. PTK involves 50 microns ablation in the PRK mode followed by CXL and BCL application which can be removed after 3 days.

2. Discuss corneal topography. (10) (RGUHS MS 2021)

Introduction
- Corneal topography is graphical representation of geometrical properties of cornea
- Keratometer measures only anterior curvature of central 3 mm of cornea along 2 principle meridian based on the principle that anterior surface of cornea acts like a convex mirror and the size of image formed varies with its curvature
- Therefore, keratometer is not sufficient in cases of refractive surgeries and diagnosing corneal ectasia where accurate analysis of whole anterior as well as posterior surface is required

Corneal topography techniques are based on 3 principles
- *1st generation:* Placido disc-based devices that took into account only the anterior corneal curvature into account
- *2nd generation:* Tomographer Orbscan combines placido disc and slit scanning technologies
- *3rd generation:* Uses the Scheimpflug principle with rotating camera Pentacam (Oculus, Germany), TMS-5 (Tomey Corporation, Japan), Sirius (CSO, Italy), Galilei (Ziemer, Switzerland) **(Table 1)**

TABLE 1: Types of corneal topography.

Topographer	*Pentacam*	*Galilei*	*Sirius*
Principle	Single Scheimpflug	Dual Scheimpflug with placido	Single Scheimpflug with placido
Acquisition speed/2 s	25	25-50	25
Points mapped	25,000	122,000	21,632 anterior, 16,000 posterior

Placido Disc Technique

Based on the principle that cornea works as a convex mirror and the reflected image is directly viewed and analyzed as mires, Shape and orientation of mires gives idea about the shape of cornea, but posterior corneal surface cannot be characterized.

Videokeratoscopes—practical instruments that display concentric rings at the slit lamp for quick assessment of topographical changes (e.g., astigmatism induced by sutures), provide a computerized quantitative assessment of the same.

Slit Scanning Technique

- Slit scanning and triangulation are used to derive actual special location of thousands of points on the surface
- Uses a series of light slits (40 slits) passing over the cornea at an angle of 45°to the camera
- Each of the slit has 240 data points (data for points in between is extrapolated) and acquisition time is 1.5 sec
- Orbscan II combines both slit scanning and placido disc system

Scheimpflug Technique

The Scheimpflug law says - to get a higher depth of focus, move the three planes, provided that the picture plane, the objective plane and the film plane has to cut each other in one line or one point of intersection. The typical Scheimpflug corneal tomographer is pentacam.

Advantages of Pentacam

- Pentacam goes beyond topography and pachymetry and enables 3D corneal reconstruction which evaluates anterior as well as posterior curvature and creates a pachymetry map
- Based on Scheimpflug technique, it maintains the central (thinnest) point of each meridian.
- Thus, can re- register these central points and compensates for involuntary eye movements.
- So, it is 10 times more accurate than Orbscan which takes vertical image separate slice having no common point, thus can't register for any eye movement.

Examination of Corneal Tomography Maps

1. Elevation maps
   - Relative elevation measures height difference from a best fitting reference sphere
     - Green is the reference surface or zero level
     - Red is high (anterior) and positive
     - Blue is low (posterior) and negative
   - Normal cornea is prolate, so it rises centrally above the reference sphere and results in a central hill
   - And immediately surrounding the central hill is an annular sea where the cornea dips below the reference surface
   - In the far periphery, prolate cornea again rises above the reference surface , producing peripheral highlands
2. Curvature maps
   - Mean K value
   - Inferior-superior asymmetry
   - Skewing of axis in sagittal curvature
   - Anterior and posterior maps: Constructed in relation to a reference shape such as a best fit sphere or ellipsoid are values to detect ectasia, namely >12 microns in anterior float and >15 microns in the posterior float
3. Thickness maps
   - Pachymetry is important as at least 350 to 400 microns thickness of corneal tissue should be left behind after ablation by refractive surgery procedures
   - Corneal thickness spatial profile: It is a graph showing corneal thickness from center to periphery as lying with respect to±2 SD of normal
   - Percentage thickness increase: It is a graph showing
     - Vertical axis - percentage of thickness increment
     - Horizontal axis - location as circle centered on thinnest location

- Red color – curve of examined cornea
- Black dashed line – result of standard value study
- The upper and lower line represents the double standard deviation (95%) of corneal thickness

Uses of Corneal Topographers/Tomographers

- Screening for corneal ectasia
- Corneal ectasia monitoring and treatment
- Refractive surgery screening and monitoring
- Pre-operative intraocular lens selection
- Post-keratoplasty astigmatism evaluation and management
- Ocular surface disorder evaluation

Pentacam in Ectatic Corneal Disorders

- Pentacam captures a 3-D image of the cornea in 2 seconds over 25,000 elevation points
- It is important to rule out possibility of ectasia post refractive surgery by detecting contraindications to corneal refractive surgery such as forme fruste or overt keratoconus.
- In the Pentacam, there is the Belin Ambrosio Enhanced Ectasia display where detection of a cone is enhanced by enhancing the reference surface relevant indices are: total deviation (BAD-D)
- Ambrosio relational thickness (ART) values
- It also displays Corneal Thickness Spatial Profile (CTSP), Percentage Thickness index (PTI) and pachymetric progression index (PPI).
- Belin Ambrosio enhanced ectasia display II
- Newer Pentacam Random Forest Index uses artificial intelligence or machine learning to detect ectasia possibility.

3. Write briefly on corneal vascularization. (5) (TN MGRMU MS)

Cornea is supplied by anterior conjunctival branches of anterior ciliary arteries. A perilimbal plexus supplies minute arcades 1 mm into the limbus. Rest of the cornea is avascular for transparency.

Inflammation or ulceration of the cornea can lead to corneal vascularization due to disturbed balance of angiogenic and anti-angiogenic factors, namely upregulation of cytokines and VEGF secretion which, in turn upregulates matrix metalloproteinases. Causes may be infection, chemical injury, trauma, contact lens related hypoxia, post corneal transplant, allergy and autoimmune conditions.

If the scarring is minimal and the lesion heals, deep corneal vessels get obliterated and appear as ghost vessels. Often, it is accompanied with corneal scarring. Extensive scarring can lead to conjunctivalization of the cornea and serious threat to vision. Vascularization is also a prominent component of corneal rejection.

Types of Vascularization

Vascularization of the cornea may be superficial or deep. Difference between the two are as follows in **Table 2**.

TABLE 2: Types of corneal vascularization.

Superficial vascularization	*Deep vascularization*
Bright red	Dull red
Branches of ant conjunctival arteries	Branches of ciliary artery
Cross limbus	Seen to arise from limbus
Arborizing pattern seen	Oriented radially, brush-like or in tufts

Treatment

- Medical management: Steroids and anti VEGF agents are effective in early stages.
  - Steroids inhibit chemotaxis and cytokines IL-1 and IL-6, cause lymphocyte death and inhibits vascular dilatation. Combined with heparin and cyclodextrin they cause degradation of basement membrane of blood vessels.

- Anti VEGFs inhibit endothelial proliferation and topical or sub-conjunctival bevacizumab has been found to be safe and effective in early stages. It is more effective at treating acute rather than established or chronic corneal neovascularization

- *Laser photocoagulation:* Argon or Nd:YAG laser coagulate blood vessels and ablate tissue as hemoglobin in blood vessels absorbs the laser energy. Hence it can be used in case of established blood vessels in lipid keratopathy and graft rejection where medical therapy fails. However, titration of the amount of therapy is difficult and excessive treatment with this modality itself leads to an inflammatory response, increasing vascularization. Obliterated vessels may reopen and new shunt vessels may form
- Mitomycin intravascular chemoembolization (MICE) is a novel surgical technique for the treatment of visually significant corneal neovascularization and lipid keratopathy.
- *Photodynamic therapy:* Although effective, this is costly and can cause production of reactive oxygen species.
- Diathermy and cautery of limbal feeder vessels carry risk of damaging limbal stem cells.
- Deep anterior lamellar keratoplasty or even keratoprosthesis may be required in certain cases.

4. Write briefly on Fuchs' endothelial dystrophy. (10) (WBUHS DO)

It is a non-inflammatory endothelial dystrophy involving the endothelial layer of cornea.

Inheritance: Most commonly, unknown or sporadic, some cases show autosomal dominant inheritance, heterogenous, variable expressivity and incomplete penetrance.

Epidemiology

- Early onset (1st decade): Chromosome 1p 34.3-p32, collagen type VIII, COL 8A2 gene
- Late onset (4th decade): Chromosomes 13p, 18q,20p, 5q, 10p, 9p and 15q TCF4 gene
- Male-female ratio is 2.5-3.1, most common in 5th to 6th decade

Pathology

- Diffusely thickened and laminated Descemet membrane, especially anterior banded part in early onset disease. Endothelial cells are sparse or atrophic with or without buried or confluent guttae.
- There is increased waviness of stromal collagen lamellae

Symptoms

- Intermittent diminished vision, especially in morning due to corneal edema.
- Glare
- Earliest symptom is reduced contrast sensitivity
- Pain due to ruptured bullae
- Photophobia
- Lacrimation
- Significant decreased vision is result of epithelial and stromal edema and fibrosis in later stage.

Stages

Stage 1

1. Guttata - small excrescences of Descemet's membrane called guttae seen in the endothelial surface of cornea. It starts centrally, progress peripherally, larger in late-onset
2. Endothelial mosaic appearance is noted in specular microscopy.
3. Beaten metal appearance – In progressive stages, it is associated with melanin deposition called endothelial dusting.

Stage 2

1. Endothelial decompensation—leads to central stromal edema causing morning blur vision.
2. Epithelial edema - when stromal thickness is increased by 30% epithelium edema develops.
3. Descemet membrane folds are visible

Stage 3

- Persistent epithelial edema (Bullous keratopathy) - results in microcyst and bullae. Its painful when bullae rupture as naked nerve endings are exposed.
- Late primary open angle glaucoma and nuclear cataract are associations.

Signs

Slit lamp biomicroscopy:

- Epithelial microcyst
- Epithelial bullae
- Guttae on Descemet's membrane
- Stromal edema
- Stromal scar
- Endothelial folds
- Vascularization into the cornea

Differential Diagnosis

Anything that causes endothelial deposits and or corneal edema will be included in differential diagnosis.

- Pigment dispersion syndrome
- Chronic Iridocyclitis
- Herpetic stromal keratitis
- Bullous keratopathy
- TASS
- Congenital hereditary endothelial dystrophy
- Posterior polymorphic membrane dystrophy

Treatment

Medical

- Hypertonic sodium chloride drops and ointment.
- Control of with anti-glaucoma medications.
- Hair driers are used to decrease corneal edema.
- Bandage contact lens is used in ruptured bullae

Rho-kinase inhibitor eye drops with or without prior transcorneal endothelial cryotherapy can stimulate endothelial cell proliferation and function.

Surgery

Indications—when medical treatment fails:

- PKP is done in advance stages of Fuchs dystrophy
- DSEK/DSAEK (Descemet's stripping automated endothelial keratoplasty) – For mild to moderate cases.
- DMEK (Descemet's membrane endothelial keratoplasty)
- DWEK - Descemetorhexis without endothelial keratoplasty is a latest surgical technique for Fuchs where guttae is located in central cornea and peripheral endothelium is healthy.
- Conjunctival hooding and amniotic membrane transplantation can be done

Cataract surgery in advance cases causes loss of endothelial cells resulting in more decompensation. Triple procedure (Cataract surgery + IOL implantation + DSEK/DMEK) are preferred in such scenario.

Follow-up: 3 monthly in case of corneal edema till surgery is performed or 6-12 monthly where IOP control is needed

5. Briefly describe herpes simplex epithelial keratitis. Outline the management. (5+5) (WBUHS DO 2018)

- Herpes simplex keratitis is one of leading cause of corneal blindness
- Mostly unilateral, rarely bilateral.

- HSV is a double-stranded DNA virus with two subtypes HSV-1 affects mostly eyes, face and lips and HSV 2 causes venereal disease. Virus resides in all neuronal ganglia.
  Incidence - around 1 million people in world are affected by herpes simplex epitheliitis each year.
- *Mode of infection* - oral infection or direct contact with infective secretions- the viruses can penetrate the cornea via trigeminal nerve.

Symptoms

- Pain in eye is hallmark sign
- Redness
- Diminished vision
- Photophobia
- Lacrimation

Signs

- Diminished vision
- Epithelial cells become swollen and opaque appears as stellate pattern.
- Desquamation of epithelial cells leads to dendritic ulcer. The small branching epithelial dendrites with terminal bulb over central cornea is a classical feature.
- The virus laden cells present over the margins of the ulcer can be stained with rose Bengal and the bed of ulcer is stained by fluorescein.
- Reduced corneal sensation is diagnostic of viral etiology.
- Mild AC cells are seen.
- Acute follicular conjunctivitis may be associated.
- Persistent punctuate epithelial erosion and irregular epithelium can be a feature of inactive stage.
- Mild subepithelial haze may persist for weeks. Corneal scarring may enlarge after each attack of HSV infection which leads ocular morbidity.
- Frequent infection causes stromal scarring may leads to corneal transplantation.
- Vesicular eyelid lesions along with epithelial ulceration can be seen simultaneously.
- Increased IOP due to AC cells is a feature.

Complications

Nonhealing neurotrophic ulcers, severe dry eyes and corneal perforation.

Management

Investigations

- Laboratory tests - conjunctival scrapings, impression cytology and scrapings from vesicular skin lesions may be useful.
- Serum HSV antibody may not be positive.
- Scrapings with transport medium for culture can establish presence of virus.
- PCR and immunocytochemistry can detect HSV-DNA.
- Tzanck smear scraping shows presence of HSV infection
- Giemsa staining confirms multinucleated giant cells in corneal smears.
- Papanicolaou stain shows intranuclear eosinophilic inclusion bodies of Lipschutz (Cowdry type A)
- ELISA is used for rapid test and detects by mononuclear antibody.

Treatment

Medical

- Though it resolves spontaneously treatment with antivirals shortens the duration of disease.
- Antiviral medication interferes with DNA synthesis which stops viral DNA polymerase and first line of drug.
- Ganciclovir 3% or 15% can be applied for five times a day till the ulcer resolves afterward three times a day is applied for another week.

- Topical antibiotic may be applied to prevent secondary bacterial infection.
- Cycloplegics to reduce pain.
- Topical steroids is contraindicated.
- Epithelial debridement can be done to decrease the viral load.
- Amniotic membrane promotes epithelial healing and reduces the scar formation.
- Long term Acyclovir therapy 400 mg twice per day for one year subside the epithelial and stromal herpetic keratitis
- Herpetic Eye Disease Study (HEDS) proves that long term prophylaxis of oral acyclovir reduces the recurrence rate.
- Frequent follow-up may be needed to observe the recurrence.

Surgical

- Penetrating keratoplasty may be needed in corneal scarring. Oral antiviral therapy may be continued to prevent graft as Recurrence is common causing graft failure.
- If scarring is central in visual axis lamellar keratoplasty may be an option.
- In ocular morbid case, boston keratoprosthesis is the only choice.

  Prognosis—good but depends upon recurrences.

6. Discuss interstitial keratitis. (10) (WBUHS MS 2023)

Nonsuppurative and non-ulcerative inflammation of corneal stroma with cellular infiltration and vascularization without involving epithelium and endothelium. It is Immune mediated process against stromal antigens, residual infectious antigens or both.

Causes

- Bacterial, e.g., syphilis lyme ds, tuberculosis.
- Viral, e.g., herpes simplex, Epstein–Barr virus, HTLV-1
- Parasitic, e.g., onchocerciasis, *Acanthamoeba*
- Autoimmune causes like cogan syndrome, sarcoidosis.
- Herpes simplex virus and syphilis are the leading cause.

Clinical Features

Symptoms

Decreased vision depending upon the extent of location of involved cornea.

Significant photophobia and pain

Slit-lamp Findings

- Conjunctival injection
- Corneal haze, ground glass appearance obscuring iris, lipid keratopathy.
- Stromal infiltration, edema, presence of immune ring in active interstitial keratitis
- Deep vascularization leads to salmon-patches.
- Anterior uveitis in syphilis.
- Inflammation begins to subside after 1-2 months leaving behind opacity resulting in mild to moderate visual impairment.
- Inactive interstitial keratitis: Here is mid-to-posterior corneal scarring, deep vascularization giving rise to ghost vessels, and sometimes reduplication of the Descemet's membrane

Congenital Syphilis

- Bilateral (80%), diffuse stromal disease with deep vascularization occurs between 5 to 20 years of age, peak 9 to 11 years, associated with iris atrophy, posterior synechiae, salt and pepper fundus.
- Systemic manifestations as a part of Hutchinson's triad with deafness and anomalous teeth, saddle-like nose, frontal bossing and maxillary overgrowth
- Acquired syphilis
- Unilateral, sectoral stromal disease, mild vascularization 10 years after infection

- Episcleritis, scleritis, iritis, iris papules, chorioretinitis, papillitis, retinal vasculitis, exudative RD are the features with may be associated with syphilis.

Mycobacterial: (Unilateral, Sectoral)

- Herpes simplex virus: Unilateral diffuse or sectoral vascularization with iritis, decreased corneal sensation, corneal edema, radiating corneal infiltration i.e., "sunburst" appearance and iris atrophy.
- Cogan's syndrome: Associated acute tinnitus, vertigo, deafness. Ciliary congestion with diffuse/sectoral anterior stromal, sub-epithelial infiltrates 0.5–1 mm. In atypical cases, scleritis and retinal vasculitis can be associated.
- Investigations: HLA B17, A9, leukocytosis, elevated ESR and CRP, MRI of inner ear shows calcific bony and soft tissue obliteration of labyrinth fluid spaces.
- T/t steroids: Systemic and topical, cycloplegics.

Diagnosis If IK

- It is basically clinic based on the findings of non-ulcerating stromal keratitis with deep stromal neovascularization and associated symptoms and proper history of patients.
- Slit lamp biomicroscopy – Helps in determining the depth and pattern of stromal infiltration.
- Corneal pachymetry
- Applanation tonometer
- Confocal microscopy in suspected atypical infections.
- Assessment of pupillary function and visual acuity
- Dilated fundus examination – for posterior pole and peripheral retina.
- History taking
- Lab test
- For syphilis – RPR, VDRL, FTA-ABS, MHA-TP

Treatment

- Treatment of underlying condition, e.g., Systemic penicillin in syphilis.
- Topical steroid prednisolone acetate eye drops six times a day and tapered gradually over several weeks are the mainstay of the treatment.
- In case of herpes simplex or herpes zoster, the treatment should be topical steroids in conjunction with topical or oral antiviral.
- The use of corticosteroid is controversial in *Acanthamoeba* and other parasitic mediated interstitial keratitis. And they need specific systemic antiparasitic medication.

Surgery

- Rarely, dense cornea scarring necessitates keratoplasty to be done only if the inflammation has subsided to prevent rejection or failure
- 6 monthly to yearly follow-up is required.

7. What is keratoconus? Describe its clinical signs and recent management.

(1+4+5) (WBUHS MS 2023, DO 2018)

Keratoconus is a progressive bilateral ectatic condition characterized by cone-like steepening of the cornea, central or paracentral stromal thinning and progressive vision loss.

The condition may be:

- Congenital (autosomal dominant with variable penetrance) or acquired as a result of eye rubbing in vernal catarrh, contact lens wear or associated Down's syndrome. Young male children, typically beginning in puberty and progressing into the mid-30s.

Symptoms—progressive n frequent change in vision not corrected by glasses

Clinical Signs

Early

- Initially there may be no clinically visible signs in an asymptomatic patient.
- Typically affects both eyes, it may be asymmetric.
- Asymmetric refractive error with progressive astigmatism shown by keratometry
- Retinoscopy shows scissoring reflex.
- *Charleaux sign:* Direct ophthalmoscope from a distance of 1 foot shows oil-droplet reflex.
- *Corneal thinning:* Posterior thinning may be the first detectable sign on topography. This can be followed by steepening of the cornea, especially inferiorly, with thin apex.
- *Vogt striae:* Deep vertical striae in stroma when lids are pressed.
- *Pachymetry:* Thinnest pachymetry at apex <10 microns, asymmetry between the two eyes < 30 microns are suggestive of Keratoconus.
- *Fleischer ring:* Hemosiderin in epithelium at base of the cone seen best with cobalt blue filter
- *Rizzuti sign:* When light beam shown from temporal side conical reflection seen in nasal cornea.

Late

- *Munson's sign:* V-shaped configuration of lid on looking down
- Breaks in Bowman's membrane
- Acute hydrops is a complication due to sudden rupture in Descemet's membrane allowing aqueous in Stroma resulting in corneal edema. This heals in 6-10 weeks with stromal scarring.
- Stromal scarring- after healing of acute hydrops resulted scar increase the vision due to reduction in steepening.

Management

Goal of treatment is to restore visual acuity and control the progression of disease

- Spectacles and soft toric contact lenses in mild cases. Rigid gas permeable contact lenses used in distorted corneas. Rose-K contact lenses, PROSE lenses are special lenses used in keratoconus.
- Collagen cross-linking (*CXL*): Progression of keratoconus can be halted by cross-linking corneal stromal collagen using the classical Dresden protocol where de-epithelialized cornea is exposed to 0.1% riboflavin eye drops once every 3 minutes for 30 minutes for photosensitization. De-epithelization is assisted by application of a drop of alcohol every 5 minutes for 30 minutes followed by debridement of the central 2-9 mm. This is followed by photo-oxidation with 3mW/cm^2 ultraviolet A light after which a bandage contact lens or soft contact lens is put till the epithelium heals. This technique requires a corneal thickness of 380-400 microns after epithelial removal.
- *Stromal lenticule assisted CXL or contact lens assisted CXL:* Where a lenticule or contact lens is soaked in riboflavin solution for 20 minutes and applied onto the cornea, thereby allowing conventional CXL to be used in a corneal thickness of 350 microns.
- *Accelerated/high-fluence CXL:* Takes into account the fact that the total energy required for effective CXL is 5.4 mN/cm^2. This can be achieved by new protocols of 9 mW/cm^2 over 10 minutes or 18 mW/cm^2 over 5 minutes. Any further acceleration would be ineffective due to depletion of oxygen. Prior enrichment with oxygen can lead to better outcomes.
- *Asymmetrical CXL* is customized to target areas of ectasia for stabilization.
- Early CXL in 18-19 year olds can be done with pachymetry less than 450 microns without waiting for actual progression. A CXL calculator has been developed to assist in such decisions.

Surgery

- Intracorneal Ring Segment implantation (ICRS) for mild to moderate cases who are contact lens intolerant. Advantage is that this process does not require any removal of corneal tissue. Corneal thickness >450 microns is required.
- Corneal Allogenic Intracorneal Ring segment (CAIRS) implantation has been recently introduced to flatten the conical in mild to moderate cases. It can be combined with collagen cross linking.
- Combined modalities of treatment like SMILE with CXL or femtosecond laser assisted INTACS with CXL are also being used.

- *Keratoplasty:* Deep anterior lamellar keratoplasty (DALK) has 95% success rate with advantage of no risk of endothelial graft rejection
- *PKP:* Used in full thickness scar and have high success rate.

Acute hydrops is managed by

- Topical measures like lubricants, hypertonic saline, steroids, antibiotics, cycloplegic agents and IOP control by AGM.
- 2/3rd of the anterior chamber can be filled with intracameral SF6 or C3F8
- Compressive sutures can be put oriented at right angles to the initial tear
- Endothelial keratoplasty
- PKP/DALK

8. Write briefly on peripheral ulcerative keratitis (PUK). (10) (TN MGRMU MS 2019)

It is a vision threatening inflammatory condition which causes progressive thinning of peripheral part of cornea characterized by epithelial defects and stromal lysis.

Two subdivisions:

1. Associated with systemic disease
2. Without systemic association disease, i.e., (Mooren's ulcer)

Incidence

0.2–3 persons per million populations. Middle and old aged females are more affected in this disease.

Etiology

Half of noninfectious cases of PUK are associated with connective tissue disorder, RA being most common

- *Systemic causes*
  - Infection – e.g., Varicella zoster virus n Syphilis
  - Autoimmune – e.g., Rheumatoid arthritis n GPA
- *Ocular causes*
  - Infection – e.g., *Staphylococcus*
  - Autoimmune disease – Mooren's ulcer n Allograft rejection
  - Trauma –
  - Neurological – xerophthalmia
  - Iatrogenic – post trabeculectomy, post-LASIK.
- Pathophysiology of PUK –
  - Both humoral and cellular immune mechanism plays a key role in pathogenesis. In contrast to central cornea, peripheral cornea has a rich vascular and lymphatic supply as blood vessels from limbus extends 0.5 mm on to peripheral cornea making it prone for immune reaction.
  - An imbalance between collagenase and tissue inhibitor results in increased matrix turnover.

Peripheral corneal endothelial cells are rich in high mitogenic activity –

↓

Corneal matrix turnover increased-

↓

Matrix metalloproteinase level elevates-

↓

Destroy extracellular matrix and keratolysis results.

Clinical Features

Systemic evaluation – is very helping in approach towards diagnosis Systemic features like subcutaneous nodules in upper and lower limbs associated with rheumatoid arthritis. Malar facial rash suggestive of SLE. Saddle nose can suggest for relapsing polychondritis.

Symptoms

1. Pain with decrease vision
2. Redness
3. Lacrimation
4. Photophobia

Signs

On slit-lamp examination

- Crescent shaped thinning at juxta-limbal
- Superimposed epithelial defect
- Loss of corneal stroma
- Conjunctival and limbal hyperemia
- Limbal infiltration with an overhanging edge
- Episcleritis
- Scleritis
- Corneal perforation
- Prolapse of Iris tissue
- Anterior uveitis or grade IV uveitis (hypopyon) may be present.

Staging of PUK

- Mild stage – localized PUK with less than 2-3 O'clock.
- Moderate – it is more extensive with 3-5 O' clock extension of peripheral cornea. Thinning of cornea is moderate.
- Severe - >5 O'clock hours corneal thinning with Impended corneal perforation.
- Perforated stage – present as an ophthalmic emergency.

Laboratory Tests

- Complete blood count
- Serum for ANA, Rheumatoid factor, Anti-citrullinated protein antibodies ACPA.
- CRP, ESR defines presence of inflammatory markers and indicate systemic vasculitis and autoimmune disease.
- CXR-PA view shows hilar lymphadenopathy in TB or sarcoidosis.
- CT-orbit and sinus is useful in GPA cases.
- AS-OCT – shows the depth of corneal thinning
- Corneal topography detects areas of corneal thinning.

Management

Medical Management

- Combination of topical lubricants, oral steroids and collagenase inhibitors with vitamin C rebuilds collagen in cornea and it is the mainstay of treatment.
- Preservative free lubricants and ointments are mostly preferred.
- Closure of puncta with punctual plug given in associated dry eye and helps in re-epithelialization of ulcer
- Topical cyclosporine promotes to reduce inflammation.
- Topical corticosteroids are controversial to apply.
- Topical antibiotic, topical acyclovir is used to address bacterial and herpes infection.

Systemic Medications

- Aim is to reduce ocular inflammation in PUK associated with systemic autoimmune disorder.
- Prednisolone (1 mg/kg/day) or methylprednisolone (1 g/day for 3 days)
- Steroid sparing agents i.e. antimetabolites such as methotrexate, azathioprine, mycophenolate mofetil, T-cell inhibitors like cyclosporine, tacrolimus, alkylating agents like chlorambucil, cyclophosphamide and biologic agents infliximab and rituximab are indicated to prevent from impending perforation.

Surgery—done only after inflammation subsided
High risk of recurrence
Melting of graft

Indications

- Corneal thinning
- Impending perforation
- Perforated cornea
  - Cyanoacrylate adhesive is applied to prevent from perforation
  - Lamellar, penetrating or crescentic keratoplasty and sclera-corneal keratoplasty with partial thickness scleral resection with scleral melting are possible options.
  - To reduce inflammatory load from conjunctiva, conjunctival resection or recession may be performed.

Prognosis

Depends upon severity of DS

9. Stains in fungal corneal ulcer—write short note. (5) (WBUHS MS)

Stains in fungal corneal ulcer can be used as follows:

In Vitro Staining

To diagnose fungal corneal ulcer, base and edges of the ulcer in anaesthetized cornea are scraped with a no. 15 blade or Kimura's spatula. Scrapings are spread thinly over a slide and can be stained with the following stains.

- *Potassium hydroxide (KOH):* A wet mount of KOH is the commonest in vitro stain to detect fungi in corneal scrapings. This has 90% sensitivity
- *Gram's stain* identifies yeast
- *Giemsa stain* is useful in detecting yeast and dimorphic fungi. The above two stains are only 50% sensitive.
- *Calcofluor white:* Fungal hyphae fluoresce bright greenish- yellow
- *Lactophenol cotton blue:* A mixture of methyl blue and lactophenol, this stains the chitin in walls of fungi blue
- *Gomori Methenamine silver:* Stains fungi grey or black and helps identify yeast or hyphae
- Periodic Acid Schiff: Stains fungal cell wall pink and helps identify yeast from filamentous ulcers

In Vivo Staining

- *Fluorescein:* Used to stain de-epithelized area of ulcer to demarcate extent of ulcer. Staining is done by placing a drop of sterile saline on a fluorescein strip, pulling the lower lid downwards and gently touching the bulbar conjunctiva with the strip. It is retained by underlying stroma and appears green in color when viewed under cobalt blue light.
- *Rose Bengal:*
  - Diagnostic use is to stain infected tissues but causes irritation. Hence fluorescein staining is preferred.
  - For augmented treatment of ulcers, Rose Bengal is a photochrom activated dye. Rose Bengal 100, 120 and 150 is applied and the ulcer subject to ultraviolet rays in the technique of PACK-CXL. It can also be used in combination with photodynamic therapy to act as antimicrobial. Although, the role of this augmented treatment in fungal corneal ulcers is not yet clear.

SUGGESTED READING

1. American Academy of Ophthalmology, 2023-2024 BCSC Section 8: External disease and Cornea. [online] Available from https://store.aao.org/basic-and-clinical-science-course-section-08-external-disease-and-cornea.html [Last accessed March, 2025].
2. Salmon JF. Kanski's Clinical Ophthalmology, 9th edition. Philadelphia: Elsevier; 2019. pp. 205-69.
3. Weiss JS, Moller HU, Aldave AJ, Seitz B, Bredrup C, Kivelä T, et al. IC3D classification of corneal dystrophies-edition 2. Cornea. 2015;34(2):117-59.

CHAPTER

Refractive Surgery

Prateek Nishant, Sony Sinha

QUESTIONS

1. **What are the criteria for good donor cornea? Discuss graft failure and graft rejection.** **(3+7) (WBUHS MS 2023)**
2. **Discuss corneal graft rejection, its management and prevention.** **(10) (DNB 2018)**
3. **DSEK: Discuss the procedure in brief—indications, advantages, and complications.** **(10) (WBUHS MS 2014, 2019)**
4. **Discuss artificial cornea.** **(10) (DNB)**

1. What are the criteria for good donor cornea? Discuss graft failure and graft rejection.

(3+7) (WBUHS MS 2023)

Criteria for a Good Donor Cornea: Include the following parameters:

- Optimal death-preservation time <6 hours in summer season, less than 8 hours in winter season in tropical country like hours. In colder countries it is prolonged to <12–18 hours.
- A donor not at extremes of age has better tissue, among which the younger ones have better tissue due to age-related endothelial cell apoptosis.
- No contraindications to cornea retrieval, namely:
  - Death of unknown cause
  - *Disease:* Cruetzfeld-Jakob disease, subacute sclerosing pan-encephalitis, active meningitis, encephalitis
  - *Infections:* Viral hepatitis, rubella, septicemia, fungal endocarditis, syphilis, suspected rabies, Chikungunya, dengue, H1N1, HIV, HCV infection
  - Active miliary tuberculosis
  - Leukemia and disseminated lymphomas
  - Ocular malignancy or inflammation

Evaluation of Donor and Tissue is done

- At the place of retrieval:
  - Torch and loupe examination or a portable slit lamp is used before and after removal to ensure that intra removal damage to the cornea did not occur.
  - Medical records are examined
  - Blood for serological examination taken from donor postmortem
- In the eye bank:
  - Slit lamp examination
  - Specular microscopy
  - Microorganism culture
  - Serotyping

Corneas are Best Used when

- For optical grade cornea:
  - Endothelial count >2,000/mm^2
  - Cornea is optically clear
  - Preservation time <14 days for cold storage donor tissue. >1500/mm^2 is considered adequate to cover for almost 50% loss of endothelial cells after corneal transplantation
- *For tectonic and therapeutic purposes:* Endothelial count criteria are not so stringent and lower counts are acceptable. Only medical exclusion criteria still apply.

Graft Failure

Primary corneal edema that fails to clear from the immediate postoperative period in the absence of severe hypotony or intense inflammation

Cause: Inherent deficiencies in the donor graft (prolonged death-enucleation time, poor endothelial count, extremes old age), surgical trauma or improperly stored tissue

Prevention: Proper donor selection as outlined above, good technique of tissue harvesting, good handling and preservation, early surgery minimizing preservation time.

During keratoplasty, liberal use of dispersive viscoelastic substance, minimal distortion during tissue handling and suturing, minimal contact with surgical instruments and avoidance of excessive irrigation of the anterior chamber help preserve endothelial cells.

Management: Early regrafting after 3–4 weeks of conservative treatment. A thorough review of and avoidance of the causative factor is essential.

2. Discuss corneal graft rejection, its management, and prevention. (10) (DNB 2018)

Graft rejection is specific immunological response of the host tissue to the donor corneal tissue. Rejection of graft corneal tissue occurs in 21% cases after penetrating keratoplasty, 10% in case of DSEK and 1% in DMEK.

Duration: Occurs after 2 weeks to years after primary graft. The incidence of rejection is highest in first year after surgery.

Cause: Donor-specific lymphocytotoxic antibodies are produced that lead to antibody-dependent complement-mediated lysis.

Risk Factors in PKP for Rejection

- Very young or old recipient age
- Previous graft failure
- Large or eccentric grafts
- Massive blood transfusion
- Preoperative inflammation
- Corneal neovascularization
- Loose sutures
- History of glaucoma medication and surgery

For DSEK, Risk Factors

- Preexisting glaucoma
- Steroid responders resulting in high IOP
- African American race

Symptoms

- Diminution of vision
- Photophobia

- Mild pain
- Irritation
- Redness

Signs of Graft Rejection

- Corneal edema
- KPs on graft but not on the recipient peripheral tissues.
- Deep vascularization in ≥2 quadrants of cornea
- *Stromal rejection:* Full thickness haze with DV
- *Epithelial rejection:* Rejection line which can stain with fluorescein or Rose Bengal begins in the periphery progresses across graft as epithelial cells get destroyed. Eye may be quiet or mildly inflamed.
- Subepithelial infiltrates or Kaye's dots are 0.2–0.5 mm white infiltrates seen below Bowman's membrane usually close to a suture in asymptomatic patients.
- Endothelial rejection—is the most common, occurring in 50% of rejection episodes. Khodadoust line originates at a vascularized area of peripheral donor cornea or at junction of anterior synechiae with the endothelium. It advances across cornea leaving behind damaged endothelium and pigmented keratic precipitates
- Diffuse rejection with KPs scattered throughout, edema (increasing thickness by 10%), Descemet folds and anterior chamber reaction may also occur.

Treatment

- Topical steroids are mainstay of treatment for acute graft rejection.
- For epithelial and subepithelial rejection where chances of reversibility is more, topical steroids can be used 6 times per day with gradual tapering over 6–8 months. Prednisolone acetate or difluprednate eye drops, dexamethasone eye ointment can be used.
- In endothelial rejection, topical corticosteroids are used hourly in combination with systemic therapy, either oral in 40–80 mg/day or single or three pulse IVMP therapy (500 mg). It can be combined with subconjunctival betamethasone (3 mg in 0.5 mL).
- As a corticosteroid-sparing agent, tacrolimus and cyclosporine are options. Tacrolimus can be used both topically and orally and help in both treating and preventing the graft rejection.
- Later clinical and intraocular pressure monitoring is done with tapering doses of steroids.

Prevention

The CCTS (Collaborative Corneal Transplantation Study) suggested that ABO blood matching may be effective in reducing the risk.

- Topical cyclosporine may be considered in high-risk grafts, repeated rejection episodes, one-eyed patients with large or eccentric grafts along with oral dose in selected cases.
- Corneal graft performed in eyes with active inflammation is more likely to reject.
- Tacrolimus, rapamycin, and anti-gamma interferon antibody are some of the new additions for treatment or prevention.
- Study showed that subjects with preoperative (pre-PKP) subconjunctival intrastromal injection of bevacizumab (5 mg in 0.2 mL) experienced no graft rejection in 26 months of follow-up.

3. DSEK: Discuss the procedure in brief—indications, advantages, and complications.
(10) (WBUHS MS 2014, 2019)

Endothelial keratoplasty (EK) refers to selective surgical replacement of corneal endothelium and adjacent corneal tissue, which retains healthy portions of a patient's cornea while replacing diseased innermost corneal layer(s) with healthy donor tissue. Briefly, EK encompasses removal of the posterior lamellar corneal tissue (lenticule) of the recipient cornea by a maneuver called Descemetorhexis, its displacement into the anterior chamber (AC) and removal through an incision in the peripheral cornea. A donor posterior lenticule is then inserted into the AC and apposed to the recipient bed using a large air or gas bubble filling the AC. A peripheral iridotomy fashioned inferiorly prevents pupillary block.

Descemet-stripping EK (DSEK) or automated EK (DSAEK) technique utilizes dissection of the posterior-most 100–130 microns of donor corneal tissue manually or by use of an automated microkeratome respectively, thereby providing a donor lenticule consisting of the endothelium, DM and some amount of pre-Descemet tissue for transplantation.

Donor corneoscleral button is mounted on artificial anterior chamber which is filled with air to create an interface for reference. With dissection spatulas, manual dissection is done at 95% stromal depth using the reference. Once complete, tissue is placed endothelial side up on a Teflon block and desired size of tissue trephined.

In the recipient, after conjunctival peritomy, a 5-mm sclerocorneal tunnel is made with 2 side ports at 10 and 2 O'clock positions. After injecting cohesive viscoelastics, Descemet membrane is scored with a reverse Sinskey hook and removed. After doing a peripheral iridectomy, viscoelastics are removed. Donor tissue is folded into a taco in 60:40 ratio, held with Utrata forceps at the edge with 60% side up and inserted through the tunnel into the anterior chamber. Anterior chamber is filled with balanced salt solution when tissue gets unfolded. With a 30-gauge cannula, air is injected to unfold the tissue and interface venting performed. After 10–15 minutes, 40% of the bubble is replaced by balanced salt solution.

Anterior segment OCT after a successful procedure clearly demonstrates a thick donor lenticule attached to the posterior stroma, tamponade by the residual gas bubble in the AC. Thus, although DSEK yields a thicker graft.

Indications

- Fuchs' endothelial dystrophy
- Congenital hereditary endothelial dystrophy and other dystrophies
- Aphakic and pseudophakic bullous keratopathy
- Failed penetrating keratoplasty (following endothelial rejection)

Advantages

- Minimally invasive, small incision procedure
- Low incidence of irreversible graft detachment and failure
- Repeatable
- Can use pre-cut and automatically dissected tissues thereby improving cornea utilization
- Good visual and anatomical outcomes
- Can be combined with cataract surgery and IOL implantation, or other surgical procedures.

Complications

- Graft inversion—reversed graft orientation during implantation leads to a graft that does not adhere to the underlying stroma. Reorientation and rebubbling of the graft corrects this complication.
- Graft detachment—poor graft adherence leads to detachment of large areas of the graft which can be observed on anterior segment optical coherence tomography and rebubbling done to tamponade it. Strategies that promote EK graft attachment include meticulous incision construction to avoid postoperative wound leaks, a firm air or gas tamponade, and ask patients to avoid eye rubbing, which could dislodge the graft.
- *Immunologic rejection:* Younger recipient age, African-American race and preexisting glaucoma or ocular hypertension are some of the significant risk factors for immunologic rejection of DSEK grafts. Subjects who continue using even a weak steroid eye drop once daily experience no rejection episodes, whereas those who discontinued topical steroids have 6% cumulative risk of rejection episodes. In most cases (70%), the rejection episodes are asymptomatic, mild, and discovered by slit lamp examination.
- *Intraocular pressure elevation:* It is a common complication after keratoplasty procedures. The risk of IOP elevation is significantly associated with steroid dosing, frequency and duration and controlled using glaucoma medications and steroid reduction.
- Lamellar interface abnormalities are a concern with EK but can usually be avoided with careful surgical technique. Fragments of the host Descemet membrane with guttae can distort vision and impair graft attachment if left in the interface.

- *Refractive abnormalities:* Irregular posterior graft surface will produce higher order aberrations that impair vision. There are 2 principal causes of posterior surface irregularity. The first is an irregular microkeratome cut or manual dissection during DSEK donor tissue preparation resulting in an irregular posterior corneal surface. Secondly, mismatch donor and recipient curvature will result in wrinkling of the donor tissue as it is applanated against the host cornea.

4. Discuss artificial cornea. (10) (DNB)

These are synthetic corneas meant to augment the shortfall in supply of donor corneas for keratoplasty. They are also the last option for patients who had multiple graft failures or rejections or those who are not suitable to undergo corneal transplantation using natural tissues.

An ideal prosthesis should have a moist surface, permit a good blink without exposure or immunological complications.

Classification

1. Collar-stud type
2. Soft optic and skirt from polymers with an intracorneal securing of the skirt within stromal layers
3. Device secured on external cornea and sclera with a central clear optical core

Boston KPro type 1 keratoprosthesis: Since its FDA approval in 1992, it is the most widely implanted device globally. It has a front plate with central optical stem, a backplate, and a donor cornea button sandwiched in between. The plates are made of PMMA and the power determined by the radius of curvature. Click on and Lucia models that have a two-piece design were also subsequently approved by FDA. However, long-term retroprosthetic membrane formation, sterile keratolysis and glaucoma limited application of these devices.

Boston KPro type 2 keratoprosthesis (1992) has a longer optic cylinder protruding through closed eyelid, although with less field of vision.

Boston mi-KPro: Has ultra-thin titanium backplate implanted anterior to the Descemet membrane while the optic penetrates the anterior chamber. The material permits limited biointegration while its flexibility helps to avoid microtrauma during blinking unlike previous devices and hence leads to less inflammation.

Osteo-odonto keratoprosthesis (OOKP): After intracapsular cataract extraction, anterior vitrectomy, and penetrating keratoplasty, the optic cylinder is fitted over the canine tooth of the patient and implanted under the buccal mucosa for 3 months. After this the implant with tissue skirting is taken out and placed in the previous graft area to replace anterior segment structures. It has good integration and less inflammation or dry eye. Hence, it is suitable for patients of Sjogren's syndrome, Steven-Johnson syndrome, chemical burns, Lyell's syndrome or ocular pemphigoid. Nowadays, tibial bone is being used in edentulous patients.

AlphaCor 2003 was the first approved fully synthetic prosthesis having poly-2-hydroxyethylmethacrylate but led to stromal melts and hence, is no longer used.

CorNeat has a central full thickness PMMA optic placed with central corneal trephination. Its polyurethane fiber skirt placed under and integrates with the host conjunctiva, the vascularity of which minimizes device extrusion although its rigidity and lack of bio integration pose limitations. Multicentric study for long-term outcomes is ongoing in France, Canada, Israel, and Netherlands.

EndoArt (Eye Yon Medical, Israel): 50 microns thick, flexible hydrophilic acrylic partial thickness 6-mm disc designed to function as endothelium. Implantation technique is the same as DMEK with the device held in place by an air bubble. Indicated for multiple endothelial graft failure or a bridge therapy while waiting for surgery. Early human transplantations are promising with reduction in corneal thickness and improved visual acuity.

GORE Synthetic Cornea Device: Has central optic with skirt of perfluoroalkoxy alkane with expanded polytetrafluoroethylene lining skirt and optic wall to enhance biointegration into recipient corneal stroma by placing it in a circumferential pocket. After animal tests, initial human tests are being planned.

Recombinant LinkCor, is a bioengineered corneal implant containing 95% collagen that recruits host cells for biointegration. Gene regulating natural production of collagen is introduced into specially programmed yeast cells. It can be implanted into the stroma by femtosecond laser assisted techniques such as FLISK or FLAP-FALK and held in place by full thickness suture.

Prognosis

- *Good prognosis:* In pediatric cases and chemical burns.
- *Poor prognosis:* After failed grafts, post viral keratitis, silicone oil filled eyes, aniridia and limbal stem cell deficiency.

SUGGESTED READING

1. American Academy of Ophthalmology. 2020-2021 BCSC Section 13: Refractive Surgery. [online] Available from https://www.slideshare.net/slideshow/aao-bcsc-20202021-13refractive-surgey/250613827. [Last accessed March, 2025]
2. Salmon JF. Kanski's Clinical Ophthalmology, 9th edition. Oxford, UK: Elsevier; 2019. pp. 277-89.

CHAPTER 11

Lens

Smiti Rani Srivastava, Rituparna Ghosh, Erum Hayet

QUESTIONS

1. **Short note on Toric IOL implantation.** **(5) (DNB)**
2. **Enumerate the options to overcome small pupil in cataract surgery. Risks and complications of phakic IOLs implantation.** **(5+5) (DNB 2020)**
3. **Write briefly on Phakonit.** **(10) (DNB 2021)**
4. **What are the types of pediatric cataract? Challenges in biometry of pediatric cataract and visual rehabilitation.** **(3+3+4) (DNB 2019)**
5. **Discuss management of pediatric cataract.** **(10) (WBUHS MS 2024)**
6. **Ophthalmic viscosurgical devices (OVDs)—what are they? Describe classification, uses and side effects.** **(10) (WBUHS MS 2024)**
7. **Optical biometry-short note.** **(5) (BHU MS 2020)**
8. **Discuss the Management of subluxated lens.** **(10) (WBUHS DO 2019)**
9. **Femto-laser assisted cataract surgery—discuss principle, advantage and disadvantage.** **(3+7) (WBUHS MS 2018)**
10. **Evaluation and management of postuveitic cataract /complicated cataract.** **(10) (DNB, WBUHS MS 2024)**
11. **Enumerate the types of secondary IOLs implantation in aphakia.** **(10) (DNB 2018)**
12. **Extended depth of focus (EDOF) IOL: short note.** **(5) (TNMGRMU MS 2020)**
13. **Write briefly on PCR management.** **(10) (WBUHS DO 2018)**

1. Short note on Toric IOL implantation. (5) (DNB)

Toric IOL Implantation

To remove cataract with refractive error like astigmatism toric IOL is the ultimate modality of current situation in anterior segment surgery.

Indications

- The ideal candidates for toric IOL are those with preexisting corneal astigmatism greater than 1D (1 to 6 D) with no corneal pathology
- *Corneal ecstatic disorders:* Mild to moderate keratoconus patients and other ecstatic disorders with regular astigmatism are considered as fit for cataract surgery with Toric IOL
- Postpenetrating keratoplasty patients.

Contraindications

- Patients with weak zonules
- Corneal scars and irregular astigmatism are relative contraindications.

- Poor dilating pupils prevent the visualization of Toric marks on IOL obscuring the proper alignment so surgery might be difficult.
- Patients with pre-existing retinal pathologies, postvitrectomized eye are not ideal for toric IOL implantation as visual outcomes are compromised.
- Intraoperative PCR.

Toric IOL Design (Fig. 1)

- Single piece hydrophobic acrylic IOL with dot or line axis markings are noted on posterior surface of IOL.
- Flatter axis is indicated by their markings and is to be aligned with pre-operative corneal markings.
- Toric IOLs can be monofocal, multifocal, extended depth of focus and phakic toric IOLs.

Preoperative Measurement

For Toric IOL implantation apart from patient selection SIA (surgery induced astigmatism) of surgeon is very important. Proper biometry and Toric IOL calculation done in taking considerations of SIA. Preoperative manual marking over cornea is done under topical anesthesia with patient in sitting position. Intraoperative alignment of the horizontal axis is done by using a Mendez gauze and finally marking of the desired axis is done along with IOL marking will be aligned. FLACS assisted marking can be done for more accuracy.

Well centralized round continuous curvilinear capsulorhexis of 5 mm is the choice to prevent the post-operative rotation. Complete viscoelastic removal from the anterior chamber and behind the IOL is must step to prevent rotation.

Wound is hydrated before the final alignment of IOL is considered. Patient is asked to maintain supine position after an hour of surgery.

Challenges (Figs. 2 and 3)

1. IOL misalignment—various issues are liable for IOL misalignment
   - Corneal marking technique
   - Size of capsulorhexis
   - The amount of capsulorhexis margin covering IOL edge
   - Sealing of corneal incision
   - Rotational stability of IOL
   - Surgeon experience
2. Misalignment ≥30°—In this case the cylindrical power got a new meridian. One degree of misalignment leads to 3% loss of effective power and 30° misalignment results in the loss of toric effect.

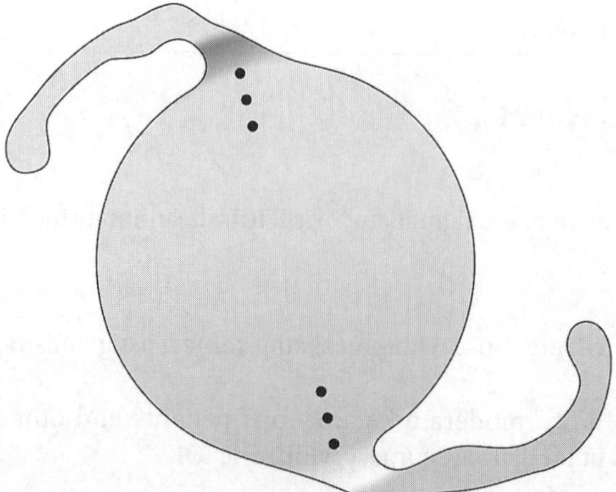

Fig. 1: Toric IOL.

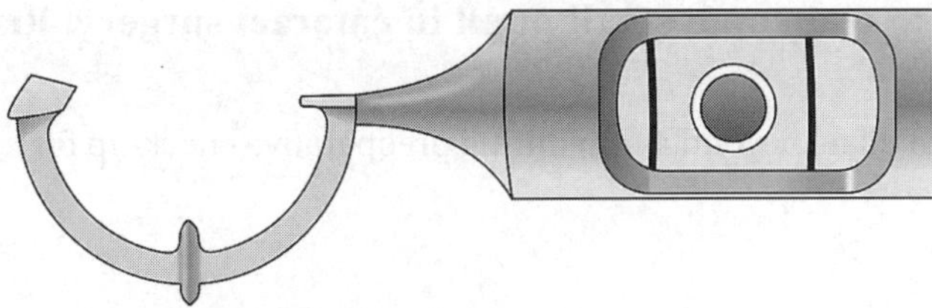

Fig. 2: Nuijts Solomon bubble marker.

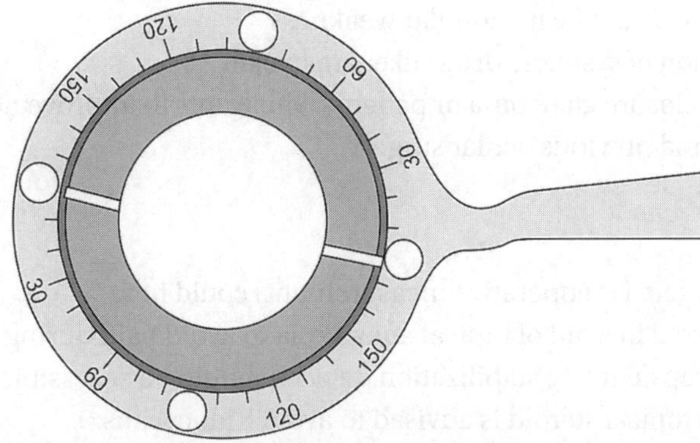

Fig. 3: Cionni toric axis marker.

Equipment for various measurements are mentioned in **Box 1.**

BOX 1: Equipment.

- Computing total corneal astigmatism
  - Swept-source imaging devices, AS-OCT
- Spherical power calculation
  - Optical biometry (IOL master/Lenstar)
    - Measures K readings using manual instruments
    - Axial measurement using A scan / B scan
- Pre-planning of Incision and IOL alignment
  - Online toric calculators are installed to plan the IOL alignment and precise incision like:
    - Barrett calculator
    - Alcon
    - Amos toric IOL calculator
- Pre-operative axial marking
  - Manual reference marking:
    - Marking thread
    - Geuder–Gotth pendulum marker
    - Nuijts–Solomon bubble marker
- Intra-operative alignment of IOLs
  - Manual marking
  - Intraoperative:
    - Mendez gauge
    - Boresch gauge
    - Nuijts-Solomon bubble marker
    - Clarity Toric Marker
  - FADES guided marking
  - Image guided marking systems—Verion, iTrace
- Phacoemulsification/ FLACS for implantation of IOL
  - Phacoemulsification machine
  - FLACS
    - Marks the incisions, capsulorhexis, and segmentation of nucleus

2. Enumerate the options to overcome small pupil in cataract surgery. Risks and complications of phakic IOLs implantation. (5+5) (DNB 2020)

A small pupil denotes a failure to dilate beyond 4 mm during preoperative check-up for cataract surgery.

It can be associated with:

- Diabetes mellitus
- Uveitis
- Senile miosis
- Pseudoexfoliation syndrome associated with zonular weakness
- Atonic pupil due to consumption of systemic drugs like tamsulosin
- Patients is on miotics in angle closure glaucoma or patients who wants to improve near vision
- Anterior segment dysgenesis and previous ocular surgery
- Laser or iris sphincter fibrosis.
- Iridoschisis

Precautions to be taken before surgery (Preoperative measurement) could be:

- Peribulbar anesthesia is preferred instead of topical anesthesia to avoid pain during manipulation of iris.
- Pupil expanding devices and capsular bag stabilization devices should be accessible.
- A short course of preoperative topical steroid is advised to avoid iridocyclitis.
- Miotics could be switched into another IOP lowering drugs.
- Topical NSAID thrice a day a week before surgery.

Intraoperative Measurement

The goal is to dilate pupil at least 6 mm to perform capsulorhexis and phacoemulsification.

Pharmacological Techniques

- Intracameral phenylepinephrine; phenocaine injection causes pupil dilatation.
- Intracameral lidocaine;
- Omidria; is a combination of phenylepinephrine 1.0% and ketorolac injection 0.3% added to BSS
- NSAIDs prevent intraoperative miosis.

Mechanical Stretching

- High molecular viscoelastic substances can be used as a pupil expander.
- Pupil sectoral iridectomy (previously used) which is sutured later after IOL implantation.
- Kuglen hooks or Sinskey's hook can be used for mechanical stretching of iris towards opposite direction.
- Beehler's pupil dilator is also considered as options for mechanical stretching.
- Cresentic cuts over iris by Vannas scissors leads to micro sphincterotomies.
- Iris hook–is basically made up of nylon with silastic sleeve hook.
- Pupil expander rings **(Figs. 4 to 6)**—cause expansion of pupil by stabilizing and protecting the iris tissue, e.g., the Perfect pupil, the Morcher pupil dilator ring, Bhattacharjee pupil expansion ring etc.
- Malyugin ring is most popular square foldable device made up of polypropylene which is injected into anterior chamber and removed from the eye with the injection system.

Risks and Complications of Phakic IOLs Implantation

Phakic IOL are IOLs implanted in the eye without removing the natural lens. They come into two categories (1) AC pIOLs which is further subdivided into angle supported AC pIOLs and iris fixated AC pIOLs. (2) PC pIOLs- ICL (intracameral lens).

- Risks of phakic IOLs implantation:
  - *Loss of corneal endothelial cells:* Angle supported pIOLs have highest risk of chronic endothelial loss which further causes endothelial decompensation.

- *Raised IOP:* Inserting pIOL near or at angle causes pupillary block.
- *Cataract formation:* Chronic inflammation and pIOL – lens touch induces cataract formation.
- *Pigment dispersion syndrome:* Rubbing of the eyes releases iris pigments over angle and endothelium. Pigment deposition in angle raises IOP results pigmentary glaucoma.
- *Retinal detachment:* High myopic patients may develop RD
- *Infection:* Larger wound incisions are the reason for infection.
- *Bleeding:* Due to iatrogenic trauma to iris causes bleeding.
- Severe inflammation (severe iridocyclitis)
- CSCR due to chronic postoperative inflammation
- May need additional surgeries like IOL repositioning, replacement or removal of IOL.

Complications of Phakic IOLs Implantation

- Glare – glare and halos in low light. Nowadays better ICLs are available to reduce the chances of glare and halos.
- Pupil ovalization
- *Corneal decompensation:* pIOL-corneal touch causes endothelial cell loss which contributes endothelium decompensation.
- *Bullous keratopathy:* Endothelial trauma or compensation of endothelial cells causes bullae over cornea.
- *Chronic subclinical inflammation:* It is a common complication as pIOL rubbing the posterior surface or cornea.
- Anterior subcapsular cataract.
- Pigment dispersion and pupillary block glaucoma
- Rhegmatogenous retinal detachment.
- *Endophthalmitis:* Large scleral and corneal incisions leads to endophthalmitis.

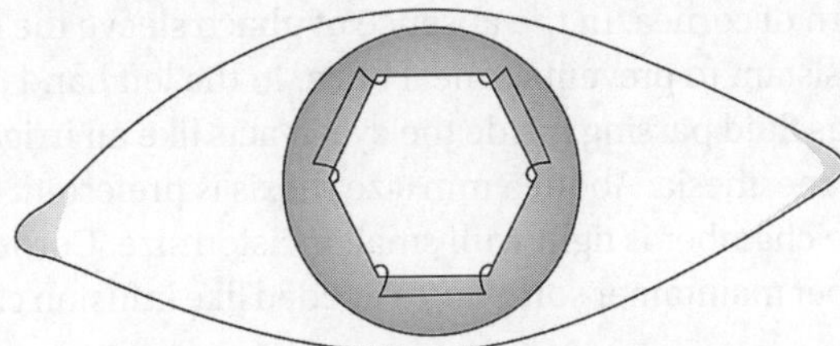

Fig. 4: Small pupil with B-Hex pupil expander.

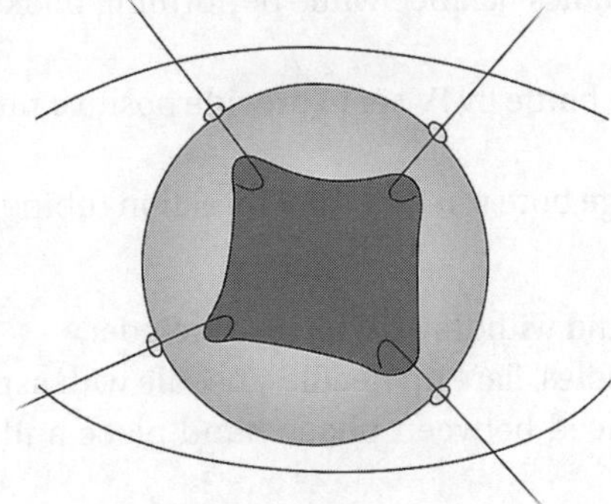

Fig. 5: Small pupil with four iris hook pupil expanders in a diamond shape (1.5 mm radial stretch at 4 contact points).

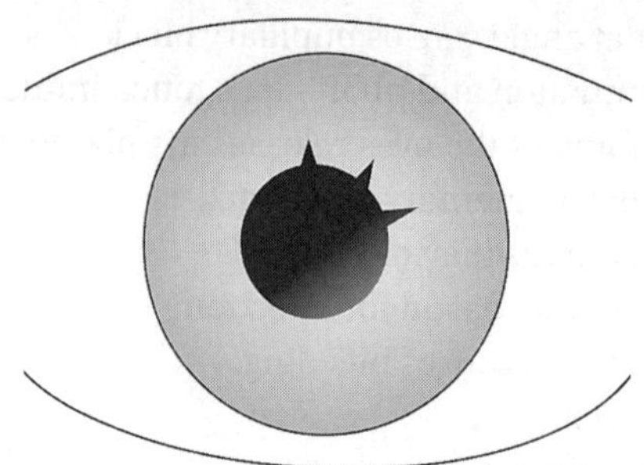

Fig. 6: Small pupil with mini sphincterotomy.

3. Write briefly on Phakonit. (10) (DNB 2021)

It is also called bimanual phaco, sleeveless phaco, and MICS.

It is a procedure of phacoemulsification using an incision of just 0.9 mm 1st performed by Amar Agarwal in1998. Word came from phacoemulsification with (N) needle opening via an (I) incision with the phaco tip. It is increasingly popular due to following reasons.

- Stabilization of refraction occurs in just 4–5 days compared to 2 weeks in phaco
- Less astigmatism
- Development of Rollable IOL
- Development of advanced instrument such as cold phaco to prevent corneal burns

Procedure: Phaco tip which has a diameter of 0.9 mm is introduced into the eye through clear corneal incision which is created by MVR blade without the infusion sleeve surrounding it. The infusion sleeve serves the purpose of cooling the phaco tip to prevent the thermal burn of cornea. In the absence of phaco sleeve the site of incision has to be constantly irrigated by cold BSS at 4^0 c by an assistant to prevent corneal burn. In the left hand through side port a bend needle (at present 18 gauge) was held which has fluid passing inside the eye. It acts like an irrigating chopper.

Mostly the cases done in topical anesthesia. About 5 mm size rhexis is preferred. Hydro dissection should be carried out with small amount of fluid as the chamber is tight with small incision size. Cortical wash is done with the bimanual irrigation aspiration. Anterior chamber maintainer sometimes needed like infusion cannula in a three-port phakectomy.

How to Maintain AC

Destabilization of anterior chamber in bimanual phaco is basically due to the fact that more fluid is moving out of the eye than entering at a given moment. Fluidics balance while performing phakonit is critical. Methods by which inflow can be increased include:

- Air pump is connected to the infusion bottle by IV set to provide positive pressure
- Gas forced internal infusion
- Two IV bottles are connected with large bore transurethral resection tubing instead of normal IV tube.
- Use of anterior chamber maintainer.

Conversely, methods which reduce the fluid withdrawn from eye include:

- Special phaco needles-micro flow needles, flare tip needles, needle with aspiration bypass system.
- Disposable flow restrictor device placed between phaco hand piece and aspiration tubing which restricts fluid outflow
- A small disposable device fitted on the aspiration port of phaco hand piece called vacuum surge suppressor which control egress fluid outflow

How to Prevent Thermal Burn

- Use of cold BSS at 4° C.
- Microflow needles—phaco needles with external grooves which allows fluids to flow.
- Two infusion bottles, one with regular phaco but with cut sleeve and one for the irrigating choppers.
- Cold phaco—Whitestar version 6.0

IOL – perfect IOL yet not available

- ThinOptx rollable IOL- these are made of hydrophobic material. They are ultrathin and carefully inserted through 1.4 mm incision. The natural warmth of the eye cause the lens to open gradually.
- Acri Tec IOL- Consists of hydrophobic acrylate. Introduced via injector through 1.5 mm incision.
  - If Rollable IOLs are available, the incision can be kept small. But these are not widely manufactured. One has to extend the incision to 2 mm, which is the lowest available diameter of commercial foldable lenses.

4. What are the types of pediatric cataract? Challenges in biometry of pediatric cataract and visual rehabilitation. (3+3+4) (DNB 2019)

Pediatric cataract is treatable childhood blindness. Early detection and management may restore visual outcomes.

Pediatric cataract may be:

- Congenital – present at birth
- Acquired – develop as an infant child or adolescent

Types of cataract as per morphology

Punctate Cataract

- Most common type
- Multiple blue spots are scattered over cortical lens.
- Variant – cataracta centralis pulverulenta
- Autosomal dominant (AD), nonprogressive

Zonular Cataract

- 50%
- Congenital or developmental
- Zone around embryonic nucleus become opacified.
- Opacity sharply demarcated and area of lens within and around opaque zone is clear.
- Linear opacities i.e., riders may run outwards.
- Autosomal dominant
- Associated hypovitaminosis D or hypocalcemia

Coronary Cataract

- Occurs at the age of puberty
- Situated in deeper layers of cortex and superficial layers of adolescent nucleus
- Corona or club shaped opacities near periphery of lens
- Nonprogressive
- Cataract doesn't affect the vision.

Nuclear Cataract

- It is associated with rubella
- When mother contracts rubella virus in 1st trimester of pregnancy.
- Associated with microphthalmos, nystagmus, strabismus, glaucoma, iris hypoplasia and pigmentary retinopathy.

Anterior Capsular Cataract

- Developmental
- Acquired – after perforation of ulcer in ophthalmia neonatorum.
- Three types:
  1. Anterior polar cataract
  2. Anterior pyramidal cataract
  3. Reduplicated cataract

- Associated with:
  - Aniridia
  - Peter's anomaly
  - Anterior lenticonus
  - Persistent papillary membrane (PPM)

Posterior Polar Cataract

It is associated with persistent hyaloid remnants, posterior lenticonus and persistent anterior fetal vasculature.

Other Types

1. Sutural cataract:
   - Opacity follows anterior or posterior surface of the lens.
   - Y suture.
   - Associated with other opacity
2. Membranous cataract:
   - Rare
   - Associated with Hallermann–Streiff Francois syndrome.

Challenges in Biometry

- Patients are not cooperative and its difficult to measure accurate parameters so GA is preferred.
- Eye is growing even after surgery which makes proper IOL calculation more challenging.

Biometry Parameters

- Axial length; in case of children axial length at birth is 17-17.5 mm which increases until 18 months of age rapidly followed by a slow growth.
  AL is estimated by immersion A Scan or indentation A Scan technique
  B -Keratometry; hand held keratometer can be used under GA in smaller children.
  C -Optical biometer can be used in older children for calculating AL and Keratometry.
  IOL power calculation: As these eyes are growing after surgery so a myopic shift is expected. To compensate that, hyperopia in immediate postoperative period is aimed.
- Dahan and Drusedau formula – children <2 years are under corrected by 20% and 10% under correction is suggested children between 2-8 years.
- *Prost formula:*
  - 20% under correction - between 1 and 2 years of age
  - 15% under correction – between 2 and 4 years.
  - 10% under correction - between 4 and 8b years.
    - Enyedi – IOL power calculation for the target refraction is (age + postoperative refraction) = 7
- *IOL formula:* Theoretical formulas that is SRK-T, Holladay 1 and 2 and Haigis are preferred over regression formula as they have least predictive error.
- *Criteria for IOL implantation:*
  1. Axial length > 17 mm
  2. Corneal diameter >10 mm.
- *Choice of IOL:*
  1. Hydrophobic acrylic lenses with square edges – prevent lens epithelial cell migration and posterior capsular opacification.

Types of pediatric cataract **(Flowchart 1)**.

Flowchart 1: Types of pediatric cataract.

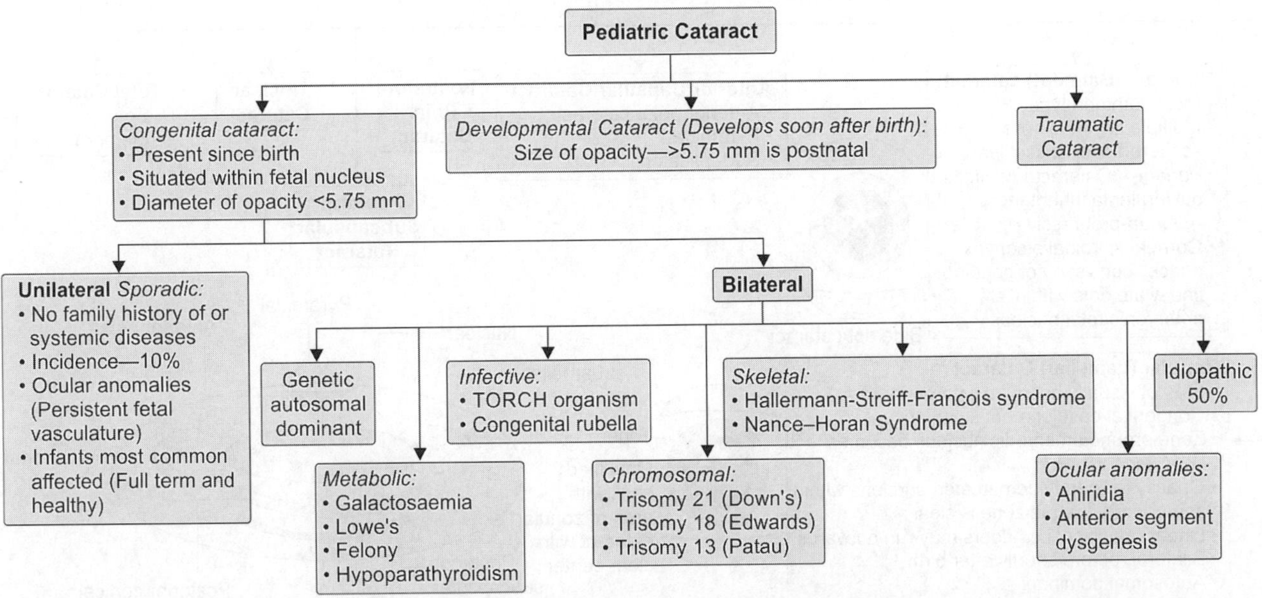

Visual rehabilitation after pediatric cataract surgery involves a combination of methods which includes;

1. *Glasses and contact lenses:* To correct refractive error and to prevent amblyopia as child is generally kept hyperopic. Refraction is repeated as the eye is growing and patient is asked for a regular follow-up till 8 years of age.
2. *Amblyopia therapy:* Regular patching and penalization with atropine in noncooperative patient with good counseling of parents required to achieve desirable vision.
3. *Management of aphakia:*
   - Spectacles- in bilateral aphakia, most children adapt well and develop good visual responses.
   - Contact lenses- in unilateral/bilateral aphakia. Better optical correction and long term result is comparable to primary IOL implantation.

   Rigid gas permeable lens/silicone/hydrogel lenses are the options of CL available.
3. *Management of pseudophakia:*
   - Single vision correction for young infants with near add of +3.00
   - Bifocals for toddlers aged 3 years and above
   - Progressive glasses for older children
   - Secondary IOL implantation in the sulcus for aphakic cases when child in 4-5 years of age.

The morphological classification of pediatric cataract is mentioned in **Flowchart 2** and **Figures 7**.

Flowchart 2: Morphological classification of paediatric cataract.

Morphological Classification

Punctate (Blue dot) cataract:
- Most common type
- Multiple tiny blue spots scattered over critical lens
- Variant— Cataracta centralis pulverulenta inheritance
- AD, non-progressive
- Corneal spiroidal/biconvex opacity consisting of ponding fine white dots within embryonic/fetal nucleus

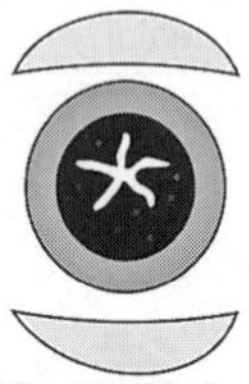

Blue dot cataract

Anterior Capsular Cataract
- Anterior polar cataract
- Pyramidal
- Reduplicated

Posterior Polar Cataract

Posterior Subcapsular Cataract

Nuclear Cataract

Total Cataract
- Soft
- Membranous

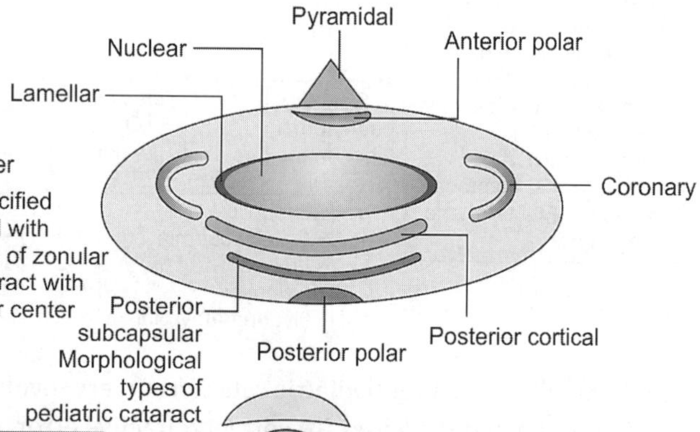

Zonular (Lamellar) Cataract
- 50% of visually deprived cataracts
- Congenital/developmental can occur
- Zone around embryonic nucleus becomes opacified
- Opacity is sharply demarcated and lens within and around opaque zone is clear
- Linear opacities, i.e., riders may run outwards
- Bilateral, before/shortly after birth
- Autosomal dominant
- Associated with hypovitaminosis D and hypocalcemia

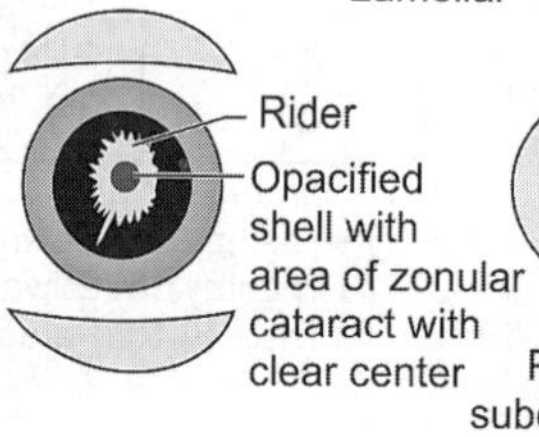

Rider
Opacified shell with area of zonular cataract with clear center

Pyramidal
Nuclear
Anterior polar
Lamellar
Coronary
Posterior subcapsular
Posterior polar
Posterior cortical

Morphological types of pediatric cataract

Coronary Cataract
- Puberty
- Situated deeper layers of cortex and superficial layers of adolescent nucleus
- Corona/club shaped opacities near the periphery of lens
- Non-progressive and does not interfere with vision

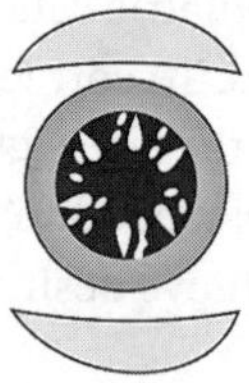

Coronary cataract

Polar Cataract

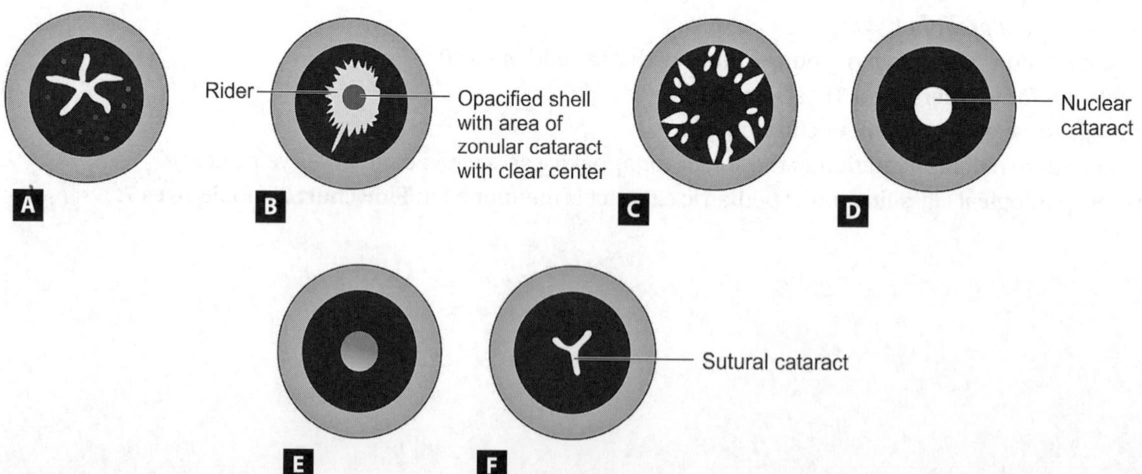

Figs. 7A to F: Types of pediatric cataract. (A) Blue dot cataract; (B) Zonular cataract with clear center; (C) Coronary cataract; (D) Nuclear cataract; (E) Posterior polar cataract; (F) Sutural cataract.

5. Discuss management of pediatric cataract. (10) (WBUHS MS 2024)

Pediatric cataract is a treatable cause of childhood blindness. Unlike adult cataracts, management of pediatric cataract is relatively challenging in terms of planning surgery, decision regarding implantation of intraocular lens, visual rehabilitation as well as lifelong follow up for early detection of any associated complications.

Common Causes of Pediatric Cataract

- Idiopathic
- Rubella
- TORCH
- Hereditary – familial/autosomal dominant
- Metabolic
- Traumatic
- Steroid induced

History Taking

A detailed history taking is very important. The points which should be remembered are:

- Antenatal infection
- Family history of childhood cataract- examine parents and siblings
- Drug intake/steroid use
- Birth and developmental history
- Metabolic disorder
- History of trauma

Ocular Examination

- Assessment of visual response in terms of C/S/M, preferential looking, fixation behavior, how briskly child follows light with each eye.
- Morphology of cataract
- Associated nystagmus, strabismus
- Dilated fundus examination if cataract is not dense.
- Assessment of red glow using Distant Direct Ophthalmoscope with an undilated pupil to determine if cataract is visually significant.

Investigations

- USG- B scan – done in dense cataract and Unilateral cataract to rule out persistent hyperplastic primary vitreous (PHPV)
- In bilateral and non-familial cataracts, the following investigations are done – TORCH screening, urine analysis for reducing substances and amino acids, karyotyping for genetic counseling.
- These investigations are not done in unilateral cataracts.
- Besides this, investigations for general anesthesia clearance include routine blood hemogram, BT, CT, APTT, stool for OPC, chest x-ray, 2-D echocardiography in syndromic children.

Role of Conservative Management

- Indicated in case of focal lenticular opacity where some part of clear lens is within the pupillary axis.
- A trial of mydriatic with patching of the better eye can be tried.
- Close follow up is essential in these cases to look for development of amblyopia

Indication of Surgery

- Location at posterior pole, posterior sub-capsular
- Presence of nystagmus, strabismus
- Bilateral dense cataract
- Unilateral dense cataract

Timing of Surgery

- U/L Cataract – as early as 4-6 weeks, as soon as anesthesia clearance can be given
- B/L cataract – 6-8 weeks. The other eye should be operated in quick succession, preferably within a week.

IOL Versus No IOL

Depends on the following factors:

- Age of the child – IOL is not implanted in children less than 7 months of age in view of unreliable biometry and myopic shift
- Anatomical factors - axial length < 19 mm and corneal diameter < 10 mm , anomalies in the angle – IOL is not implanted

Choice of IOL

- Single piece or multipiece PMMA lens
- Hydrophobic acrylic single piece (in-the-bag)
- Hydrophobic acrylic 3-piece (in sulcus)

Target Refraction

An ideal power should aim at prevention of amblyopia in childhood and least possible residual refractive error when the child becomes an adult.

- The various formulas used are – SRK-T, SRK -II, Hoffer -Q
- Age >4 years, 2-4 years: Undercorrection by 10%
- Age <2 years: Undercorrection by 20%

Examination under Anesthesia

A thorough examination is very important. It includes the following:

- Measurement of corneal diameter (vertical and horizontal)
- Axial length
- Pachymetry
- Intraocular pressure
- Gonioscopy
- Fundus examination if cataract is not dense
- Biometry for IOL calculation
- Anterior segment evaluation

Surgical Techniques

1. Lens aspiration + primary posterior capsulorhexis + anterior vitrectomy + intraocular lens implantation (LA + PPC+ AV + IOL)
2. Lensectomy with vitrectomy (via limbal/pars plana route); when primary IOL is not an option

Surgical Steps

1. General anesthesia, antiseptic dressing and draping
2. Scleral tunnel/superior clear corneal tunnel 2.8-3 mm in size
3. Anterior capsulorhexis – at least 6 mm in size. This is one of the most challenging step of the surgery as the anterior capsule is very elastic and has a tendency to run out. Staining the capsule with trypan blue, use of high molecular weight viscoelastic and capsulorhexis forceps helps to overcome the challenge.
4. Cortical aspiration
5. Posterior capsulorhexis at least 4 mm in size. It should be done in all children <8 years of age and also in mentally challenged children who will not allow YAG capsulotomy later.
6. Limited anterior vitrectomy – intact anterior hyaloid phase acts as a scaffold for lens epithelial cells to grow; hence chance of visual axis opacification is higher. Can be deferred if child is over 6-8 years of age.
7. Placement of Intraocular lens in the bag.

8. Section closure – all wounds including side-ports should be sutured with 10-0 MFN because less corneal and scleral rigidity in children.

Postoperative Management ***(Flowchart 3)***

- Topical steroids hourly which is tapered gradually
- Topical broad spectrum antibiotics for 2 weeks
- Topical cycloplegics for 2 weeks
- Oral steroids in selected cases.

Visual Rehabilitation

Timely correction of residual hyperopia with near add and amblyopia management with patching as long as needed.

1. *Management of aphakia:*
   - Spectacles- in bilateral aphakia, most children adapt well and develop good visual responses.
   - Contact lenses- in unilateral/bilateral aphakia. Better optical correction and long term result is comparable to primary IOL implantation.

     Rigid gas permeable lens/silicone/hydrogel lenses are the options of CL available.
2. *Management of pseudophakia*
   - Single vision correction for young infants with near add of +3.00
   - Bifocals for toddlers aged 3 years and above
   - Progressive glasses for older children
   - Secondary IOL implantation in the sulcus for aphakic cases when child in 4-5 years of age.

Complications

- Postoperative inflammation
- Glaucoma
- Posterior capsular opacification
- Retinal detachment
- Secondary membrane formation
- Pupillary capture of IOL/ IOL decentration.

The need for regular follow up and the risk of associated complications needs to be discussed with the parents pre-operatively. They should be educated about the importance of compliance to glasses and amblyopia therapy postsurgery.

Follow-Up

- Initially the follow up is done frequently in the immediate postoperative period to look for any signs of inflammation.
- There after it can be done every 6 months, and later annually when the child is older
- At every follow-up visit, detailed evaluation of anterior segment to look for development of posterior capsular opacification, IOL decentration, IOP measurement, cycloplegic refraction, fundus examination is done.
- Look for myopic shift in refraction and co-relate with the axial length along with IOP and optic disc changes to detect development of glaucoma in the earliest stages.

Flowchart 3: Management of pediatric cataract.

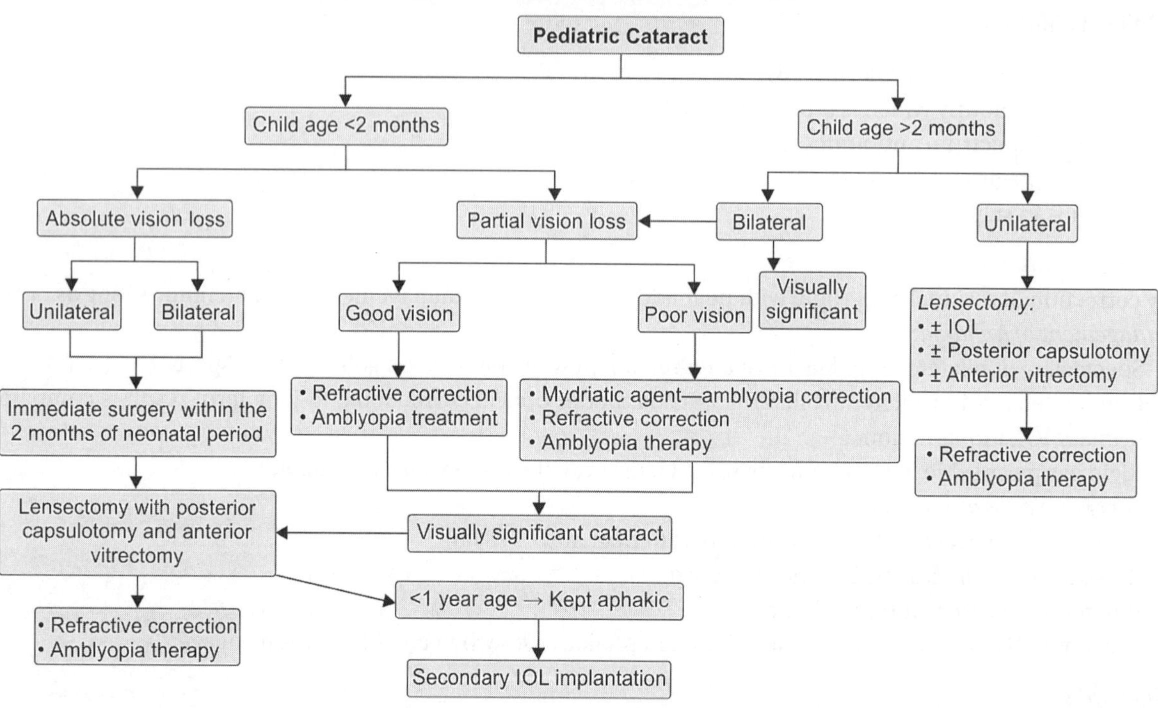

6. Ophthalmic viscosurgical devices (OVDs)—what are they? Describe classification, uses and side effects. (10) (WBUHS MS 2024)

Ophthalmic Viscosurgical devices are sophisticated biopolymers whose main constituents are glycosaminoglycans and hydroxy propyl methyl cellulose.

They are of various types:

1. *Cohesive:* It is a property by which the molecules of viscoelastics adhere to one another and form a clump. Higher the molecular weight, higher the surface tension, higher the pseudo plasticity, higher the cohesiveness of a viscoelastic. They are of:
   - Long chain and high molecular weight and high viscosity.
   - Used to create and maintain intraocular space during capsulorhexis.
   - Easy to remove.
   - Causes raised IOP, if not removed and tends to iris prolapse in shallow AC.
   - Minimal coating capacity

   E.g., Healon, Healon GV
2. *Dispersive:* They have less tendency to adhere to each other. They are of:
   - Low molecular weight, low surface tension, short chain and low viscosity
   - Low pseudoplasticity.
   - Used to coat and protect endothelium.
   - More difficult to remove than cohesive.
   - Can cause raised IOP by obstructing angle if not removed properly.

   e.g., Viscoat, ocu coat
3. *Viscoadaptive:* It is the property where it changes from a supraviscous state at a low shear rate to a pseudo dispersive at a higher shear rate.

They have properties of both cohesive and dispersive.
They are more viscous and cohesive at lower flow rate
They should be removed completely at the end of surgery otherwise can increase IOP
E.g., Healon 5

Physical Properties

- *Viscosity:* It means resistance to flow of a substance. Higher the viscosity of a viscoelastic, better is its ability to maintain a uniform shape and difficult to displace it from anterior chamber.
- *Elasticity/Viscoelasticity:* It is the property of a substance to return to its original shape after it has been stretched and deformed.
- *Psedoplasticity:* It refers to the ability of a viscoelastic to change from gel to a liquid under pressure. It is also defined as the ability to pass from a state of high viscosity at rest to low viscosity at high shear rates.
- *Surface tension:* It is the property by which a viscoelastic can coat the substance. It is governed by contact angle formed by a drop of viscoelastic on a flat surface. Lower the surface tension and low contact angle better coatability.

Uses

- Cataract surgery
    - *Cohesive OVDs:* Viscomydriasis is done in poorly dilating pupil.
        - Can be used to break posterior synechiae.
        - Maintain anterior chamber during running out of CCV
        - Blood from iris or angle, prolapsed iris tissue at incision site can be held back by cohesive OVDs
        - Deepen anterior chamber in hypermetropic eyes.
        - Intraoperative floppy iris syndrome (IFIS) occurs in patients treated with α-adrenergic blockers for prostate. Viscoadaptives are helpful to mechanically dilate and stabilize the pupil during surgery.
        - Dispersive OVDs- coat endothelium and protect cornea.
        - It is very useful in phaco surgery with compromised endothelium, e.g., endothelial dystrophy
        - Plugs PCR area and prevents vitreous prolapse in anterior chamber.
        - Magnification and clarity when cornea is coated with OVDs.it prevents dryness too.
        - Helps in separating the cortex from capsule - viscodissection

Soft Shell Technique

This technique reduces endothelial cell loss during phaco surgery in hard cataracts.

At the beginning of surgery dispersive agent is injected in AC followed by cohesive OVD beneath it thus pushing the dispersive OVD upward which is now coating the endothelium.

When nucleus and cortex is removed cohesive OVD is injected first followed by dispersive OVD. Cohesive OVD is now pushed against periphery of AC stabilize iris capsule and AC depth.

Viscoanesthesia- with intracameral lignocaine

3. Other Uses

- Viscocanalostomy in glaucoma surgery. In trabeculectomy it prevents endothelial trauma and maintain anterior chamber depth.
- *Corneal surgeries:* In penetrating keratoplasty it maintains anterior chamber before trephining and coat the donor corneal button while suturing to prevent endothelial damage.
- As a buffer agent in gonioscopy.
- During pan retinal photocoagulation procedure.

Side Effects

- Postoperative IOP spike and secondary glaucoma—OVDs especially Dispersive OVD can increase IOP by blocking angle if not removed completely.
- Cohesive OVDs can cause iris prolapse in shallow anterior chamber.

- Capsular block syndrome
- Crystallization of IOL surface
- Hypersensitivity reaction
- Corneal edema and decompensation

7. Optical biometry–short note. (5) (BHU MS 2020)

Optical biometry is a non-contact procedure which measures the distance from corneal tear film to retinal pigment epithelium in contrast ultrasound biometers measures axial length from anterior surface of the cornea to ILM of retina **(Flowchart 4)**.

Optical biometer also measures

- Central corneal thickness (CCT),
- Anterior chamber depth (ACD),
- Lens thickness (LT),
- Retinal thickness
- Radii of curvature of flat and steep meridian,
- Axis of flat meridian,
- White to white measurement (WTW) and
- Pupillometry.

Advantages of Optical Biometry

- It measures true AL of eye. Each subject has varied retinal thickness so an arbitrary value is added in measuring the biometry which is a source of false positive value in ultrasound biometry method.
- Optical biometry measures axial length from the Centre of cornea to macula along the visual axis providing more accuracy
- In case of posterior staphyloma optical biometers truly measures AL of eye.
- In silicone oil filled eyes the media changes. So the ultrasound biometers have to change the velocity of sound waves but optical biometers doesn't have to change it.
- As optical biometers is faster and noncontact procedure so it is more comfortable for patients.
- In ultrasound biometry more compression over cornea produces erroneous measurement but optical biometer is noncontact.
- The narrow wavelength of PCI measures much more accurate AL than broad wavelength of ultrasound biometers.

Disadvantages of Optical Biometry

1. The procedure and machine is much more costly than ultrasound biometers.
2. Limitation are dense cataract.

Flowchart 4 summarizes the important points about optical biometry.

Flowchart 4: Optical biometry.

Optical Biometry

Partial Coherence Interferometry (PCI)
- It has 180 nm Infrared laser in a dual beam setup
- Eye and photodetector are kept at each end of interferometer
- Partial beams are reflected at corneal surface of RPE
- Two beams of light which have a mutual time delay equal to twice the arm length difference of interferometer are introduced and light reflected from tissue interfaces
- The beam gets reflected at the anterior corneal surface and RPE due to position of interferometer mirror
- The interferometer detects a partial coherence interferometry signal which detects highly accurate axial length measurements and other refractive indices of ocular media with a resulting resolution of 12 μ
- Devices are:
  – IOL Master 500 from Carl Zeiss
  – AL scan from Nidek and Pentacam AXL from Oculus

Optical Low Coherence reflectometry (OLCR)
- It has 820 nm superluminescent diode in a standard Michelson interferometer setup
- The light divides into two beams by a coupler, one beam enters the eye, and the other is directed towards a scanning reference mirror
- Light is reflected at each tissue interface, and it is detected by the detector
- The emitted and reflected light travel coaxially
- The reference beam is scanned to produce an interference signal, and the exact location of the reflected light is detected
- Devices are:
  – Lenstar LS 900 (Haag Streit)
  – Aladdin (Topcon)

Swept Source Optical Coherence Tomography (SS-OCT)
- The source is a swift-sweeping laser.
- Interference signal detected by detector which under goes Fourier transformation
- No rotation of reference, mirror facility is noted
- Devices are:
  – IOL master 700 (Carl Zeiss)
  – Argos (Movu)
  – Eyestar 900 (Haag Streit)

8. Discuss the management of subluxated lens. (10) (WBUHS MS 2024, DO 2019)

When the lens is partially displaced but remain in hyaloid fossa it is called subluxated and when it is completely outside of hyaloid fossa and freely floating in vitreous, retina or anterior chamber it is defined as luxated or dislocated.

Diagnosis

- *History*
  - Recent history of trauma is most common cause.
  - Family history of cardiovascular diseases and Skeleto muscular abnormality in atraumatic cases.
- *Symptoms*
  - Reduced visual acuity of distant vision due to astigmatism and myopia.
  - Poor near vision due to loss of accommodation and monocular diplopia.
  - Reduction in degree of visual acuity depends on degree of subluxation or dislocation.
- *Slit lamp examination*
  - Phacodonesis
  - Iridodonesis
  - Vitreous in AC
  - Subluxated lens
  - Megalocornea
- *Retinoscopy*/refraction in both phakic and aphakic zone.
- *IOP measurement:* IOP may be elevated due to pupillary block or traumatic angle recession
- *Ultrasound biomicroscopy and anterior segment OCT* for zonular and angle assessment.
- *Gonioscopy for* pseudo exfoliation material and trauma.
- *Full dilated fundus examination* to see lattice, RD etc.
- *USG B Scan* if fundus view is obscured.
- Systemic examination/lab test

- Complete physical examination
- Total plasma homocysteine level for homocystinuria
- Cardiac evaluation for Marfan' syndrome.

Management

Medical management:

- Management of associated systemic conditions
- Refractive correction and amblyopia treatment if required.
- Pupillary block glaucoma treated with laser PI
- IOP elevation treated medically.

Surgical

Indications for surgeries are:

- Anisometropia or refractive error not amenable to optical correction
- Lens-induced glaucoma
- Lenticular opacity with poor visual function
- Lens-induced uveitis
- Impending dislocation of the lens
- Lens in the anterior chamber specially touching corneal endothelium
- In younger children to prevent amblyopia.
- Retinal detachment.

Management Protocol

See **Flowchart 5** in next page.

If capsule support is insufficient then slow motion phacoemulsification is done in low parameters and Capsular hook, CTR or CTR segments can be used. CTR is avoided if anterior capsule is torn or interrupted.

Vitreoretinal surgeon may be enlisted for pars plana lensectomy approach in severe zonular insufficiency. Premium IOL, e.g., Toric, Trifocal should be avoided here. If surgeon fails to implant single piece IOL then following options are there-

- 3 piece IOL can be placed in sulcus with or without optic capture.
- 3 piece IOL with haptics placed where there is zonular weakness.
- Scleral fixated IOL
- Posterior chamber iris claw lens
- ACIOL

Precautions During Surgery

- Excessive massage after peribulbar block should be avoided
- If possible, main incision should be given away from area of zonular weakness
- Stable anterior chamber – before leaving the anterior chamber Viscoelastics should be injected.
- Capsulorhexis - should be started away from zonular dialysis, creation of flap is most difficult step, large rhexis (6 mm) is preferred.
- Hydro dissection- gentle and in multiple locations preferred.
- Slow motion phaco- low vacuum with low aspiration rate with low bottle height.
- In area of zonular weakness, viscodissection to be done to remove nuclear fragments.
- If vitreous is present, it should be completely removed by anterior vitrectomy
- Slow irrigation and aspiration is the choice.
- Removal of cortical matter in tangential manner rather pulling directly towards center giving less stress to zonules.
- IOL implantation with large optics and large overall diameter is recommended with the haptic in the area of dehiscence so as to provide support.

Postoperative Complications

- PCR
- Nucleus drop
- IOL decentration and dislocation
- Capsular contraction syndrome
- Malignant glaucoma

Flowchart 5: Choice of capsular bag support.

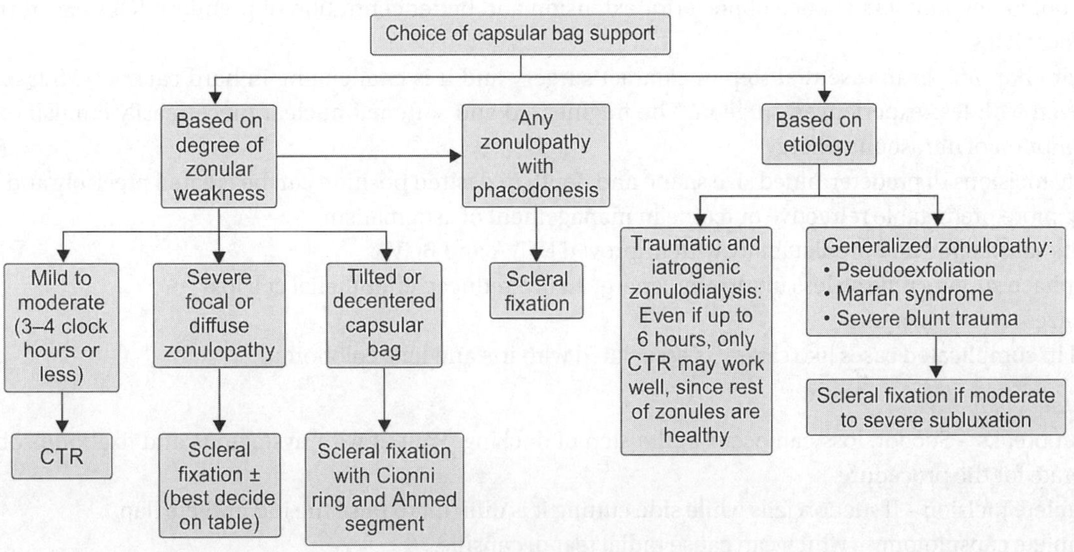

(CTR: capsular tension ring)

9. Femto-laser assisted cataract surgery—discuss principle, advantage and disadvantage. (3+7) (WBUHS MS 2018)

- Femtosecond laser is an infrared laser with wavelength of 1053 nm and pulse duration of femtosecond range i.e., 10^{-15} sec. Reduced duration causes reduced collateral damage of tissues i.e., 106 times less than Nd YAG laser. FSL is a focused infrared laser that uses ultrafast pulses with duration of 100 fs. It creates cleavage planes by photo disrupting transparent or translucent tissues **(Fig. 8)**.
- Focused laser energy is absorbed by tissues and plasma is formed.

↓

- The plasma of free electrons rapidly expands and induces shock wave, cavitations and bubble formation.

↓

- Force of cavitation and bubble cause separation of tissues.

  It creates very precise planes for:
  - Wound
  - CCC plane
  - Fragmentation of nucleus
  - Arcuate keratotomies for incisional astigmatism management.
- Before heading to the procedure, the settings of the machine to be done like corneal relaxing incisions, capsulotomy size, and the pattern of lens fragmentation.
- Patient is kept under laser unit after dilating the eye. The 3D-OCT assesses the anterior segment measurements, astigmatic axis direction etc.
- The laser is augmented by pressing foot pedal. Corneal incision created by docking. During pneumodissection, gas is released from cavitation bubbles between lens fragments.

- Corneal incisions are completed by separating preplanned programmed tri planer incision by FSL and capsulotomy flap has been removed. After doing hydro dissection and nuclear rotation, the softened lens emulsified by phacoemulsification.

Advantages of FLACS

- Precise thin uniplanar, biplanar, and triplanar corneal incision creation at desired site minimizing the chances of endophthalmitis.
- Good centration and predetermined size and shape of CCC – Round central symmetrical capsulorhexis causes better visual outcomes with less chance of posterior extension and better centration of premium IOLs e.g., toric IOL and multifocal IOLs.
- Nuclear chopping is an essential step in cataract surgery and it is challenging in hard cataract. FS laser makes it easy even with less experienced surgeon. The fragmented and softened nuclear pieces easily emulsified with less consumption of ultrasound energy.
- Arcuate incisions of predetermined size shape and depth in desired position can be created precisely and helping in getting more predictable refractive outcome in management of astigmatism.
- Patients satisfaction and predictability with Improved UCVA and BCVA
- Short phaco surgery time so less ultrasound energy hence reduced endothelial cell loss
- Minimizes stress to zonules
- Useful in complicated cases like cataracts associated with iris and lens coloboma.

Disadvantages of FACS

- Suction breaks – Suction loss can occur at the step of docking. Patient with nystagmus and fixation problem can't cooperate for the procedure.
- Incomplete incision – If suction fails while side cutting it is difficult to raise the incomplete flap.
- Incomplete capsulotomy – which can cause radial tear of capsule.
- Capsule tear- FSL induced CCC it is not technically a CCC but an advance form of can opener capsulotomy which can lead to tear.
- Persistence of bubble in stroma or anterior chamber – Intraocular gas formation within the tissue may dislodge behind the lens nucleus in the capsular bag can cause IOP rise followed by posterior capsular tear and lens drop. Removal of trapped bubbles by tapping over the lens with the blunt instrument before starting phacoemulsification is suggested.
- Intraoperative capsular block syndrome –it is a dreaded complication which may lead to PCR and posterior dislocation of crystalline lens.
- Poor papillary dilatation – As iris obstructs the capsular view, capsulotomy becomes difficult in this scenario. Pupil size more than 5 mm required.
- Expensive procedure
- High maintenance of machine

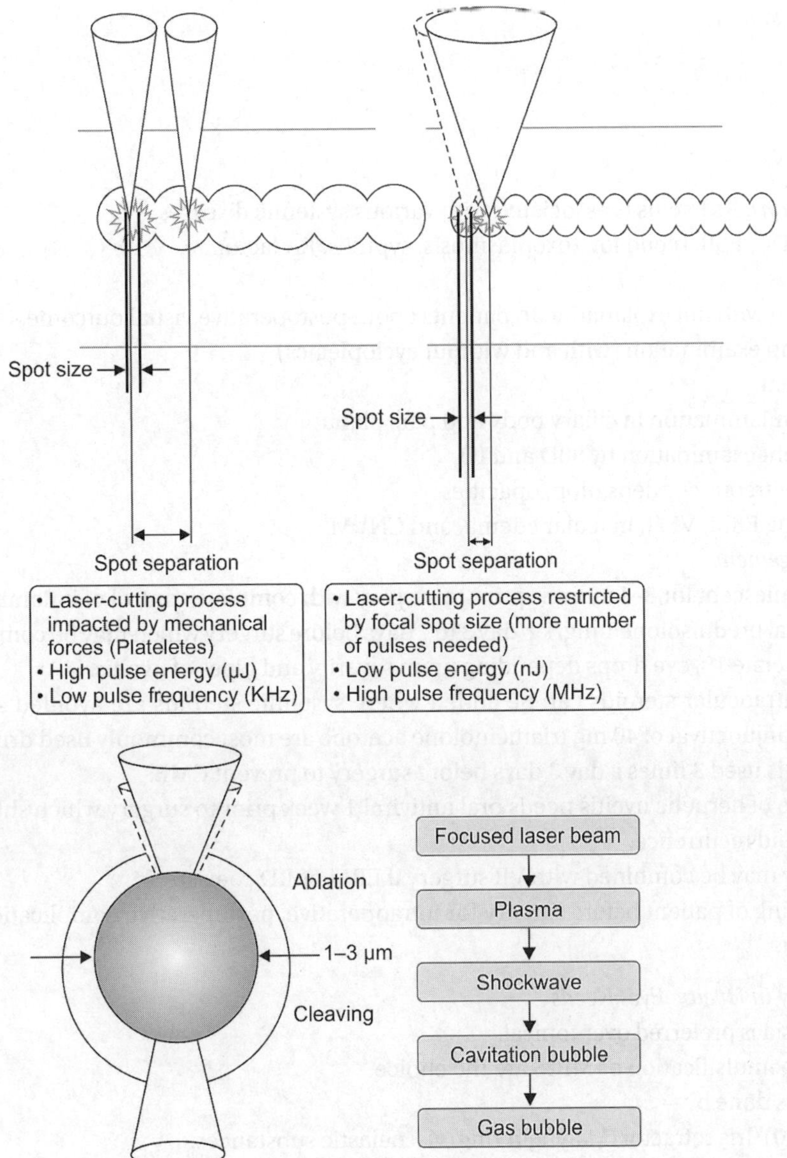

Fig. 8: Principle of FLACS.
Courtesy: Alcon Laboratories

10. Evaluation and management of postuveitic cataract/complicated cataract.

(10) (DNB, WBUHS MS 2024)

Cataract formation in uveitis is caused due to recurrent intraocular inflammation and prolong use of topical, periocular and systemic corticosteroid. Cataract surgery in uveitis is challenging and postoperative complications affect the final visual outcome so it is important to do a proper work up before surgery.

Challenges with Uveitic Eyes

- Small and irregular pupil,
- Pupillary membrane formation
- Posterior synechiae,
- Peripheral anterior synechiae.

- Shallow anterior chamber
- Vitreous haze
- CME
- Weak zonules.

Preoperative Work up:

- *Systemic examinations:* As uveitis is associated with various systemic diseases.
  - FBS, PPBS, TC, DC, ESR, blood for Toxoplasmosis, syphilis, RA factor.
- *Ocular examinations*
  - VA and PH vision with full explanation to patients about postoperative visual outcome.
  - Detailed slit lamp examination (with and without cycloplegics)
  - IOP measurement.
  - UBM to detect inflammation in ciliary body and pars plana
  - Posterior segment examination by 90D and IO
  - USG B scan for vitreous condensation, opacities
  - OCT for detecting ERM, VMT, macular edema, and CNVM
- *Preoperative management*
  - Eye should be quiescent for 3–4 months prior to surgery with complete control of inflammation.
  - Perioperative oral prednisolone 1 mg/kg/day 3 to 7 days before surgery which may be complemented with topical prednisolone acetate 1% eye drops depending upon severity and types of uveitis.
  - Periocular or intraocular steroids can be added where systemic steroids are avoided as in diabetes patients. Subtenon, subconjunctival of 40 mg triamcinolone acetone are most commonly used drug.
  - Topical NSAIDs is used 3 times a day 3 days before surgery to prevent CME.
  - Cataracts in case of herpetic uveitis needs oral antiviral 1 week prior to surgery which should be continued till 4 to 6 weeks to avoid recurrence.
  - Cataract surgery may be combined with VR surgery if ERM or RD coexist.
  - Proper counselling of patient before surgery for intraoperative, postoperative complications and possible visual outcome is must.

Intraoperative—Surgery in Uveitic Eyes Needs

- Peribulbar anesthesia is preferred over topical.
- Clear corneal phacoemulsification or MICS are the choice
- Pupil enlargement is done by—
- Adrenalin inj (1:1000)/Iris retractor/Malyugin ring/viscoelastic substances.
- Synechiolysis,
- Removal of pupillary membranes by rhexis forcep and viscoelastics.
- Pupillary relaxing incision
- Micro sphincterotomies
- Adequate size capsulorhexis of 5–6 diameter. Smaller size leads to capsular contraction and IOL displacement and posterior synechiae.
- Phaco emulsification in low parameter. Intact posterior capsule and keeping IOL in bag is must in uveitic cataract to prevent further inflammation and complications.
- Single piece foldable hydrophobic acrylic IOL is the choice.
- Minimum intraoperative manipulation is needed to have a good postoperative outcome.

Postoperative Care

- Topical corticosteroids – intensive use is indicated in immediate postoperative period i.e., prednisolone acetate 1% hourly
- Topical NSAIDs 8 hourly

- Broad spectrum topical antibiotics - 6 hourly
- Short acting mydriatics to avoid posterior synechiae e.g., tropicamide 6 hourly for 10–15 days.
- Corticosteroid eye ointment at night time.
- Oral corticosteroids in tapering doses if required in severe cases.

Complications

Intraoperative:

Due to irregular small pupil surgery is very challenging.

- Incomplete capsulorhexis,
- Iris prolapse,
- Zonular dehiscence due to long standing inflammation
- PCR
- Amsler sign—bleeding from filiform iris vessels (Air tamponade and intra cameral adrenaline can be used)
- Hypotony

Postoperative:

- Severe intraocular inflammation (topical steroid hourly, cycloplegics i.e., atropine and oral steroid in tapering doses are often required)
- IOP spikes/secondary glaucoma-managed with (Antiglaucoma medications i.e., β blockers and carbonic anhydrase inhibiter).
- Miotics, Alpha adrenergics and prostaglandin analogues should be avoided.
- Uveitis flare up (oral corticosteroid 1 mg/kg body weight.
- PCO- commonly seen in spite of uneventful surgery, managed by ND-YAG laser capsulotomy after inflammation is subsided.
- CME- managed with subtenon injection of 40 mg Triamcinolone Acetonide or intravitral steroids. In refractive cases oral prednisolone or immunosuppressives can be required.
- Hypotony-Rare and grave complication due to ciliary shut down.

11. Enumerate the types of secondary IOLs implantation in aphakia. (10) (DNB 2018)

Phacoemulsification with IOL implantation into the capsular bag and SICS are done routinely nowadays. Adequate support of IOL bag complex is a necessary for endocapsular placement of IOL, but if capsule is not intact, other IOLs with different surgical methods are to be considered **(Flowchart 6)**.

Indications

- After congenital cataract removal in children <1-2 years of age.
- Following PCR during cataract surgery with no or insufficient capsular bag
- Iatrogenic.
- Trauma with loss of crystalline lens.

IOLs and Technique

- Single piece or 3 piece foldable IOL in the bag.
  - A. 3 piece IOL in sulcus
  - B. Iris claw lenses
    - Anterior
    - Retro pupillary
  - C. Scleral fixation IOL

Flowchart 6 depicts the steps to manage aphakia.

Flowchart 6: Management of aphakia.

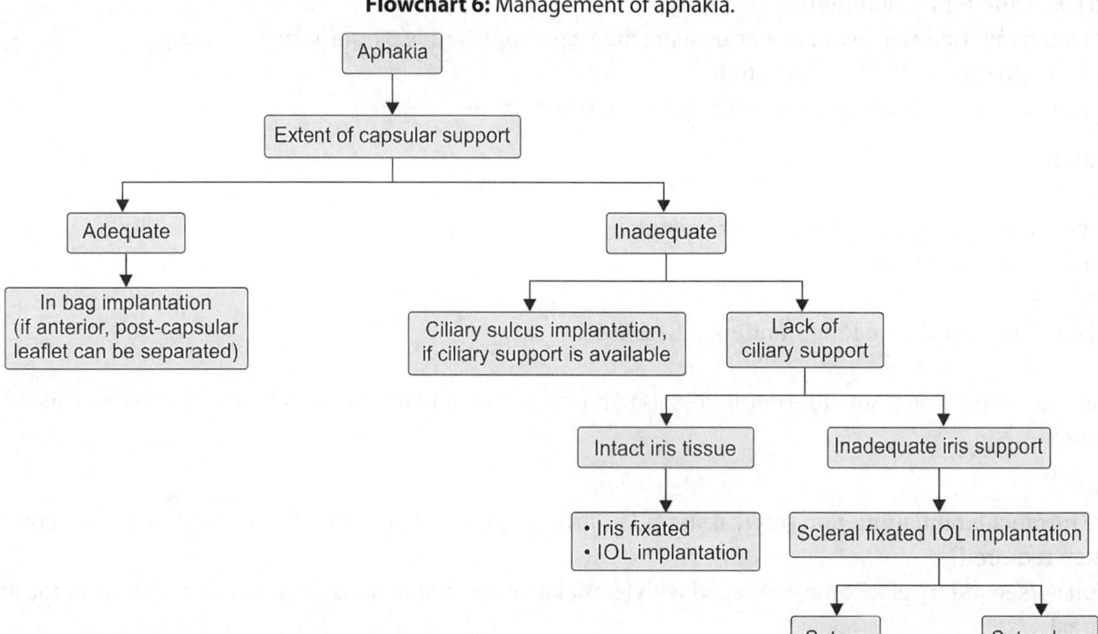

I. Single Piece or Three Piece Foldable IOL in the Bag

- Secondary IOL implantation in the bag is preferred choice in pediatric aphakia.
- Soemmering's ring or proliferating epithelial cells create a space between anterior and posterior capsule which is opened by a MVR 360° in small can opener movement and residual cortical matter if any is aspirated by vitrectomy cutter. Single or three piece foldable IOL implanted in capsular bag.

II. Three Piece IOL Implantation in Sulcus

The presence of intact anterior capsulorhexis rim is necessary for implantation of three piece IOL implantation in sulcus with or without optic capture. Optic capture gives stability to the IOL and prevents vitreous prolapse anteriorly and gives good centration of IOL and cause less myopic. The most definitive technique is placement of haptics in the ciliary sulcus with optic capture through CCC. The advantages are the long-term IOL stability, risk of reduced capsular phimosis and prevent zonular damage.

III. Iris Fixated IOL

Before implantation of iris claw lenses, AC should be free from vitreous so a meticulous anterior vitrectomy should be performed. Anterior chamber depth should be more than 3 mm is required to avoid endothelial loss.

Two types:

A. *Ante pupillary*
B. Retropupillary
   - It is effective in aphakic eyes with no capsular support.
   - It has quicker and better visual recovery.
   - It has fewer complications than the other secondary IOL implantation.
   - As it has lower invasive procedure and shorter surgical time there is reduced risk of photic retinal damage.
   - PI is required.
   - Retropupillary technique has more chance of posterior dislocation but deep anterior chamber and less endothelial damage are advantages.

Complications

- Endothelial cell loss due to shallow AC and closeness of IOL to endothelium.
- IOP rise due to iritis, iris chaffing and pupillary block.
- Ovalization of pupil
- Dislocation of IOL
- CME

IV. Scleral Fixated IOLs

Indications

- Insufficient iris tissues or capsular bag
- In case of a decompensated cornea
- Shallow anterior chamber.

It may be suture less or sutured.

Suture related complications like suture knot erosion followed by endophthalmitis can be avoided in suture less techniques like glued IOL. Yamane developed an easy technique where haptics of 3 piece IOL is externalized by using 27 gauge needle and then cauterized them forming bulbs at the end of haptics giving them more stability in scleral pocket.

- Intraoperative complications SFIOLs:
  - Unequal flaps may lead to unstable IOLs.
  - Hyphema
  - Iridodialysis
  - Improper tucking of haptics may lead IOL tilt and decentration.
  - Vitreous prolapse and iris peaking may occurs if vitrectomy is not done properly leading to vitreous and retinal traction in further future.
  - Thin flaps cause extrusion of haptics.
  - CME

V. Anterior chamber IOLs

- Nowadays it is an almost obsolete procedure.
- Complications –
  - ↑IOP
  - PBK
  - Uveitis glaucoma hyphema syndrome
  - Corneal decompensation
  - Chronic uveitis

Approached to fix scleral IOL are given in **Flowchart 7**.

Flowchart 7: Approaches for scleral fixation IOL.

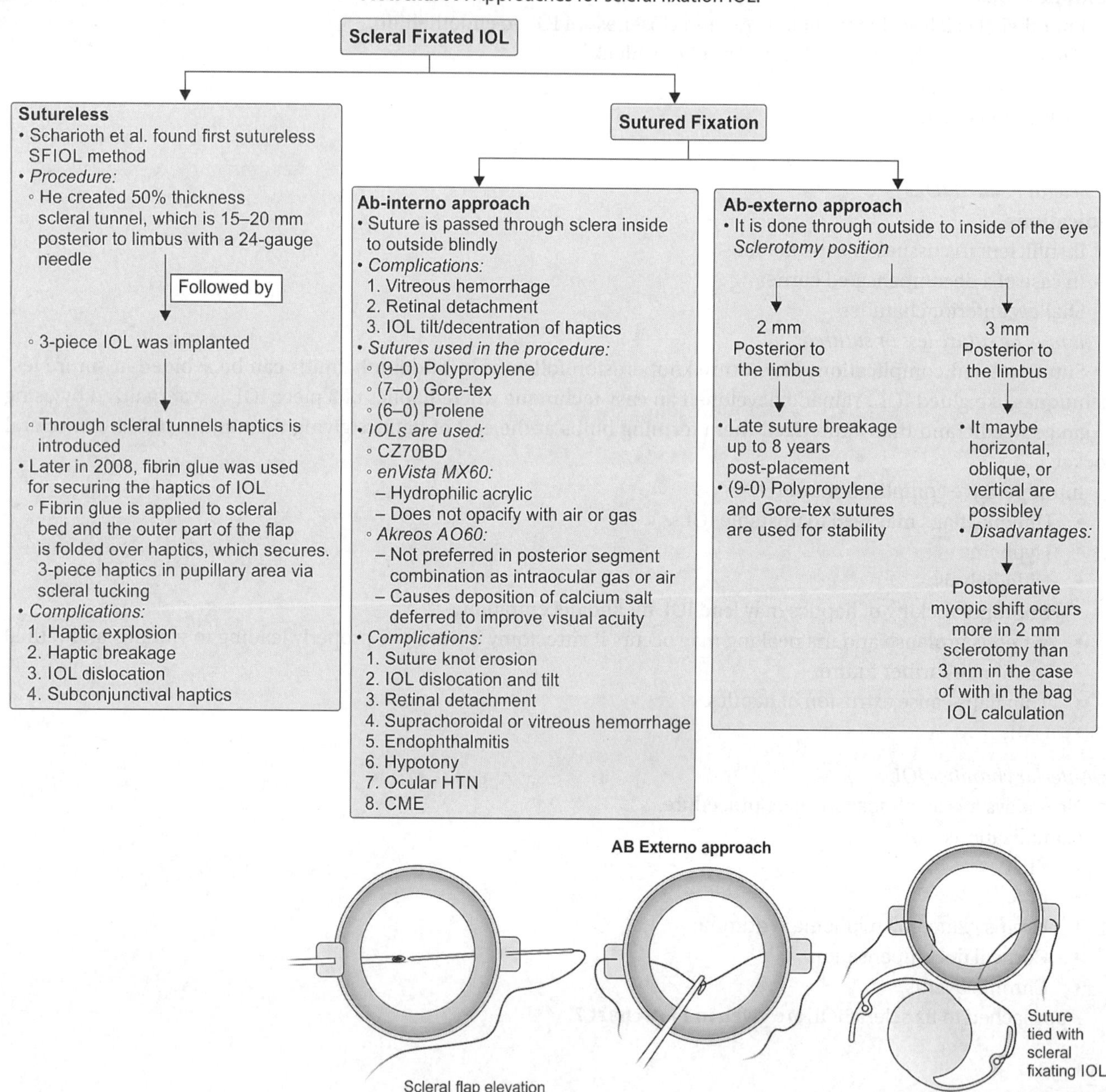

12. Extended depth of focus (EDOF) IOL: short note. (5) (TNMGRMU MS 2020)

These are enhanced mono focal presbyopia correcting IOLs which changes the power from center to periphery either by increasing the central power of lens or by elongating the focus by a wavefront modulation effect. This single elongated focal point enhance range of vision and depth of focus giving distant n intermediate vision **(Fig. 9)**

Advantages of EDOF IOL

- Good range of vision from distance to intermediate.
- Reduced glare, halo and dysphotopsia as compared to multifocal IOLs.

- Loss of contrast sensitivity is less than MFIOLs.
- Night vision is better than MFIOLs.

Disadvantages of EDOF IOL

- Provide inadequate near vision to read fine print. Surgeons can make non dominant eye for mild residual myopia (-0.5D) and dominant eye for emmetropia for better near vision in nondominant eye. So patients counselling is critically important.
- Unwanted photic phenomenon like glare halos.

Criteria to be Fulfilled for Good Visual Outcome

- Patient selection is very important considering age and occupation.
- Accurate biometry is must. Immersion technique or optical biometer preferred
- Round, well centered CCC of 5 to 5.5 mm with removal of all viscoelastics from bag and behind the IOL is must.
- Patient counselling is must regarding spectacle independence. Over expectations should be counseled.

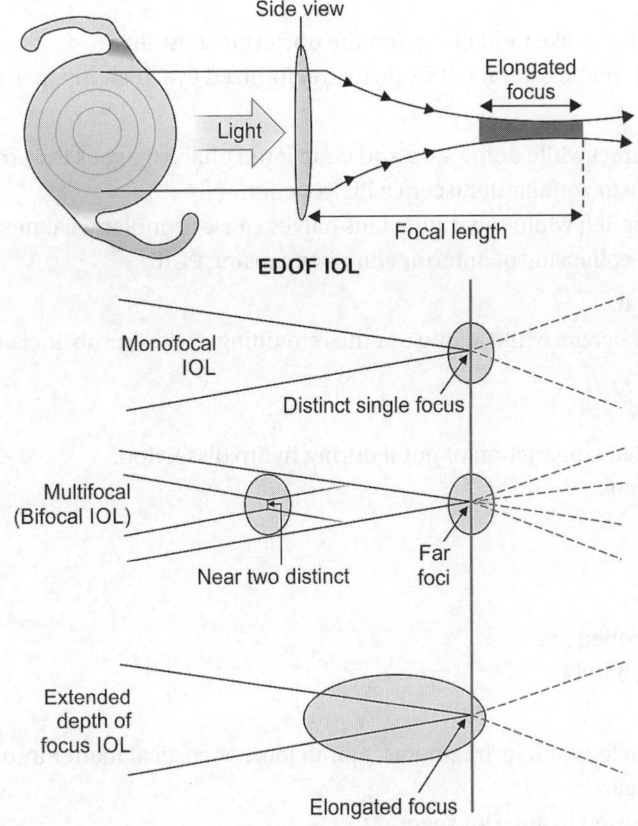

Fig. 9: Principle of EDOF.

13. Write briefly on PCR management. (10) (WBUHS DO 2018)

Iatrogenic breach in the continuity of posterior capsule is posterior capsular rent or posterior capsular tear.

It is a common intra-operative complication in cataract surgery which may be combined with vitreous loss, CME, RD, nucleus drop and IOL drop.

Predisposing Factors for PCR

- Poorly dilating pupil
- Excessive Shallow and deep anterior chamber

- Intumescent or hard cataract
- Fibrous capsule
- Pseudoexfoliation syndrome
- Poor visibility of media
- History of vitreous loss due to posterior segment surgery or repeated intravitreal injection.
- Inexperienced surgeon

PCR in Different Steps of Cataract Surgery

- Wound construction – Leaky wound leads unstable and shallow AC.
- Rhexis margin tear – It is two types curved/tangential and radial.
  - Curved RMT occurs mainly in young and pediatric patient as capsule and capsular zonules are highly elastic.
  - Radial – In morgagnian or intumescent cataract, rhexis runs out towards periphery.

Hydro Dissection

- *Blockage in outflow:* It occurs due to increase resistance by viscoelastic in anterior chamber or small pupil or small CCC.
- *Due to excessive fluid force:* Excessive fluid blows out the posterior capsule.
- *Inherent weakness:* PPC, traumatic cataract, PXF, postvitrectomized eye, high myopes are more prone for PCR.

During Nucleotomy

- *While trenching:* In soft cataract while doing stop and chop if the phaco tip goes towards periphery PCT can occur at the site. In hard cataract due to zonular dehiscence PCT occurs.
- *Splitting:* Excessive force applied while separating lens halves causes zonular weakness causing PCR
- *Chopping:* Sudden surge or collapsing of anterior chamber causing PCR.

During epinuclear plate removal.
During cortical aspiration: PCT occurs while taking out the remaining cortex in sub-incisional area.

Diagnosis and Confirmation of PCR

- Sudden deepening of AC.
- Snap sign of pupil i.e., sudden constriction of pupil during hydro dissection.
- Loss of followability of nucleus.
- Loss of nuclear fragments.
- Tilting of nucleus

Signs of Hyaloid Phase Rupture

- Posterior capsule torn and rolled up.
- Irregular depth of anterior chamber

Aim of PCR Management

- To prevent dislocation of nucleus and its fragments, epinucleus, or cortical matter into vitreous cavity.
- Prevention of extension of tear
- Prevention of vitreous prolapsed in anterior segment

Management of PCR

- *First step:* When PCR noticed, recede phaco foot pedal to position 1 (i.e., irrigation mode) from position 3. Ask the assistant to lower all parameters and meanwhile instrument in left hand is taken out from side port and OVD preferably viscoat is injected to the area of PCR (viscotamponade) then phaco probe is taken out slowly.

  If there is no vitreous loss (do staining with triamcinolone acetonide 4 mg/mL)

- 2nd Step – removal of nuclear fragment-
- After reducing all fluidics setting, nuclear fragments are emulsified slowly at the area away from PCR (viscoshield strategy).

- IOL scaffold technique -may be tried by experienced surgeon where multipiece IOL is inserted anterior to PCR creating a barrier and nuclear fragments are emulsified above it taking protection of endothelium by repeated injection of dispersive OVD.
- A posterior continuous curvilinear capsulorhexis can be considered in PCR without vitreous loss with the help of micro forceps which limits the extension of PCR and can allow foldable IOL in capsular bag.
- If nuclear fragments are large and if PCR getting extended, it is wise to convert into SICS or conventional ECCE .if patient is under topical anesthesia, subtenon or peribulbar block is preferred.

If vitreous strand is present in anterior chamber, stained positive by triamcinolone acetate.

↓

- Phacoemulsification should be avoided as it aspirate vitreous resulting more vitreous traction leads to RD. Bimanual anterior vitrectomy is performed with highest cut rate and low bottle height, vacuum and AFR in ICA mode (irrigation -cut-aspiration) Nowadays, 23G trocar-cannula system is used for vitrectomy to minimize too much vitreous removal.
- At first the vitreous at the site of PCR is cut to disconnect it with rest of the vitreous humor in posterior chamber then the loose vitreous is removed from anterior chamber.
- Excessive vitrectomy is avoided so bimanual pars plana vitrectomy is advised by many surgeons.
- Cortex is aspirated in IAC mode (irrigation-aspiration-cut) with low flow and irrigation to be kept far from PCR site. Cortex removal from PCR site should be done last. Controlled cortical removal can be done by bimanual IA.
- Surgical PI can be created by vitrectomy cutter.

IOL Preference

- In case of small PCR, where PCCC is performed, single piece IOL can be implanted in capsular bag.
- In large or peripheral PCR, after limited anterior vitrectomy 3-piece IOL is placed in sulcus. (0.5 D less)
- Iris fixated IOL, scleral fixated IOL is advocated in absence of capsular support. That can be done in second sitting after 4 to 8 weeks.

Postoperative Management

- Frequent topical steroids,
- IOP lowering agents,
- Cycloplegics,
- Topical NSAIDs for 3 months are prescribed postoperatively to prevent inflammation, CME.

SUGGESTED READING

1. AAO. AA0-2021-2022 BCSC Section11, lens and cataract. [online] Available from https://store.aao.org/basic-and-clinical-science-course-section-11-lens-and-cataract.html#:~:text=Section%2011%20of%20the%20Academy%27s%20Basic%20and%20Clinical,overview%20of%20cataract%20surgery%2C%20including%20in%20special%20situations[Last assessed March, 2025].
2. AAO. Eyewilki. [online] Available from Eyewiki.aao.org [Last assessed March, 2025]. Nema HV, Nema N. Current concept and recent updates of optical biometer. Recent Advances in Ophthalmology, Volume No. 14. New Delhi: Jaypee Brothers; 2017. p. 117.0
3. Al Shamrani M, Al Turkmani S. Update of intraocular lens implantation in children. Saudi J Ophthalmol. 2012;26(3):271-5.
4. Chakrabarti A, Kasturi N. Ten pearls for the management of posterior capsular rupture. [online] Available from https://www.eophtha.com/posts/ten-pearls-for-the-management-of-posterior-capsular-rupture#google_vignette [Last assessed March, 2025].
5. Chakraborty A, Nazm N. Posterior capsular rent: Prevention and management. Indian J Ophthalmol. 2017;65(12):1359-69.
6. Chang D. Bimanual phaco chop. In: Chang D. Textbook on Phaco chop. USA: Slack; 2004. pp. 239-50.
7. DOS. DOS times, Vol. 11, No. 3, September 2005, page 169. [online] Available from https://www.dosonline.org/about-dos-times [Last assessed March, 2025].
8. DOS. DOS Times Vol 12, no 7. [online] Available from https://www.dosonline.org/about-dos-times [Last assessed March, 2025].
9. DOS. DOS Times Vol 9, No 6, page no 390. [online] Available from https://www.dosonline.org/about-dos-times [Last assessed March, 2025].

10. DOS. DOS times – Vol. 13. No.1. July 2007 Page – 57. . [online] Available from https://www.dosonline.org/about-dos-times [Last assessed March, 2025].
11. DOS. DOS times – Vol. 16, No. 7, January 2011. . [online] Available from https://www.dosonline.org/about-dos-times [Last assessed March, 2025].
12. Harbansh Lal. Management of posterior capsular tear. [online] Available from https://docslib.org/doc/7440112/management-of-posterior-capsular-tear [Last assessed March, 2025].
13. Kanski J. Chapter 10. Textbook on clinical ophthalmology, 9th edition. Philadelphia: Elsevier; 2019.
14. Kim DH, Kim JH, Kim SJ, Yu YS. Long-term results of bilateral congenital cataract treated with early cataract surgery, aphakic glasses and secondary IOL implantation. Acta Ophthalmol. 2012;90(3):231-6.
15. Medsinge A, Nischal KK. Pediatric cataract: challenges and future directions. Clin Ophthalmol (Auckland, N.Z.). 2015;9:77-90.
16. Mohankumar A, Mohan S. Toric Intraocular lenses. Study Guide from Treasure Island (FL): StatPearls Publishing; 2023.
17. Nema HV, Nema N. Current concept and recent updates of optical biometer. Recent Advances in Ophthalmology, 1st edition. New Delhi: Jaypee Brothers; 2017.
18. Pandey SK, Werner L, Apple DJ, Agarwal A. Agarwal S, Agarwal AT. No anesthesia cataract surgery. In: Agarwal, eta l (Eds). Phacoemulsification, Laser Cataract surgery and foldable IOL, 1st edition. India: Jaypee; 1998. pp. 144-54.
19. Rojas B, Foster CS. Cataract surgery in patient with uveitis. Curr Opin Ophthalmol. 1996;7:11-16.
20. Wilson E. 2015. Pediatric Cataracts: Overview. [online] Available from https://www.aao.org/pediatric-center-detail/pediatric-cataracts-overview [Last accessed March, 2025].

CHAPTER

Glaucoma

Sandip Samaddar, Niranjan Karthik, Rituparna Ghosh, Arun Kumar Singh

QUESTIONS

1. **Ocular hypertension: Clinical features, evaluation and management.** **(3 + 3 + 4) (DNB 2020)**
2. **Write short notes on—Pre-perimetric glaucoma.** **(10) (RAN MS 2023)**
3. **Glaucomatous field loss. Discuss.** **(WBUHS DO 2019)**
4. **Normal tension glaucoma. Management and differential diagnosis.** **(10) (WBUHS MS 2019)**
5. **What is pathophysiology of Glaucoma? Describe the role of neuroprotectors in a case of Glaucoma. What is the role of Rho-kinase inhibitors in management of Glaucoma?** **(3 + 4 + 3) (DNB 2021)**
6. **Describe changes in Optic disc in Glaucoma. How will you differentiate from non-glaucomatous optic atrophy?** **(10) (WBUHS MS 2021)**
7. **What is meant by angle closure suspect? Outline of management.** **(10) (WBUHS MS 2021)**
8. **Describe the clinical features, evaluation, differential diagnosis and management of Pigment Dispersion Syndrome** **(2 + 2 + 3 + 3) (DNB 2019)**

   Gonioscopy findings of Pigmentary glaucoma and its management. **(RGUHS MS 2020)**
9. **Pseudoexfoliation syndrome: clinical features, evaluation and management.** **(2 + 2 + 3) (DNB 2023)**
10. **Neovascular Glaucoma-causes, clinical features and management enumerate the stages of NVG.** **(2 + 3 + 5) (2) (DNB 2021, 2023)**
11. **Angle recession glaucoma—short note.** **(5) (DNB)**
12. **Write Briefly on Aqueous misdirection syndrome.** **(10) (DNB)**
13. **Postpenetrating keratoplasty glaucoma—Short note.** **(5) (DNB 2023)**
14. **Indications, techniques and adverse effect of laser iridotomy, selective laser trabeculoplasty and argon laser trabeculoplasty.** **(3 + 4 + 3) (DNB 2020)**
15. **Discuss the Advances in trabeculectomy.** **(10) (DNB)**
16. **A patient with chronic angle closure undergoes a trabeculectomy and has a shallow AC on a first postoperative day. Describe the process by which you would discern the cause of postoperative AC shallowing and how you would manage this situation.** **(5 + 5) (DNB 2019, 2022, 2023)**
17. **Indications, pressure lowering effect, advantages, disadvantages and complications of iStent in glaucoma.** **(2 + 2 + 2 + 2 + 2) (DNB 2021)**
18. **Discuss briefly on Micro-invasive glaucoma surgery (MIGS).** **(10) (DNB 2020, WBUHS MS 2024)**
19. **Enumerate various implant drainage devices in glaucoma surgery. Indications and adverse effects of Ahmed Glaucoma Valve.** **(10) (DNB)**
20. **Goniotomy–short note.** **(5) (DNB 2022)**

21. **Classify the various non penetrating glaucoma surgeries. What are their indications, advantages and disadvantages over conventional glaucoma surgeries.** **(2 + 3 + 3 + 2) (DNB 2021)**
22. **Discuss Glaucoma Shunt procedures.** **(10) (RGUHS MS 2020)**
23. **Discuss Tube vs Trabeculectomy study.** **(5) (DNB 2019)**
24. **What is megalocornea? Difference between megalocornea and buphthalmous.** **(5) (DNB 2021)**

1. Ocular hypertension: Clinical features, evaluation and management. (3 + 3 + 4) (DNB 2020)

Ocular hypertension is defined as the condition where IOP raised >21 mm Hg which is two standard deviation among the population along with normal visual fields and optic nerve measured by standard test and open angles on gonioscopy. 1 in 10 will develop glaucoma in a 10-year period.

Risk factors:

- *Central corneal thickness (CCT):* CCT <555 μ were at greater risk of POAG than eyes with CCT >588 μ.
- Elevated IOP
- Increasing age
- *Pattern standard deviation (PSD):* Greater PSD correlated with increased risk of progression to POAG.
- *Cup-to-disc ratio:* Increase in cup–disc ratio leads to higher risk of progression to POAG.
- African race
- Males
- History of heart disease

Genetics:

- In white population it has been noticed that single nucleotide polymorphism in TMC01 is probably associated with OHT which may lead to glaucoma.
  Around 112 genetic loci have been found to relate with IOP which has a role for angiopoietin-receptor tyrosine kinase signaling, lipid metabolism and mitochondrial function.

Clinical features:

- *Symptoms:*
  - Usually no visual symptoms present
  - Sometimes patient may complain pain in the affected eye.
- *Signs:*
  - Elevated IOP: Consistently more than 21 mm Hg by explanation tonometry.
  - No glaucomatous disc changes usually seen (like asymmetric cup disc ration, notching or narrow of neuroretinal rim)
  - No visual field changes

Diagnosis:

- OHT is a diagnosis of exclusion.
- No visual symptoms and signs are noted in these patients.
- Family history may be present.
- Past history of DM, HTN, trauma, myopia, or oral contraceptive pills are noted.
- Use of systemic medications influencing IOP like steroids or beta-blockers should be rule out.
- History, slit-lamp examination and gonioscopic examination are done to diagnose glaucoma.
- Thorough ocular examinations to be done including tonometry, gonioscopy, optic disc assessment and visual field evaluation at periodic intervals.

Management:

- Raised IOP is a risk factor for development of glaucoma.
- According to OHTS trial, around 1–2% of patients are progressed to POAG during annual follow-up.

- Patients are stratified according to the risk of progression to POAG into:
    - High risk: Treatment is advocated, and at least 20% of IOP is recommended for lowering.
    - Moderate risk: Annual follow-up is needed. Treatment is resumed whenever earliest sign of glaucomatous change have been seen.
    - Low risk: IOP monitoring and optic nerve evaluation every 2 years.
- Prostaglandin analogs or topical beta blockers are the first line of treatment.
- Monotherapy is desirable with maximum of 2 medications.
- Frequency doubling perimetry (FDP) or short wavelength automated perimetry (SWAP) help detect glaucomatous damage at very early stages than white-on-white perimetry, and are useful in initiating therapy.

2. Write short notes on—Pre-perimetric glaucoma. (10) (RAN MS 2023)

Pre-perimetric glaucoma is described as the change in optic disc and RNFL damage in the absence of visual field defects in standard automated perimetry.

The individuals have elevated IOP, doubtful optic disc appearance, and visual field associated with risk factors.

Risk factors:

- Long-standing IOP elevation
- African or American race
- Family history of glaucoma
- Old age
- Central corneal thickness (CCT) <556 µm
- Cup disc ratio >0.4
- More than the average PSD in standard automated perimetry.
- Ocular and systemic risk factors are DM, HTN, high myopia, CVD and migraine.

On slit-lamp biomicroscopic examination:

- Anterior chamber depth
- Any association with secondary cause of glaucoma
- Gonioscopic examination—shows open angles frequently.
- *On fundus examination:*
  Classical signs are:
    - Increased or asymmetric cupping with diffuse or focal narrowing of disc margin
    - Recurrent disc hemorrhages
- The difference between glaucomatous and nonglaucomatous disc are tilted discs, large oval-shaped optic nerve head with thin rims and abnormal disc.
  Diagnosis of PPGs is given in **Flowchart 1**.

Flowchart 1: Diagnosis of PPGs.

Diagnosis of PPGs

Functional analysis:
- SAP
- SWAP
- FDT
- High motion perimetry
- Motion detection perimetry

Structural analysis:
- Ophthalmoscopic examination
- Stereoscopic photography
- CSLO
- SLP
- OCTA

Investigations:

- Stereo-photography of central fundus: It registers the baseline disc appearance, progression, and follow-up.

- *Automated perimetry:* Standard achromatic perimetry is used to evaluate the visual field loss. Short wavelength automated perimetry (SWAP) and frequency doubling technology can detect early visual field changes. Pattern standard deviation and mean deviation assess the between the healthy eyes and glaucomatous eyes. SWAP test examines the blue cone mechanism and the small bistratified ganglion cells which tracks progression. STATPAC points out the each point of visual field. GHT is an important parameter to detect PPG. Anderson Patella's criteria are followed to establish glaucoma progression.
- *High pass resolution perimetry:* It measures the P ganglion cells function which specifies the resolution of visual field.
- Frequency doubling perimetry is used to detect VF changes conventional standard automated perimetry. It targets the function of M ganglion cells carries information like flicker and motion, detects small amount of redundancy.
- OCTA measures ocular blood flow. Optic nerve head blood flow impairment confirms glaucoma progression.
- *Scanning laser polarimetry with GDx VCC:* It is a scanning laser polarimeter which measures nerve fiber layer thickness. It measures TSNIT standard deviation and nerve fiber indicator which quantifies the abnormal retardation patterns (ARP) may determine the glaucoma progression.
- *Scanning laser polarimetry with ECC (enhanced corneal compensation):* It also has a better performance than GDx-VCC. It provides quality images which indicate the lower point of RNFL thickness and higher NFI, gives a better correlation to perimetric values.
- Laser speckle flowmetry (LSFG) measures ocular blood flow in ONH. Mean blur rate is an index of relative blood flow velocity which is used for ocular perfusion.
- Abnormal circumpapillary RNFL thickness (cpRNFL) at least one clock hour in 6–12 o'clock establish the glaucoma diagnosis.

Conclusion: Observation and monitoring are the only choice of treatment.

Limitations:
- Stereographs cannot determine the subtle distinction between the glaucoma and healthy eyes.
- Abnormal disc fails to prove PPGs.
- These advanced tests cannot replace the gold standard tests for functional and structural tests.

3. Glaucomatous field loss. Discuss. (WBUHS DO 2019)

Introduction: Glaucoma is a chronic optic neuropathy that causes characteristic patterns of visual field (VF) loss.

Characteristics of visual field loss:
- VF changes are usually localized at first, but become wider, deeper, and more numerous as the disease progresses.
- The rate and mode of worsening vary greatly between patients.
- Visual field defects near fixation have a greater impact on function than peripheral changes.
- The initial defect may be located in the center of the visual field, not just in the periphery.

Pattern of field loss in glaucoma ***(Figs. 1A to F)****:*
- Field defects in glaucoma follow a pattern according to the extent of damage. The characteristic defect in glaucoma is the retinal nerve bundle defect that results from damage in the optic nerve head.
- The damaged nerve fiber bundle will correspond to the specific defect in visual field.
- Classical visual field defects nomenclature are derived from the appearance when they plotted on a kinetic visual field chart.
- *Earliest changes:* Suggestive of glaucoma consists of increased variability of responses in areas that subsequently develop defects; alternatively there may be slight asymmetry between two eyes.
- *Paracentral (B):* Small relatively steep depression, most commonly superonasally, constitute approximately 70% of early glaucomatous field defects. Since the defects respect the distribution of the retinal nerve fiber layer they terminate at the horizontal midline.
- *Nasal/Roenne/Step:* Represents a difference in sensitivity above and below the horizontal midline in the nasal field. It is commonly associated with other defects.

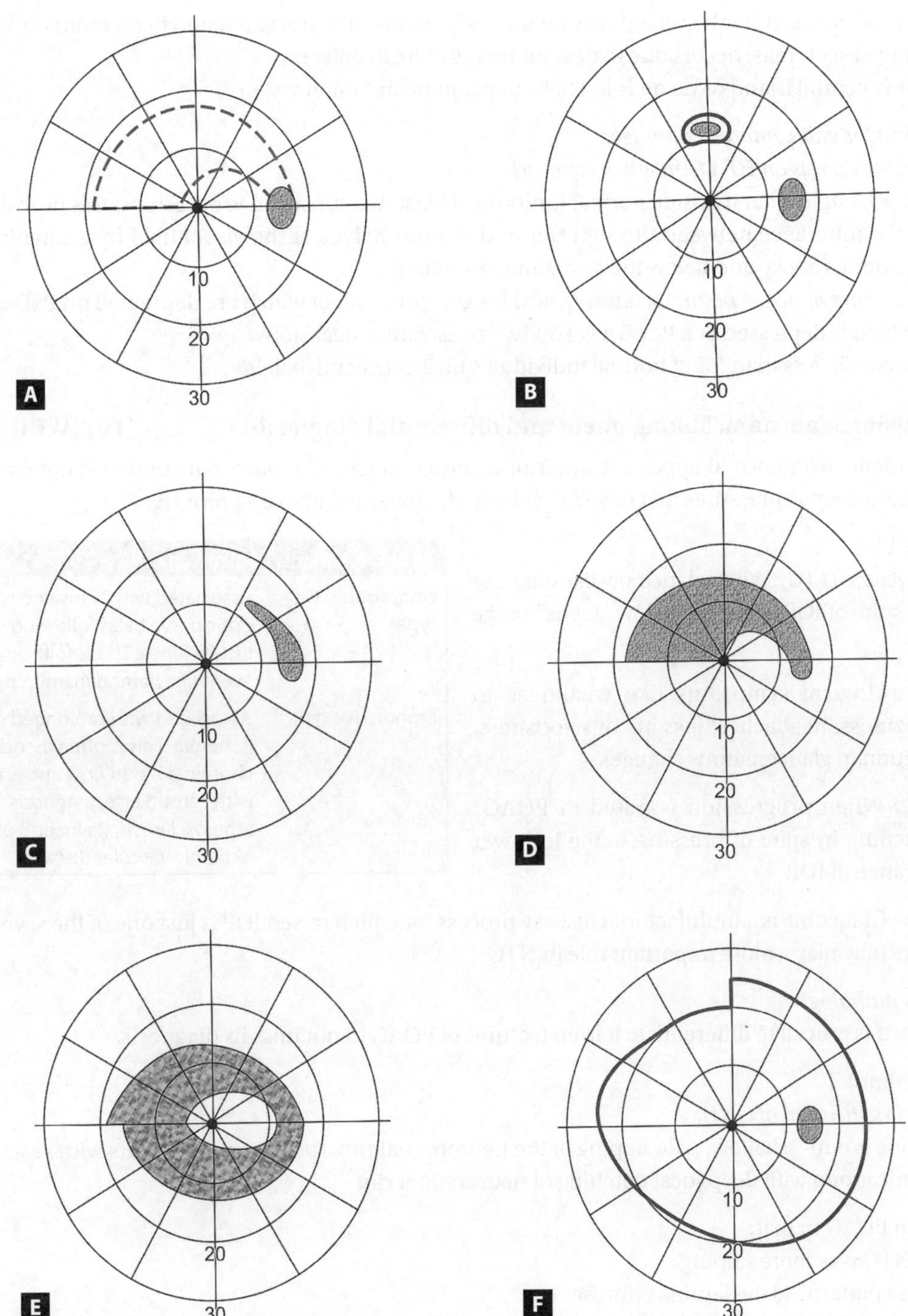

Figs. 1A to F: The patterns of field loss in glaucoma.

- *Arcuate-shaped:*
  - Formed from coalescence of paracentral scotomas
  - Develop between 10° and 20° of fixation in areas that constitute downward or more commonly upper extension from the blind spot around fixation (Bjerrum area).
  - Elongate circumferentially along the distribution of arcuate fibers (Seidel scotoma—C),
  - Connect with the blind spot (arcuate scotoma—D) reaching to within 5° fixation nasally.

- Arcuate scotoma on either hemifields simultaneously results in double arcuate/ring scotoma (E)
- Deepening of scotomas: occurs due to developments of fresh defects.
- Finally only central island of vision is left behind resulting in tunnel vision

Diagnostic criteria for glaucomatous damage:
One of the following defects on HFA (Anderson criteria):

- *Glaucomatous hemifield test:* Outside normal limits on at least two consecutive occasions; this provides information concerning the difference between the superior and inferior halves of the visual field by evaluating threshold at mirror image points above and below the horizontal meridian.
- *Cluster of 3 or more nonedge point:* location typical for glaucoma, all of which are depressed on PSD at a P<5% Level and one of which is depressed at a P<1% level on two consecutive occasions.
- CPSD that occurs in less than 5% of normal individuals on 2 consecutive fields

4. Normal tension glaucoma. Management and differential diagnosis. (10) (WBUHS MS 2019)

Introduction: Patients with normal appearing anterior chamber angle, who have glaucomatous optic nerve head and visual field changes despite pressures that have never been documented above 21 mm Hg.

Variants (Table 1)

Low tension glaucoma (LTG): When glaucoma-like changes are observed in spite of IOP being in the low "teens" range of normal value.

LTG plus: Neurological symptoms like weakness in extremities, dizziness, headaches, loss of consciousness, diplopia in addition to glaucomatous changes.

LTG equivalent: When progression is noted in POAG/ exfoliative glaucoma in spite of pressure being in lower side of normal range of IOP.

TABLE 1: Variants of glaucoma.

Nonprogressive type	Associated with transient ischemia of optic nerve head following vascular insufficiency. This is following an acute event like hemodynamic crisis
Progressive type	Associated with prolonged worsening ischemia. This is often associated with poor choroidal blood flow and is associated with carotid artery stenosis following atherosclerosis, Raynaud's phenomenon, ischemic vascular diseases

Pathophysiology: Glaucoma is a multifactorial disease process for which raised IOP is just one of the several risk factors. The other factors may play a more important role in NTG.

Ocular vascular pathology
Clinical features: It is crucial to differentiate it from features of POAG to not miss its diagnosis.

Fundus examination:
Morphological classification of ONH:

- Senile sclerotic group—shallow, pale sloping of the neuroretinal rim. (primarily in patients with vascular disease)
- Focal ischemic group with deep focal notching of neuroretinal rim

NTG differs from POAG in that:

- Cupping in NTG was more sloping
- An "hourglass pattern" to the lamina cribrosa
- Recurrent hemorrhages around optic nerve head (Drance hemorrhages)
- Nerve fiber layer defect is more localized in the NTG group as compared to more diffused loss in the POAG
- Large parapapillary atrophy particularly in Zone ß

Investigations:

- *Applanation tonometry:*
  - Characteristically bilateral but offer asymmetric
    - Studies have indicated that in glaucomatous eyes with normal but asymmetric IOP, worse damage usually occurs in the eye with higher IOP. To exclude NTG diurnal variation is must.

- *Gonioscopy:*
  - Performed to rule out angle closure, angle recession, or evidence of previous intraocular inflammation or pigment dispersion
- *Perimetry:* Visual field defects
  - Field defects tend to be closed due to fixation, deeper, sleeper and more localized.
  - NTG tend to present with more advanced damage in POAG.
    - Owing to delay in diagnosis
- *Other characteristic diagnostics:*
  - Reduced blood flow velocity in ophthalmic and ciliary arteries can be demonstrated with color Doppler.

Differential diagnosis of NTG ***(Table 2):***

TABLE 2: Differential diagnosis of NTG.

Undetected glaucoma	• POAG with diurnal variation • *Intermittent IOP elevation*: – Angle closure suspect – Glaucomatocyclitic crisis • *Previously elevated IOP*: – Old secondary glaucoma • Normal IOP in an eye with previously elevated IOP
Nonglaucomatous optic nerve disease	• Congenital anomalies • Compressive lesion of optic nerve and chiasma • Shock optic neuropathy • Anterior ischemic optic neuropathy • Optic nerve drusen

Treatment ***(Flowchart 2):***

Indications:

- Visual field threatening fixation
- IOP higher ranges 16–20 mm Hg
- *Splinter hemorrhages:*
  - Documented progression of field defects or optic disc cupping
- Risk factors like female and history of migraine

Flowchart 2: When to start treatment for NTG.

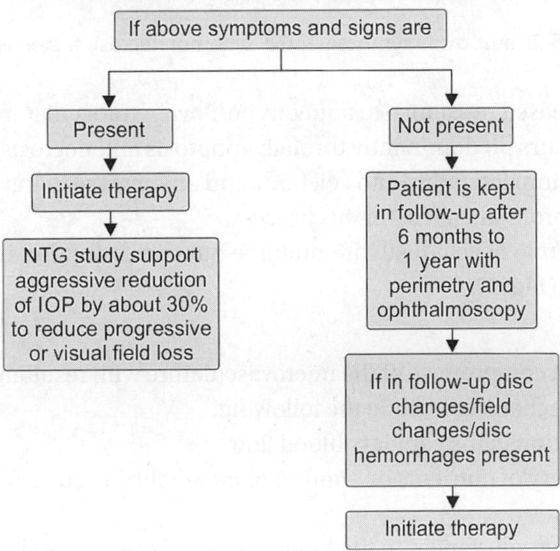

Medical treatment:
- Topical therapy is the most common initial approach in management of Normal tension glaucoma (prostaglandin analogs to have a greater ocular hypotensive effect in eyes)
- Treatment in a progressive case may include betaxolol because of its beneficial effect on the optic nerve blood flow in addition to its IOP lowering action.

Other modalities:
- *Laser trabeculoplasty:* Should be considered in one eye if the progression of visual field loss occurs despite IOP lowering medications
- *Glaucoma filtering surgery:* Should be considered if medical management fails

5. What is pathophysiology of Glaucoma? Describe the role of neuroprotectors in a case of Glaucoma. What is the role of Rho-kinase inhibitors in management of Glaucoma? (3 + 4 + 3) (DNB 2021)

Glaucoma is chronic optic neuropathy characterized by progressive damage to the optic nerve, death of the retinal ganglion cells and ultimately visual field loss. It is one of the leading cause of irreversible loss of vision worldwide. The most important trigger of glaucomatous damage is elevated eye pressure.

Pathophysiology of neuronal death **(Flowchart 3)**

Flowchart 3: The complex interplay of primary and secondary factors leading to RGC apoptosis in glaucoma.

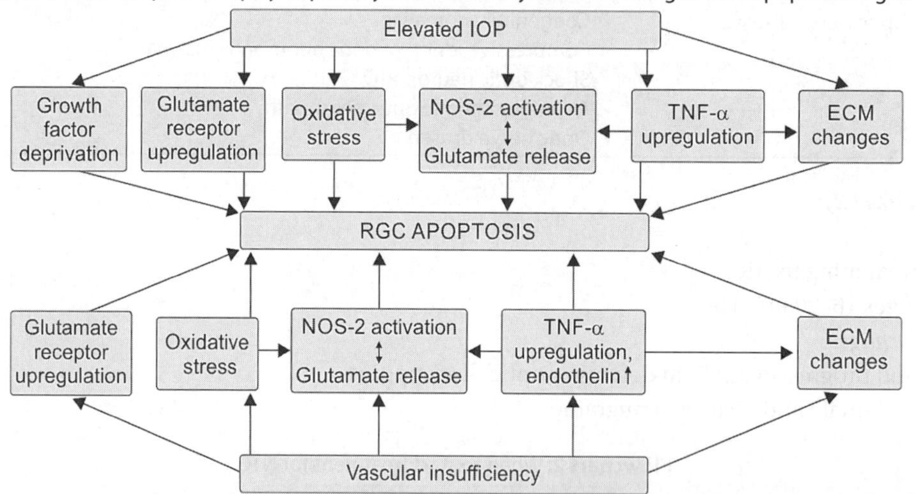

(ECM: extracellular matrix; NOS-2: nitric oxide synthase-2; TNF-α: tumor necrosis factor alpha; RGC: retinal ganglion cell)

- Elevation in IOP is due to increased resistance to aqueous outflow in trabecular meshwork.
- Retinal ganglion cell death occurs predominantly through apoptosis and necrosis as shown in **Figure 2.**
- The predominant event is calcium ion influx into cell body and an increase in intracellular NO.
- Glutamine metabolism has a profound effect on this process.
- The factors that influence the role of cell death are multiple but current option is polarized between ischemic and mechanical causes of damage **(Fig. 3)**.

Theories of pathogenesis:
1. *Ischemic theory:* Postulates that compromise of the microvasculature with resultant ischemia in the optic nerve head is responsible. The possible mechanism include the following:
   a. Loss of capillaries or alteration in the capillary blood flow
   b. Interference with the delivery of nutrients or removal of metabolic products from axons
   c. Failure of blood flow regulation
   d. Delivery of hostile vasoactive substances to the blood vessels of optic nerve head

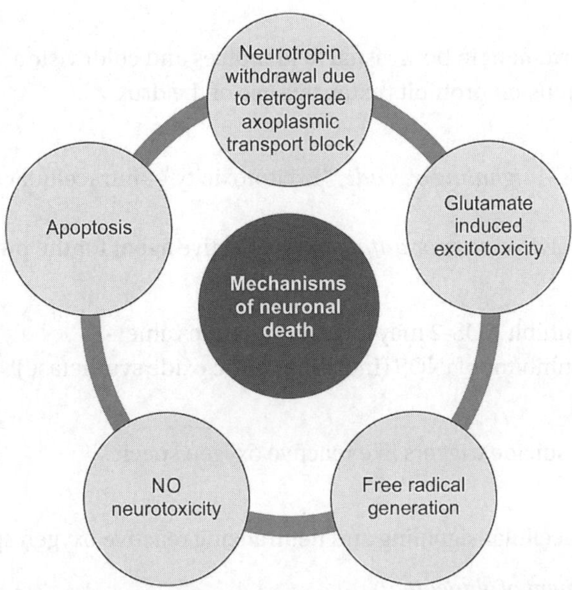

Fig. 2: The different mechanisms leading to neuronal death.

2. *The direct mechanical theory:* Suggests that increase in IOP directly damages the retinal nerve fibers as they pass through lamina cribrosa
3. *Optic nerve head remodeling:* May be a primary or secondary response to local factors such as elevation of IOP, ischemia, and axonal loss

Neuroprotection in glaucoma

Introduction: Neuroprotection is a therapeutic regime that can prevent or delay neuronal cell death and maintain neural function and in many cases of glaucoma where there is progressive structural and functional loss in spite of excellent IOP control. This can help to maintain visual function and prevent optic nerve damage.

Stages of neuronal cell death ***(Flowchart 4)***

Flowchart 4: Stages of neuronal death.

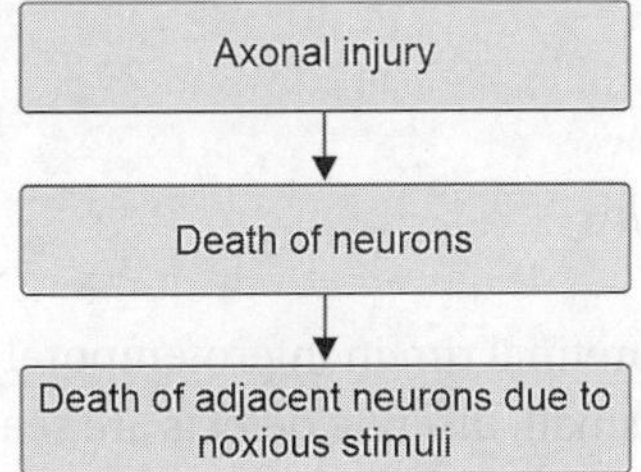

Mechanism of action: By correcting the imbalance between cellular death and survival signals. They target the targets mentioned in **Figure 3**.

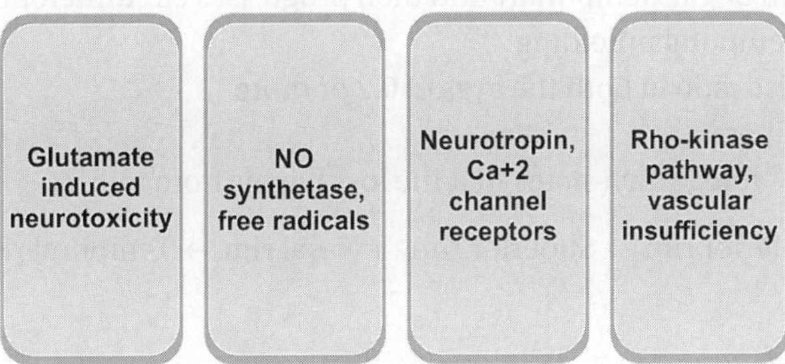

Fig. 3: Mechanism of action.

Calcium channel blockers:
- *Nimodipine:* Significant improvement in both visual field indices and color vision.
  - Drawback: Systemic hypotension prohibits extensive use of the drug

NMDA antagonists:
- *Excessive activation of the NMDA signaling cascade:* "Excitotoxicity"—intracellular calcium overloads neurons a-cell death by apoptosis
- *Memantine (noncompetitive NMDA receptor antagonist):* Effective agent for the prevention of progression

Nitric oxide synthetase inhibitors:
- Pharmacological agents that inhibit NOS-2 may have therapeutic value
- Aminoguanidine, a selective inhibitor of iNOS (inducible nitric oxide synthetase)

Antioxidants:
- These agents neutralize other suicide triggers like reactive oxygen species

Ginkgo biloba extracts:
- Ginkgo Biloba influences intracellular signaling and neutralizing reactive oxygen species

Rho-kinase inhibitors in management of glaucoma:
- Rho-kinase inhibitors can be used in combination with other ocular hypotensive medications or alone; netarsudil, ripasudil
- *Mechanism of action:* These drugs lowers IOP mainly by relaxing the cytoskeleton of trabecular meshwork and Schlemm's canal there by reducing the cell stiffness and increasing the conventional outflow.

They increase corneal endothelial cell proliferation—help with healing and migration.
- *Preparations:* Approved for clinical use are Ripasudil 0.4% to be used twice daily and netarsudil 0.02% to be used once daily
- *Indications:* Primary open angle glaucoma, ocular hypertension

6. Describe changes in Optic disc in Glaucoma. How will you differentiate from non-glaucomatous optic atrophy? (10) (WBUHS MS 2021)

There are three major categories of optic disc changes in glaucoma:
1. Disc patterns
2. Vascular signs
3. Peripapillary changes

1. *Disc patterns of glaucomatous optic atrophy:*
   a. Focal atrophy:
      i. There will be selective loss of neuroretinal rim in inferotemporal region
      ii. Inferior or polar notching which is small, discrete defects are seen.
   b. Concentric atrophy:
      i. Less common
      ii. Loss of neuroretinal rim begins temporally and then progresses circumferentially towards the pole
      iii. This is referred to as "temporal unfolding"
   c. Discrepancy in the cup disc ratio in both the eyes of 0.2 or more
   d. Loss of neuroretinal rim fibers:
      i. This follows the "ISNT" rule, which states that the loss begins from:

      Inferior rim → Superior rim → Nasal rim → Temporal rim

   e. Pallor of neuroretinal rim
   f. Saucerization of the disc:

i. Diffuse, shallow cupping which extends to the disc margin with retention of central pallor of the cup at the center.
ii. The retention at normal rim column area of focal saucerization is called "tinted hollow".

g. Bean pot cupping:
  i. Total cupping with complete loss of NRR and vessels emerging from the disc margins.
h. Lamellar dot sign:
  i. Optic disc passes through a sieve-like structure known as the lamina cribrosa. Due to the stretching of the optic nerve head, these pores enlarge and later on become slit-like called lamellar dot sign.

2. *Vascular signs of glaucomatous optic atrophy:*
  a. Optic disc hemorrhages:
    i. These are usually seen near the margins of the optic nerve head (Drance hemorrhage)
    ii. More common in patients with normal tension glaucoma
    iii. Most common location in in the inferior quadrant
    iv. May be the first sign of glaucomatous damage, preceding RNFL defects
  b. Tortuosity of retinal blood vessels:
    i. Seen in advanced glaucomatous optic atrophy
    ii. These are loops of collateral vessels formed in response to chronic central retinal vein occlusion
  c. Baring of the circumlinear vessels:
    i. With glaucomatous enlargement of the cup, vessels may be bared from the margin of the cup
    ii. It is characterized by a space between the neuroretinal rim and the superficial blood vessels
  d. Bayonetting of vessels:
    i. Characterized by double angulation of the blood vessels
    ii. With progressive NRR loss, vessels entering the disc angle sharply backwards and then turn towards its original direction to run across the lamina
3. *Peripapillary changes associated with glaucomatous optic atrophy:*
  a. RNFL defects:
    i. These are dark stripes or wedge-shaped defects of varying width in the peripapillary area
    ii. These often follow disc hemorrhages and correlate highly with visual field changes
    iii. Useful parameter in early detection of glaucoma
    iv. Seen in red free examination as dark stripe/wedge-shaped defects
  b. Peripapillary atrophy occurs more frequently and increases with decreasing area of NRR and correlates with maximum rim loss

  Early signs:
  - Polar notching
  - Splinter hemorrhage at margin
  - Discrepancy in CDR of both eyes
  - Pallor of NRR
  - Loss of ISNT rule
  - RNFL loss (wedge-shaped)

  Late signs:
  - Enlargement of CDR to 0.7 or more
  - Lamellar dot sign
  - Bean pot cupping
  - Nasal shifting of vessels
  - Bayonetting sign
  - Baring of circumlinear vessels
  - Pulsation of retinal arterioles: Pathognomonic of glaucoma

Table 3 outlines the differences between glaucomatous and nonglaucomatous optic atrophy.

TABLE 3: Difference between glaucomatous and nonglaucomatous optic atrophy.

Features	*Primary*	*Secondary*	*Consecutive*	*Glaucomatous*
OD appearance	Chalky white	Dirty gray-white	Waxy pallor	Pale
OD margin	Well defined	Ill defined	Well defined	Deep wide cupping of OD
Lamina cribrosa	Well seen	Observed	Well seen	Laminar dot sign seen
Vessels	Normal	Peripapillary slanting	A herniation	Nasal shifting of blood vessels
Surrounding retina	Healthy	Hyaline bodies present	Pathological scars	Healthy

7. What is meant by angle closure suspect? Outline of management. (10) (WBUHS MS 2021)

Introduction:

- An anatomical description only where a retrospective diagnosis is only made with any degree of certainty in one eye during an attack of acute congestive angle closure in the other eye.
- An eye classified as angle closure suspect has an "occludable or narrow", anterior chamber angle but no overt signs of PAC (IOP elevation or PAS) or glaucomatous optic nerve damage.
- Feature at least 2 quadrants of iridotrabecular contact.
- Only a small percentage of eyes with a shallow anterior chamber develop PAC **(Fig. 4)**.

Clinical features:

- Patients are asymptomatic
- Slit-lamp examination
  - Axial anterior chamber length is less than normal and iris-lens diaphragm is convex
  - Close proximity of the iris to the cornea.
- *Gonioscopy:*
  - Shows an occludable angle in which the TM is not visible (Shaffer grade 1 or 0) without indentation or manipulation in at least three quadrants.

Natural course:

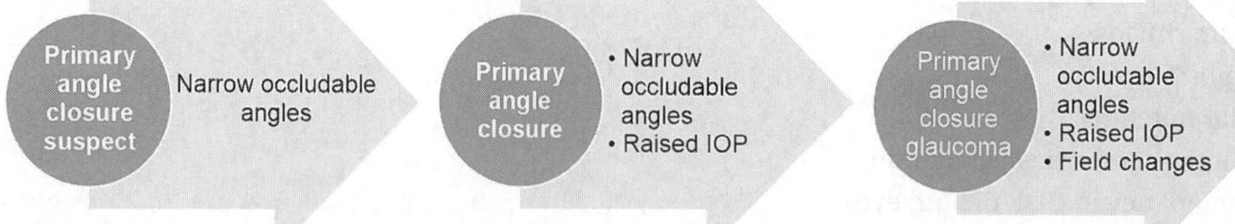

Fig. 4: Natural course of primary angle closure glaucoma.

- IOP may remain normal.
- Acute or subacute angle closure may ensure.
- Angle closure may develop without passing through the subacute or acute stage.
  - Most common conversion was from PACS to PAC due to the development of PAS.
  - Singapore Asymptomatic Narrow Angles Laser Iridotomy Study (ANA-LIS)
    - Untreated PACS eyes had twice the risk of developing end points over 5 years compared with eyes that underwent prophylactic LPI.

- Zhongshan Angle Closure Prevention (ZAP) trial
    - LPI useful in managing special groups of patients anxious about PAS formation, PACS patients taking medications that may provoke pupillary block, or patients who have difficulty accessing ophthalmic care.
- If both eyes have occludable angles, there is no parameter or provocative test that is sufficiently sensitive or accurate to determine whether acute attack will later develop.

Treatment:

- *Prophylactic peripheral iridotomy:*
    - If one eye has had acute or subacute angle closure, fellow eye should undergo peripheral laser iridectomy.

8. Describe the clinical features, evaluation, differential diagnosis and management of Pigment Dispersion Syndrome (2 + 2 + 3 + 3) (DNB 2019)
Gonioscopy findings of Pigmentary glaucoma and its management. (RGUHS MS 2020)

Introduction: Pigmentary glaucoma (PG) is one of the iris or ciliary body disorders characterized by disruption of the iris pigment epithelium (IPE) and deposition of the dispersed pigment granules throughout the anterior segment.

Pathophysiology:

- In pigment dispersion syndrome, zonular fibers rub the posterior iris pigment epithelium, resulting in release of pigment granules through the eye.
- Posterior bowing of the iris with "reverse pupillary block" configuration is noted.

Clinical features

Classic triad is shown in **Figure 5**.

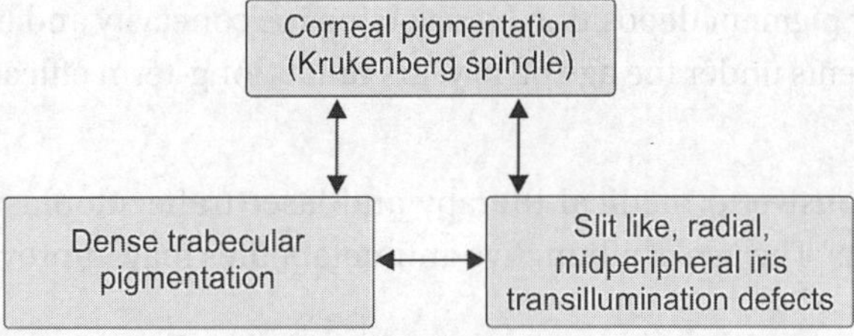

Fig. 5: Classic triad.

- Pigment dispersion syndrome classically presents with pigment deposits on corneal endothelium, trabecular meshwork and lens periphery, and mid peripheral iris; transillumination defect in a "Spoke like pattern".
- The pigment deposits on corneal endothelium are typically in vertical spindle pattern, referred to as Krukenberg Spindle.
- The midperipheral iris transillumination defect are a result of contact between fibers and posterior iris pigment epithelium.
- Elevation of IOP appears due to pigmentary obstruction of the intertrabecular spaces and damage to the trabeculae secondary to denudation, collapse and sclerosis.
- Stages are mentioned in **Table 4**.

Gonioscopy:

- Widely open angle , with a homogeneous, dense hyperpigmented band on the trabecular meshwork
- Peripheral iris approach is often concave, maximum in mid periphery
- Trabecular meshwork commonly appears as homogenous and densely pigmented with speckled pigment at or anterior to Schwalbe line, often forming "Sampaolesi line".
- Pigment deposited on the zonules and on the posterior capsule: Zentmeyer line or Scheie stripe

TABLE 4: Stages of PDS.	
Stage 1	Most common in young myopic eyes, large eyes with deep a/c, concave bowing of peripheral iris
Stage 2	Early tissue changes, IOP still in normal range, Krukenberg's spindle
Stage 3	Initial elevation of IOP
Stage 4	Glaucomatous optic neuropathy
Stage 5	Progressive visual field loss

Differential diagnosis:
- Pseudoexfoliation syndrome which us usually unilateral but PDS is usually bilateral.
- Uveitis
- Iris or ciliary body cyst
- Iris or ciliary body melanoma

Treatment:

Medical:
- Topical carbonic anhydrase inhibitors, brimonidine, prostaglandin analogues are effective.
- Miotics may theoretically be of particular benefit because they decrease irido-zonular contact in addition to facilitate aqueous outflow. They, however carry disadvantage of exacerbating myopia.

Laser trabeculoplasty: Often effective initially and in younger patients appear to respond better. It is important to not overtreat eyes with heavily pigmented angles and to start at a relatively low power laser setting.

Laser iridotomy:
- Effective in preventing further pigment deposition by reversing iris concavity and eliminating irido-zonular contact. It appears to work best in patients under the age of 40 years but its long-term efficacy is not known.

Trabeculectomy:
- Required in patients unresponsive to medical therapy and laser trabeculoplasty. Although the results are less predictable in younger patients. The use of adjunctive antimetabolites may improve surgical outcome.

9. Pseudoexfoliation syndrome: clinical features, evaluation and management.

(2 + 2 + 3) (DNB 2023)

It is the most common cause of secondary open-angle glaucoma also known as capsular glaucoma.
- Pseudoexfoliation material (PXF) is a grayish-white fibrillary material which is obtained from abnormal extracellular matrix metabolism in ocular and other tissues, deposited over the lens capsule, zonular fibers, iris, trabecular meshwork and conjunctiva.
- Pseudoexfoliation syndrome (PXS) is an ocular manifestation which has a systemic entity.
- Pseudoexfoliation glaucoma (PXG)
- Incidence—the risk of glaucoma during diagnosis is 15–30%. 60% of cases may require medical treatment within 5 years.
- Age—5th decade
- Gender—more commonly seen in females.
- Pathogenesis—It is associated with *LOXL1* gene on chromosome 15. The gene has single nucleotide polymorphism due to which it produces an enzyme causes cross-linking of tropoelastin and collagen maintains elasticity and extracellular matrix. Due to disruption of elastin metabolism, pseudoexfoliative material deposits in different systems.
- Due to exposure of chronic infrared radiation (glassblower's cataract) true capsular exfoliation deposits.

Clinical features:

- Symptoms:
  - Most of the patients are asymptomatic and incidental findings confirm the disease.
  - Unilateral eye involvement is noted frequently.
  - Pain
  - Redness
  - Distant vision loss
- Signs:
  - Eyeball may be deep seated or normal.
  - Conjunctiva—normal or ciliary congestion
  - Cornea:
    - White small flakes over endothelium
    - Scattered iris pigment deposits are common with PXF.
    - Endothelial cell abnormalities i.e. corneal decompensation is more common.
  - Anterior chamber:
    - Shallow AC may be due to forward displacement of lens.
    - Floated PXF material may be seen
    - Raised flare due to impaired blood-aqueous barrier.
  - Iris:
    - Granular PXF material deposits over pupillary margin are the characteristic sign.
    - Patchy transillumination defects at pupillary margin leads to "moth-eaten" appearance.
    - Iridodonesis, sphincter muscle degeneration, posterior synechiae are the features of PXS.
  - Lens:
    - A central disc and radially indented peripheral layer of PXF material separated by clear zone maintained by pupillary abrasion is seen on anterior lens capsule
    - Peripheral capsular deposition, often visible on pupillary dilation, which may be flaky with scrolled edges
    - Phacodonesis due to zonular weakness
  - Anterior chamber angle:
    - Patchy trabecular and Schwalbe line hyperpigmentation is noticed inferiorly.
    - Sampaolesi line is an irregular band of pigment anterior to the Schwalbe line.
    - Dandruff-like deposits noted in angle on gonioscopic examination.
    - Zonular laxity may cause angle closure.
  - IOP:
    - Glaucomatous damage occurs due to elevated IOP
    - Chronic open-angle glaucoma develops, usually unilateral at first.
    - Occasionally the IOP may rise acutely despite a wide angle, mimicking acute angle closure.
- *Management:*
  - Medical treatment is similar to that of POAG, but failure is more common.
  - Laser trabeculoplasty is more effective than in POAG, with mean IOP reduction around 30% following SLT.
  - Phacoemulsification alone may significantly lower IOP, though it may give better control combined with trabeculectomy. There is a higher risk of complications, due to poor mydriasis, increased fragility of the zonule and lens capsule, and endothelial deficiency. There is also an increased risk of a postoperative IOP spike, postoperative corneal oedema, capsular opacification, capsulorrhexis contraction (capsular phimosis) and late IOL decentration or dislocation.
  - Filtration surgery in PXG has a similar success rate to POAG.
  - Trabecular aspiration alone seems to confer at least a short-term benefit, and can be performed at the same time as other intraocular procedures.

Q 10. Neovascular Glaucoma–causes, clinical features and management enumerate the stages of NVG. (2 + 3 + 5)

(2) (DNB 2021, 2023)

- Neovascular glaucoma (NVG) is a potentially blinding secondary glaucoma, characterized by the development of fibrovascular proliferation of tissue in iris and angle causing elevation of IOP, often associated with and/or secondary to retinal ischemia.
- *Risk factors:*
  - Diabetic retinopathy (33%)
  - Ischemic CRVO (33%)
  - Ocular ischemic syndrome (13%)
  - Central retinal artery occlusion
- *Etiology of NVG:*
  - Retinal ischemic causes:
    - Diabetic retinopathy
    - Ischemic CRVO
    - CRAO
    - Retinopathy of prematurity
    - Sickle cell retinopathy
    - Coats disease
    - Eales disease
    - Retinoschisis
  - Ocular inflammation:
    - Chronic uveitis
    - Chronic retinal detachment
    - Retinal vasculitis
    - Traumatic eye
    - Endophthalmitis
  - Neoplasms:
    - Malignant melanoma
    - Retinoblastoma
    - Ocular lymphoma
    - Metastatic carcinoma
  - Systemic disease:
    - Systemic vascular diseases—carotid occlusive disease, carotid-cavernous fistula
    - SLE
    - NF-1

  Stages and classification of NVG are mentioned in **Tables 5 and 6**, respectively.
- *Clinical features:*
  - Symptoms:
    - Depend upon the cause the symptoms may vary
    - Painful red eye with significant loss of vision
  - Signs:
    - On slit-lamp biomicroscopic examination shows:
      - Lid—either normal or edematous lid due to elevation IOP.
      - Conjunctiva—congestion
      - Cornea—edematous if IOP elevated
      - Iris—neovascularization of iris and angle can be visible

TABLE 5: Stages of NVG.

Stage	Features
Pre-rubeosis stage	• It is associated with retinal ischemic conditions • Normal IOP and anterior segment examination appears normal • NVI/NVA should be observed
Pre-glaucoma or rubeosis iridis	• Iris neovascularization appears at pupillary margin, iris surface and angles • IOP is normal • Patient is asymptomatic usually unless patient does not have preexisting glaucoma • NVA can be present along with NVI
Open angle glaucoma	• Mild pain, redness, photophobia • New vessels are encroaching the angle • IOP elevation is noted • Florid NVI along with anterior chamber cells may be detected • Due to leakage of blood vessels hyphema may be associated • Gonioscopy reveals open angle
Angle closure glaucoma	• Marked IOP elevation (>50 mm Hg) • Florid NVI causes contraction of fibrovascular membrane in the angle which leads to angle closure, ectropion uvea • Gonioscopy—PAS • Conjunctival congestion and corneal edema is noted • Moderate to advance GON • Loss of vision

TABLE 6: Weiss and Gold classification of iris and anterior chamber angle neovascularization.

	Grade 1	*Grade 2*	*Grade 3*	*Grade 4*
NVI	IRIS new vessels at pupillary zone <2 quadrants	IRIS new vessels at pupillary zone >2 quadrants	IRIS new vessels at ciliary zone and/or ectropion uveae 1–3 quadrants	Surface new vessels at ciliary zone and/or ectropion uveae ≥3 quadrants
NVA	Angle vessels cross SS and ramify on TM <2 quadrants	Angle vessels cross SS and ramify on TM ≥2 quadrants	Angle vessels at TM and PAS 1–3 quadrants	PAS ≥8 quadrants

- AC—shows cells, flare, posterior synechiae, hyphema
- Pupil—RAPD, fine superficial vessels are present near pupillary margin, ectropion uvea noted.
- IOP—initially normal, extremely high in late stages.
- Lens—after initiation of NVI cataract formation occurs; pseudophakia, aphakia promotes NVI
- NVI: Thin, tortuous vessels, randomly oriented, usually begins at pupillary margin
- NVA: Appears as thin vessels crossing the scleral spur, branching and arborizing over the TM
- Gonioscopy: NVA along with partial or complete angle closure (PAS)
- On fundus examination—CRVO, PDR, CRAO causes retinal ischemia. In end stages, glaucomatous optic neuropathy is inevitable.

▪ *Investigations:*
- Systemic investigations—BP, FBS, PPBS, HBA1C for ruling out HTN, DM
- Carotid doppler test for OIS.
- CECT scan/MR venogram is to detect CCF.
- PET scan is used to look for any tumor or metastasis
- HLA B-27 is for uveitis.
- Retinal vasculitis
- Blood dyscrasia—Hb, ESR, CRP, ANA, VDRL, serum protein electrophoresis and immunoelectrophoresis
- FFA: Gold standard procedure which confirms the etiology, CNP areas, presence of NVE and NVD
- Anterior segment FA shows leakage from the new vessels over iris.

- B scan—In hazy media, it finds the underlying associated pathology like long-standing RD or any intraocular tumors.
- UBM—shows any presence of ciliary body tumors
- OCT angiography is a rapid, noninvasive modality, is used to reveal neovascularization, new vessels formation and monitoring after PRP.

▪ *Differential diagnosis of NVG:*
  - Acute angle closure glaucoma (no NVI/NVA, no ectropion uveae, no membrane over angles)
  - Uveitic glaucoma (KPs on endothelium, AC cells, complicated cataract)
  - Chronic angle closure glaucoma (shallow AC, pupillary block)
  - Iridocorneal endothelial syndrome (corneal decompensation, pseudopolycoria, iris atrophy, corectopia)
  - Fuchs heterochromic iridocyclitis (white eye, stellate KPs, iris heterochromia, Amsler sign)

Flowchart 5: Treatment of NVG.

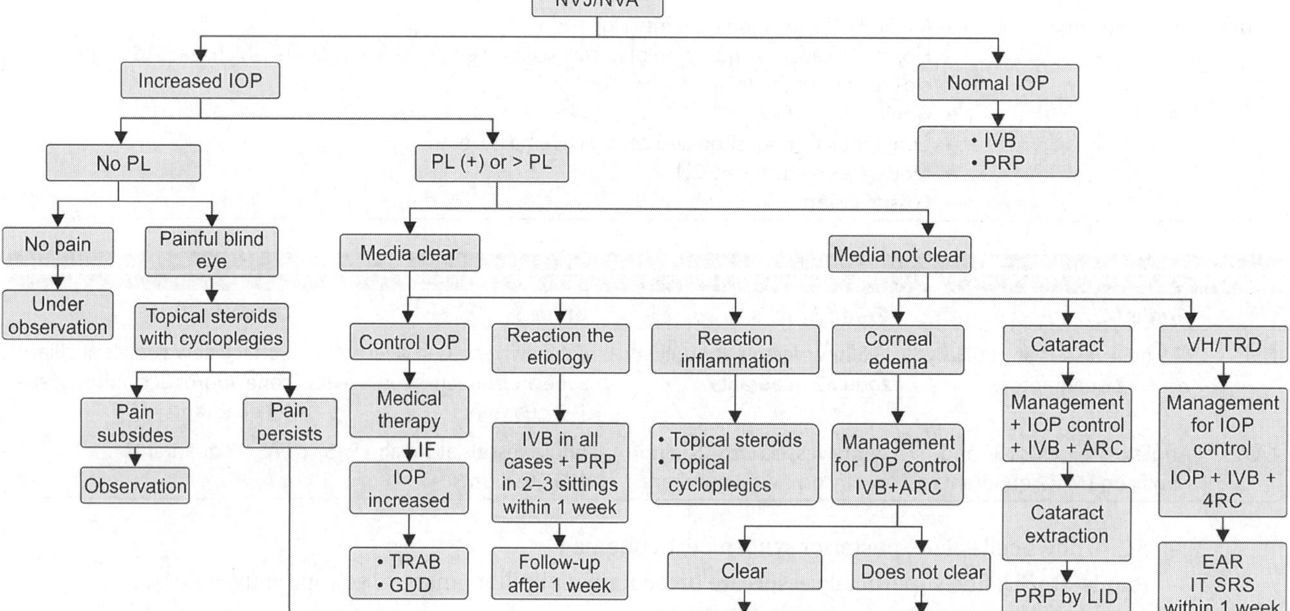

▪ *Management of NVG* ***(Flowchart 5)***:
Aim to achieve—Reduction of anti-inflammatory and angiogenic factors to prevent retinal ischemia.
  - Intravitreal anti-VEGF agents—reduces the NVA/NVI
  - PRP
  - Treatment for systemic diseases
  - IOP reduction
  - Reducing inflammation

Early diagnosis is the key to success.

Medical management:

▪ Topical steroids are used to treat inflammation and cycloplegics like atropine 1% for synechiolysis.

▪ Anti-glaucoma agents—CA inhibitors (oral and topical), beta-blockers, and alpha-2 agonists are advised to reduce aqueous production.

Miotics use is avoided due to raise inflammation and can deteriorate synechial angle closure.

In acute condition IV mannitol is needed.

- Pan-retinal photocoagulation (PRP):
    - First-line therapy in all cases of NVG with retinal ischemia.
    - Causes regression of anterior and posterior segment neovascularization by reducing oxygen demand.
    - The parameters should be 1,200–1,600 burns, size – 500 μm spot size and one spot apart which will be accomplished with a week by 3 sessions.
- Anti-VEGF:
    - Intracameral and intravitreal can be given simultaneously.
    - It is an adjunctive to PRP or bevacizumab (1.25 mg/0.05 mL) alone application helps to clear media haze, i.e., hemorrhage.
    - Provide temporary measure to reduce NVI and NVA leading to lowering of IOP.
- Filtration surgery: Indications for surgery are to reduce inflammation, IOP reduction, in GON, presence of visual potential.
    - It has more failure rate due to presence of inflammatory cells.
    - The favorable outcome of TRAB with MMC is around 60–80%. The success rate of trabeculectomy may be increased if bevacizumab or PRP may be added along with it (around 95%).
    - Adjunctives can be used in glaucoma like glaucoma drainage devices, trabeculectomy with mini-shunt implantation and postoperative sub-conjunctival 5-fluorouracil.
    - Active NV should be treated pre-operatively with Anti-VEGF and PRP.
    - Aggressive post-operative anti-inflammatory treatment should be stated, which may include systemic steroids.
- Glaucoma drainage devices:
    - Valved GDDs are preferred over non-valved GDDs due to their immediate IOP lowering potential and less risk of hypotony.
    - Molteno implant, Baerveldt implant and Ahmed valve are used to control IOP in NVG cases.
    - PPV with preoperative endolaser and anti-VEGF at an early stage along with GDD may give fruitful outcome.
- Cyclodestructive procedure:
    - Trans-scleral cyclophotocoagulation (TSCPC) or diode laser cyclophotocoagulation are useful for lowering pain in refractory NVG cases.
    - Hyphema, hypotony, chronic iritis, phthisis bulbi are noted as complications.
- Retinal detachment repair
- Enucleation or evisceration can be accounted if all the standard treatments becomes failure.

Prognosis—Around 25–50% patients sustain their visual potential.

11. Angle recession glaucoma—short note. (5) (DNB)

Definition: Rupture of the face of ciliary body resulting a tear in between the longitudinal and circular muscles of scleral spur following blunt trauma.

It is a secondary open angle glaucoma which develops after ocular trauma.

Patients may be symptomatic or asymptomatic.

Around 20–94% blunt trauma patients have angle recession glaucoma.

Mechanism of angle recession – Closed globe injury → anteroposterior axial compression of globe equatorial expansion of sclera → indentation of cornea → increasing sclerocorneal limbal ring → shock waves traverses in the globe weakening the roots of iris → atrophy of inner muscles of circular muscles of ciliary body → obliteration of intertrabecular spaces and Schlemm's canal hyaline membrane is grown in the trabecular meshwork decreased aqueous outflow IOP elevation.

Symptoms:

- Diminished vision
- Redness

- Deep eye pain
- Symptoms may occur after years of trauma

Diagnosis:

- Unilateral chronic glaucoma
- Slit-lamp evaluation: Signs of blunt trauma
    - Deep anterior chamber
    - Hyphema, Vossius ring
    - Iris sphincter tear
    - Mydriasis
    - Iridoschisis
    - Iridodonesis
    - Phacodonesis
    - Ectopia lentis
    - Focal subcapsular cataract
    - Recessed angle 180°–240°
    - Elevation of baseline IOP
- *Gonioscopy:*
    - Tear between the longitudinal and circular muscles of ciliary body.
    - Irregular widening of the ciliary body band.
    - Whitening of scleral spur due to iris process tear or PAS.
    - Recession may get obscured by fibrosis.
    - Hyperpigmentation may be present in angle.
    - PAS may present at the border of the recession.
    - More than two quadrants are involved in angle recession are prone for glaucoma

Treatment:

- *Medical:*
    - Topical aqueous suppressants like β blockers, CA anhydrase inhibitors and α agonists are choice of treatment.
    - Prostaglandin analogues are avoided as anterior segment reaction is more in acute cases. It may be applied in chronic phases.
    - Pilocarpine is strictly avoided in angle recession.
    - Dislocated lens may raise IOP due to pupillary block. Cycloplegics are helpful till extraction of lens.
- *Surgical:*
    - Argon laser trabeculoplasty can be done in few cases but it proved to be failed for controlling glaucoma.
    - Trabeculectomy with ant-metabolites like MMC, 5-FU is generally effective.
    - Chances of failure rate are high in these cases after trabeculoplasty without antimetabolites.
    - Glaucoma drainage devices have more success rate in these cases than other types.
    - Cyclodestructive procedures are the last resort for painful blind eyes.
    - Follow-up: Yearly IOP evaluation and progression to be noted after trauma.

12. Write Briefly on Aqueous misdirection syndrome. (10) (DNB)

Introduction: Aqueous misdirection is a type of secondary angle closure causes raised intraocular pressure (IOP), shallowing of the central and peripheral anterior chamber in spite of the presence of a peripheral iridotomy.

Etiology and risk factors:

- *Etiology:*
    - Cataract surgery
    - Laser/surgical iridotomy

- During early postoperative days, overfiltration causes shallow AC. Due to rotation of anterior ciliary body causes posterior chamber shallowing.
- Rising pressure in posterior chamber causes forward movement of lens iris-diaphragm results to balance anterior chamber.

- *Risk factors:*
  - Axial hyperopia and a history of chronic angle closure with peripheral anterior synechiae are the chief risk factors to develop aqueous misdirection syndrome.
  - Partial or complete closure of AC angle associated with or without iridectomy may be a reason for ciliary block glaucoma.

Pathogenesis:

- *Theories:*
  - Chandler and Grant theory:
    - Axial shallowing of AC can be due to weakness or laxity in the zonules with posterior chamber pressure.
  - Shaffer theory:
    - Accumulation of aqueous humor in the posterior chamber behind a posterior vitreous detachment (PVD) culminates in anterior displacement of the iris-lens diaphragm.

Mechanism involved is shown in **Flowchart 6** as follows.

Flowchart 6: Mechanism.

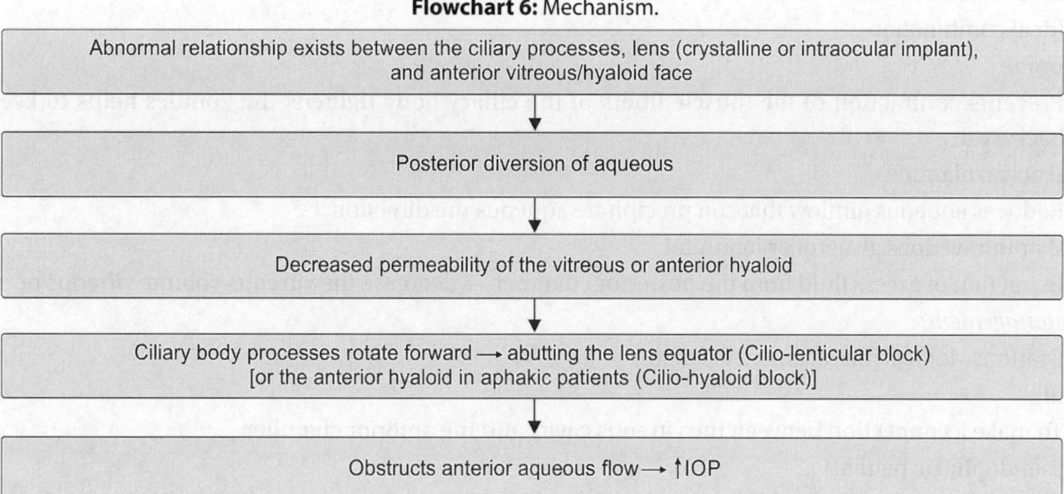

Clinical features:

- *Symptoms:*
  - Redness
  - Pain in eyes
  - Diminishing of vision

  The symptoms are due to suffering from chronic angle symptoms, past h/o any eye procedures, inflammation or any infection.
  - Short-term improvement of near sight is caused by myopic shift from forward rotation of the lens–iris complex.
- *Signs:*

  On slit-lamp examination:
  - Raised intraocular pressure
  - Shallowing of both the peripheral and central anterior chamber

- Through lens iridotomy the ciliary body can be evident during examination of anterior chamber during disease process.

On fundus examination:
- Presence of choroidal detachment and suprachoroidal hemorrhage should be examined.

Investigations:
- *B-scan ultrasonography:*
  - Detection of choroidal detachments and suprachoroidal hemorrhage should be ruled out if media haze is present.
  - Ultrasound biomicroscopy (UBM)
    - The state of anterior chamber angle, iris configuration, and lens configuration are examined.
- *Anterior segment optical coherence tomography (OCT):*
  - In absence of corneal haze anterior chamber depth measurement and configuration are noted.

Management:
- *Aim:*
  - Restoring the normal anatomic relationship between the ciliary body, lens and iris
  - Restoring anterior flow of the aqueous and controlling IOP.
- *Medical management:*
  - Concomitant use of cycloplegics–mydriatics, aqueous suppressants, and hyperosmotics
    - In few situations this combined medications are ineffective.
    - Ideal combination
  - Atropine
    - Prevents contraction of the muscle fibers of the ciliary body tightens the zonules helps to keep the lens backward.
  - Oral acetazolamide
    - Reduces aqueous outflow that can precipitate aqueous misdirection
  - Oral or intravenous glycerol or mannitol
    - Extraction of excess fluid from the posterior chamber → decrease the vitreous volume vitreous permeability.
- *Laser management:*
  - Indication: Medical management is failed.
  - Goal:
    - To make a connection between the vitreous cavity and the anterior chamber.
  - In pseudophakic patient:
    - Nd:YAG laser disrupts the anterior vitreous face and helps to escape misdirected aqueous from AC to the posterior chamber.
- Laser cyclophotocoagulation:
  - It uses argon laser to photocoagulate ciliary processes.
  - It reduces the size of the ciliary processes which decreases further cilio-hyaloidal apposition and posterior aqueous flow.
- *Surgical management:*
  - Indication—In refractory cases which are nonresponsive to both medical and laser management
  - Pseudophakic patient:
    - Transcorneal needling is performed through a patent iridotomy during slit lamp examination.
    - Posterior sclerotomy causes interruption in anterior hyaloid. A small amount of fluid extracted and air injected into AC.
    - Anterior vitrectomy via pars plana approach with or without AC reformation with air helps to release the entrapped fluid from posterior chamber.

- Phakic patient:
  - Vitrectomy-phacoemulsification-vitrectomy (with zonulohyaloidectomy-iridectomy) is done to get successful outcome in these patients.
  - In refractory cases PPV with lensectomy is required to reduce IOP by creating iridectomy-hyloidectomy-zonulectomy.
- *Differential diagnosis:*
  - *Pupillary block glaucoma:* Moderately deep central anterior chamber with bowing of the peripheral iris in pupillary block which is released by iridotomy.
  - *Choroidal detachment:* Hypotony is associated with a shallow anterior chamber and a serous choroidal detachment
  - *Suprachoroidal hemorrhage:* Dilated fundus examination shows elevated choroidals with reddish-brown hemorrhage.
  - Secondary angle closure: Patients may be associated with choroidal effusion.
- Prognosis—Highly challenging cases may require early diagnosis, prompt action are required. Many of these cases result as sight-threatening conditions.
  - Phakic eye—needle aspiration of vitreous via pars plana vitrectomy.
  - Pseudophakic eye—by Nd:YAG laser
  - Aphakic eyes—managed by vitrectomy and hyloidectomy ± Nd:YAG laser.

13. Postpenetrating keratoplasty glaucoma—Short note. (5) (DNB 2023)

Postpenetrating glaucoma is a condition in which raised IOP >21 mm Hg or elevation of IOP >20% of baseline associated with or without changes in optic nerve and visual field loss which may require medical or surgical intervention.

Incidence:
- Early postoperative cases was found with glaucoma around 9–31%.
- Late postoperative glaucoma was associated with glaucoma around 18–35%.

Types of keratoplasty:
- *Penetrating keratoplasty:* Corneal pathology or corneal opacity involves all the layers of cornea. The cornea is replaced by the full thickness of donor's cornea.
- *Lamellar keratoplasty:* corneal pathology is lying over the stromal area which is replace by an analogous corneal layer called partial or lamellar keratoplasty; e.g., superficial anterior lamellar keratoplasty (SALK) and deep anterior lamellar keratoplasty (DALK).

Risk factors **(Table 7)**:

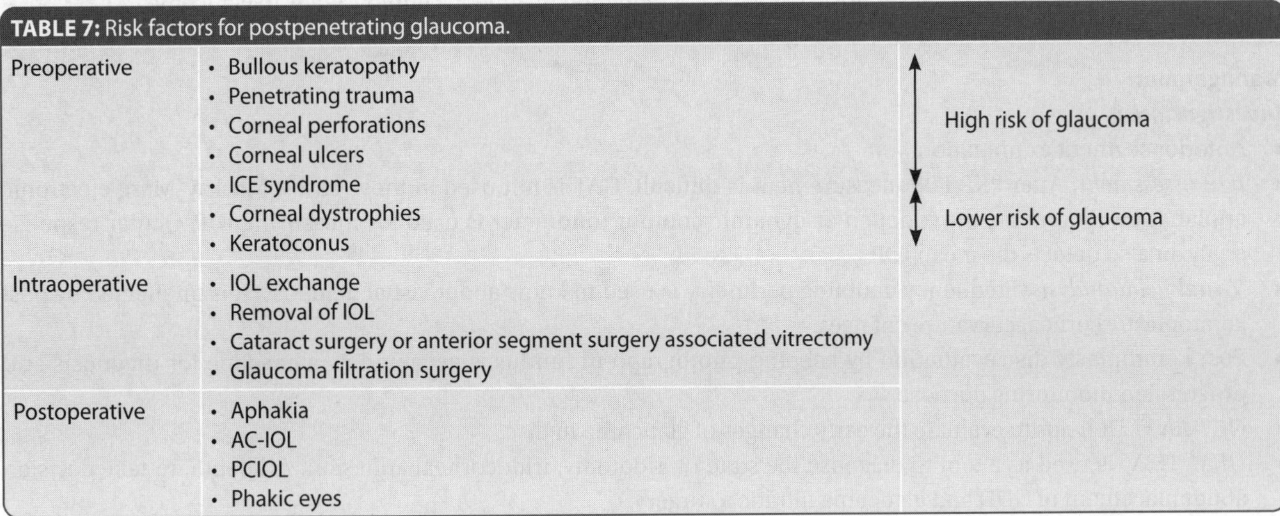

TABLE 7: Risk factors for postpenetrating glaucoma.

Preoperative	• Bullous keratopathy • Penetrating trauma • Corneal perforations • Corneal ulcers • ICE syndrome • Corneal dystrophies • Keratoconus	High risk of glaucoma ↕ Lower risk of glaucoma
Intraoperative	• IOL exchange • Removal of IOL • Cataract surgery or anterior segment surgery associated vitrectomy • Glaucoma filtration surgery	
Postoperative	• Aphakia • AC-IOL • PCIOL • Phakic eyes	

Pathogenesis ***(Flowchart 7):***

Flowchart 7: Pathogenesis.

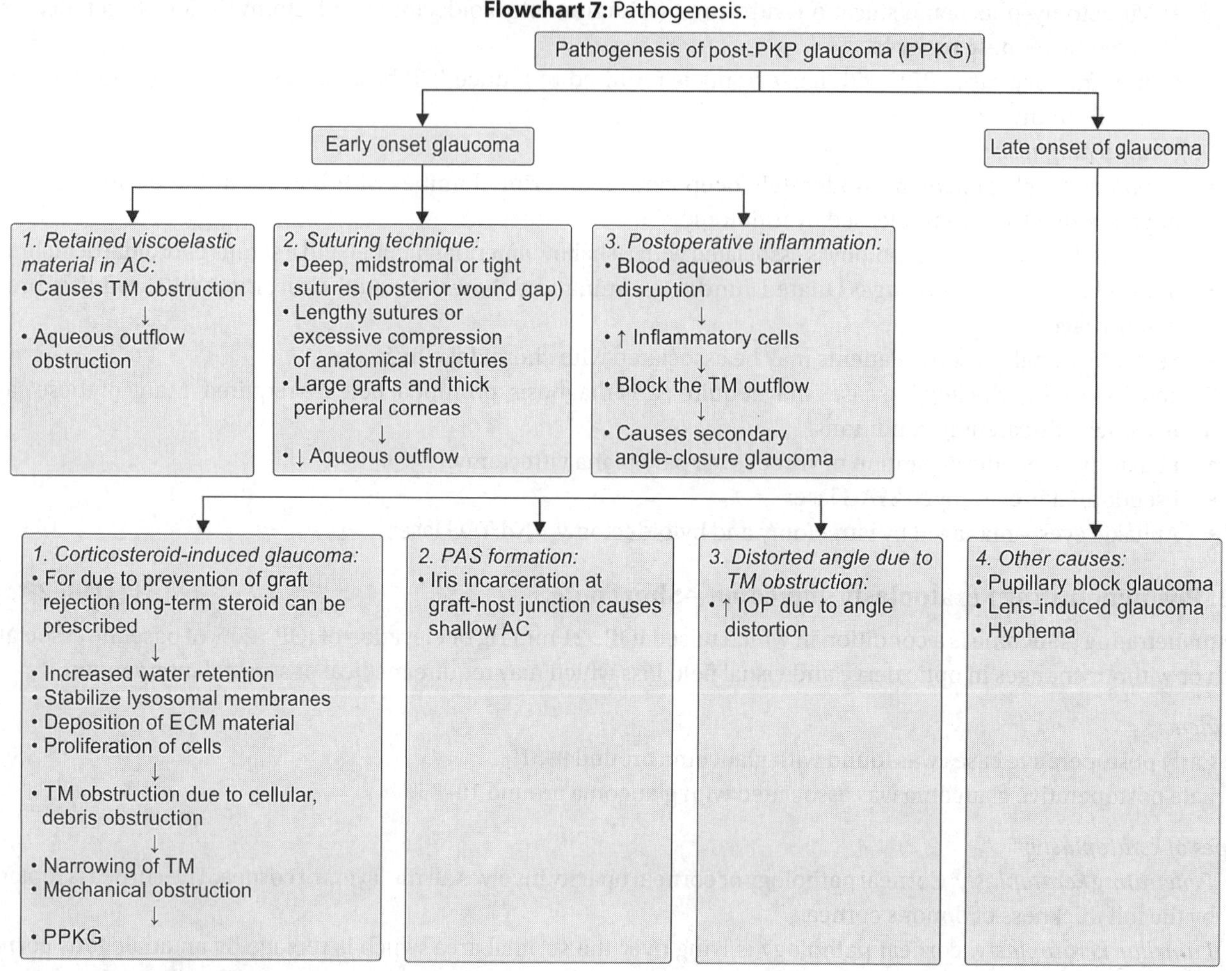

Pathogenesis of glaucoma after post DALK, DSEAK:

- In big bubble technique, pupillary block glaucoma occurs due to escaping the air through TM or air behind the iris leads to shallow AC.
- Inflammatory cell blockage causes obstruction of TM reduction of aqueous outflow leads to glaucoma.
- Steroid also induces glaucoma and its progression.

Management:

Investigations:

- Anterior segment examination
- *IOP assessment:* After PKP IOP measurement is difficult. GAT is not used in these cases. Mackay-Marg electronic applanation tonometer, the tonopen or dynamic contour tonometer is used for measuring IOP. Ocular response analyzer also detects the mean IOP.
- *Visual field analysis:* Frequency doubling perimetry is used to know about visual field loss. It is unaffected by post keratoplastic corneal curvature changes.
- Post keratoplasty disc evaluation by keeping photograph of fundus is accepted as a baseline for diagnosis and progression monitoring purpose.
- *OCT-RNFL:* It helps to evaluate the early changes of glaucoma in disc.
- *UBM:* UBM is used as a tool to diagnose the state of iridotomy, iridocorneal adhesion, AC depth, to take decision about placement of GDD and glaucoma filtration surgery.

Management ***(Flowchart 8):***

Flowchart 8: Management of PPKG.

Management of PPKG

Preoperative measurement:
- Pre-existing glaucoma needs attention
- IOP-lowering agents is administered prior to the surgery

Intraoperative measurement:
- Donor graft size should exceed <0.5–1 mm develops glaucoma
- *Suturing technique:* The length of suture should be short and equal less distortion of corneal tissue
- Removal of viscoelastic substances before completion of surgery
- In DSAEK/DMEK, only 80% of AC should be filled with air to prevent pupillary block
  ↓
  For prevention of pupillary block, inferior peripheral iridotomy should be done as air may block 12 o'clock PI

Postoperative measurement
Medical treatment:
- Topical AGM: Beta2-blockers, adrenergic agonist and CA inhibitors and aqueous humor production
- Brimonidine tartrate (0.15% or 0.2%) can be applied thrice daily
- Newer Rho-kinase inhibitors can be used certainly
- Oral CA inhibitors should be administered in immediate postoperative
- In chronic cases, other AGMs should be used as adjunctive
- SLT is implemented in PPKG cases which acts on TM to control IOP
- Nd:YAG laser iridotomy is applied to prevent pupillary block glaucoma*

***Surgical treatment:**
1. *Trabeculectomy:*
- In progressive and refractory cases, trabeculectomy is the last option. It is helpful in post-DSAEK eyes than post-PKP
- Ahmed Glaucoma Valve (AGV) is more efficient in penetrating keratoplasty cases
- TRAB with MMC have excellent outcome in PPKG

2. *GDDs (Glaucoma Drainage Devices):* GDDs are applied in post-keratoplasty cases when after trabeculectomy fails to control IOP
3. *Cyclodestructive procedures:*
- Cyclophotocoagulation is effective in PPKG patients with painful blind eye
- Micropulse trans-scleral cyclophotocoagulation (TSCPC) is administered in post-keratoplasty eyes

Prognosis
- It is challenging to manage secondary glaucoma
- Assessing the risk factors, managing the cases, determining the choice of surgery, and severity of the case management is often tricky

14. Indications, techniques and adverse effect of laser iridotomy, selective laser trabeculoplasty and argon laser trabeculoplasty. (3 + 4 + 3) (DNB 2020)

Laser iridotomy

Introduction: The most common procedure for angle closure is YAG LPI to make an iridotomy make equal pressure in anterior and posterior chamber.

Principle/mechanism: PAC causes resistance to increase aqueous flow through pupil to AC which increases IOP pushes the posterior surface of iris forms a bow like structure. Iridotomy helps to release aqueous from posterior to anterior chamber by creating an alternate pathway.

Indications: The various subgroups of angle closure disease in its various forms constitute the main group of diseases which benefits from laser iridotomy. It is frequently performed as a prophylactic procedure.

Prophylactic indications:
- *Primary angle closure suspect (PACS):*
  - Patients with high risk of progression to angle closure disease
  - Positive on provocative test in occludable angles
  - Occludable angles with chronic features of attack
  - One eyed with PACS
  - Family history of PAC/PACG
- Fellow eyes of established PAC or PACG

- Primary angle closure (PAC)—iridotomy prevents to develop PACG on further future.
- Primary angle closure glaucoma (PACG)—it helps to reduce IOP to prevent further progression.

Therapeutic indications:

- Phacomorphic glaucoma with pupillary block
- Subluxated lens
- Aphakic/pseudophakic pupillary block
- Plateau iris syndrome
- Pigmentary glaucoma
- In cases of secondary angle closure with iris bombe, iridotomy is the first line of treatment of choice to prevent further an acute angle closure attack and reduces IOP.
- Aqueous misdirection syndrome
- Phakic IOLs

Contraindications:

- *Neovascular glaucoma (NVG):* Likely to result in hyphema if neovascularization of the iris is present
- *Nonpupillary block mechanism:* Lens-induced narrowing of the angle and drug-induced secondary angle closure (such as antipsychotic drug therapy).

Technique:

- *Preprocedural preparation:*
  - H/o intake of anticoagulants—excessive bleeding during/after an iridotomy
  - IOP well controlled using systemic medications like mannitol or acetazolamide
  - One drop of pilocarpine 2% instilled—15 minutes before treatment
  - Informed consent taken
- *Procedure:*
  - Consent for laser is extremely important before starting the procedure.
  - IOP measurement should be done before the procedure. If it is raised Tab acetazolamide or mannitol is introduced in treatment chart to reduce the IOP.
  - Patient is comfortably seated in front of laser machine and the eye is anesthetized with 0.5% proparacaine eyedrops.
  - One drop of pilocarpine 2% is applied in 15 minutes before laser treatment.
  - An Abraham's contact lens with a coupling fluid or gel is used which provides a 1.5× image magnification and concentrates the laser power.
  - Site of choice:
    - Superior part of peripheral one-third of the iris is best choice for LPI as it is covered by the lid.
  - Energy requires around 3–9 mJ which is completed in 3–4 shots.
  - The full thickness of iris orifice formation shows sudden release of aqueous along with posterior surface of iris pigment.
  - Special technique for thicker iris:
- Argon pretreatment: A coagulative laser, i.e., argon/double-frequency YAG is implemented in a circular manner. (spot size of 300–500 µm, duration of 0.2–0.3 s, power of 0.3–0.5 W). A drumhead is created and central stretched our iris is easily pierced by Nd:YAG.
  - End point of YAG PI:
    - Fresh gush of aqueous through iridotomy
    - Waterfall-like dispersion of iris pigments from laser site
    - Transillumination positivity through PI

Complications/adverse effects:

- *Mild bleeding from iris:*
  - Inevitable side effect—often insignificant
  - Applying a little pressure with the iridotomy lens serves enough
- Transient IOP elevation
- Cataract formation
  - Progression of cortical cataract following LPI is reported
- Visual disturbances like diplopia, transient blurring, glare, shadows, lines and ghost images.
- *Endothelial damage:*
  - It is due to direct focal injury, thermal damage, mechanical shock waves, iris pigment dispersion and transient rise in IOP.
- *Lens subluxation and lens dislocation:*
  - Predisposing condition, e.g., pseudoexfoliation→ weak the zonular fibers→ further zonular damage following shock wave from LPI → lens dislocation

Selective laser trabeculoplasty (SLT)

Introduction: SLT works on selective photothermolysis, it releases thermal mediated radiation to TM without any collateral damage.

Principle/mechanism:

Van Buskirk theory:

Mechanical theory suggests that the argon laser produces electromagnetic energy gets converted to thermal energy in proximity of trabecular meshwork.

Biochemical theory says the laser stimulating cellular activity releases thermal energy. After application of ALT, the number of macrophages increases in the trabecular meshwork.

Cellular theory says laser energy stimulates increased cell division and trabecular meshwork repopulation.

Indications:

- Primary open angle glaucoma
- Ocular hypertension
- Few types of angle closure glaucoma
- POAG in pregnancy

Procedure:

- *Parameters:*
- SLT device has Q-switched, frequency-doubled, 532 nm Nd:YAG laser, 400 μm diameter spot size which delivers energy in 3 ns.

Procedure:

- After taking consent from patient topical anesthesia is applied.
- Patient seated in front of laser machine
- SLT single mirror goniolens with OVD coupling media is placed on the eye.
- By using the helium-neon (He-Ne) aiming beams, laser is focused on the TM.
- Initially it uses 0.7–0.8 mJ afterward it reduces to 0.4–1.2 mJ.
- The degree of TM pigmentation SLT titrate its energy level.
- Cavitation bubbles ("champagne bubbles") → energy is reduced by 0.1 mJ increments until no bubble formation → treatment is continued at this energy level.
- If there is no cavitation bubble formation pulse energy is increased by 0.1 mJ till the bubble formation happens then decreases as previously.

- Energy is maintained below the bubble formation occurs.
- Confluent spots give the best results.
- 360 of TM is lasered (100 spots, 25 spots per quadrant is filled).
- Success rate of ST is 60% after five years it becomes 50%.
- It reduces IOP around 3–6 mm Hg.

Complications/adverse effects:

- *Common:*
  - Redness, discomfort, and AC reaction at first week
- *Transient rise in IOP:*
  - Iritis
  - Hyphema
  - Macular edema
- *Uncommon:*
  - Transient corneal thinning
  - Reduction of endothelial cells
  - Foveal burn
  - Corneal haze

Argon laser trabeculoplasty: It is a low grade coagulative laser burn, which targets anterior trabecular meshwork.
Mechanism: It causes TM tension circumferentially which pulls outer layer of TM helps in aqueous outflow.

- The exact mechanism is unknown.
- There are mechanical, cellular and biochemical theories which facilitates aqueous outflow for lowering IOP.
- Based on mechanical theory, laser electromagnetic energy is converted to thermal energy which causes contraction of TM. Further scar formation causes stretching of TM improves aqueous outflow.

Indications:

- Primary open angle glaucoma
- Ocular hypertension
- Few types of angle closure glaucoma
- POAG in pregnancy
- Secondary glaucoma, i.e., PXF, pigmentary glaucoma
- Steroid induced glaucoma

Procedure:

- Alpha adrenergic agonist is applied before 30 minutes of procedure.
- After taking consent from patient topical anesthesia is applied.
- Patient seated in front of laser machine.
- ALT single mirror goniolens with OVD coupling media is placed on the eye.
- Argon green laser is set at 50 µm spot size, in 0.1 s duration, power 300–1,000 mW.
- It targets at the junction between ATM and PTM.
- Laser blanches TM by producing small amount of bubble.
- IOP reduces by treating 180° TM angle.

Complications:

- Raised IOP
- PAS formation

15. Discuss the Advances in trabeculectomy. (10) (DNB)

Introduction: Trabeculectomy is considered the gold standard surgery till date. A number of modifications have reduced complications from increased understanding of wound healing, the development of antimetabolites regimens, and modifications in surgical techniques.

Modifications in trabeculectomy
Anesthesia:

- Shifting to topical anesthesia based trabeculectomy:
  - Limitation: Lack of akinesia; orbicularis oculi be paralyzed to prevent globe compression in patients who have prominent eyelid squeezing
- Intracameral unpreserved 1% lidocaine—supplements topical anesthesia
  - Limitations: Risk of damaging the phakic lens, and inadvertent dilation may cause the peripheral iridectomy to be excessively large.

Traction suture: Superior rectus suture may decrease surgical access, put tension on the conjunctiva, and cause scarring from hemorrhage or tissue damage. A corneal traction suture is more firmly fixed and therefore exerts a more consistent vector force

Choice of surgical site:
Ideal bleb position: Totally under the upper lid—provides additional protection from infection and exposure in the interpalpebral area—risk of repeated massage—like action while blinking—hypotony and recurrent SCH.

Tenon dissection:
Small incision trabeculectomy (SIT): Minimizes tenon dissection; a 2.5-mm conjunctival incision is made at the limbus, avoiding Tenon dissection—a scleral pocket is dissected posteriorly—subconjunctival space is entered via the pocket to form a bleb.

In chronic angle closure patients, SIT surgery, even without enhancement has been comparable in success to trabeculectomy with mitomycin-C.

Table 8. Difference between Limbus and fornix based flaps.

TABLE 8: Limbus versus fornix-based flaps.

	Fornix-based conjunctival flap	***Limbal-based conjunctival flap***
Technical difficulty	Easier and faster to perform	More difficult and takes longer to perform
Exposure of operative field	Good exposure allowing good visualization of sclerostomy and easier 'releasable' suture placement	Not as good, less visualization of sclerostomy and reflected conjunctiva may make releasable sutures difficult
Area to be dissected	Smaller	Larger
Antifibrotic application	Need great care on insertion, may need more sponges	Easier antifibrotic application
Re-operation	Easier	More difficult due to extensive scarring
Bleb morphology	More diffuse posteriorly draining blebs	May get more cystic blebs and "ring of steel" with more anterior drainage

- *Flap size:*
  - Strategies to maximize posterior flow:
    - Leaving the sides of the flap intact 1 mm posteriorly to the limbus, to encourage posterior flow.
    - Thickness of the flap should be enough (half scleral thickness) preventing dehiscence (and anterior drainage) and cheese wiring of sutures.
    - Adequate size:
      - Large flap with a large mitomycin C treatment area - less cystic and well-tolerated diffuse bleb.

- *Flap handling:*
  - Sutures can be manipulated transconjunctivally with noncutting forceps Duckworth and Kent. Advantages include fine and smooth edges to prevent button-holing and minimal discomfort under topical anesthesia at the slit lamp

Peripheral iridectomy:

- Intraocular infusion at the time of iridectomy—can be used to present the iris, avoiding intraocular manipulation.
- *Horizontal iridectomy:*
  - creates a short broad defect, achieving the necessary effect
  - reduces the chance of the iridectomy encroaching on the visual axis.

Suture-based modifications:

Adjustable/releasable sutures:

- Sutures provide resistance to flow across the flap in the early postop period before wound healing
- *Principle of releasable sutures:*
  - Use of releasable sutures reduced the incidence of shallow anterior chamber and hypotony in the early postoperative period.
  - Once the wound and anterior chamber stabilize, the sutures are released to enhance the outflow of aqueous humor.
- *Technique in **Figures 6A to C**:*
  - Common technique

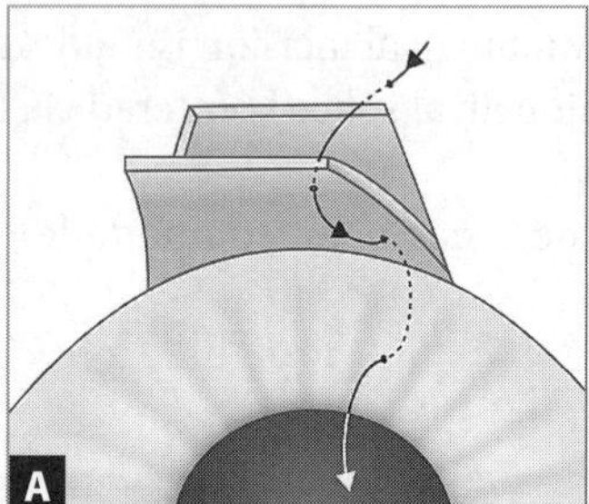

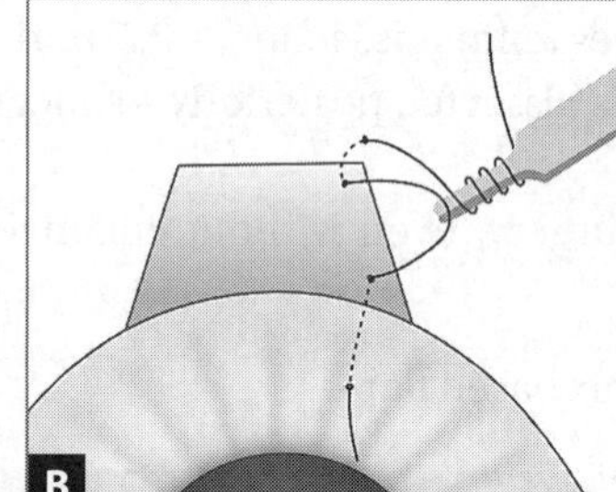

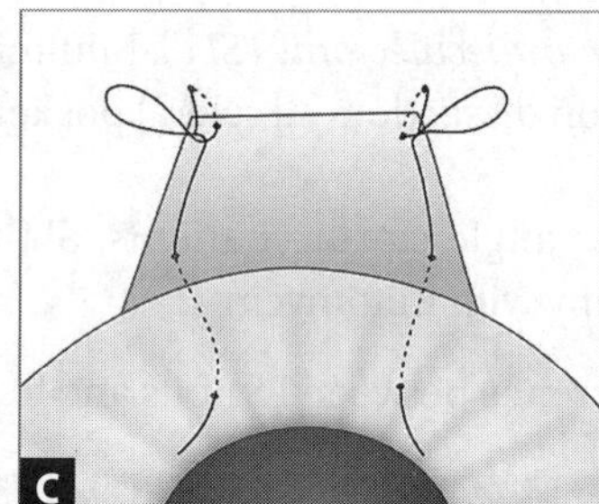

Figs. 6A to C: (A) The needle is passed into sclera and through flap. After passing the needle through base of scleral flap, beneath the conjunctival insertion, it is taken through the peripheral cornea; (B) The suture is tied with a quadruple throw slipknot; (C) The rectangular scleral flap is sutured with two releasable sutures.

- Wilson technique **(Fig. 7)**:
  - Mattress type scleral suture, externalized with the knot on the cornea.
  - Postoperatively, the suture could be cut or removed.
- *Complications:*
  - Windshield wiper keratopathy:
    - Wedge-shaped keratopathy due to the rubbing of suture on cornea with the movement of lids.
  - Risk of bleb infection:
    - A track remains when the suture is trimmed—increased risk of infection.

*Stitchless trabeculectomy **(Figs. 8A to E)**:*

- *Procedure:*
  - Similar to SICS, valved fistula is created for drainage of aqueous without need for sutures.

Wilson's releasable

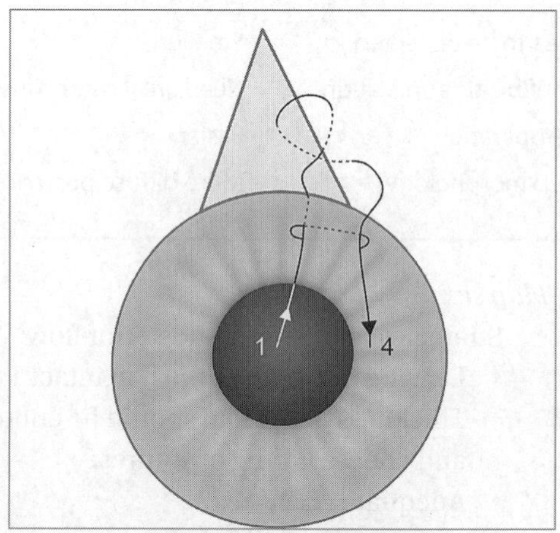

Fig. 7: Wilson releasable suture.

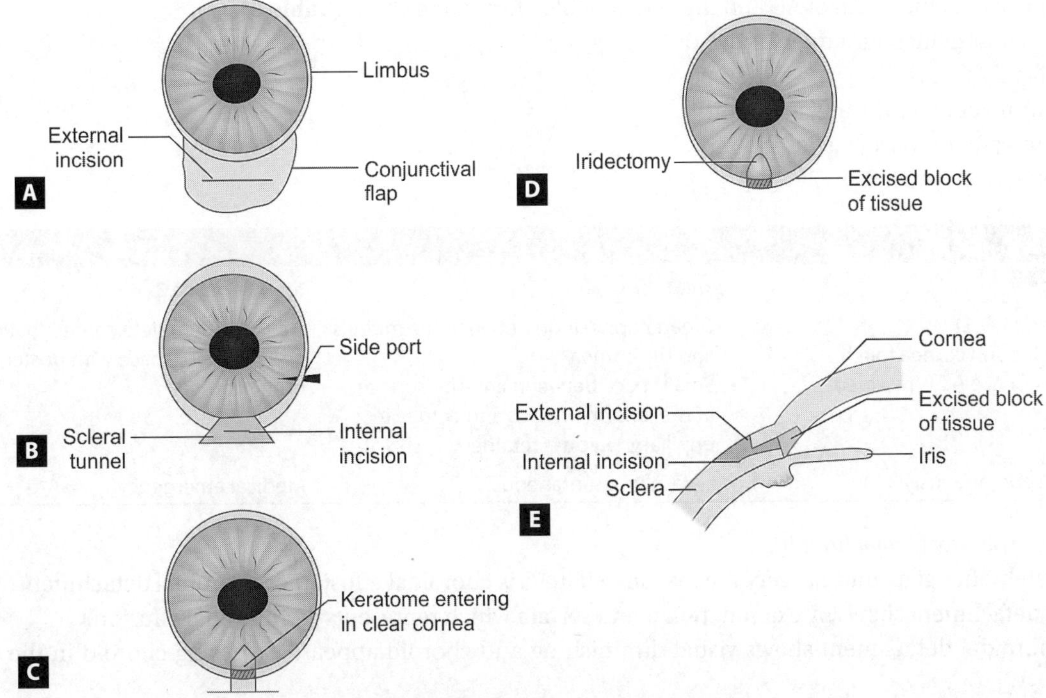

Figs. 8A to E: Steps of stitchless trabeculectomy.

- *Advantages:*
  - Single-visit surgical manipulation unlike adjustable suture techniques
  - Significantly reduced chances of postoperative infection because of there being no stitches.
  - No irritation and other discomforts of the stitches.
  - Lesser visits by the patient because suture removal is not required.
  - A diffuse and noncystic bleb.
  - Lesser chances of postoperative uveitis just like in "phaco".

Maintenance of anterior chamber: A simple anterior chamber infusion with a three-way tap can maintain a near constant pressure intraoperatively.

Conjunctival closure:

- Anchoring corneal suture technique seals the conjunctiva under tension with no mattress sutures.
- Clear cornea grooves are preplaced 2 mm from the limbus, with 10-0 nylon passed through the groove and conjunctiva, with the knots buried in the corner

Use of antimetabolites:

- *Physiologic antiscarring agents:*
  - Target-specific mediators of scarring, such as inflammatory mediators, transforming growth factor ß (TGF-ß), and matrix metalloproteinases
  - Delivered with minimal risk of hypotony
- Postoperative injections of 5-fluorouracil—better postoperative

Prognosis—Combined with viscoelastics to improve delivery and minimize complications

16. A patient with chronic angle closure undergoes a trabeculectomy and has a shallow AC on a first postoperative day. Describe the process by which you would discern the cause of postoperative AC shallowing and how you would manage this situation. (5 + 5) (DNB 2019, 2022, 2023)

Trabeculectomy is an antiglaucoma surgery in which lamellar scleral flap is excised from Schlemm's canal, produces flirting bleb through subconjunctival space.

Based on few factors, the depth of AC and the extent of bleb formation occur **(Table 9)**:

- If full thickness glaucoma surgery is done
- Scleral flap tightness
- Using antimetabolites during operation
- Using intracameral viscoelastics
- The tightness of eyepatch

TABLE 9: Spaeth grading.

Spaeth grade 1	*Spaeth grade 2*	*Spaeth grade 3*
• Flat peripheral ACD • Peripheral iris and cornea touch • At pupillary space AC is reserved	• Greater apposition between the mid-iris and the cornea • Small space between anterior surface of the lens or vitreous and cornea in pupillary region is retained.	AC is flat; complete contact between iris and pupillary space with posterior surface of the cornea
May resolve spontaneously	May resolve spontaneously	Medical emergency

Flat AC with hypotony ***(Flowchart 9)****:*

- Immediately after glaucoma surgery the reason of flat AC is choroidal effusion or choroidal detachment.
- Annular detachment shows by examination of ora serrata which represents as choroidal effusion.
- Large choroidal detachment shows visual diminishing and choroid appears as kissing choroid in the midvitreal cavity.

Flowchart 9: Shallow and flat AC.

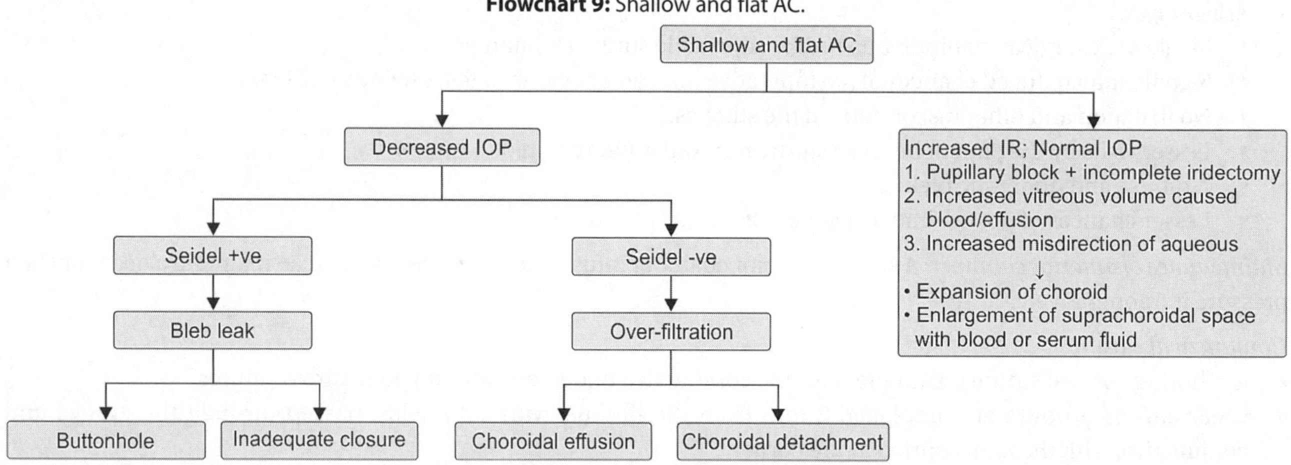

Management:

- *Medical management:* Seidel's test rules out the presence conjunctival leakage. In absence of conjunctival leak the surgical intervention does not need.

Surgical intervention:

- It is needed in kissing choroid to reduce the bullous detachment. To reduce inflammatory cells steroid and atropine.
- Severe shallow ACD leads to aqueous misdirection syndrome.

Bleb leak:

- Soft contact lens or Simmon's shell can be introduced to prevent aqueous leak and promotes healing of buttonhole.
- Using antimetabolites during glaucoma surgery prevents buttonhole formation; may be treated with cyanoacrylate, fibrin glue and compression suture.

- "X "like suture is given in wound leak site and attached to episcleral tissue.
- If the lens or IOL push the posterior cornea—viscoelastic injection or intraocular gas introduction. Introduction of 30 gauge needle can be passed in AC.
- If the injected material comes out through sclerotomy site—AC is reformed with BSS or OVD. Suprachoroidal effusion drainage should be done by maintain AC.

Aqueous misdirection syndrome:
Refer to question 12.

Suprachoroidal hemorrhage:
- It occurs frequently with glaucoma surgery with antimetabolites and glaucoma shunt procedures.
- *Risk factors:*
  - Aphakia—most common cause
  - Traumatized eyes
  - Vitrectomized eyes
  - Pathological myopia
  - Megalocornea with congenital glaucoma eyes with significant post-operative hypotony
  - Patients under systemic anticoagulants
- *Clinical signs:*
  - Severe pain with sudden onset loss of vision on 4th or 5th postoperative days.
  - In severe hemorrhage, IOP gets high.
  - Patient having nausea and vomiting.

Treatment:
Medical treatment:
- Aqueous suppressants
- Hyperosmotic agents
- If the IOP is low then BSS, OVD or air reform AC; AC maintaining device is applied.
- If IOP is high enlargement of sclerotomy can be done.

17. Indications, pressure lowering effect, advantages, disadvantages and complications of iStent in glaucoma. (2 + 2 + 2 + 2 + 2) (DNB 2021)

Introduction: iStent is a group of devices employed in minimally invasive glaucoma surgery.

The device evolved over time and is divided into three generations

iStent (Glaukos, Laguna Hills, CA): First and the tiniest (photograph inset)

Design: GlaukosiStent is a lightweight, titanium, L-shaped device placed inside Schlemm's canal. It is coated with heparin, rendering it biocompatible, has thrombolytic activity and prevents stenosis **(Fig. 9)**. A small, snorkel shaped tube (0.5 mm) is lodged in the peripheral anterior chamber. This part of the tube is 1 mm in length and is shaped like a half pipe. It is designed to fit within the lumen of the canal, with the curved convex side lying against the inner wall of Schlemm's canal. The role of the barbed ridges is to prevent loosening and provide a secure placement of the stent in the canal. Stents are designed as either right-handed or left-handed for ease of insertion into the canal.

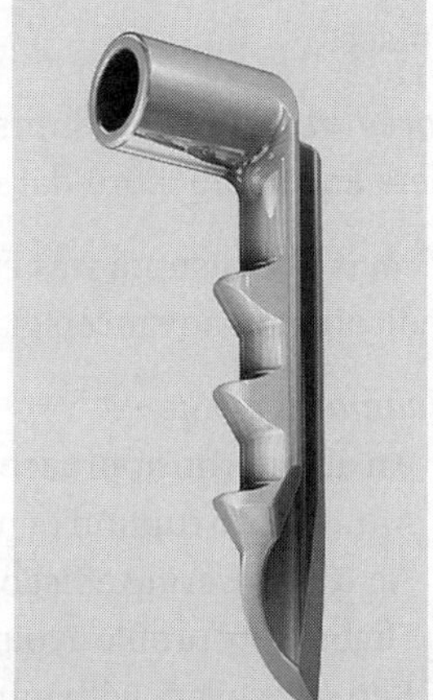

Fig. 9: Glaukos iStent.

Mechanism of action: This tube allows aqueous to bypass the inner wall of Schlemm's canal and the juxtacanalicular trabecular meshwork.

Surgical procedure: The surgical procedure is explained in **Figure 10**.

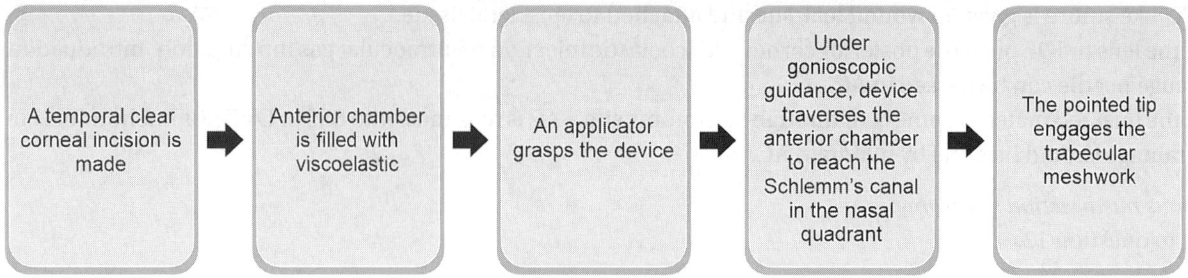

Fig. 10: Surgical procedure.

Efficiency: iStent implantation resulted in an IOP reduction of more than 20%(around 25%) in 70% of the patients in most of the studies with significant decrease in the number of medications used at 1 year.

iStent inject (Glaukos, Laguna Hills, CA): Second-generation **(Fig. 11)**

Design: Smallest medical implant approved for use in the human body during surgical procedures. It is a heparin-coated, non-ferromagnetic titanium stent, 360 microns in height by 230 microns in diameter with a central lumen of 80 microns.

Procedure: Delivered via ab interno approach under gonioscopic visualization. The single use injector (G2-M-IS injector system) comes preloaded with two stents, which are to be placed nasally into the TM and Schlemm' s canal with 30°–60° apart.

Efficacy: IOP reduction of 35–39% with improved medication burden following iStent inject, where 65–75% subjects were completely off medication at 1 year.

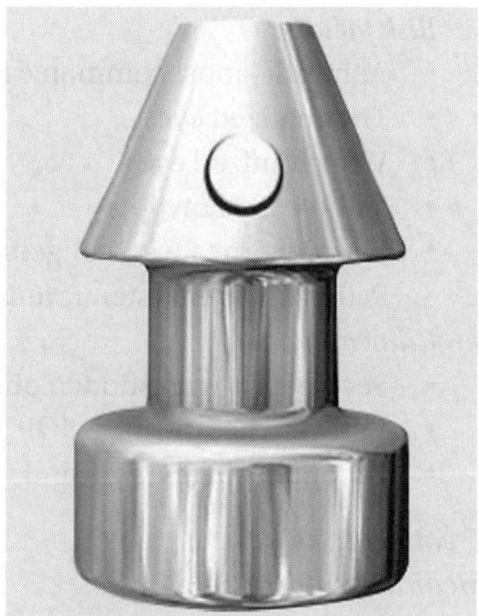

Fig. 11: Second-generation iStent.

iStent Supra (third generation)
It is different from previous iStents in being a suprachoroidal shunt rather than just a trabecular bypass shunt **(Fig. 12)**.

Design: Heparin-coated, 4 mm curved tube with a 0.16–0.17 mm lumen, made of biocompatible polyethersulfone (PES) with a titanium sleeve and retention ridges to hold it in place.

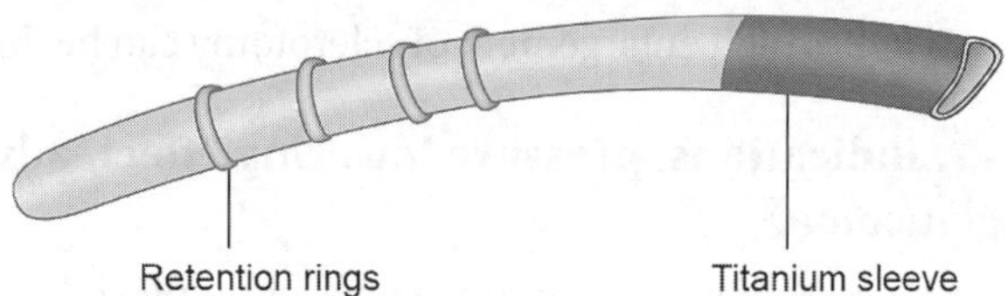

Fig. 12: Third-generation iStent.

Procedure: The iStentSupra is guide mounted. This guide is used to direct the device between the anterior chamber/ sclera and suprachoroidal space via an ab interno approach under direct gonioscopy.

Efficacy: iStent supra was effective along with Travoprost eye drops in reducing more that 20% IOP with reduction in 1 medication in advanced glaucoma.

Advantages of iStent:
- An ab interno approach through a clear corneal incision which spares the conjunctiva of incision.
- Minimal disruption of normal anatomy.
- An IOP lowering efficacy that justifies the approach.
- High safety profile avoiding serious complications compared to other glaucoma surgeries.
- Rapid recovery with minimal impact on the patient's quality of life.

Disadvantages of iStent:
- Less comparable in efficacy to conventional filtration surgeries.
- Steep learning curve in handling surgeries under direct gonioscopy

Complications:

- *Intraoperative:*
  - Inadvertent damage to adjacent structures like corneal endothelium, iris
  - Dislodging of stent-free floating stent in AC
- *Postoperative:*
  - Failure to reduce IOP
  - Late dislodgement of the stent
- *Indication:*
  - Mild to moderate primary open angle glaucoma
  - Combined with cataract surgery in patients with mild to moderate open angle glaucoma
  - Ocular hypertension
- *Contraindications:*
  - Angle closure glaucoma
  - Uveitic glaucoma
  - Neovascular glaucoma

18. Discuss briefly on Micro-invasive glaucoma surgery (MIGS). (10) DNB 2020, WBUHS MS 2024

Shunt procedures/minimally invasive glaucoma surgery

- *Introduction/definition:*
  - American Glaucoma Society and US Food and Drug Administration (FDA) definition: Implantation of a surgical device intended to lower IOP via an outflow mechanism with either an ab interno or ab externo approach, associated with very little or no scleral dissection.
- *General characteristics of MIGS procedure:*
  - An ab interno approach through a clear corneal incision- spares the conjunctiva of incision.
  - Minimal disruption of normal anatomy.
  - An IOP lowering efficacy that justifies the approach.
  - High safety profile avoiding serious complications compared to other glaucoma surgeries.
  - Rapid recovery with minimal impact on the patient's quality of life.
- *Classification:*
  - The three main approaches of reducing IOP by MIGS are included in **Flowchart 10**.

Flowchart 10: Approaches to reduce IOP by MIGS.

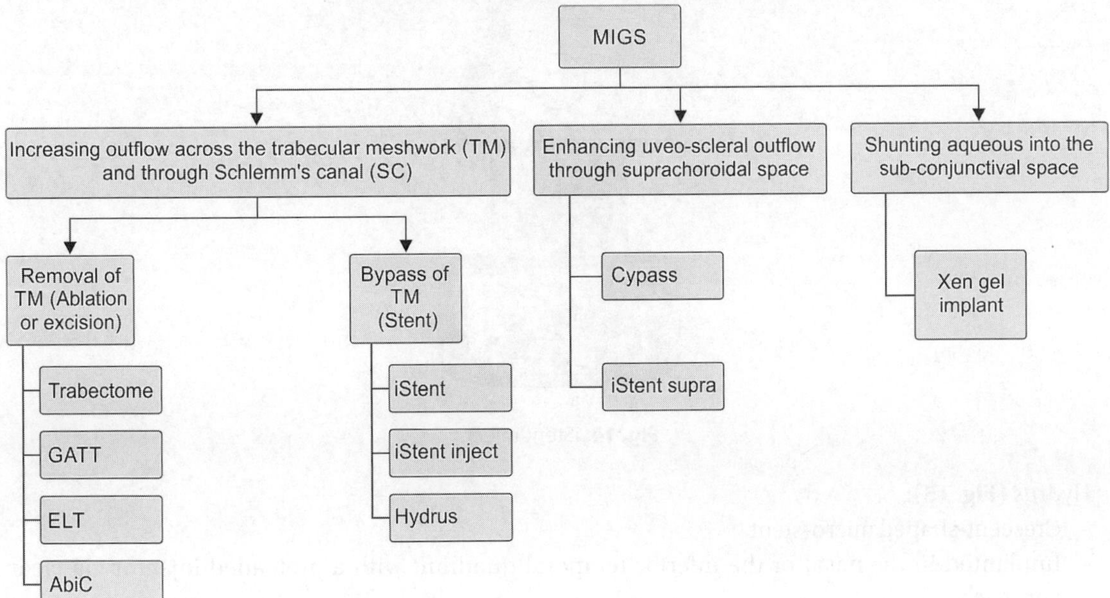

- *Trabecular meshwork-based procedures:*
  - Aims:
    - To remove (by ablation and excision) or bypass (through stents) the aforementioned tissue, allowing more direct access to aqueous humor
  - Indications:
    - Mild to moderate primary open-angle glaucoma, pigmentary glaucoma, pseudoexfoliation glaucoma, ocular hypertension with modest IOP target of 15–16 mm Hg
  - Contraindications:
    - Eyes with primary or secondary angle closure glaucoma.
    - Eyes with active neovascularization.
    - Eyes with hazy cornea and angle dysgenesis
    - Patients with elevated episcleral venous syndrome such as retrobulbar tumor, thyroid eye disease, Sturge-Weber syndrome.
  - Adverse effects:
    - Hyphema (most common), stent malposition or temporary obstruction, focal peripheral synechiae, transient increase in IOP.
- *Types of procedures:*
  - Stent placement-based procedures:
    - iStent **(Fig. 13)**:
      - Heparin-coated, non-ferromagnetic titanium stent with a ridged snorkel design.
      - Efficacy was modest but allowed a prolonged reduction in IOP and medication burden
    - iStent inject **(Fig. 14)**:
      - Smallest medical implant approved for use in the human body.
      - Implantation of 2 iStent injects is comparable to treatment with two agents (latanoprost and timolol) in reducing IOP at 1 year.

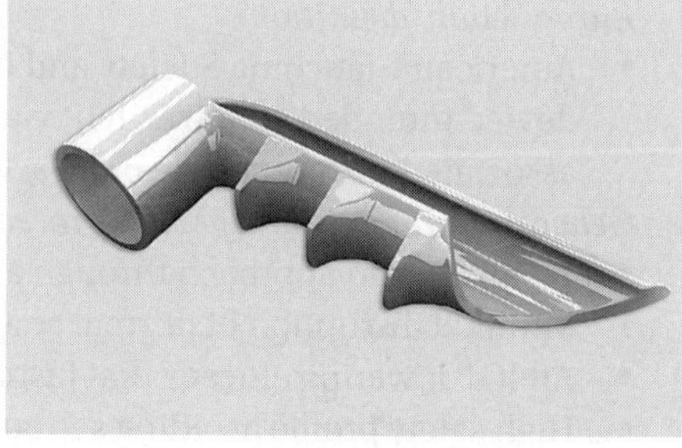

Fig. 13: iStent.

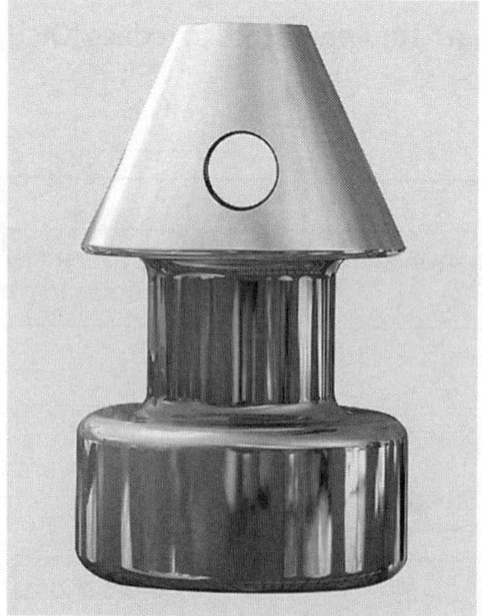

Fig. 14: iStent inject.

    - Hydrus **(Fig. 15)**:
      - Crescent-shaped micro-stent.
      - Implanted in the nasal or the inferior temporal quadrant with a preloaded injector via clear corneal approach.

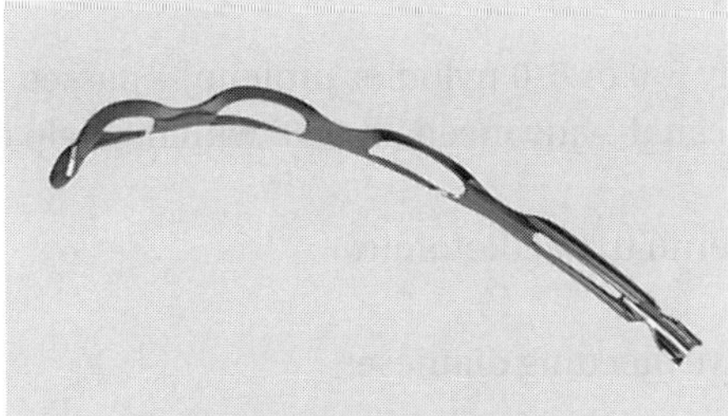

Fig. 15: Hydrus device.

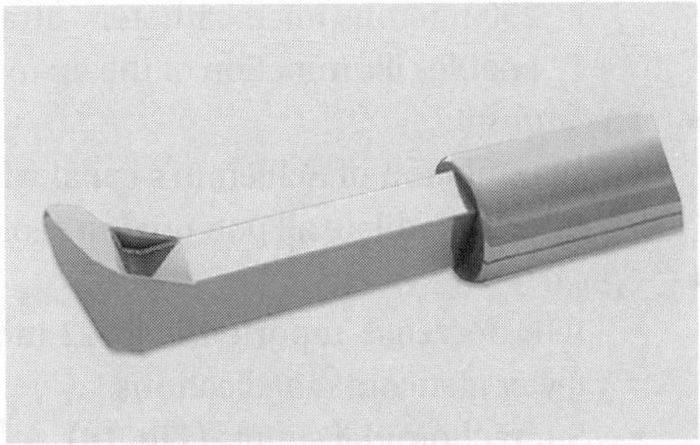

Fig. 16: Kahook blade.

- *Mechanism:*
  - Works on the trimodal mechanism—allowing aqueous humor to bypass the trabecular meshwork.
  - Dilating Schlemm's canal 4–5 times the natural width
  - Countering the collapse of the canal induced by increased IOP.
  - Enable outflow through more collector channels.
- *Efficiency:*
  - COMPARE study, comparing Hydrus with iStent showed better efficacy of Hydrus.
  - Trabecular meshwork bypass by tissue excision (trabeculotomy)
    - Kahook Dual Blade Goniotomy **(Fig. 16)**:
      - Stainless steel disposable, dual blade with a sharp tip.
- *Mechanism:*
  - Causes near complete removal of trabecular meshwork with negligible surrounding tissue damage and less fibrosis.
- *Efficacy:*
  - KDB has also shown better results compared with Trabectome and iStent
    - Trabectome **(Fig. 17)**:

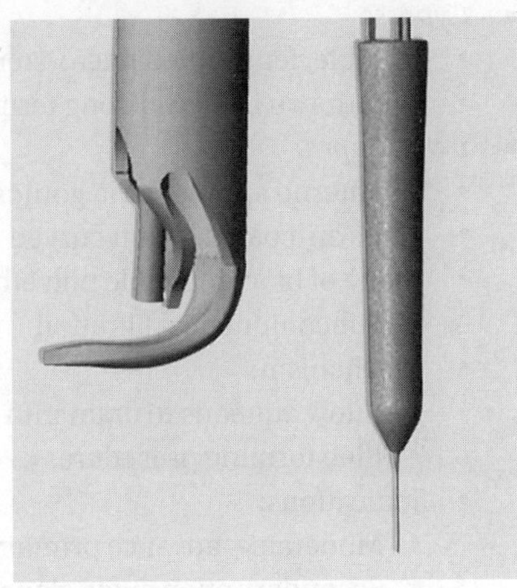

Fig. 17: Trabectome.

- *Components:*
  - Disposable 19.5 gauze handpiece, console
  - Automated irrigation and aspiration and
  - Electrocautery generator with foot pedal.
- *Principle:*
  - Tip has a bipolar 550 KHz electrode
  - Generates plasma that ionizes and ablates TM—opening from AC into Schlemm's canal.
  - Up to 40% fewer medications at 2 years.
    - Excimer laser trabeculostomy:
- *Principle and working:*
  - An ab interno procedure performed under direct visualization of gonioscope or endoscope.
  - 1.2 mJ at the fiber tip, the laser pulse duration is between 10 and 60 ns and the repetition rate is 20 Hz.
- *Efficacy:*
  - Moderate IOP lowering, decrease in 1 glaucoma medication.
    - Gonioscopy-assisted transluminal trabeculotomy (GATT)
- *Components:*
  - Microsurgical forceps
  - iTrack microcatheter with a 200-micron diameter shaft
  - Lubricating coating and an illuminated distal tip (to monitor catheter location).

- *Procedure:*
  - Microcatheter or suture (typically 5-0 or 6-0 nylon or prolene)—passed through a 1–2 clock hour goniotomy in the nasal quadrant—Schlemm's canal—advanced for 360° with the help of microforceps.
- *Efficacy:*
  - Similar in effectiveness as ab externo trabeculotomies
- *Contraindication:*
  - Requiring anticoagulation, or have bleeding diatheses
  - Ab interno canaloplasty:
- *Components:*
  - iTrackmicrocatheter system
    - 250 microns microcatheter—atraumatic bulbous tip and a greasy coating for easier passage + fiber optic that enables illumination of the tip to monitor + visco-injector
- *Mechanism:*
  - Cannulation of Schlemm's canal with the microcatheter—withdrawn as an ophthalmic visco-surgical device is injected—dilate all potential sites of outflow resistance
- *Efficacy:*
  - IOP decrease reported is at 12 months with at least 2 fewer glaucoma medications.
  - Suprachoroidal shunts **(Fig. 18)**
    - Mechanism: Direct aqueous outflow in a controlled fashion to suprachoroidal space essentially increasing physiological uveoscleral pathway.

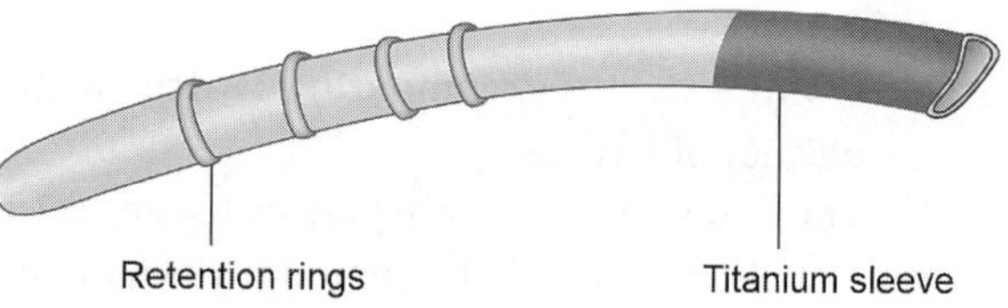

Fig. 18: Suprachoroidal shunts.

- *Cypass:*
  - Flexible, fenestrated micro-stent sized with a lumen and composed of biocompatible, polyimide material.
  - Withdrawn in view of long term adverse effect of endothelial cell loss.
- *iStent Supra:*
  - Ab interno approach via gonioscopy
  - Heparin-coated, 4 mm curved tube
  - Made of biocompatible polyethersulfone (PES) with a titanium sleeve and retention ridges to hold it in place.
    - Subconjunctival filtration
  - Mechanism:
    - Allow aqueous to drain into the subconjunctival space.
    - Bleb forming procedures
  - Indications:
    - Moderate—advance primary
    - Secondary open angle glaucoma
    - Refractory glaucoma in whom maximal medical therapy is not sufficient
  - Contraindications:
    - Angle closure glaucoma Patients with conjunctival scarring
  - Types:
    - Xen gel stent **(Fig. 19)**:
  - Structure:
    - Hydrophilic tube, composed of porcine derived gelatin cross-linked with glutaraldehyde.

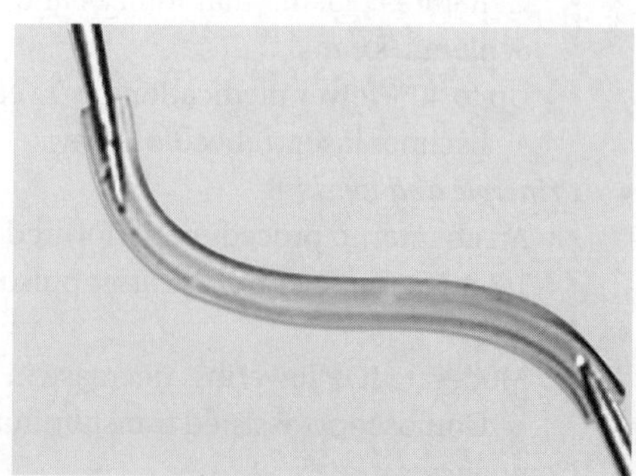
Fig. 19: Xen gel stent.

- Relatively straight and rigid when dry, flexible, and soft when hydrated.
- Principle:
  - Hagen–Poiseuille equation
  - Very small lumen versus its length leads to outflow resistance—less risk of hypotony
- Procedure:
  - Via an ab interno approach,
  - Superonasal/superior quadrant and tunneled through sclera
  - After implantation, stent creates a filtering bleb—can be augmented with Mitomycin-C.
- Efficacy:
  - 45% decrease in average IOP, 45% being medication free.
  - Adverse effects:
  - Exposure of the stent
  - Obstruction of the stent with blood, lens fragments or visco-elastics

19. Enumerate various implant drainage devices in glaucoma surgery. Indications and adverse effects of Ahmed Glaucoma Valve. (10) DNB

Introduction: Implant surgery has founds its unique place in the management of difficult cases in glaucoma management and offers the option of Glaucoma drainage devices.

Principle/Mechanism: These aim to create an alternate pathway for aqueous outflow by rerouting aqueous from the anterior chamber (AC) through the long tube of the implant towards the subconjunctival space of the equatorial region of the globe.

Classification **(Flowchart 11)**

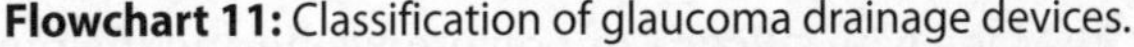

Flowchart 11: Classification of glaucoma drainage devices.

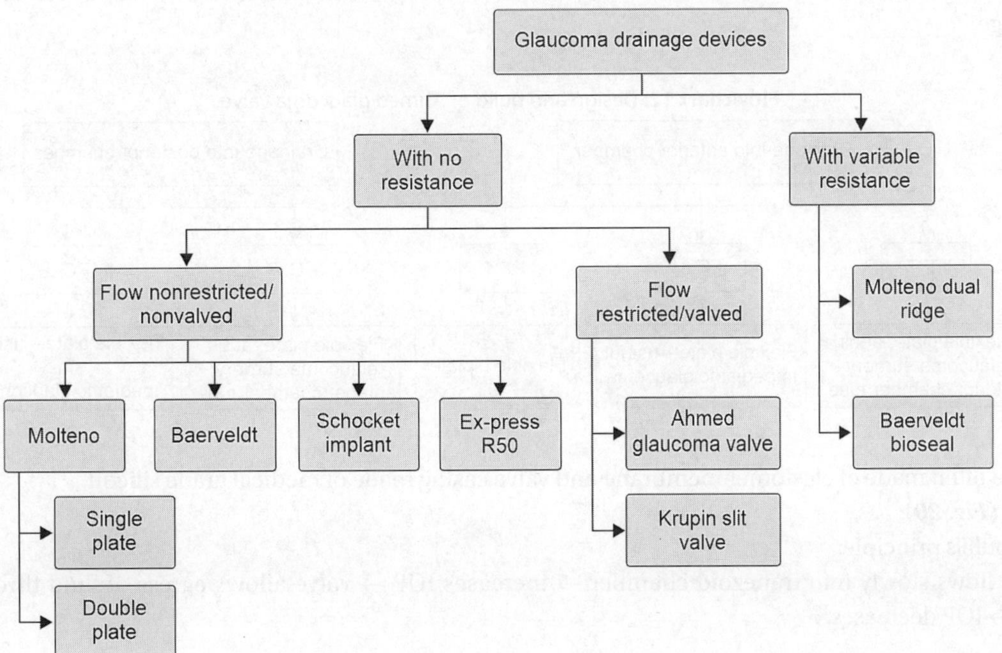

Indications:

- Reserved for refractory glaucoma cases and those not responding to a conventional filtration surgery
- Neovascular glaucoma
- PKP with glaucoma
- Uveitic glaucoma
- Retinal detachment surgery with glaucoma
- ICE syndrome
- Traumatic glaucoma
- Sturge-Weber syndrome
- Open-angle glaucoma with failed trabeculectomy
- Epithelial downgrowth
- Refractory infantile glaucoma
- Contact lens wearers who need glaucoma filtration surgery

Contraindications:

- *Absolute:*
  - Ciliary block glaucoma
  - Extensive fibrosis of conjunctiva
  - Eyes with severe scleral and or sclerolimbal thining.
- *Relative:*
  - Vitreous in anterior chamber
  - Intraocular silicone oil—implant if required is placed in inferotemporal quadrant

Ahmed glaucoma valve

- *Introduction:* Valved drainage device which utilizes patented venturi valve mechanism for control of aqueous drainage.
- *Design and build **(Flowchart 12)**:* Made with silicone or polypropylene and the models vary depending on the area of drainage

Flowchart 12: Design and build of Ahmed glaucoma valve.

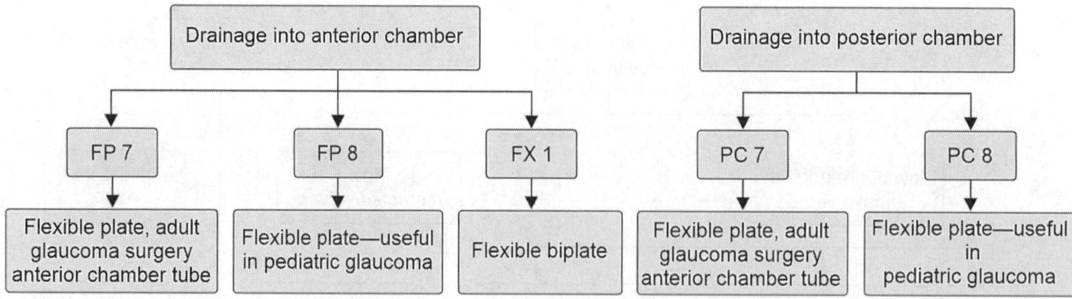

Valves are often made of elastomer membrane and valve casing made of medical grade silicon.

- *Principle **(Fig. 20)**:*
  - Bernoulli's principle:

Aqueous flows slowly into trapezoid chamber → increases IOP → valve allows egress of fluid through silicone membrane → IOP decreases.

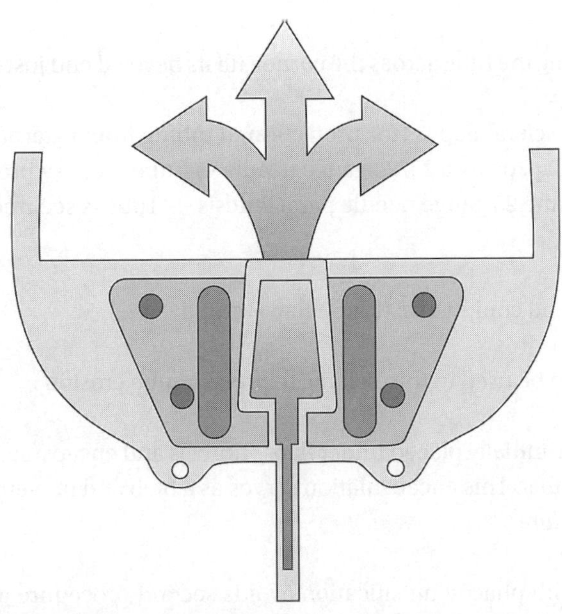

Fig. 20: The patented trapezoidal valve mechanism of Ahmed Glaucoma Valve.

Comparison with Molteno implant is shown in **Table 10**.

TABLE 10: Difference between AGV and Double Molteno.

	AGV	*Double Molteno*
Ideal	Minimal optic nerve damage	Advanced glaucomatous damage
Surgical techniques	1-quadrant dissection	extensive dissection
Complications		
Hypotony	Low incidence of hypotony	High incidence of hypotony
Postoperative care		
Need for stent to prevent hypotony	No	Yes
Additional glaucoma meds/needling of bleb	May be needed	Not needed

Surgical technique

- *Priming/preparation:*
  - All devices are primed with balanced salt solution to check it's patency before insertion.
  - Nonvalved implant the glaucoma drainage device is disabled before insertion to prevent an excessive early IOP drop by ligating it using an absorbable or a prolene suture (*Latina suture)*
- *Procedure:*
  - A fornix-based conjunctival flap with radial relaxing incisions/ limbal based flap is made. Plate part of the glaucoma drainage device is inserted beneath the Tenon's capsule preferably in the superotemporal followed by the superomedial quadrant if the former area is scarred.
- *Anchoring and positioning:*
  - Anterior edge of the implant – at least 8 mm away from the limbus.
  - Nonabsorbable- 8-0 or 10-0 nylon sutures are used to anchor the implant plate to the sclera through the fixation holes.

Tube placement:

- Length is then assessed by laying the tube across the cornea till its beveled end just enters 2–3 mm inside the anterior chamber.
- Partial thickness limbal based scleral flap is (for protection of tubing from external exposure) → Anterior chamber is entered beneath the scleral flap, using a 23/24 gauge needle → Tube is cut → proximal end beveled, and placed in the anterior chamber through the 23 gauge needle paracentesis → Tube is secured to the sclera with a two to three 9-0/10-0 nylon sutures.
- *Closure:*
  - Scleral flap approximated and conjunctiva-Tenon flap sutured
- *Technical modifications:*
  - Donor sclera/fascia lata can be used in thin sclerae to prevent tube erosion
- *Two staged approach:*
  - Non valved implants—Tube initially placed under flap—fibrosis and encapsulation allowed for 4 weeks then tube inserted into anterior chamber. This encapsulation serves as a bleb and prevents hypotony.
- *Combination with other procedures:*
  - In coexisting cataract cases
    - Combined procedure with phacoemulsification avoids second procedure and imminent cataract formation following GDD procedure.
  - Prior PPV/buckle placement
    - Buckle placement—360° conjunctival peritomy and scarring
    - Superotemporal quadrant—first choice
    - If silicon oil present—inferotemporal quadrant preferred
    - Oil is lighter than fluid it migrates upward/superiorly—chance of egress of silicone oil into subconjunctival space if GDD is superotemporal
- *Postoperative care:*
  - Topical steroids, antibiotics and occasionally systemic steroids.
- *Complications:*
  - Early
    - Hypotony results from excessive flow/leakage through the tube
      - If temporary occlusion does not work → Reform AC with paracentesis → does not work → Remove tube and suture
    - Elevated IOP
      - Early causes due to obstruction of the tube by fibrin, blood, iris tissue, or vitreous while late *causes are* due to an excessively thick fibrous capsule.
      - Less common ones include hyphema and corneal endothelial touch
  - Late complications—occurring within weeks or months
  - Increased IOP
  - Tube exposure/migration/extrusion
    - Migration is usually due to slippage of anchoring sutures.
    - Treatment is initially by rotating an adjacent partial; thickness flap to cover the tube but ultimately a fresh site needs to be selected.
  - Others are ocular motility disturbance and epithelial down growth.

20. Goniotomy – short note (5) DNB 2022

Indications:

- Primary congenital (infantile) glaucoma
- Congenital ectropion uveae with open angles

- Aniridia with open angles or limited angle closure
- Congenital iris hypoplasia with open angles
- Sturge–Weber syndrome
- Uveitic glaucoma

Preoperative consideration:

- Examination under anesthesia (EUA):
  - Extent of glaucoma
  - Ocular health: Corneal diameter, IOP, axial length, dilated fundoscopy, B-scan, pachymetry
- One or both eyes to be decided
- If IOP is high and cornea is hazy
  - Medical management with topical medication, e.g., β blockers, CAI, PGs to be used first to clear the cornea to facilitate goniotomy
  - Short course of systemic acetazolamide at 25 mg/kg body weight may be needed

Contraindications:

- Eyes with corneal scarring or cloudy cornea
- Older children with advanced disease
- High risk of bleeding due to dilated vessels
- Very large eyes: Schlemm's canal and aqueous outflow channels may be obliterated

Principles of goniotomy:

- Ab interno angle surgery
- Angle structures are visualized directly using surgical goniolens like Swan Jacob
- Nonfunctional TM sliced using a knife or blade
- Provides a conduit for the aqueous to bypass the TM and exit through the Schlemm's canal and connector channels

Steps:

1. Microscope tilted at 45°
2. Head of the patient tilted to the opposite side
3. Surgeon sits directly opposite the angles to be operated
4. Child under GA
5. Side port made with MVA blade 180° away from the angle to be operated
6. Nasal angle is preferred for initial goniotomy
7. 2% Pilocarpine injected in AC
8. Angles visualized with goniolens
9. AC deepening with viscoelastic
10. Goniotomy performed with MVR knife/gonioknife/24 G needle by cutting the TM in the middle
11. Successful goniotomy shows formation of goniocleft and falling back of iris
12. Side port sutured with 10-0 MFN

Complications of goniotomy:

- Hyphema
- Injury to iris and lens
- Iridodialysis and cyclodialysis

21. Classify the various non penetrating glaucoma surgeries. What are their indications, advantages and disadvantages over conventional glaucoma surgeries. (2 + 3 + 3 + 2) DNB 2021

Introduction:

- Nonpenetrating glaucoma surgery is a group of procedures which aim to safer than the standard filtering operation.
- There is no intraoperative entry into the anterior chamber and there is no resultant bleb formation which eliminates the possibility of bleb related complications.

Principle:

- Aqueous outflow resistance is believed to be in the juxtacanalicular meshwork and the inner wall of the Schlemm's canal.
- The goal of nonpenetrating glaucoma surgery is to improve the outflow facility but it retains some residual outflow resistance by maintaining a membrane between the anterior chamber and the sclera dissection—trabeculo-descemetic's membrane (TDM).

Classification ***(Flowchart 13)***

Flowchart 13: Classification of nonpenetrating glaucoma surgery.

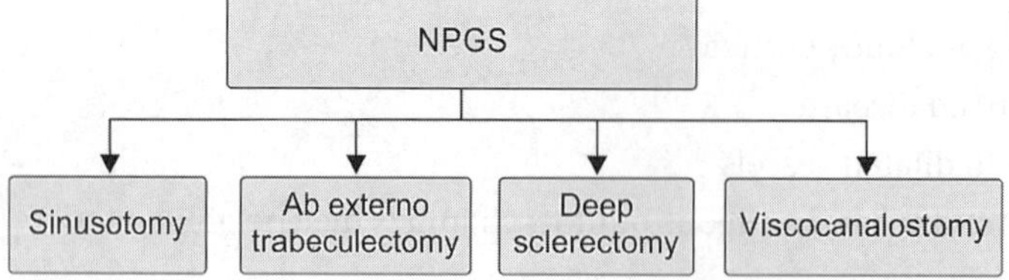

Indications:

- Pigmentary glaucoma
- Glaucoma with high myopia
- Open angle glaucoma
- PXF glaucoma
- Aphakic and pseudophakic glaucoma
- Congenital and juvenile glaucoma
- Sturge-Weber syndrome
- Aniridia and anterior segment digenesis
- Glaucoma secondary to uveitis

Contraindications:

- Absolute:
  - Neovascular glaucoma
- Relative:
  - Narrow angle glaucoma
  - Post ALT
  - Angle recession glaucoma
  - Late congenital glaucoma where the mesoderm remnants reach Schwalbe line

Procedures:

- *Sinusotomy:*
  - Pioneer work of Krasnov
  - Lamellar band of sclera is removed.
  - At 10 to 2 o'clock position, an opening in Schlemm's canal is made over 12 o'clock position **(Fig. 21)**
  - Inner wall of Schlemm's canal is left intact with overlying conjunctiva closed as in **Figure 22**

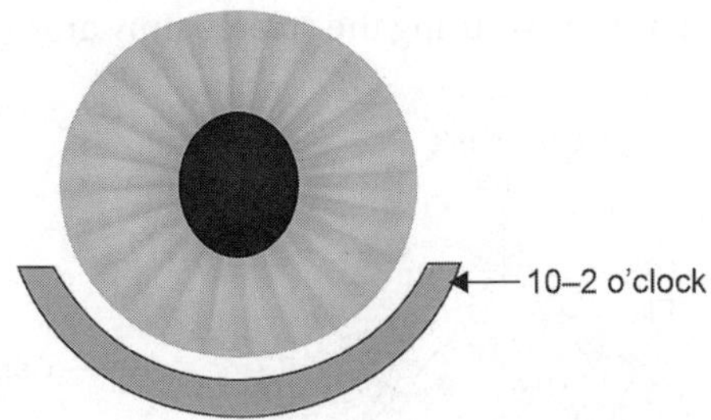

Fig. 21: 10 to 2 o'clock Schlemm canal opening site.

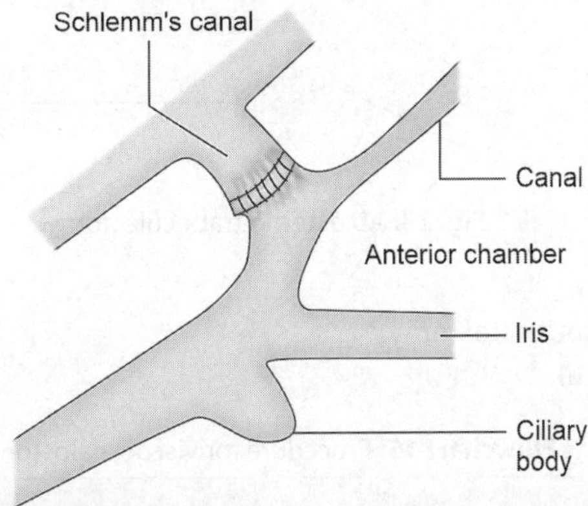

Fig. 22: Inner wall of Schlemm's canal is left intact with overlying conjunctiva closed.

- *Deep sclerectomy:*
  - **Procedure is given in Flowchart 14.**

Flowchart 14: Procedure for deep sclerectomy.

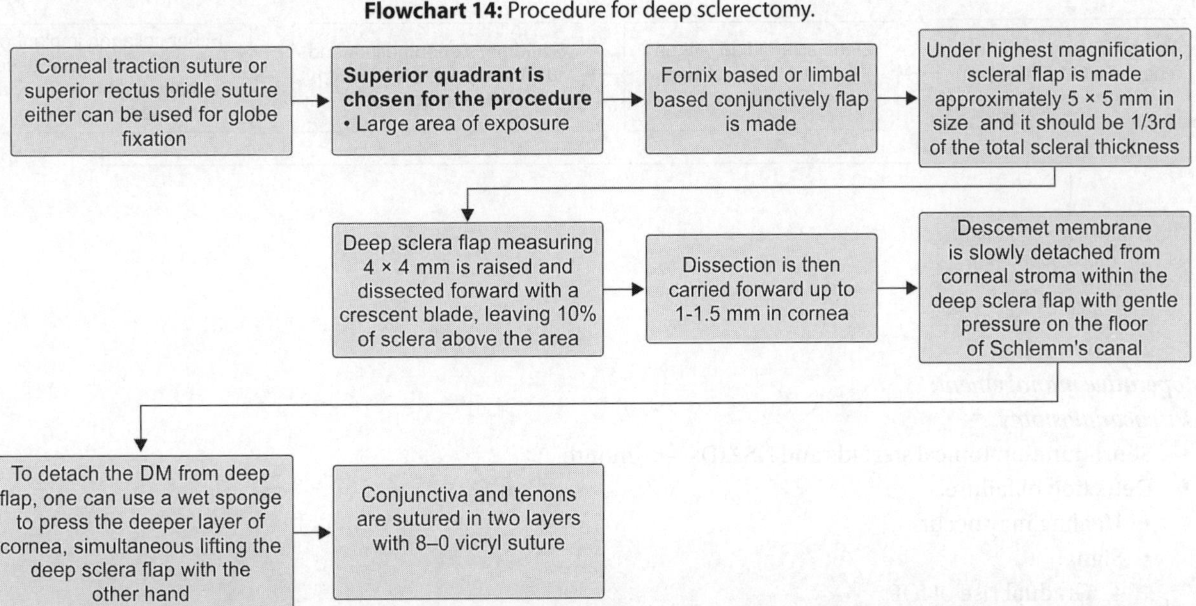

Ab externo trabeculectomy:

- Zimmerman described this procedure
- Deep sclerectomy along with unroofing of Schlemm's canal is done followed by the inner wall of Schlemm's canal and juxtacanalicular trabeculum were removed.

- Thin superficial sclera flap is used to cover by suturing the sclerectomy area **(Fig. 23)**.

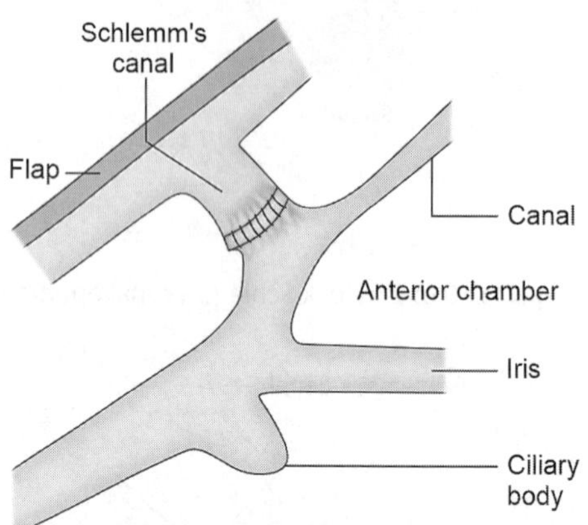

Fig. 23: Ab externo trabeculectomy.

Viscocanalostomy:
- Stegmann (1995) introduced viscocanalostomy.
- Procedure is given in **Flowchart 15**.

Flowchart 15: Procedure for viscocanalostomy.

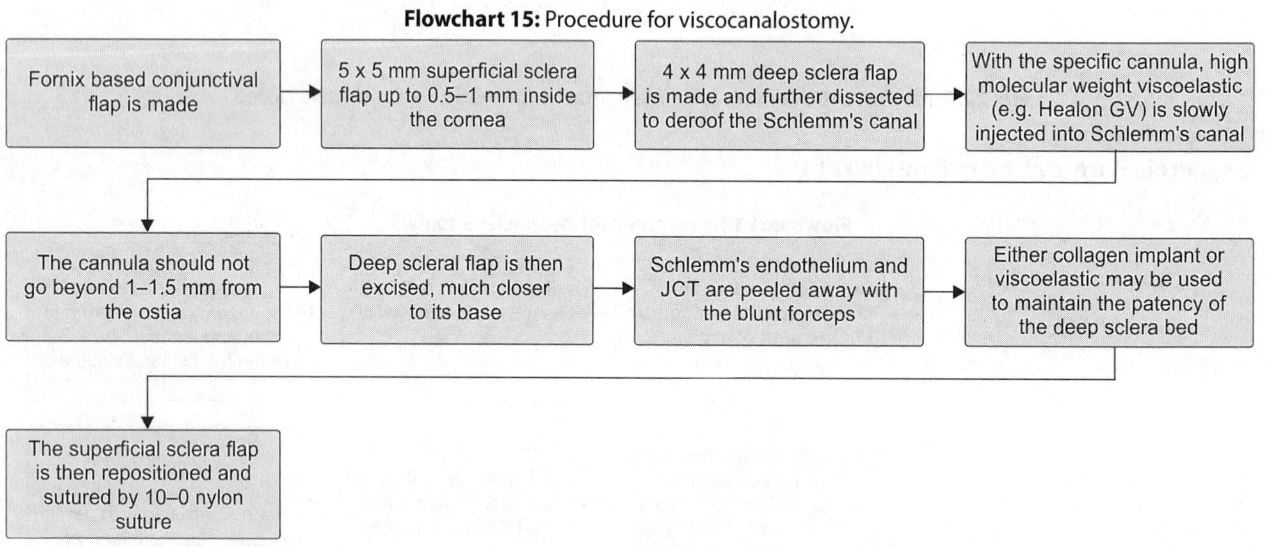

Postoperative management:
- *Viscocanalostomy:*
  - Short duration topical steroids and NSAIDs—<1 month
  - Detection of failure:
    - Healing may occur
    - Signs:
      - Gradual rise of IOP
    - Site:
      - Between the scleral bed and flap
      - Cut ends of the SC

- Management:
  - Nd:YAG laser goniopuncture (LGP)
  - Less effective in the absence of a bleb
- *Deep sclerectomy:*
  - Minimal postoperative management.
  - Topical steroids are every 2 hours for the first week and then the frequency is decreased
  - Early bleb failure is uncommon
  - Managed aggressively like a trabeculectomy.
  - Increasing frequency of topical steroids, subconjunctival steroids, Avastin (Bevacizumab) and 5-FU is warranted.
  - Laser goniopuncture should be delayed for 1–2 months.
  - When the IOP starts increasing over the target range, usually 16–20 mm Hg, laser goniopuncture should be done.
  - If the IOP doesn't decrease after LGP, needle revision with antimetabolites is indicated.
  - Gonioscopy is recommended regularly and especially after laser and needle revision.
  - Done to check whether iris is covering the TDM.

Complications:

- *Intraoperative complication:*
  - Perforation of trabeculo-descemet's membrane
  - Smaller perforation without iris prolapsed—observation and overlying sclera flap is tightened with 10-0 nylon suture.
  - Marginally large perforation—If iris prolapse is present, high molecular weight OVD is injected in perforated area followed by deep sclera flap is sutured with a collagen graft for sealing. The superficial scleral flap is then closed tightly.
  - Larger perforation usually treated with peripheral iridectomy. Sometimes it may be converted to conventional filtering surgery.
  - Hemorrhage: During flap formation or deep flap excision
  - Malignant glaucoma: Rare complication
- *Postoperative complications:*
  - Wound leak
    - Positive Seidel's test
    - Observation
    - Resuturing
  - Hyphema:
    - Microhyphema resolves spontaneously
  - Choroidal detachment:
    - Shallow detachment—treated with cyclopedia and NSAIDs
    - Large detachment—treated with draining suprachoroidal fluid
  - Hypotony:
    - On first postoperative day—IOP < 5 mm Hg
    - Early hypotony is a sign for successful surgery.
  - Blebitis
  - Shallow AC
  - Decompression retinopathy
  - Implant displacement
  - Decreased visual acuity

22. Discuss Glaucoma Shunt procedures. (10) RGUHS MS 2020

Tube shunt implantation: There are many types of devices that aid angle filtration shunting aqueous to a site away from the limbus, such as the equatorial subconjunctival space.

Tube shunt implantation generally involves placing a tube in the anterior chamber, in the cilliary sulcus, or through the pars plana into the vitreous cavity.

The tube is connected to an extraocular plate, which is attached to sclera in the equatorial region of the globe, between the extraocular muscles, and in some cases tucked under the muscles.

Aqueous flows out through the tube into the subconjunctival space in the region of the extraocular plate.

Tube shunts can be classified into:

- Nonvalved devices (no flow restrictor)
- Valved devices (flow restrictor present)

Most commonly used nonvalved devices are:

- Molteno (Molteno Ophthalmic Ltd., Dunedin, New Zealand) and Baerveldt (Abott medical optics, Santa Ana, CA) designs.

  The most widely used valved device is the Ahmed design (New World Medical, Inc, Rancho Cucamonga, CA).

  Two multicenter RCT comparing Ahmed Glaucoma valve (AGV) and Baerveldt Glaucoma Implant (BGI) found that the average IOP after 3–5 years was slightly higher in AGV pts; however there were lower vision-threatening complication associated with use of AGV > BGI

  The surface area of the plate of each tube shunt varies and can influence IOP control and complications post-operatively.

Indications:

The devices mentioned and similar type of implants are generally reserved for difficult glaucoma cases in which trabeculectomy has failed or likely to fail.

- However tube shunt can be primary procedure.
- The eyes follow-up results of trabeculectomy versus tube study showed that tube shunt surgery with Baerveldt implant had a higher success rate compared with trabeculectomy with MMCin eyes with prior intraocular surgery.
- Both procedures were associated with a similar reduction in IOP and use of supplemented medications , but tube shunts require fewer additional surgical procedure.

A tube shunt should be considered in the following clinical settings:

- *Failed trabeculectomy with antifibrotics:* It may be appropriate to perform a second trabeculectomy in some clinical situations. However, when the factors that
  - Precipitate the initial failure cannot be modified or when it is not technically possible to repeat the trabeculectomy implantation of a tube shunt may be the procedutre of choice.
- *Acute uveitis:* Although few randomized prospective studies have been performed comparing trabeculectomy with antifibrotics to tube shunts in active uveitis, the success of trabeculectomy is disappointingly low in most cases of active inflammation. In certain types of uveitis (e.g., young patients with juvenile idiopathic arthritis), the success rate of trabeculectomy is low and tube shunt implantation is offer the primary surgical treatment.
- *Neovascular glaucoma:* When possible panretinal photocoagulation anti-VEGF therapy should be administered prior to glaucoma surgery in case of neovascular glaucoma when the IOP level is such that urgent surgery is required, or when the neovascular glaucoma does not respond to panretinal photocoagulation a tube shunt is implanted.
- *Inadequate conjunctiva:* In patients who have undergone severe trauma or previous surgery involving conjunctiva (e.g., retinal detachment surgery), the likelihood of trabeculectomy success may be reduced because these patients may have excessive conjunctival scaring.

  A tube shunt can be implanted, even in presence of scleral buckle. When a complete vitrectomy has been performed, the tube can be placed through pars plana.

Aphakia: The success of conventional filtering surgery in aphakic eyes is low, even when MMC is used.

Contraindication: Tube shunt may have a complicated postoperative lower *borderline corneal endothelial function* is a relative contraindication for anterior chamber placement of a tube.

Preoperative consideration: States of conjunctiva, health of sclera at the anticipated sites for the tube and external plate, the location of PAS near possible tube insertion sites, and the location of vitreous in the eye should be examined.

Techniques:

The superotemporal quadrant is preferred first quadrant for all model of tube shunt.

Subsequent tube shunts can be placed in any quadrants, but the inferonasal quadrants tends to be used for larger plates models. Implantation in supranasal quadrant may be associated with restricted eye movement of the superior oblique tendon.

If there is silicon oil, or if it is anticipated an inferior quadrant is preferred.

Valved devices must be primed before implantation.

The extraocular plate is sutured between vertical and horizontal rectus muscles, posterior to the muscle insertions.

The tube portion is then routed in 1 of 3 ways:

1. Anteriorly to enter the anterior chamber angle parallel to the iris.
2. Into the ciliary sulcus in a pseudophakic eye with a posterior facing bevel 2.5 mm from limbus
3. Or through pars plana, 4 mm from the limbus for posterior implantation in eyes that had undergone complete vitrectomy
4. Typically the tube is covered with tissue such as sclera and cornea to help prevent erosion through conjunctiva
5. Corneal patch graft are particularly useful in cases with inferiorly placed tubes because of its better cosmetic reason

A confounding of cause of hypotony can be leakage of aqueous around the tube at its entry site.

In general tubes should be introduced into the anterior chamber via needle incision that is no larger than the diameter of tube (23 G or most tubes). When the patients eye has thin sclera or when the tube is introduced under a partial thickness scleral flap, a tighter entry site, e.g., 25 G may be required.

Complication ***(Table 11):***

TABLE 11: Complications.

Complication	***Prevention/Mx***
Tube cornea touch	• Insert tube in anterior chamber parallel to the iris plane • Use tube occlusion technique to avoid flat chamber with nonvalved shunts
Flat chamber and hypotony	• Valved devices can decrease overfiltration leading to these complications • With nonvalved devices, occlusion of the tube by ligature or suture within tube can decrease early hypotony • Use of viscoelastic agents if flat chamber develops • Ensure entry site of tube is watertight around the tube • Correct overdrainage early • Consider drainage of suprachoroidal affusions
Tube occlusion	• Bevel the tube away from uveal tissue or vitreous • Generous vitrectomy if needed; Nd:YAG laser can be used to clear an occlusion; however surgical intervention is often required
Valve malfunction	• Test valves patency before insertion
Plate migration or tube retraction	• Secure the plate tightly to sclera with nonabsorbable suture • If the plate migrate, the intraocular tube may become longer or retract • Plate migration toward the limbus reduces repositioning of the plate in equatorial subconjunctival space

23. Discuss Tube vs Trabeculectomy study. (5) DNB 2019

Introduction:

- Tube versus trabeculectomy (TVT) study is a multicenter randomized clinical trial which differentiates the safety and efficacy of tube shunt surgery to trabeculectomy with mitomycin C (MMC) in eyes with prior cataract or glaucoma surgery.

Study design:

- Prospective comparative study

Inclusion criteria:

- Age 18–86 years
- Uncontrolled IOP > 18 mm Hg till < 40 mm Hg on maximum tolerated medical therapy.
- Previous cataract extraction with intraocular lens implantation, trabeculectomy or both.

Exclusion criteria is given in ***Flowchart 16***.

Flowchart 16: Exclusion criteria for the study.

Patient related
- Unwilling or unable to give consent, unwilling to accept randomization, or unable to return for scheduled protocol visits
- Pregnant or nursing women
- Unwilling to discontinue contact lens use after surgery
- Need for glaucoma surgery combined with other ocular procedures (i.e. cataract surgery, penetrating keratoplasty, or retinal surgery) or anticipated need for additional ocular surgery

Ocular comorbidities
- Active iris neovascularization or active proliferative retinopathy
- Chronic or recurrent uveitis
- Epithelial of fibrous downgrowth
- Aphakia
- Iridocorneal endothelial syndrome
- Conjunctival scarring precluding a trabeculectomy superiorly

Study methodologies are shown in **Flowchart 17**.

Flowchart 17: Study methodology.

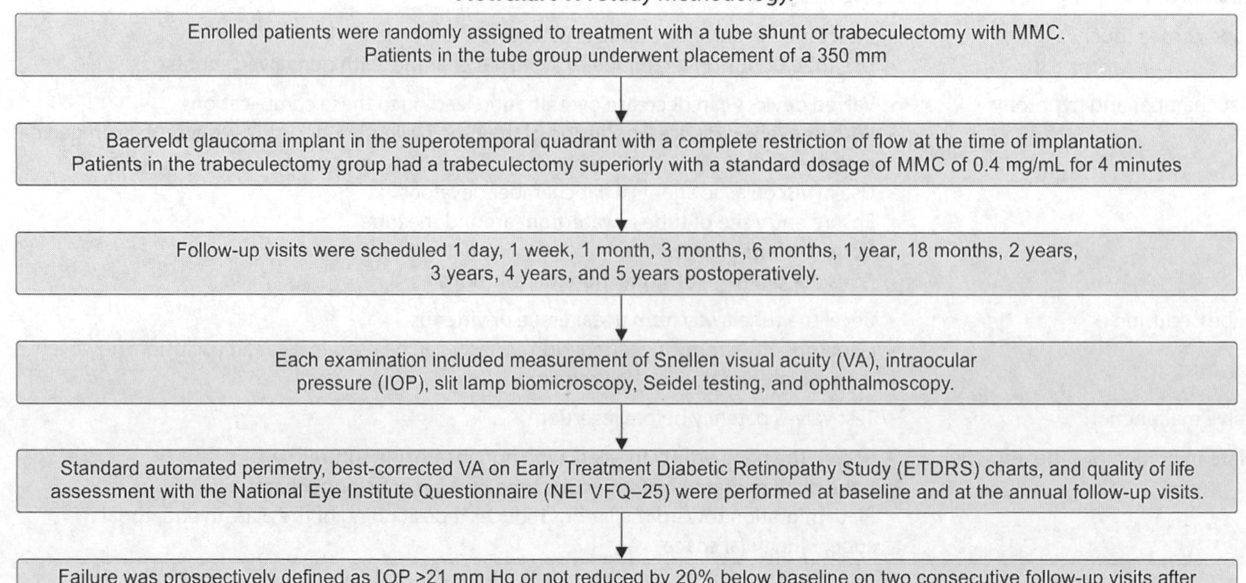

- *Outcomes of the study:*
  - At the end of three years:
    - Both surgical procedures were associated with similar IOP reduction and use of supplemental medical therapy
    - Rate of vision loss after trabeculectomy with MMC and tube shunt surgery was not significantly different
    - Tube shunt surgery—more likely to maintain IOP control and avoid persistent hypotony, loss of light perception vision, or reoperation for glaucoma than trabeculectomy with MMC.
  - *Incidence of postoperative complications:*
    - Higher after trabeculectomy with MMC compared with tube shunt surgery
    - Cataract progression—similar frequency with both surgical procedures.
    - Serious complications associated with reoperation and/or vision loss—similar with both
  - *Limitations to the study:*
    - Very narrow criteria for inclusion and exclusion and hence results should not be generalized to different patient group.
    - Variations in surgical technique are expected with different surgeons.
    - No standardized definitions or quantification of surgical complications.

24. What is megalocornea? Difference between megalocornea and buphthalmous. (5) DNB 2021

Megalocornea: It is nonprogressive symmetric enlargement of the cornea (>13 m in horizontal diameter) without a significant change in corneal thickness or contour unlike keratoglobus where corneal diameter is normal but thickness is reduced.

- Horizontal diameter of cornea is of adult size at birth or 13 mm or greater after the age of two years.
- At birth, horizontal diameter of cornea is about 10 mm.
- Adult size of about 11.7 mm is attained by of two years.
- Differences between megalocornea and buphthalmous are listed in **Table 12**.

TABLE 12: Difference between buphthalmos and megalocornea.

	Buphthalmos	*Megalocornea*
Laterality	Usually bilateral (75%)	Almost always bilateral
Sex	Males (65%)	Males (90%)
Hereditary	Autosomal recessive	X-linked recessive > AD
Vision	Impaired due to photophobia, corneal edema and folds in Descemet's membrane	Not impaired
Eyeball	Increased axial length may be seen	Usually normal
Sclera	Bluish discoloration of sclera d/t stretching, it becomes thinner and translucent	Normal
Cornea	Corneal edema, corneal opacities due to tears in DM (Haab's striae)	Normal
Anterior chamber	As ocular enlargement continues the AC deepens	Normal
Lens	In advance cases zonular fiber may stretch lens may subluxate usually normal	Clear
IOP	Raised	Normal
Optic disc cupping	• Usually normal • Very few may have • Cup disc ratio >0.3 which may regress once • IOP is normalized	Physiological cupping
Clinical features	Triad of photophobia, epiphora and blepharospasm	Usually asymptomatic
Diagnosis	• IOP—measured with Perkin's tonometer or tonopen • Gonioscopy—performed with a Koeppe lens or direct goniolens	By measuring corneal diameter
Treatment	• Gonioscopy—c/o sufficient corneal clarity and angle can be visualized • Trabeculotomy—it creates direct communication between AC and Schlemm's canal • Trabeculectomy—usually done ≥1 angle procedure has failed • Combined trabeculectomy and trabeculotomy • GDD	• Does not need any treatment • It may be a/w – Myopia – Astigmatism – Krukenberg's spindle – Mosaic corneal dystrophy

SUGGESTED READING

1. Agarwal R, Gupta SK, Agarwal P, Saxena R, Agrawal SS. Current concepts in the pathophysiology of glaucoma. Indian J Ophthalmol. 2009;57(4):257-66.
2. American Academy of Ophthalmology. EyeWiki. [online] Available from https://eyewiki.org/Main_Page [Last accessed March 2025].
3. American Academy of Ophthalmology 2019-2020 BCSC Section 10: Glaucoma.
4. Chakravarti T. Pigment Dispersion Syndrome. DOS Times. 2011;17(3).
5. Devi S. Newer Glaucoma Surgeries. DOS Times. 2009;15(2).
6. Gedde SJ, Heuer DK, Parrish RK 2nd; Tube Versus Trabeculectomy Study Group. Review of results from the Tube Versus Trabeculectomy Study. Curr Opin Ophthalmol. 2010;21(2):123-8.
7. Gupta S, Jeria S. A review on Glaucoma Drainage Devices and its Complications.
8. Han Y. Evolution of management on primary angle-closure suspect: observation versus laser peripheral iridectomy. Ophthalmology. 2022;129(2):159-60.
9. Jones E, Clarke J, Khaw PT. Recent advances in trabeculectomy technique. Curr Opin Ophthalmol. 2005;16(2):107-13.
10. Kumar H, Mansoori T, Warjri GB, Somarajan BI, Bandil S, Gupta V. Lasers in glaucoma. Indian J Ophthalmol. 2018;66:1539-53.
11. Lasers on Glaucoma- DOS Times- Volume 26. Number 4, January- February 2021.
12. Menon MG. Minimally Invasive Glaucoma Surgery (MIGS). Shalini- Delhi J Ophthalmol. 2021;31:26-34.
13. Patyal S, Baranawal VK, Kumar S. Neuroprotection in Glaucoma. DOS Times. 2010;15(8):39-42.
14. Post Keratoplasty Glaucoma- DOS Times- Volume 26, Number 4, January-February 2021.
15. Salmon JF. Glaucoma. Kanski's Clinical Ophthalmology: A Systematic Approach, 10th edition. Philadelphia: Elsevier; 2024.

CHAPTER

Uvea

Sangeeta Roy, Smiti Rani Srivastava

QUESTIONS

1. **Acute posterior multifocal placoid pigment epitheliopathy (APMPPE)—etiology, clinical features, investigations, management and prognosis. (2 + 2 + 2 + 2 + 2) (DNB 2020)**
2. **Differential diagnosis of white dot syndrome. What are the clinical features evaluation and management of serpiginous choroiditis? (10) (DNB 2019, 2021)**
3. **Discuss anterior uveitis—methods of examination. (10) (RGUHS MS 2020)**
4. **Bechet's disease—etiology, clinical features and management. (10) (MS 2018)**
5. **Coats' disease—short note. (5) (DNB 2022)**
6. **Fuchs' heterochromic iridocyclitis—short note. (5) (DNB 2022)**
7. **Intermediate uveitis—clinical features and management. (10) (MS 2020)**
8. **What is juvenile idiopathic arthritis (JIA)—discuss its ocular manifestations and management. (2 + 4 + 4) (DNB 2019)**
9. **Write a short note on Masquerade syndromes in uveitis. (5) (WBUHS MS 2021, 2024, DNB 2023, RGUHS MS 2020)**
10. **Ocular manifestations of sarcoidosis. (5) (DNB 2023, WBUHS MS 2021, RGUHS MS 2020)**
11. **Toxoplasmosis—ocular manifestations, investigations and management. (10) (WBUHS MS 2019)**
12. **Vogt-Koyanagi-Harada syndrome—describe various stages, clinical features and management. (10) (WBUHS DO 2018)**

1. Acute posterior multifocal placoid pigment epitheliopathy (APMPPE)—etiology, clinical features, investigations, management and prognosis. (2 + 2 + 2 + 2 + 2) (DNB 2020)

Acute posterior multifocal placoid pigment epitheliopathy (APMPPE): It is rare acute but self-limiting inflammatory disorder which is bilateral. The inflammation occurs in choriocapillary layer and causes hypoperfusion of RPE leading to ischemia of RPE and photoreceptors. This affects young to middle aged person and the ratio of male and female is 1:1.

Etiology

- Idiopathic
- Infective causative organism—influenza like virus (50%), *Streptococcus*-A, adenovirus-5, TB, Lyme disease
- Non-infective of systemic conditions—APMPPE has been described in cases of thyroiditis, erythema nodosum, granulomatosis with polyangiitis, polyarteritis nodosa, nephritis, sarcoidosis, scleritis, ulcerative colitis, central nervous system (CNS) vasculitis, and post vaccination.
- Genetics may play a role in an individual's risk for APMPPE as several associations have been reported including HLA-B7 and HLA-DR2 genetic haplotypes.

Clinical Features

- *Symptoms:*
  - Rapid onset of blurred vision associated with central and paracentral scotomas
  - Photopsias and metamorphopsia have been reported prior to vision loss.
  - Symptoms are usually bilateral, asymmetric and can occur several days apart
  - Visual acuity can range from 20/40 to count-fingers depending on the extent of foveal involvement.
  - Headache and other neurological symptoms such as sensorineural hearing loss may be noted and may appear months after the ocular involvement
- *Signs:*
  - Anterior chamber cells and flare may be present but many times there is no anterior chamber reaction
  - A total of 50% of cases might have vitritis
  - Fundoscopic examination typically shows multiple bilateral creamy yellow-white placoid lesions at the level of RPE and choroid 1–2 disc diameters throughout the fundus located posterior to the equator (generally within the posterior pole).
  - The lesions gradually fade over the course of 1–2 weeks.
  - Papillitis may occur, but cystoid macular edema is uncommon.
  - Older lesions are replaced with RPE atrophy or hyperpigmentation.

Investigations

- *Fundus fluorescein angiography:* Active lesions exhibit early hypofluorescence (blockage) corresponding to the placoid lesions followed by late, irregular hyperfluorescent staining. Early hypofluorescence may represent poor perfusion of the choriocapillaris or signal attenuation from overlying outer retina and/or RPE thickening. Late hyperfluorescence may be a result of vascular leakage, which resolves in subacute or healed lesions.
- *Indocyanine green angiography:* Active placoid lesions manifest as early and late hypofluorescence, which is thought to occur due to poor perfusion of the choriocapillaris. Normalization of the ICG signal may occur as the lesions resolve
- *OCT:* Hyperreflectivity from the outer plexiform layer to the RPE in acute lesions, with normal retinal thickness. Absence of the ellipsoid zone may also indicate foveal involvement and correlate with the loss of visual acuity. Hyperreflectivity of outer layers disappears, the EZ reemerges, and focal photoreceptor/RPE atrophy occurs during resolution of the placoid lesions.
- *OCT-A:* Hyperreflectivity of outer layers disappears, the EZ reemerges, and focal photoreceptor/RPE atrophy occurs during resolution of the placoid lesions.
- *Fundus autofluorescence (FAF):* Placoid lesions generally appear hypoautofluorescent and may have edges that are hyperautofluorescent. Hypoautofluorescence may persist at borders after lesion resolution.
- Additionally, *CNS imaging* should be performed to rule out CNS vasculitis in all patients with a new diagnosis of APMPPE.

Treatment

- No therapy has been proven to be useful in the management of APMPPE. It is mostly a self-limiting disease.
- Few cases might need systemic steroids especially when there is CNS involvement.
- Rarely CNV can develop which might need anti-VEGF treatment.

Prognosis

- APMPEE is self-limiting with a generally good prognosis with the majority of affected patients achieving a visual acuity of 20/40 or better.
- Visual recovery typically takes 4 weeks, but can extend to 6 months in some patients.
- Foveal involvement confers a worse visual prognosis.
- Other atypical features, including age older than 60 years, unilaterality, an interval before involvement of the second eye of at least 6 months, recurrence of the disease, and leakage from choroidal veins may also portend a poorer prognosis.

2. Differential diagnosis of white dot syndrome. What are the clinical features evaluation and management of serpiginous choroiditis? (10) (DNB 2019, 2021)

It is a group of inflammatory diseases in which white, multiple, discrete lesions involves deeper layers of choroid and retina.

Differential Diagnosis of White Dot Syndrome

- Acute posterior multifocal placoid maculopathy
- Birdshot chorioretinopathy
- Serpiginous choroiditis
- Relentless placoid chorioretinopathy
- Persistent placoid maculopathy
- Multifocal choroiditis and panuveitis (MFC)
- Punctate inner choroidopathy
- Progressive subretinal fibrosis and uveitis syndrome
- Multiple evanescent white dot syndrome
- Acute zonal occult outer retinopathy
- Acute idiopathic blind spot enlargement
- Acute macular neuroretinopathy

Serpiginous Choroiditis

Clinical features: Serpiginous choroiditis is a rare, bilateral, idiopathic inflammatory disorder that results in geographic destruction of the retinal pigment epithelium, retina, and choriocapillaris. It is a chronic, recurrent, and progressive disease that typically affects patients 30–60 years of age.

Symptoms

- Although a bilateral disease it has an asymmetric presentation
- Patients are usually asymptomatic till fovea is involved.
- Small central or paracentral scotomas may be preset.
- The scotomas are absolute in their acute stages and relative when healed.

Fundus findings: There are two variants of serpiginous choroiditis: Classical variant seen in 80% of the cases and macular serpiginous choroiditis.

1. *Classical variant:* Starts as geographical patches of gray or creamy yellow patches of placoid lesions in the peripapillary region and it generally progresses centrifugally like a serpentine fashion. Extensive chorioretinal scarring and fibrosis happens after healing. The recurrences start at the edges of the healed lesions.
2. *Macular serpiginous choroiditis:* similar gray or creamy white lesion in the macular area. It has poorer prognosis because of early macular involvement. Vision loss may also be due to secondary CNVM.

Investigations

- *Fundus fluorescein angiography:* Acute lesions appear hypofluorescent, with irregular and poorly defined borders in early phases of the study. In the later phases, hyperfluorescent borders are seen, representing leakage of fluorescein from the surrounding intact choriocapillaris. Inactive lesions are hypofluorescent with sharp borders in early phases of the study and become progressively hyperfluorescent with variable levels of staining.
- *Indocyanine green angiography:* Lesions appear hypofluorescent on ICGA throughout all phases of the study, representing disruption in choroidal perfusion. Early subclinical lesions may be better appreciated on ICGA than on funduscopic examination or FA. ICGA may also be useful in differentiating active new lesions, which are hypofluorescent, from CNV, which appears hyperfluorescent during the middle to late phases of the study.
- *Fundus autofluorescence:* Newer lesions appear hyperautofluorescent and older lesions appear hypoautofluorescent. Recurrences are characterized by hyperautofluorescent borders at the edges of old hypoautofluorescent lesions.

- *OCT:* Acute lesions primarily affect the outer retinal layers and choriocapillaris and appear as increased reflectivity localized to the outer retina and disruption of the photoreceptor bands. OCT of older lesions demonstrates outer retinal atrophy and RPE disruption.
- *OCT-A:* Choriocapillaris flow disruption is an early sign of the disease, preceding structural involvement of the outer retinal layers. Prompt treatment at this early stage may allow for resolution without chorioretinal scarring.

Management

- *Systemic workup:* TB skin test, chest X-Ray, Quatiferon gold TB test, ACE, VDRL, fluorescent treponemal antibody absorption test, *Toxoplasma* titers, and a viral screen.
- *Steroids are the mainstay of treatment:* Oral steroids to be started at the dose of 1 mg/kg body weight with slow tapering. Posterior subtenon triamcinolone can also be used. Intravenous methylprednisolone can be considered for macular lesions.
- For recurrent cases corticosteroids can be used along with other immunosuppressives like cyclosporines, azathioprine, and cyclophosphamides.
- Biologic therapy with a tumor necrosis factor α (TNF-α) inhibitor such as adalimumab has been found effective in patients who progressed despite therapy with other immunosuppressants. Now, adalimumab is also frequently used as a first-line agent for serpiginous choroiditis. It is imperative to rule out TB before starting a TNF-α agent.

3. Discuss anterior uveitis—methods of examination. (10) (RGUHS MS 2020)

Anterior uveitis: Inflammation of anterior uveal tissue consists of iris and anterior part of ciliary body (pars plicata).

Methods of examinations include:

- AT
- Ophthalmoscopy
- Imaging test
- Laboratory test
- Analysis of aqueous and vitreous cells
- Diminished vision, pain, redness, photophobia are the common symptoms of anterior uveitis.
- VA

Slit-lamp Examination

- Ciliary injection is pattern of circumcorneal congestion as deep conjunctival vessels are involved.
- Miosis is due to pupillary sphincter spasm which can predispose to posterior synechiae.
- Endothelial dusting of cornea
- Presence of anterior chamber cells confirms the diagnosis. Slit beam should be kept as 1 × 1 mm with ample intensity and magnification. In this small area the amount of anterior chamber cells is to be evaluated. The anterior segment examination for anterior chamber cells should be done prior dilation.
- Aqueous flare is haziness of aqueous humor caused by protein released is due to breakdown of blood–aqueous barrier. By seeing flare the severity of uveitis is detected.
- *Types KPs*: Inflammatory cells consist of lymphocytes, macrophages and plasma cells are deposited over corneal endothelium. Due to gravity and convection current the inflammatory cells precipitates inferior part of corneal endothelium, this pattern of KPs deposition in inferior cornea is inverted triangle this is called Arlt's triangle.

  KPs can be classified into five categories:
  Type I (small, round)
  Type II (stippled)
  Type III (dendriform)
  Type IV (large, smooth-rounded)
  Type V (globular)

In Fuchs' uveitis, the KPs are smaller but in granulomatous diseases the KPs are like mutton fat appearance, i.e., large.

- Hypopyon—seen in severe cases

HLA-B27 has immobile hypopyon and Behçet disease has hypopyon.

- *Fibrinous exudates in AC:* It can be seen in severe iridocyclitis associated with HLA B27.
- Iris nodules—mainly seen in granulomatous ds
  - Busacca nodules are present over iris stroma.
  - Koppe nodules are present in pupillary margin.
  - Yellowish nodules seen in syphilis
  - Iris pearls seen in leprosy
  - Iris crystals can be seen Fuchs' uveitis. The pattern of iris nodule can give idea about the disease.
- *Iris atrophy*: Diffuse iris atrophy is noted in Fuchs while in herpes it is the patchy sectorial
- Heterochromic iridis is seen in Fuchs.
- Pseudo-rubeosis can be found in few cases. New iris vessels can be seen but it does not occlude the angular structure.

Applanation tonometry: Due to impaired aqueous secretion the IOP is reduced.

Fundus examinations: By IO/90 D—usually normal but must be checked to rule out any spill over anterior uveitis.

Imaging Tests

- Chest X-Ray for tuberculosis and sarcoidosis
- Sacroiliac joint X-Ray for spondyloarthropathy
- CT and MRI of brain and thorax for sarcoidosis, MS, etc.
- OCT macular scan to detect macular edema

Laboratory Test Includes

- HLAB27 typing
- FTA/RPR
- Serum ACE/lysozyme
- Quantiferon gold
- Analysis of aqueous and vitreous cells in patients presenting with hypertensive uveitis to test for herpetic uveitis

4. Bechet's disease—etiology, clinical features and management. (10) (MS 2018)

Bechet's disease: It is an idiopathic, systemic vasculitis that affect multiple organs mainly consists of recurrent oral aphthous ulcers, genital ulcers and uveitis. Uveitis with sterile hypopyon is the most commonly seen. Vasculitis involves small medium large veins and arteries.

Etiology

- The cause is idiopathic.
- Exact etiology is not known genetic and environmental factors may play a role.
- It frequently associated with HLA B51/B5 carriers.
- HLA B51 is the common genetic factor which is found in Japanese, middle eastern area and Turkish people.
- It has been suggested that hypersensitivity to *Streptococcus sanguinis* antigens can be a causative factor.
- Other pathogens like *Staphylococcus aureus*, herpes simplex, and *Escherichia coli* can trigger Behcet's disease.
- Recent belief is that the exposure of infectious organisms or external agents induce autoinflammatory reaction to already genetically predisposed patients.

Clinical Features

- Bilateral presentation
- Young males are mainly affected.
- Severe vision loss

- Redness
- Pain
- Photophobia

On Examination
- Bilateral acute anterior uveitis with transient mobile hypopyon is classical. Eye is relatively white (cold hypopyon)
- Posterior uveitis
- Severe vitritis is common in active disease.
- *Retinitis:* Transient superficial white infiltration which heals without scarring is noted in acute stage of the disease.
- *Vasculitis:* Affecting both retinal veins and arteries resulting in occlusion.
- Retinal detachment is the complications of the disease.
- Inflammatory cells deposits are present in inferior part of extreme periphery of retina.
- Arteritis, phlebitis can be associated with sheathing, perivascular hemorrhages and occlusion.
- Due to perfusion of choriocapillaries, diffuse retinal edema and CME occurs in many cases.
- Due to increased intracranial pressure optic disc swelling and atrophy resulting in visual impairment and impaired color vision
- Inflammation and ischemia lead to NVD and NVE.
- End-stage disease includes optic atrophy, gliosis, sheathing, attenuation, and ghosting of affected vessels.

Complications
- Macular edema—common complication
- Angle closure of glaucoma
- Cataract
- Episcleritis
- Scleritis
- Conjunctival ulcers
- Corneal immune ring
- BRVO
- Vitritis
- vasculitis
- NVG/NVE
- Optic papillitis
- Secondary optic atrophy
- Phthisis bulbi

Investigations
- Complete blood count may show leukocytosis.
- Raised serum inflammatory markers, i.e., ESR, CRP, complement levels, WBC
- Serum HLA-B51 and AECA are most common biomarkers.
- Pathergy test—pricking the skin with needle and observing for red spot within next day
- X-Ray for arthritis
- CT scan is used to look for aneurysms of vessels.
- Lumbar puncture detects the presence of meningitis.
- FA detects ischemic areas of retina. It is also for disease monitoring and inflammation.
- Superficial lesion biopsy, synovial fluid aspiration can establish the presence of disease.
- Laser flare photometry detects inflammation.

International Criteria for Bechet's Disease (ICBD): If a patient scores at least 4 points he is said to have the disease. A score of 3 indicates probable Bechet's disease and a score less than 3 denies Bechet's disease.

1. Oral aphthosis—2 points
2. Ocular lesion—2 points

3. Genital aphthosis—2 points
4. Skin aphthosis—1 point

Vascular lesions like phlebitis, large vein thrombosis, aneurysm, arterial thrombosis—1 point
1. CNS involvement—1 point
2. Positive pathergy test—1 point

Treatment
- *Topical steroids* in high frequency doses, cycloplegics are the treatment for isolated AAU.
- *Systemic steroids* used in acute posterior uveitis in high doses (IVMP) 250–1,000 mg for 3 days then oral 1 mg/kg/day can be tapered till the disease gets resolved.
- *Subtenon* triamcinolone acetonide injections are useful in unilateral cases
- Intravitreal steroids—dexamethasone implant or fluocinolone acetonide used in macular edema and retinal inflammation.
- *Laser panphotocoagulation* used in retina periphery
- *Immunosuppressants* are advised together with CoS; azathioprine (2.5 mg/kg daily) used along with steroids
- Cyclosporine (2–5 mg/kg daily) is combined with azathioprine and systemic steroids.
- *Biological treatment*, i.e., infliximab as single dose can be injected in posterior uveitis as a second line of treatment.
- Infliximab or adalimumab is used in vision-threatening cases.
- *Tumor necrosis factor alpha*: TNF-α inhibitors and interferon-α with or without steroids are advised in severe cases.

5. Coats' disease—short note. (5) (DNB 2022)

Coats' disease is usually characterized by unilateral (95%), progressive development of abnormal vessels in the retina of the affected individuals. It's more frequent in males (at least 3:1) than females, and in patients younger than 8 years old, even though it has been observed in infants as well as older patients.

Clinical Features
- Usually presents in the first decade but one-third of cases present at 30 years of age.
- Usually children are referred as a case of leukocoria with a differential diagnosis of retinoblastoma
- The patients present with loss of vision, strabismus and leukocoria.
- Visual acuity on presentation can vary from 20/200 to PL negative.
- *Fundus picture*: Mild disease presents with focal telangiectasia and microaneurysm in the temporal side of the macula with or without mild exudations.
- The moderate disease ranges from cystoid macular edema with significant exudation around to extensive aneurysms to massive exudation.
- Severe forms may present with exudative retinal detachment.

Fluorescein Angiogram

The features include:
- Telangiectatic vessels
- Aneurysms appearing like light bulb
- Early and progressive perivascular leak
- Peripheral capillary nonperfusion
- Capillary dropout

There are many staging systems but the most commonly used is the shield's classification which is as follows:

Stage 1: Retinal telangiectasia only

Stage 2: Telangiectasia and exudation

A—Extrafoveal exudation

B—Foveal exudation

Stage 3: Exudative retinal detachment
A—Subtotal detachment—(1) Extrafoveal, (2) foveal
B—Total retinal detachment
Stage 4: Total retinal detachment and glaucoma
Stage 5: Advanced end-stage disease

Differential Diagnosis

- Retinoblastoma
- Retinopathy of prematurity
- Toxocariasis
- Familial exudative vitreoretinopathy
- Retinal metastatic lesions
- Noorie disease
- Pars planitis

Treatment

- *Observation:* In minimal telangiectatic vessels with little or no exudation and no imminent threat to vision, or in painless and comfortable blind eyes.
- Laser or cryotherapy aiming at the lesions to decrease exudates and preserve vision.
- For severe exudative retinal detachment external drainage can be performed followed by cryotherapy to the abnormal vessels.
- Sectoral panretinal photocoagulation may be used for the nonperfusion area.
- Vitreoretinal surgery—for extensive retinal detachment not allowing cryo or laser
- *Enucleation*: Painful blind eye or when retinoblastoma cannot be ruled out by imaging and clinical examination
- Repeated anti-VEGF therapy has been seen to reduce exudation but the safety profile for children is as yet unclear.

6. Fuchs' heterochromic iridocyclitis—short note. (5) (DNB 2022)

Fuchs' Heterochromic Iridocyclitis

- It is a chronic unilateral non-granulomatous uveitis which has a triad of iris discoloration, cataract and glaucoma.
- Occurs mostly in 3rd to 4th decade affecting both sexes
- HSV, CMV, RV, and chikungunya are associated with FHI.

Clinical Features

- *Symptoms:*
  - Blurring of vision
  - Complaints of floaters
  - Colored haloes surrounding the light
- *Signs:*
  - Heterochromia of iris—affected eye is hypochromic; reverse heterochromia is seen in blue eyes where it is hyperchromic.
  - Iridocyclitis—not responding to steroid
    - Absence of posterior synechiae
    - Small to medium size white stellate KP with feathery fibrin filament scattered throughout in corneal endothelium.
    - Mild fare in AC
  - Iris—diffuse iris atrophy
    - Retroillumination shows post pigment layer atrophy
    - Iris nodules, i.e., Koppe's nodules are present on pupillary border
    - Aggregation of immunoglobulin present as Iris crystals called Russel bodies seen on anterior surface of iris

- Cataract—posterior subcapsular cataract is noted.
- Glaucoma—late manifestation
- In gonioscopy shows fine radial vessels in angle causes bleeding on anterior chamber paracentesis; Amsler sign
    - PAS
- Vitreous opacities are present.
- Posterior segment examination shows macular edema, chorioretinal scars or periphlebitis rarely.

Investigations

- Mainly clinical signs confirm the disease.
- Rubella antibodies in aqueous humor can be detected after paracentesis.
- Enhanced depth imaging optical coherence tomography shows diffuse choroidal thinning.

Treatment

- Topical corticosteroids applied for reduction of inflammatory cells not so effective.
- Antiglaucoma medications is used to control the intraocular pressure.
- Glaucoma drainage implants have more success rate than trabeculectomy with antimetabolites.
- Vitrectomy for severe floaters

7. Intermediate uveitis—clinical features and management. (10) (MS 2020)

Intermediate uveitis: It is a chronic and relapsing disease which causes inflammation of vitreous primarily. It also consists of pars planitis, posterior cyclitis, hyalitis. It may be idiopathic or may be associated with systemic disease and consists of 15% of all uveitic cases and approximately 20% of pediatric uveitis.

Symptoms: Presentation is typically bilateral and often asymmetrical. It affects younger patients aged between 15 and 40 years.

- Insidious onset of blurring of vision
- Unilateral painless floaters
- Pain, redness, photophobia are rarely seen

Signs (Table 1)

- Anterior uveitis—anterior chamber cells, few KPs are noted with linear distribution. Posterior synechiae is seen especially in inferior iris in multiple sclerosis. It is also noted in sarcoidosis and Lyme's disease where anterior uveitis is severe.
- Vitreous

Anterior Vitreous Cells

Vitreous haze: It is noted in severe retinal involvement.

Snowballs are white focal inflammatory cells, which precipitate collectively in inferior vitreous.

TABLE 1: Grading of vitreous haze.

Haze severity	*Grading*
Good view of nerve fiber layer (NFL)	0
Clear disc and vessels but hazy NFL	+1
Disc and vessels hazy	+2
Only disc visible	+3
Disc not visible	+4

Posterior Segment

- *Periphlebitis at peripheral fundus*: On peripheral fundus examination the affected eye shows mild vascular sheathing in multiple sclerosis.
- *Snowbanking*: Greyish-white plaque present in all peripheral quadrants which is mainly noted inferiorly.

Course of the Disease

- *Cystoid macular edema:* The most common complication is CME which is the reason of visual impairment (50% of cases); and related to severity and duration of the disease.
- *Neovascularization:* Due to vascular endothelial factors activity optic nerve head and peripheral fundus has neovascularization which is called NVD and NVE subsequently. Due to this vitreous hemorrhage, retinal detachment and cyclitic membrane formation are the complications. Young patients have more complications like vitreous hemorrhage.
- Optic disc swelling is present in younger individuals.
- Macular epiretinal membrane (35%)—after resolution of CME, chances of ERM formation become more.
- *Cataract formation (15–50%):* Due to inflammatory cells and steroid application chances of cataract formation is more which is mostly posterior subcapsular cataract and anterior subcapsular cataract.
- *Glaucoma formation:* Inflammation and subsequent application of steroid medication are responsible for raised IOP.
- *Retinal detachment:* Due to its etiology, tractional, rhegmatogenous and exudative retinal detachment can occur. Hypotony and phthisis bulbi are the complications of advancement of disease.
- Vitreous hemorrhage is due to neovascularization from snowbanks and optic nerve head.
- Band-shaped keratopathy

Management of IU

Investigations:

- Complete blood count, ESR, CRP confirms any presence of inflammation.
- ACE and chest X-ray to confirm for sarcoidosis
- Serology for Lyme's disease
- Treponemal and cardiolipin antibody affirm about syphilis.
- Lysozyme
- Non-treponemal and treponemal testing
- Interferon gamma release assay for tuberculosis
- OCT shows any presence subretinal fluid. Presence of ERM, CME, and macular hole can be confirmed by OCT.
- FA shows any presence of neovascularization, signs of perivasculitis and no-perfusion areas.
- *IVFA:* In early stages, filling of intralesional vascular channels occur then hypercyanescence of the lesion followed by late washout from central portion of the lesion.
- *USG-B scan:* If any media haze is present USG-B scan can be done.
- *UBM:* It is used to verify cyclitic membrane or vitreous membrane at pars plana region.
- *Diagnostic procedures:*
    - *Vitreous tapping:* Around 1 cc of vitreous is taken out from vitreous base to detect any pathology. The advantage of this procedure is less vitreous traction and less hypotony.
    - *Chorioretinal biopsies:* Bilateral involvement and rapid progression of disease are indications for this. It can be done via pars plana vitrectomy or through scleral flap.

Management:

Medical treatment: Identification of the cause and malignancy and infection must be ruled out before starting the non-specific anti-inflammatory medications. The goal is to achieve grade 0 inflammations.

Corticosteroids: Topical corticosteroid has a limited role.

Periocular steroid: Subtenon injection (0.5–1 mL) of triamcinolone (40 mg/mL) is injected for unilateral intermediate uveitic eye to reduce CME. 2–3 injects may be applied in duration of 6–8 weeks. Monitoring the baseline IOP is the must.

Intravitreal steroids (IVTA): As triamcinolone acetonide have many complications it is used in chronic cases.

Slow releasing intravitreal implants—Ozurdex (slow releasing dexamethasone 0.7 mg intravitreal implant) improves the retinal the thickness and reduce the recurrence of CME.

The MUST trial recommends sustained release fluocinolone 0.19 mg (Iiuvien) or 0.59 mg intravitreal implant (Retisert).

Systemic steroids: After ruling out the infective organisms' systemic steroids 1 mg/kg/day can be started and tapered slowly till the disease get resolved. The indications of systemic steroids are bilateral disease with severe uveitis and unilateral disease not improving with periocular steroids.

Immunosuppressants are Indicated

- Acute vision-threatening condition, RD, macular involvement, chronic and persistent disease.
- Failure of periocular and systemic steroids

Immunosuppressive agents: Methotrexate, mycophenolate mofetil, tacrolimus and cyclosporine can be used in cases of steroid complicated diseases or as a steroid sparing agent. Methotrexate is first line of treatment in children and chronic non-infectious uveitis.

Anti-tumor necrosis factor (interferon α and β): It is a third line of treatment in patients not responding to the immunosuppressive agents. They may improve macular edema.

Pars Plana Vitrectomy

Pars plana vitrectomy: It is the fourth step of therapy. The indications are:

- Vitreous hemorrhage and vitreous condensation
- Retinal detachment
- ERM causing retinal traction
- CME refractive to medical treatment

Cryotherapy may cause RD. Laser photocoagulation is considered nowadays as an adjunctive therapy to other treatment.

Management of the Complications

- Cataract surgery should be perfomed 3 months after subsiding of inflammation; oral prednisolone 1 mg/kg body weight/day should be given at least 5 days before surgery with tapering in 1 month. Acrylic hydrophobic intraocular lens is preferred.
- Uveitic glaucoma is quite common and should be taken care of.
- RD occurs in all forms so a proper follow-up is required.

8. What is juvenile idiopathic arthritis (JIA)—discuss its ocular manifestations and management. (2 + 4 + 4) (DNB 2019)

- Juvenile idiopathic arthritis is defined as arthritis for 6 weeks duration in absence of any systemic disease below 16 years of age.
- Incidence is 1:1,000.
- Most common cause of uveitis in children is JRA.
- Uveitis develops typically after arthritis but in 3–5% of cases uveitis is the first presentation.

Three types of presentations are noted:

1. *Pauciarticular:*
   a. 4 or fewer joints are involved, most common involved joint is knee.
      i. Girls predilection is seen.
      ii. ANA is positive commonly'
      iii. Uveitis is common
2. *Polyarticular:*
   a. 5 or more joints are involved here.
   b. Both small and large joints inflammation.
      i. Girls predilection
      ii. ANA positivity in half of the cases
      iii. Uveitis is found in 5%.

3. *Systemic onset:*
    a. Presents with fever, rash, lymphadenopathy
        i. Both boys and girls are equally affected.
        ii. Usually ANA is negative.
        iii. Uveitis is absent.
        iv. Still disease

Ocular Manifestations of JIA

- *Anterior uveitis:*
    - Asymptomatic. No classic sign of uveitis such as red eye, pain photophobia and blurred vision seen. Parents notice once complications set in.
    - Non-granulomatous chronic uveitis with bilateral presentation.
    - Eyes are usually white
    - Endothelial dusting seen in cornea
    - Posterior synechia
- *Posterior segment examination:*
    - Optic nerve inflammation
    - Macular edema

Management

- History
- VA assessment cycloplegic refraction
- IOP measurement.
- Slit-lamp examination for cells in anterior chamber, vitreous cells and vitreous haze
- Dilated fundus examination if required under GA for CME and optic nerve edema.

Investigations

Laboratory test depending upon systemic symptoms. Few specific tests are:

- Antinuclear antibodies (ANA)
- Complete blood count (CBC)
- Rheumatoid factor (RF)
- HLA B27 antigen

Treatment includes involvement of pediatrician and rheumatologist for the management of systemic disease. Main goal of treatment is to reduce inflammation and to reduce surgical intervention.

- Topical steroid is mainstay of treatment but glaucoma and cataract is the complication of long term steroid use so they should be monitored closely.
- Topical cycloplegics
- Periocular injection of steroid
- Oral steroid
- Systemic immunosuppressant, e.g., low-dose methotrexate first line of treatment. Azathioprine and cyclosporine are others but their use is limited due to high toxicity and resulting refractory uveitis cases.

Antimetabolites biological agents like infliximab and adalimumab are advised in children in refractory and failed therapy cases as they are well tolerated.

In severe JIA-associated uveitis new recommendation is combine therapy of methotrexate (MTX) and antitumor necrosis factor (TNF) like adalimumab.

Surgery: High rate of cataract in JIA patients needs surgery.

- *Preoperative:* At least 3 months of noninflammatory period is required.
- Postoperative control of inflammation is mandatory.

Better to keep aphakia in children less than a year specially in bilateral cataracts to avoid pupillary membrane formation while PCIOL (PMMA) implantation in bag should be considered in unilateral cases to avoid amblyopia. PCO and postoperative inflammation is very common complication in JIA.

Complications:

- Posterior synechiae
- Cataract
- Glaucoma
- Band-shaped keratopathy
- Hypotony
- Phthisis bulbi
- Optic disc edema
- Macular edema
- Epiretinal membrane
- Ciliary membrane formation and traction followed by ciliary detachment
- Amblyopia
- Male gender, early onset of uveitis and presence of synechiae at the time of presentation are associated with poor prognosis.

9. Write a short note on Masquerade syndromes in uveitis.

(10) (WBUHS 2021, 2024, DNB 2023, RGUHS MS 2020)

Masquerade syndrome: Uveitis masquerade syndrome is used to describe different noninflammatory ocular entity comes under one term which mimic intraocular inflammation.

It is associated with systemic and ocular inflammation which is not secondary to any immune-mediated or infectious disease.

It is either neoplastic or non-neoplastic. It includes mainly hematologic malignancies, chronic retinal detachment, IOFB, retinal ischemia, and other diseases.

- *Neoplastic masquerade syndromes:* Intraocular lymphoma (primary vitreoretinal lymphoma) is most common intraocular lymphoma.
  - *Primary uveal lymphoma:* It is rare intraocular lymphoma which involves is rare and involves iris, ciliary body and choroid.
  - *Leukemia:* Ophthalmic involvement commonly occurs in around 90% of patients. It is due to direct infiltration of neoplastic cells, dysplastic cells, opportunistic infection or hematologic abnormalities.
  - *Metastatic tumors:* It is most common type intraocular malignancy. It affects choroid which is highly vascular tissue.
- *Non-neoplastic masquerade syndromes:*
  - *Intraocular foreign body:* Due to penetrating injuries, foreign body insertion in ocular tissue is common. It depends upon the size, momentum, type of foreign body. Heavy metal foreign body extraction is crucial and long standing presence causes retinal degeneration and vision-threatening situation.
  - *Pigment dispersion syndrome:* Rubbing of posterior surface of iris and lens zonules release pigments and cells in anterior chamber. Pigmented debris deposits in trabecular meshwork causes raised IOP, deposits over corneal endothelium, iris or lens mimics acute anterior uveitis.
  - *Retinitis pigmentosa:* It is inherited retinal dystrophy which results progressive photoreceptor and RPE degeneration. Cataract, CME, RPE atrophy, vitreous debris is complications of RP. The combinations of features may confuse with intermediate uveitis.
  - *Ocular ischemic syndrome:* Secondary glaucoma occurs in half of cases with inflammatory cells in aqueous chamber imitates like immune mediated anterior uveitis.
  - *Retinal detachment:* Rhegmatogenous retinal detachments with PVR are associated with intraocular inflammation, hypotony and choroidal detachment can create confusion between anterior uveitis.

- *Retinoblastoma:* Retinoblastoma is a pediatric intraocular malignancy. Incidence is 1/15,000 to 18,000. The diffuse form can appear as masquerade syndrome. It combines with leukocoria, strabismus. The infiltrating subtype and uveitis may difficult to differentiate.
- *Coats' disease:* Retinal telangiectasia with exudates and hemorrhage are associate with Coats' disease. Young males around 10–20 years are commonly affected, commonly unilateral. The main differentiating points are young patient with unilateral vision loss and retinal vascular findings.
- *Juvenile xanthogranuloma:* It appears in the first year of birth. It is associated with Langerhans cell histocytosis. Iris granuloma, heterochromia, hyphema, glaucoma, and anterior uveitis are common features.

10. Ocular manifestations of sarcoidosis. (5) (DNB 2023, WBUHS MS 2021, RGUHS MS 2020)

- It is a chronic multisystemic T lymphocyte-mediated noncaseating granulomatous inflammatory disorder.
- Lung is most commonly affected.
- Other organs like skin, lymph nodes, spleen parotid glands and eyes are involved.

Ocular Manifestations (Figs. 1A to D)

- Uveitis and conjunctival nodules are commonly seen.
- It causes anterior, intermediate and posterior uveitis.
- The most common type of uveitis is bilateral anterior uveitis.
  Slit-lamp examination:
  - Granulomatous mutton fat KPs
  - Iris nodules **(Figs. 2A to D)** both Koeppe at pupillary margin and Busacca in stroma
  - Tent-shaped peripheral anterior synechia or posterior synechiae
- *Intermediate uveitis:*
  - Floaters and blurry vision are symptoms.
  - In fundus examination vitreous opacities, snow balls and snow banks are classical features.
- Posterior uveitis—usually bilateral may be symptomatic
- Nodular or segmental periphlebitis is perivenous sheathing. Candle wax dripping is perivascular retinal exudates along the retinal veins.
  - Choroid granulomas, if large may lead to RD
  - Multifocal choroiditis can lead to secondary CNVM.
  - Retinal granulomas
  - Peripheral retinal neovascularization
  - Optic nerve edema, papilledema and focal granulomas are the optic nerve involvement.

Complications are:

- Cataract due to uveitis
- Glaucoma due to inflammatory cells leading to trabecular meshwork obstruction, nodules can also be present.
- CME

Ocular Surface Manifestations

- *Conjunctiva:*
  - Conjunctival nodules
  - Acute follicular conjunctivitis
  - Chronic cicatricial conjunctivitis are seen
- *Sclera:*
  - It may be anterior diffuse, anterior nodular, or posterior scleritis.
  - Scleritis is non-necrotizing.
- *Cornea:*
  - Superficial punctate keratitis
  - Interstitial keratitis and PUK can also occur in few cases.

- Calcific band keratopathy can be noted as hypercalcemia exists in sarcoidosis patients which deposits in subepithelial layer of cornea.

- *Orbital involvement:* Sarcoidosis can affect extraocular muscles, optic nerve sheath, and orbital fat leading to ptosis, proptosis and orbital masses. They can lead to globe displacement, diplopia, compression causing CRAO and blindness.
- *Keratoconjunctivitis sicca (KCS)*—due to mass effect and inflammation of lacrimal gland, nasolacrimal sac and lacrimal drainage system.

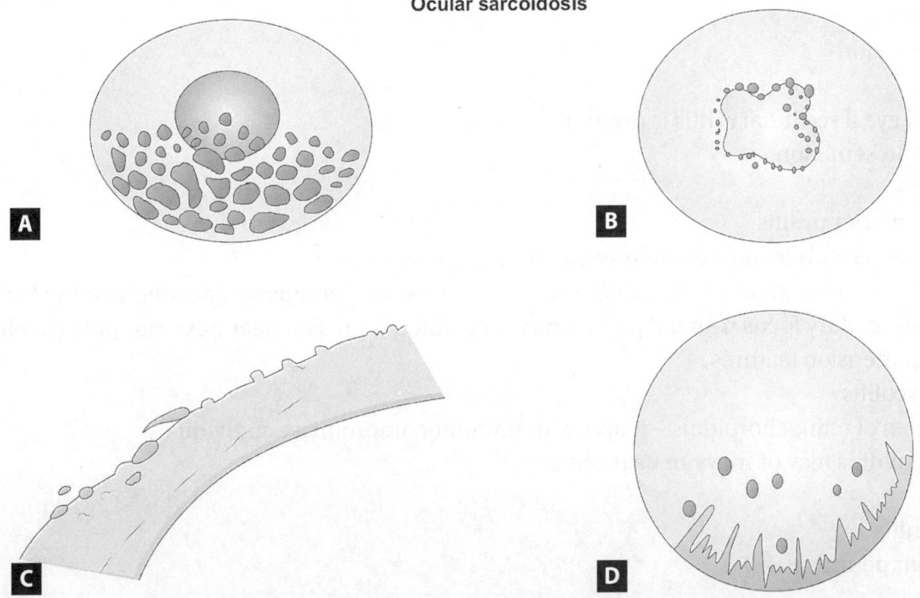

Figs. 1A to D: Diagrammatic representation of ocular sarcoidosis. (A) Very large granulomatous "mutton fat" keratic precipitates; (B) Large iris nodules; (C) Nodular involvement of the trabecular meshwork; and (D) Snowballs.

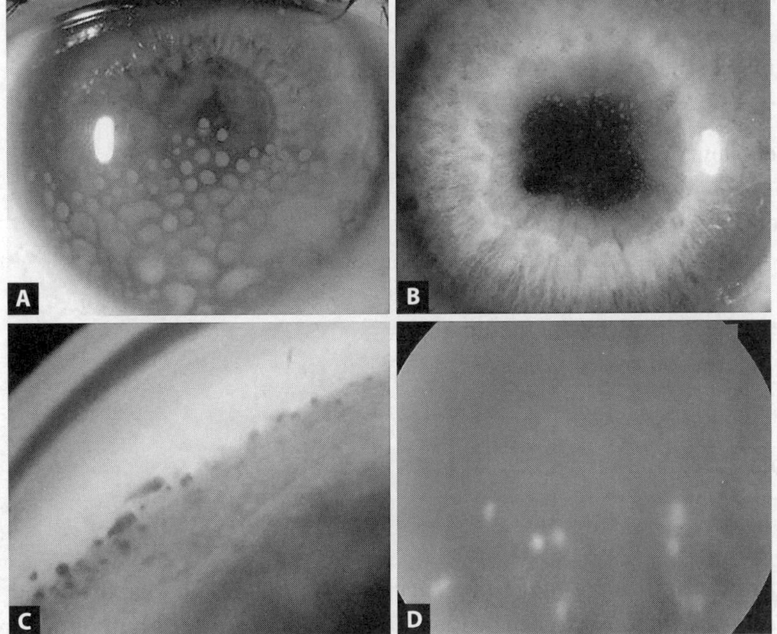

Figs. 2A to D: Ocular sarcoidosis: (A) Very large granulomatous "mutton fat" keratic precipitates; (B) Large iris nodules; (C) Nodular involvement of the trabecular meshwork; and (D) Snowballs. *(For Color version, See Color Plate 7)*

11. Toxoplasmosis—ocular manifestations, investigations and management. (10) (WBUHS MS 2019)

- *Toxoplasmosis:* The causative organism is *Toxoplasma gondii* which is an obligate protozoon. The definite host is cat, intermediate host are mice, livestock, bird. Infected cat's feces consist of oocysts, which is ingested by intermediate cysts. The water is contaminated by cat's urine which consist oocysts. The uncooked meat of intermediate host or eggs consist bradyzoites. Bradyzoites are present in muscles as inactive stage. Bradyzoite cysts rupture tachyzoites get released which is an active stage. It has also transplacental spread and spreads infection via blood or organ transfusion.
- *Ocular symptoms:*
  - Blurring of vision
  - Floaters
  - Painful red eye if secondary iritis is present
  - Unilateral presentation
- *Signs:*
  - Spill over anterior uveitis
  - Granulomatous and stellate keratin precipitates may be present
  - White focal retinitis with overlying mild to severe vitreous inflammation—"headlight in the fog" appearance.
  - Single inflammatory focus near old pigmentary scar which is present near posterior pole (satellite lesion)
  - Ocular hypertension features
  - Retinal vasculitis

  Atypical features of retinochoroiditis—it occurs in immunocompromised individuals.
  - Retinochoroiditis may or may not be present
  - Papillitis
  - Neuroretinitis
  - Retrobulbar neuritis
  - Scleritis
  - Retinal detachment
  - Branch retinal artery occlusion (BRVO)
  - Punctate outer retinitis
  - Multifocal diffuse necrotizing retinitis

  Recurrence is maximum in the first year of the disease and in old aged people.

Complications

Visual loss occurs due to following:

- *Common:*
  - Direct involvement of macula
  - Secondary optic nerve head involvement due to juxtapapillary lesion
- *Uncommon:*
  - Primary optic nerve head involvement mimic AION
    - Occlusion of major blood vessel
    - CNVM
    - Serous RD
    - Tractional RD
    - Macular edema

Investigations

- *Toxoplasma* serology confirms *Toxoplasma* by presence of *T. gondii* IgG or IgM in the blood.
- *Polymerase chain reaction: T. gondii* DNA can be identified by PCR of aqueous humor or vitreous humor.
- *Ocular fluid antibody assessment*: Goldmann-Witmer coefficient measures the ratio between specific IgG in aqueous humor and IgG of serum is sensitive investigations.

- OCT shows subtle macular edema
- USG-B scan shows RD in the presence of vitritis.

Treatment

- It is a self-limiting disease which is resolved in duration of 4–8 weeks. Aim of the treatment is to:
  - Reduce the duration and severity of acute inflammation
  - Lessen the risk of permanent visual loss
  - Reduce risk of recurrence

Indications of the treatment

- Sight-threatening lesion involving macula, papillomacular bundle, optic nerve head
- Severe vitritis causing TRD
- Immunocompromised patients
- Pregnancy

Treatment regimen:

- Oral pyrimethamine (75–100 mg for 1–2 days followed by 25–50 mg daily for 4 weeks) is combined with sulfadiazine (1 g four daily for 3–4 weeks). It is advised along with systemic corticosteroid which is also called triple-drug therapy. As pyrimethamine is a folic acid antagonist which cause dose related bone marrow suppression so folinic acid 5 mg three times per week is advised.
- Injectable clindamycin (1 mg) can be advised as an adjuvant of triple therapy.
- Intravitreal therapy with clindamycin (1 mg) and dexamethasone (400 μg) can be considered. Two to three doses may be required. Recurrently infected pregnant women are choice for intravitreal injections but it can't be given to previously immunocompromised patients or acutely.
- Azithromycin 250–500 mg daily reduces the rate of recurrence. Azithromycin, pyrimethamine, folinic acid and prednisolone can be considered as a new region. Clarithromycin can be substitute.
- Co-trimoxazole (trimethoprim 160 mg/sulfamethoxazole 800 mg), clindamycin (300 mg four times daily), atovaquone (750 mg two to four times daily) are the adjunctives.
- Topical steroid, mydriatic are used to suppress anterior uveitis.
- Antimicrobial maintenance therapy is considered for immunosuppressive patients.
- In pregnancy intravitreal injections along with systemic azithromycin, clindamycin and prednisolone can be administered in the cases of recurrence. Spiramycin alone or combination can also be applied aptly.
- In few cases, vitrectomy can acquire success to irradicate the disease.
- Surgical treatment may be required for retinal detachment.

12. Vogt–Koyanagi–Harada syndrome—describe various stages, clinical features and management. (10) (WBUHS DO 2018)

- It is an idiopathic multisystem autoimmune disorder which consists of bilateral granulomatous panuveitis with or without extraocular manifestations affecting tissues containing melanocytes like uvea ear and meninges.
- It occurs in young individual 2nd and 5th decade of life.
- It is associated with uveal infiltration of T cells and HLA-DR1 and HLA-DR4.
- It is subclassified as:
  - Vogt–Koyanagi disease—consists of skin changes and anterior uveitis
  - Harada disease—characterized by neurological features and exudative retinal detachments.
- Clinical features depends on stage of disease and consists of four phases:
  1. *Prodromal phase:* Resembles viral illness; it presents with neurological (meningitis, meningoencephalitis along with cranial nerve palsies, optic neuritis and other focal lesions) and auditory manifestations (tinnitus, vertigo, deafness). It stays for 3–5 days.

2. *Acute uveitic phase:* Presents with bilaterally blurred VA, granulomatous anterior uveitis and multifocal posterior uveitis with diffuse choroidal infiltration. Hyperemia and edema of optic disc, circumscribed retinal edema followed by multiple serous RD. Finally inflammation becomes more diffuse affecting anterior chamber becoming panuveitis.
3. *Convalescent phase:* Presents weeks after uveitic phase. It is characterized by localized alopecia, poliosis, vitiligo. Choroidal depigmentation in fundus with pale disc in bright orange choroid giving appearance of (sunset glow fundus). Sugiura sign is perilimbal vitiligo which may be earliest depigmentation. This stage remains for several months.
4. *Chronic recurrent phase:* Consists of posterior uveitis with acute exacerbation of anterior uveitis. Vision-threatening complications like cataract glaucoma, retinal neovascularization, etc. occur in this stage.

Diagnostic Criteria (as per American Uveitis Society)

- Absence of any ocular trauma or surgery
- Presence of at least three of any four signs:
  1. Bilateral chronic iridocyclitis
  2. Posterior uveitis including exudative RD, disc edema or hyperemia and sunset glow fundus.
  3. Neurologic signs—tinnitus, stiffness of neck, cranial nerve palsy or cerebrospinal fluid pleocytosis
  4. Cutaneous findings like alopecia, poliosis or vitiligo

Complete Vogt–Koyanagi–Harada Disease (Criteria 1–5 should be Present)

1. No history of penetrating ocular trauma or any history of surgery in the initial period of uveitis.
2. Clinical or laboratory findings suggesting no any other ocular disease.
3. Bilateral ocular involvement (a or b must be present):
   - Early manifestations of ds:
     - Evidence of diffuse choroiditis:
       1. Presence of focal areas of SRF
       2. Bullous serous retinal detachments
     - Both fundus findings must be present:
       1. FA shows focal areas of delayed choroidal perfusion, multifocal areas of leakage, pooling in SRF, optic nerve staining.
       2. USG-B scan showing diffuse choroidal thickening without associating posterior scleritis.
   - Late manifestations:
     1. Presence of signs 3a and signs 2, 3 below or signs of 3.
     2. Ocular depigmentation, i.e., sunset glow fundus or Sugiura sign
     3. Other ocular signs:
        a. Nummular chori retinal depigmented scars
        b. Migration or clumping of RPE
        c. Recurrent or chronic anterior uveitis
4. *Neurological diseases:*
   1. Meningismus (headache, malaise, fever, nausea, abdominal pain)
   2. Tinnitus
   3. CSF pleocytosis
5. *Integumentary signs:*
   1. Alopecia
   2. Poliosis
   3. Vitiligo

Incomplete Vogt–Koyanagi–Harada disease (Criteria 1-3 and either 4 or 5 must be present):

1. No history of penetrating ocular trauma or any history of surgery in the initial period of uveitis.
2. Clinical or laboratory findings do not suggest any other ocular disease.

3. Bilateral ocular involvement
4. Neurologic/auditory findings confirm complete Vogt–Koyanagi–Harada disease.

Or

5. Integumentary findings are present in complete Vogt–Koyanagi–Harada disease.

Probable Vogt–Koyanagi–Harada Disease

1. No history of penetrating ocular trauma or any h/o surgery in the initial period of uveitis.
2. Clinical or laboratory findings do not suggest any other ocular disease.
3. Bilateral ocular involvement as defined in complete VKH

Investigations

- *FFA:*
  - Acute stage of disease shows early patchy fluorescence of choroidal perfusion, pinpoint leakage in RPE layer.
  - In late stages the localized hyperfluorescent spots increases by coalescing with each other forming large area of leakage.
  - Optic disc shows blurred fluorescent margins with late leakage.
  - In late stage moth-eaten appearance seen.
- *ICG:* In early stage, it denotes choroidal perfusion delay and segmental or diffuse choroidal vessel hypercyanescence suggests inflammatory vasculopathy later on it shows hypocyanescent dark spots. It also used to detect and keep track of any subclinical choroidal inflammation.
- *FAF:* Hyperautofluorescence with hypoautofluorescence spots are noted in early stage which corresponds with serous detachments. Later the hypoautofluorescence spots denotes the RPE loss and chorioretinal atrophy.
- *OCT:* It detects macular edema, CNVM, serous macular detachments. EDI-OCT monitors the CNVM progression and regression pre and post treatment. Quantification of subretinal fluid with subretinal septae is typical.
- *USG:* USG A vector shows low to medium reflective thickening of posterior choroid, sclera or episcleral along with exudative RD, vitreous opacities.
- *ERG:* In full-field ERG are diffusely diminished the amplitude of scotopic and photopic phases in chronic stage.
- *Laboratory test:* Pleocytosis, high protein levels, melanin containing macrophages are noted in spinal fluid. Elevated serum ESR can indicate acute inflammatory stage association.

Treatment

- High dose oral steroid 1.5 mg/kg/day in tapering doses for minimum of 6 months augmented with 3 doses of IV methyl prednisolone 1g to run over 1 hour after excluding systemic infection and contraindications.
- Before administration of steroid any systemic infection should be ruled out and blood sugar and blood pressure should be taken care of.
- Second line of treatment is immune suppressants like azathioprine 1–2.5 mg/kg/day, cyclosporin A 3–5 mg/kg/day
- Their administration should be closely monitored.

  Prognosis depends upon no of recurrence and duration of ds.

SUGGESTED READING

1. American Academy of Ophthalmology. EyeWiki. [online] Available from https://eyewiki.org/Main_Page [Last accessed March 2025].
2. McCannel CA. 2023–2024 Basic and Clinical Science Course™, Section 12: Retina and Vitreous. San Francisco: American Academy of Ophthalmology; 2023.
3. Salmon JF. Uveitis. Kanski's Clinical Ophthalmology: A Systematic Approach, 9th edition. Philadelphia: Elsevier; 2019.
4. Sen HN. 2023-2024 Basic and Clinical Science Course™, Section 9: Uveitis and Ocular Inflammation. San Francisco: American Academy of Ophthalmology; 2023.
5. Sihota R, Tandon R. Parsons' Diseases of the Eye, 23rd edition. New Delhi: Elsevier; 2019.

CHAPTER

Ocular Tumors

Rituparna Ghosh, Rituparna Sarkar

QUESTIONS

1. **Write down the genetics, clinical features, investigation, and treatment of retinoblastoma.** **(2 + 2 + 3 + 3) (WBHUS MS 2022)**
2. **Classification, clinical features, diagnosis, and management of choroidal melanoma.** **(6 + 4) (DNB 2019) (WBHUS MS 2023)**
3. **Discuss the ophthalmic manifestations of paraneoplastic syndromes.** **(RGUHS MS 2019)**
4. **What is the differential diagnosis of leukocoria?** **(4) (DNB 2022)**

1. Write down the genetics, clinical features, investigation, and treatment of retinoblastoma. (2 + 2 + 3 + 3) (WBHUS MS 2022)

Retinoblastoma (RB) is a primitive neuroectodermal intraocular malignancy which affects young children. It is the most common intraocular tumor in children which presents as leukocoria.

- It usually affects children <5 years of age. The median age of the patient is within 18 months.
- Around 2/3rd of cases are unilateral and one third is bilateral.
- M:F = 1:1
- RB is secondary to germline or somatic mutation.

Genetics

- *RB1* is a tumor suppressor gene which regulates cellular growth. It has a protein which activates and targets the E2F family of transcription factors. It prevents the transcription of genes from G1 to S phase transition. Transcription is noted on sub band 13q14.2.
- Knudson narrated two-hit mechanism for tumor formation. Two copies of RB gene must be inactivated for retinoblastoma formation.
- The initial mutation inactivates 1 copy of the gene, in either somatic or germline cells.
- The 2nd mutation occurs in somatic cells.
- *Hereditary RB:*
    - Inherited from a patient (germline mutation)
    - Often bilateral and multifocal
    - Higher risk of secondary tumors, e.g., pinealoblastoma
    - Autosomal dominant inheritance
- *Sporadic RB:*
    - Mutations occur in the somatic cells
    - Usually unilateral
- *Genetic testing:*
    - Recommended for all cases of retinoblastoma
    - Helps determine the risk of other cancers and clinical management
    - Enables risk assessment of family members

Clinical Features

- *Symptoms:*
  - White pupillary reflex
  - Proptosis
  - Diminished vision
  - Redness
  - Painful eye
  - Rapid involuntary movement
- *Signs:*
  - Leukocoria
  - Strabismus
  - Periorbital inflammation
  - Proptosis
  - Ciliary injection
  - Pseudo-hypopyon
  - Hyphema
  - Neovascularization of iris
  - It can mimic uveitis, preseptal/orbital cellulitis
  - ± RAPD
  - Posterior segment—vitreous hemorrhage
  - endophthalmitis

Investigations

- A family history and careful examination of eye are important to conclude as retinoblastoma.
- Examination under anesthesia is needed to examine the fundus with scleral indentation. Anterior segment examination shows shallow anterior chamber with opacities confirms that vitreous seeds over iris.
  Exophytic tumor represents as subretinal lesions.
  Exudative retinal detachment can be associated with vitreous seeding.
- *USG-B scan* shows hyperechoic mass with hyperreflective foci with posterior shadowing associated with calcium. Tumor height and its thickness are essential to confirm RB. It can be associated with RD and calcification.
- CT scan confirms the calcium deposition in eye and confirms the size of tumor which is helpful for children to diagnose the cancer related syndrome.
- *MRI scan*: It is significant to state the condition of optic nerve and extraocular extension. Trilateral RB is confirmed by MRI.
- FA differentiates RB from Coats' disease. In RB it shows dilated torturous vessels with nonperfusion areas and microaneurysms.
- Bone marrow aspiration is rarely done to detect metastasis.

Management

- The aim of management is to preserve vision by minimizing the side effects and complications of surgical and adjuvant treatment.
- Enucleation is the final treatment in a case of intraocular RB.
- To salvage the eye, systemic chemotherapy with local adjuvant treatments and intra-arterial chemotherapy are necessary.
- *Intravenous chemotherapy (IVC):*
  - Nowadays systemic chemotherapy with focal destructive procedures is the globe salvaging treatment in RB.
  - In bilateral RB cases, the severely affected eye undergoes enucleation whereas the less severely affected eye undergoes with IVC with or without external beam irradiation.
  - Vincristine, high dose of carboplatin and etoposide are used. The use of subtenon carboplatin is on trial.

- *Intra-arterial chemotherapy:*
  - Anticancer agents are administered in carotid artery. The technique is modified by cannulating ophthalmic artery. The technique is called super-selective intra-arterial chemotherapy.
  - The triple therapy, i.e., melphalan, topotecan and carboplatin can be considered as IAC therapy in bilateral RB cases.
  - Trilateral RB is treated by chemotherapy than EBRT.
  - In germline RB cases systemic chemotherapy is preferred over local therapy.
- *Intravitreal chemotherapy (IVitC):*
  - Intravitreal injections 20–30 μg melphalan or 20 μg topotecan can be administered. 30–32 gauge needles with double or triple freeze thaw therapy at the injection site to prevent from vitreous seedings.
- *Radiation treatment:*
  - External beam radiation and plaque radiotherapy are used for secondary treatment after primary treatment, i.e., chemotherapy.
  - It is applied for refractory cases.
  - In plaque radiotherapy it is sutured with sclera to reduce the bulk of tumor.
- *Enucleation:*
  - In case of large tumor, enucleation is required.
  - Goal of enucleation is removal of as much area of optic nerve as possible such that the cut end is tumor-free.
  - Lateral canthotomy can be done to get better results.
  - Adjuvant therapy will be given in the cases of grossly encroaching choroidal invasion, optic nerve spread, scleral invasion and anterior segment involvement.
  - Large orbital implant can be used in growth of the pediatric orbit.

Newer Treatment

Newer drugs like MDMX-P53 antagonists (Nutin-3), histone deacetylase inhibitors (trichostatin-A), spleen tyrosine kinase inhibitors (BAY-61-3606) can be administered.

Review

Hereditary RB has more risk to develop secondary tumors. Most common secondary tumors are osteosarcoma. Patients undergone radiation therapy is more prone for secondary tumors. Long-term follow-up may be needed in patients with germline tumors.

2. Classification, clinical features, diagnosis, and management of choroidal melanoma. (6 + 4) (DNB 2019) (WBHUS MS 2023)

Choroidal Melanoma

- Most common primary intraocular malignant tumor which arises from melanocytes of uveal tissue.
- Incidence—5.1 per million.
- *Site of lesion:*
  - Uvea—90%
  - Ciliary body—7%
  - Iris—2%
- Age—around 60 years
- *Risk factors:*
  - Pale iris
  - Light-colored skin
  - Ocular melanocytic lesions (nevi, oculodermal melanocytosis)
  - UV radiation
  - North European origin

- Pathophysiology—five genes like *GNAQ, GNA11* (83–89% are involved); *BAP1, SF 3B1*, and *EIF1AX* are involved for tumorigenesis.
- *Classification:* According to modified Callender classification it is divided into three categories:
  1. Spindle-cell
  2. Epithelioid cell
  3. Mixed cell
     - Spindle cell melanomas—the best prognosis
     - Epithelioid melanomas—the worst prognosis

  According to the size of choroidal melanoma it is classified in **Table 1**.

TABLE 1: Types of choroidal melanoma.

	Apical height	*Largest basal diameter*
Small	1–2.5 mm	5–16 mm
Medium	2.5–10 mm	<16 mm
Large	>10 mm	>16 mm

- Tumor, node, metastasis (TNM) is used for tumor staging and prognosis, which is demonstrated by AJCC.
- *Clinical features:*
  - Symptoms:
    - Asymptomatic (30%)—diagnosed in routine fundus examination.
    - Dimness of vision (38%) secondary to RD
    - Photopsia (9%)
    - Floaters (7%)
    - Visual field defect (6%)
    - Pain in eye (2%)
- *Signs:*
  - A single elevated subretinal grayish-brown dome-shaped mass with irregular margin can be noted on fundus examination.
  - The margin of the lesion is around 3 mm from optic disc (60%).
  - Orange pigments scattered over the lesion in clumps.
  - Around 20% tumor breaches Bruch's membrane results mushroom-shaped or color stud appearance.
  - In few cases, subretinal hemorrhage and SRF may be present after breaching RPE. Exudative retinal detachment may be noted.
  - It can be associated with sentinel vessels, inflammation, cataract, glaucoma, NVI, and choroidal folds.
  - After erosion of retina vitreous hemorrhage and vitreous seeding are expected.
  - In large RD, shallow iris-lens diaphragm and secondary angle closure glaucoma can be seen. NVG is evident in presence of large tumors.

Diagnosis

- *Slit-lamp bio microscopy (SLB):*
  - Assessment of anterior segment
  - Gonioscopy along with slit lamp shows the tumor.
  - Indirect ophthalmoscopy—it is a gold standard technique to visualize choroidal lesions.
- *Wide-field retinal photography:* It can be a tool for monitoring and lesion.
- *Fundus autofluorescence:* Orange lipofusion pigmentation have autofluorescent properties so it becomes brighter than other lesions.
- OCT macula shows presence of any SRF or secondary retinal changes.
- *EDI-OCT:* It measures the choroid and scleral thickness.
  - Optical choroidal shadowing, SRF, subretinal lipofusion deposits, EZ loss are features of choroidal melanoma.

- *USG:*
  - It confirms the presence of choroidal melanoma.
  - It measures the basal diameter, extent, scleral extent and downward growth to monitor progression.
  - Standardized A-mode—medium to low internal activity (88%) in decrescendo pattern, i.e., positive alpha kappa angle in which the internal reflectivity decreases from apex to base of the lesion as sound attenuates through the tumor. Internal blood flow depends on fast movement of spikes. Large melanoma with necrotic tissues shows more irregular spikes. Acoustic hallowing is due to homogeneity in tumor with quiet zone at base.
  - B-mode confirms collar stud appearance associated with hallow zone in tumor, choroidal excavation, SRF and orbital shadowing.
  - FA shows dual circulation, mottled fluorescence in arterial phase, late diffuse leakage and staining.
  - UBM delineates the differentiation between iris and ciliary melanoma.
- Color Doppler ultrasound shows pulsatile blood flow at the base of tumor.
- *ICGA:* As it has less RPE interference it shows hypocyanescence throughout the fundus.
- MRI shows extraocular extension.
- PET scan shows high sensitivity in liver metastasis.
- Biopsy is demonstrated by fine needle or 25 gauge vitrectomy although the procedure is controversial.
- Immunohistochemistry for PAX8 expression—PAX8 negative is seen in melanoma cases.
- Genetic analysis—loss of chromosome 3 and chromosome 8

Management

- The aim of treatment is:
  - Prevention of metastasis
  - Preservation of useful vision
  - Tumor destruction.
- The treatment depends on the size, thickness, location, activity, status of the tumor. The thickness and size of tumor are the prognostic factors.
- Periodic observation is treatment of choice when tumor is small <2 mm, asymptomatic, associated with drusen and RPE atrophy.
- Patients with suspicious nevi should be examined every 3 months and monitored for growth. If no change is seen, examination can be done every 6 months.
- Tumors growing over a period of <2 years is highly indicative of malignancy while growth >10 years is considered benign.

Therapy

- Enucleation is the treatment of choice but metastasis rate is higher. Used in:
  - Advanced melanoma
  - Tumors invading optic nerve
  - Severe secondary glaucoma
  - Total retinal detachment
  - Gentle handling is the standard procedure during enucleation. Hydroxyapatite implants are widely used after enucleation.
- Orbital exenteration is needed when extensive extrascleral involvement is evident. Eyelid sparing exenteration has better results.
- Local resection is done in patients with small melanoma. Resection of part of retina and vitreous body are considered.
- Brachytherapy—a customized plaque containing the radioisotope iodine-125 is placed on the eye. I-125 is applied at a dosage of 0.60–0.1 Gy/h over 3–7 consecutive days. FNAC is performed before insertion of plaque brachytherapy.
  - Used for small- and medium-sized melanomas outside macula and posterior to ora serrata.
- Plaque brachytherapy can treat any size of tumor with 12 mm thickened base. It can be combined with laser therapy.

- *Radiotherapy:* 5–10% of patients undergoing radiotherapy have to proceed for enucleation later. Radiation vasculopathy is a common complication which is treated by PRP, intravitreal anti-VEGF or transpupillary thermotherapy.
- External beam therapy consists of stereotactic radio surgery and charged particle therapy.
- Charged particle radiation therapy, i.e., proton beam radiotherapy is an alternative to reduce the bulk of tumor surrounding the optic disc.
  - In stereotactic surgery, gamma knife and cyber knife are used to treat small (3 mm) melanoma.
- Laser therapies include photocoagulation, PDT and transpupillary thermotherapy. They are less used now due to:
  - High rate of incomplete control
  - Tumor recurrence
  - Extrascleral extension
- *Treatment in metastatic diseases:* Spread of disease is most common in melanoma patients. Intra-arterial chemotherapy and transcatheter intra-arterial therapy is used to treat the progression.
- Hepatic Trans Arterial Chemo Embolization (TACE) and transarterial radioembolization can be done to treat liver metastasis in uveal melanoma.
- Conventional chemotherapy, target chemotherapy and adjuvant therapy are indicated to reduce the bulk of tumor.
- Prognosis—95% patients are treated with resection and radiotherapy. Patient may survive with poor visual acuity.
- Follow-up—Patients need to undergo routine fundus examination in cases of small melanomas. PET scan can be done in metastatic patients to rule out liver and organ metastasis.

3. Discuss the ophthalmic manifestations of paraneoplastic syndromes. (RGUHS MS 2019)

Paraneoplastic syndrome is a complex disorder which forms due to altered immune complex in the systemic organs. It is secondary to occult malignancy. The incidence rate is 8%. The predilection in both genders is equal.

- *Pathophysiology:* The exact mechanism of PNS is not well defined. But cellular and humoral immune systems are responsible for PNS. Antibody formation takes place when cytotoxic T-cells detects antigen on tumor cells. The similar reaction may appear on normal cells as antigen presentation causes signs and symptoms of the disease. These are immunological or nonimmunological reactions like cancer-related retinopathy, melanoma related retinopathy, cancer associated cone dysfunction, bilateral diffuse uveal melanocytic proliferation.
- Paraneoplastic syndromes of ophthalmic significance are mentioned in **Table 2**.

TABLE 2: List of paraneoplastic syndromes of ophthalmic significance.

Features	*CAR*	*MAR*	*CACD*	*PVM*	*BCRMP*
Visual acuity	Severe DOR	Mild to severe DOR	Mild to moderate DOR	Blurring of vision is noted, Mild loss of vision	Mild to severe DOR
Visual field changes	• Central ring scotoma is seen • Peripheral scotoma	Central para central scotoma is seen	Central scotoma	Central paracentral scotoma	Nonspecific
OCT findings	Loss of outer retinal layers (central and peripheral loss)	• Macular atrophy • Inner retinal layer thinning	Loss of outer retinal layer	Submacular vitelliform deposition over pigment epithelium in neurosensory retina	• EDI-OCT scan shows diffuse thickening of choroid • Atrophy of choroidal vessels
FAF	Ring-shaped macular hyper-autofluorescence with surrounding hypo-autofluorescence	Nonspecific	NA	NA	Hypo/hyper-autofluorescence

Contd...

Contd...

Features	*CAR*	*MAR*	*CACD*	*PVM*	*BCRMP*
FFA	Normal FA or signs of periphlebitis	• Normal FA • Signs of vasculitis with vascular diffusion	NA	In late phase of FA with contrast sensitivity shows blocking effect on the choroid	• Peripheral arterial nonperfusion area is noted • RPE nonuniform RPE loss • In late phase—Exudative retinal detachment is noted
IGCA	Normal	Normal	Normal	Normal	Normal or choroidal vessels atrophy
ff-ERG	• As photoreceptors are affected; it affects a-wave • It progresses to "flat ERG"	• Normal a-wave • Due to bipolar cell loss—micro voltage or disappearance of b wave is noted	Cone receptors are affected	NA/Variable results	Reduction of a and b wave amplitude
mf-ERG	Abnormal +++	Mild Abnormal +	Abnormal + (Partial)	NA	Mild abnormal +
EOG	Normal Arden ratio	↓ Arden ratio	Normal Arden ratio	Variable Arden ratio	Normal Arden ratio

(BDUMP: bilateral diffuse uveal melanocytic proliferation; CACD: cancer-associated cone dysfunction; CAR: cancer-associated retinopathy; MAR: melanoma-related retinopathy; PVM: paraneoplastic vitelliform maculopathy)

Risk Factors

- The most common cause of cancer related underlying diseases are small cell lung cancer, non-small cell lung cancer, melanoma, breast carcinoma.
- The least causes of PNS are lymphoma, basal cell carcinoma, clear cell renal carcinoma, prostate cancer and colon cancer.

Symptoms

- Painless progressive loss of vision which is bilaterally asymmetric
- Positive visual phenomena
- Low scotopic vision
- Defective color vision
- Photopsia
- Glare
- Photosensitivity
- Scotoma
- Peripheral vision loss

Signs

- Optic disc pallor
- Retinal arterial attenuation
- May be associated with cataract, retinal detachment and retinal pigmentation.
- Constriction of visual field
- Photoreceptors dysfunction
- Low grade AC cells
- Anterior vitreous—flare is noted (vitritis)
- Atrophy of RPE
- Optic disc pallor
- Atrophy of RPE
- Macular edema

Clinical Diagnosis

Investigations

- Immunoassay
- ERG
- Western blot
- ELISA
- CT scan/PET/MRI
- CSF analysis
- Visual fields
- FFA
- FAF
- ICGA
- SD-OCT

Management

Medical Treatment

- Immunosuppressive medications like corticosteroids may improve mild to moderate vision loss.
- Intravenous immunoglobulin helps to get better results.
- Treatments like alemtuzumab, rituximab, azathioprine, cyclosporine, mycophenolate mofetil are used to improve signs and symptoms of PNS.

Surgical Treatments

- Surgical excision of tumor is needed to treat underlying malignancy.

Prognosis

- Tumor with PNS causes better prognosis.

4. What is the differential diagnosis of leukocoria? (4) (DNB 2022)

Leukocoria is a white pupillary reflex after pupillary dilatation with medication or direct illumination of fundus through pupil. The different causes of leukocoria are mentioned in **Flowchart 1**.

- The meaning of leukocoria is white pupil or cat's eye.
- Due to presence of pathology or any media opacity in posterior segment, there is obstruction of normal red reflex of fundus.

Flowchart 1: Differential diagnosis of leukocoria.

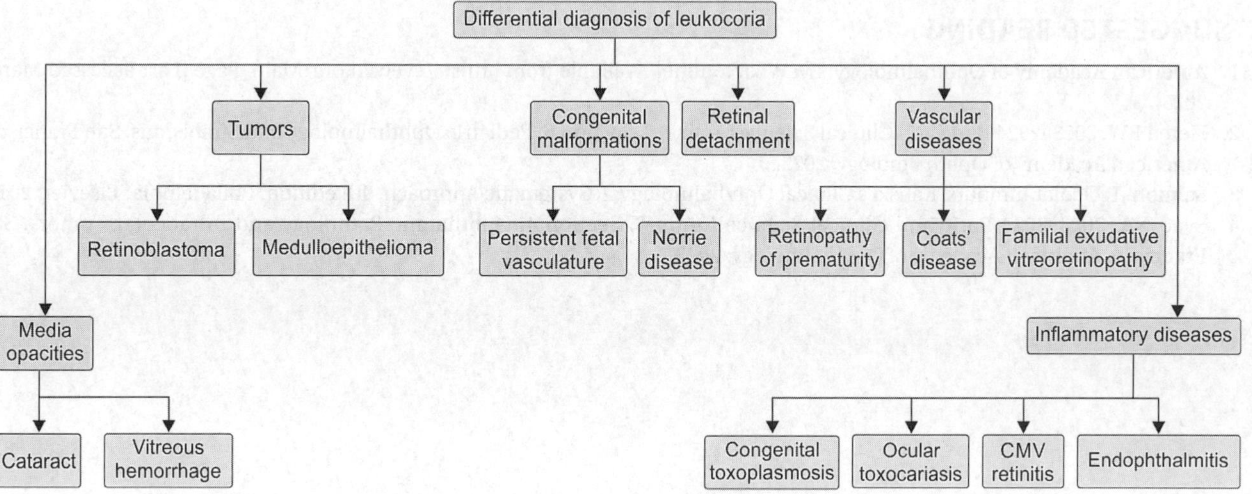

Pediatric Cataract

- Around 60% of congenital cataract occurs. Within this 18% unilateral and 42% bilateral are noted.
- The cause of unilateral cataract is mostly sporadic and bilateral cataract is related with systemic diseases, i.e., TORCH infections, metabolic diseases and chromosomal diseases.

Retinoblastoma

- Retinoblastoma has tremendous potential to convert into malignancy of primitive retinal cells.
- It has autosomal dominant transmission with 90% penetrance in 48% cases.
- The cause of RB is sporadic (95% cases).
- The *RB1* tumor suppressor gene is located on sub-band 13q14.2.
- Flexner–Wintersteiner rosette, Homer-Wright rosette, pseudo-rosettes are commonly seen in HPE reports of RB.
- Leukocoria, squint, diminished vision is common clinical features.
- Calcification is commonly seen.
- There are two types—Endophytic type starts from inner retina grows into vitreous causes endophthalmitis.
- Exophytic tumors start growing from outer retina into sclera appears as Coats' disease and traumatic retinal detachment.

Coats' Disease

- It is a retinal telangiectatic condition affecting young males.
- NVG, retinal telangiectasia, exudative RD, Leber's military microaneurysms are noted.
- NVG leads to enucleation.

Persistent Fetal Vasculature

- It is second most common cause of leukocoria.
- It is a congenital condition which causes regression of fetal vasculature.
- Mostly one eye is affected.
- It is associated with complete pupillary membrane, cataract, strabismus, glaucoma.

Toxoplasmosis

- It is due to protozoan parasite toxoplasma gondii.
- Cat is definitive host and human is intermediate host.
- White focal retinitis (headlight in fog) with surrounding pigmented scar, vitritis, secondary non granulomatous iridocyclitis, retinal vasculitis and ocular HTN are features of toxoplasmosis.
- PCR and IgG titers are helpful to diagnose.
- Systemic pyrimethamine, sulfadiazine, and corticosteroids (triple therapy) are useful toxoplasmosis treatment.

SUGGESTED READING

1. American Academy of Ophthalmology. EyeWiki. [online] Available from https://eyewiki.org/Main_Page [Last accessed March 2025].
2. Hered RW. 2023–2024 Basic and Clinical Science Course™, Section 6: Pediatric Ophthalmology and Strabismus. San Francisco: American Academy of Ophthalmology; 2023.
3. Salmon JF. Ocular tumours. Kanski's Clinical Ophthalmology: A Systematic Approach, 9th edition. Philadelphia: Elsevier; 2019.
4. Syed NA. 2023–2024 Basic and Clinical Science Course™, Section 4: Ophthalmic Pathology and Intraocular Tumors. San Francisco: American Academy of Ophthalmology; 2023.

CHAPTER

Diseases of the Retina

Rupak Roy, Soumava Mandal, Sangeeta Roy, Ekta Bharti

QUESTIONS

1. **Classify diabetic retinopathy. Mention utility of OCT and FFA in management of diabetic retinopathy. Role of HbA1c, blood pressure and blood cholesterol in prevention and management of diabetic retinopathy. (10) (DNB 2021)**
2. **DRCR.net protocols for management of macular edema. (5) (DNB 2023).**
3. **Describe the findings of fundus in proliferative diabetic retinopathy. How would you manage such a case? (10) (WBUHS MS 2021)**
4. **How will you evaluate and manage a case of central retinal vein occlusion in a 45Y male? (10) (WBUHS MS 2023/DNB 2022)**
5. **Enumerate the risk factors, clinical features, classification and management of Retinopathy of prematurity. (2 + 4 + 4) (WBUHS MS 2023)**
6. **Discuss newer anti-VEGFs. (10) (DNB 2023)**

1. Classify diabetic retinopathy. Mention utility of OCT and FFA in management of diabetic retinopathy. Role of HbA1c, blood pressure and blood cholesterol in prevention and management of diabetic retinopathy. (10) (DNB 2021)

Classifications of diabetic retinopathy are mentioned in **Tables 1 and 2.**

TABLE 1: ETDRS classification of diabetic retinopathy.

Classification	*Features*
Mild NPDR	At least one microaneurysm AND criteria not met for more severe retinopathy
Moderate NPDR	Hemorrhages/microaneurysms ≥ standard photograph 2A AND/OR cotton-wool spots, venous beading, or IRMA definitely present; AND criteria not met for more severe retinopathy
Severe NPDR	Cotton-wool spots, venous beading, and IRMA definitely present in at least two of photographic fields 4–7; OR two of the three preceding features present in at least two of fields 4–7 and hemorrhages/ microaneurysms present in fields 4–7 ≥ standard photograph 2A in at least one of them; OR IRMA present in each of fields 4–7 and ≥ standard photograph 8A in at least two of them; AND criteria not met for more severe retinopathy
Early PDR	New vessels AND criteria not met for high-risk PDR
High-risk PDR	New vessels on or within one disc diameter of the optic disc [neovascularization of the disc (NVD)] ≥ standard photograph 10A (approximately one-fourth to one-third disc area) with or without vitreous or preretinal hemorrhage; OR vitreous and/or preretinal hemorrhage accompanied by new vessels, either NVD < standard photograph 10A or new vessels elsewhere (NVE) ≥ one-fourth disc area

TABLE 2: International classification of diabetic retinopathy.

Classification	*Features*
No apparent retinopathy	No abnormalities
Mild NPDR	Microaneurysms only
Moderate NPDR	More than just microaneurysms but less than severe NPDR
Severe NPDR	One or more of the following, in the absence of PDR: • More than 20 intraretinal hemorrhages in each of four quadrants • Definite venous beading in two or more quadrants • Prominent IRMA in one or more quadrants
PDR	One or more of the following: • Extraretinal neovascularization • Vitreous or preretinal hemorrhage

OCT

- Early diagnosis of DME
- Location and extent—central or noncentral
- DME classification (based on OCT)—cystoid, spongiform, mixed, neuro-sensory detachment, taut posterior hyaloid
- *OCT biomarkers:*
  - DRIL disorganization of retinal inner layers—reliable biomarker, poor prognosis
  - Hyperreflective retinal foci–size less than 300 micron, no backshadow, reflectivity similar to RNFL; signifies retinal inflammation 16 and responds well with intravitreal steroids
  - Hyperreflective choroidal foci—poor prognosis as it signifies disruption of ELM and EZ
  - Intraretinal cystoid spaces—larger cysts in outer retinal layer can cause more photoreceptor and IS-OS junction damage, so they have poor prognosis than smaller cysts in inner retinal layers
  - Bridging retinal processes—presence of bridging processes between cystic spaces is good prognosis as they represent connecting neural elements between outer and inner retinal
  - Subfoveal choroidal thickness—greater thickness suggests good prognosis as more thickness means intact choriocapillary, so less ischemic outer retinal
  - Photoreceptor outer segment
  - Hard exudates–intravitreal steroids work better than anti-VEGFs in cases of DME with hard exudates specially subfoveal
  - Subfoveal neurosensory detachment—inconclusive
  - Integrity of ELM and EZ–intact IS-OS junction is good prognosis.
  - Taut posterior hyaloid–it is responsible for recalcitrant DME. Patients with TPH benefit more from surgical management, i.e., pars plana vitrectomy and removal of TPH.
  - Choroidal vascularity index—choroidal lumen are to total choroidal area. It is a new parameter under study and better than choroidal thickness as it is not affected by systemic and ocular factors. It correlates with the progression of DR. Eyes with DR have less CVI with unaltered choroidal thickness. Also eyes with PDR have less CVI than those of NPDR.
- Helps in surgical planning—plane of TRD, TPH assessment, presence of ERM, secondary membrane.

FFA

- NPDR—earliest sign of DR, i.e., microaneurysms can be detected on FFA even when they are not evident in clinical examination.
- DME—pattern of leakage can indicate focal or diffuse leakage and focal laser if needed can be planned accordingly.
- PDR—neovacularization can be detected, CNP areas can also be well delineated.
- Macular ischemia—unexplained loss of visual acuity due to macular ischemia can be explained by FFA.

HbA1c

HbA1c shows the average blood sugar level over the past two to three months. So it reflects the sugar control. Sugar control is the most important modifiable risk factor for diabetic retinopathy. Diabetes control and complications trial and the United Kingdom prospective diabetes study are landmark clinical trials which showed the importance of sugar control in reducing the risk of development and progression of diabetic retinopathy.

DCCT trial showed intensive therapy (mean HbA1c 7.2%) decreases the chance of developing DR by 76% and the progression of diabetic retinopathy by 54%.

UKPDS study showed patients with higher glucose level at the beginning of the trial were more likely to develop diabetic retinopathy. Intensive sugar control reduced the progression of diabetic retinopathy by 21% and the need for laser photo coagulation by 29%.

Though ACCORD study showed intensive glycemic control increased mortality but the ACCORDION study showed tight glycemic control helped in reducing the progression of diabetic retinopathy.

BP

Hypertension is another important modifiable respected for diabetic retinopathy UKPDS study showed tight blood pressure control (defined as target blood pressure less than 150/85 mm Hg) caused 34% reduction in the rate of progression of diabetic retinopathy and 47% reduction in deterioration of visual equity in patients of type 2 DM.

Cholesterol

Results of different studies regarding the role of dyslipidemia in diabetic retinopathy came to be in conclusive. A large clinical trial of fenofibrate intervention and event lowering in diabetes (FIELD) study showed that use of fenofibrate reduced the frequency for laser treatment for DME by 31% and for PDR by 30% in patients with type 2 DM. Although the subset of patients those who had high triglyceride and low serum HDL cholesterol benefited most from fenofibrate therapy.

2. DRCR.net protocols for management of macular edema. (5) (DNB 2023).

The Diabetic Retinopathy Clinical Research Network (DRCR.net) has developed several protocols for managing diabetic macular edema (DME), which is a common complication of diabetic retinopathy. These protocols are based on extensive clinical research and aim to provide evidence-based guidelines for treatment. Here's an overview of the key DRCR.net protocols related to the management of macular edema:

Protocol A: Demonstrated the efficacy of modified technique of ETDRS direct focal/grid laser photocoagulation for DME.

Protocol B: Showed that 14% of patients treated with modified focal/grid laser gained ≥15 letters, whereas approximately 18% lost ≥ 15 letters at 2 years' follow-up. Also at the 2-year primary outcome, the BCVA gain in the laser arm was significantly greater than the steroid arm.

Protocol I: Compared efficacy of intravitreal ranibizumab injection with prompt or delayed (≥24 weeks) focal/grid laser for center (fovea) involving DME (CI-DME). The followings are the key conclusions:

- Intravitreal ranibizumab with prompt or deferred (≥24 weeks) focal/grid laser is more effective through 2 years in increasing visual acuity compared with focal/grid laser treatment alone for the treatment of CI-DME
- Focal/grid laser treatment at the initiation of IVR is no better, possibly worse, for vision outcomes than deferring laser treatment for 24 weeks or more in eye with CI-DME
- At 5 years completion of follow-up: BCVA gained at 1 year was maintained to 5 years concomitant with diminishing need for treatment over time; deferring laser may be associated with more VA gain through 5 years.

Protocol T: compared aflibercept (EYLEA, Regeneron), bevacizumab (Avastin, Genentech/Roche), and ranibizumab (Lucentis, Genentech/Roche) for eyes with visual impairment due to CI-DME. *The following are the key conclusions*:

- Vision gains (from baseline) at 2 years were seen in all 3 groups with half the number of injections, slightly decreased frequency of visits, and decreased amount of laser in the 2nd year.
- At the end of the 2-year study period, there were no differences between the agents with regards to the mean change in VA from baseline, if baseline VA was between 20/32 and 20/40.

However, among patients with a baseline VA between 20/50 and 20/320, *aflibercept was superior to bevacizumab and ranibizumab at 1 year*, and *to bevacizumab only at 2 years*.

Protocol U: In patients with persistent DME, it evaluated short-term visual improvement at 6 months after the addition of corticosteroid therapy [dexamethasone intravitreal implant 0.7 mg (Ozurdex, Allergan)] to ranibizumab anti-VEGF versus ranibizumab alone. The following were the key conclusions:

- Simultaneous administration of corticosteroids with ranibizumab decreased retinal thickness on OCT at six months.
- However at 6 months, there was no difference in mean VA improvement between the two groups.

Protocol V: Evaluated three treatment strategies for patients with good vision (20/25 or better) and CI-DME: intravitreal aflibercept as frequently as every 4 weeks, focal/grid laser therapy with deferred aflibercept, or observation with deferred aflibercept. The following are the key conclusions:

- At 2 years, there was no statistically significant difference in the percentage of patients who lost at least 5 letters between the three groups.
- The researchers concluded that observation may be a reasonable initial strategy for patients with good vision and CI-DME until visual acuity worsens.

Protocol W: Evaluated the effect of intravitreal anti-VEGF aflibercept versus sham for the prevention of vision-threatening complications of moderate to severe non proliferative DR (NPDR). The following are the key conclusions:

- At 2 years, the cumulative probability of developing PDR was 13.5% and 33.2% and CI-DME with vision loss was 4.1% and 14.8% in the aflibercept and sham groups.
- Although periodic treatment with aflibercept reduced the development of vision-reducing CI-DME and PDR, it did not have any statistically significant visual acuity benefits at the end of 2 years.

3. Describe the findings of fundus in proliferative diabetic retinopathy. How would you manage such a case? (10) (WBUHS MS 2021)

Diabetic retinopathy is predominantly a microangiopathy in which small blood vessels are particularly vulnerable to damage from high glucose levels. Direct hyperglycemic effects on retinal cells, angiogenic stimulators and inhibitors are also likely to play a role.

Proliferative diabetic retinopathy (PDR) is characterized by neovascularization on or within one disc diameter of the disc (NVD) and/or new vessels elsewhere (NVE) in the fundus.

Advanced diabetic eye disease is characterized by tractional retinal detachment, significant persistent vitreous hemorrhage and neovascular glaucoma.

Signs

Microaneurysms: These are localized outpouchings, mainly saccular, of the capillary wall that may form either by focal dilatation of the capillary wall where pericytes are absent, or by fusion of two arms of a capillary loop. Most develop in the inner capillary plexus (ganglion cell layer). They tend to be the earliest sign of DR.

Signs: Tiny red dots, often initially temporal to the fovea. May be indistinguishable clinically from dot hemorrhages.

Fluorescein angiography (FA) allows differentiation between dot hemorrhages and nonthrombosed microaneurysms. Early frames show tiny hyperfluorescent dots. Late frames show diffuse hyperfluorescence due to leakage.

Retinal hemorrhages:

- Retinal nerve fiber layer hemorrhages arise from the larger superficial precapillary arterioles and assume their characteristic shape because of the architecture of the retinal nerve fiber layer.
- Intraretinal hemorrhages arise from the venous end of capillaries and are located in the compact middle layers of the retina with a resultant red "dot/blot" configuration
- Deeper dark round hemorrhages represent hemorrhagic retinal infarcts and are located within the middle retinal layers. The extent of involvement is a significant marker of the likelihood of progression to PDR.

Exudates:

These are caused by chronic localized retinal edema. They develop at the junction of normal and edematous retina. They are composed of lipoprotein and lipid-filled macrophages located mainly within the outer plexiform layer.

- *Signs*: Waxy yellow lesions with relatively distinct margins arranged in clumps and/or rings at the posterior pole, often surrounding leaking microaneurysms. With time the number and size tend to increase and the fovea may be involved. When leakage ceases, exudates absorb spontaneously over a period of months.
- FA will commonly show hypofluorescence only with large dense exudates. Although background choroidal fluorescence is masked, retinal capillary fluorescence is generally preserved overlying the lesions.

Diabetic macular edema (DMO): Diabetic maculopathy (foveal edema, exudates or ischemia) is the most common cause of visual impairment in diabetic patients, particularly type 2. Diffuse retinal edema is caused by extensive capillary leakage and localized edema by focal leakage from microaneurysms and dilated capillary segments.

Ischemic maculopathy:

- Signs are variable and the macula may look relatively normal despite reduced visual acuity
- FA shows capillary nonperfusion at the fovea (an enlarged FAZ) and frequently other areas of capillary nonperfusion at the posterior pole and periphery.

Cotton-wool spots: Cotton-wool spots are composed of accumulations of neuronal debris within the nerve fiber layer. They result from ischemic disruption of nerve axons, the swollen ends of which are known as cytoid bodies.

- *Signs*: Small fluffy whitish superficial lesions that obscure underlying blood vessels
- *FA* shows focal hypofluorescence due to local ischemia and blockage of background choroidal fluorescence.

Clinically significant macular edema the nerve fiber layer:

- Retinal thickening within 500 μm of the center of the macula
- Exudates within 500 μm of the center of the macula, if associated with retinal thickening. The thickening itself may be outside the 500 μm.
- Retinal thickening one-disc area (1,500 μm) or larger, any part of which is within one disc diameter of the center of the macula

Venous changes: Venous anomalies seen in ischemia consist of generalized dilatation and tortuosity, looping, beading (focal narrowing and dilatation) and sausage-like segmentation

Intraretinal microvascular abnormalities (IRMA) are arteriolar venular shunts that run from retinal arterioles to venules, thus bypassing the capillary bed and are therefore often seen adjacent to areas of marked capillary hypoperfusion.

- *Signs*: Fine, irregular, red intraretinal lines that run from arterioles to venules, without crossing major blood vessels
- FA shows focal hyperfluorescence associated with adjacent areas of capillary closure ("dropout") but without leakage.

Arterial changes: Subtle retinal arteriolar dilatation may be an early marker of ischemic dysfunction. When significant ischemia is present signs include peripheral narrowing, "silver wiring" and obliteration.

Proliferative retinopathy: Although preretinal new vessels may arise anywhere in the retina, they are most commonly seen at the posterior pole. Fibrous tissue, initially fine, gradually develops as vessels increase in size.

- New vessels at the disc (NVD) describe neovascularization on or within one disc diameter of the optic nerve head
- NVE describes neovascularization further away from the disc. It may be associated with fibrosis if long-standing.
- New vessels on the iris, also known as rubeosis iridis, carry a high likelihood of progression to neo vascular glaucoma.
- FA highlights neovascularization during the early phases of the angiogram and shows irregular expanding hyperfluorescence during the later stages due to intense leakage of dye from neovascular tissue.

Treatment

General

- Patient education is critical, including the need to comply with review and treatment schedules in order to optimize visual outcomes. In type 2 diabetes this also involves counselling on weight reduction programs and emphasizing the need to increase exercise.
- Diabetic control should be optimized.

- Systemic hypertension (especially type 2 diabetes) and hyperlipidemia should be controlled in conjunction with the patient's diabetologist.
- Fenofibrate 200 mg daily has been shown to reduce the progression of DR in type 2 diabetics and prescription should be considered. The decision is independent of whether the patient already takes a statin.
- Smoking should be discontinued, though this has not been definitively shown to affect retinopathy.
- Other modifiable factors such as anemia and renal failure should be addressed as necessary

Treatment of Diabetic Macular Edema

In particular, patients with good vision (6/7.5 or better) who otherwise meet criteria for treatment might prefer to be monitored once the risks of various interventions are considered.

- *Intravitreal anti-VEGF agents:* DRCR.net Protocol I concludes that intravitreal ranibizumab more effectively improves visual acuity than focal/grid laser treatment for center-involved DMO. Laser treatment should be deferred for 6 months after commencement of anti-VEGF therapy.

  Laser photocoagulation (modified ETDRS focal/grid treatment):
  - *Focal:* Diode or argon burns are applied to leaking microaneurysms, 500–3000 μm from the foveola using a spot size 50–100 μm, duration 0.05–0.1 s with sufficient power to obtain a greyish reaction beneath the microaneurysm.
  - *Grid:* Burns are applied to macular areas of diffuse retinal thickening, treating not closer than 500 μm from the foveola and 500 μm from the optic disc using a spot size of 50–100 μm and duration 0.05–0.1 s, with power adjusted to give a mild reaction. A "modified" grid includes focal treatment to foci of leakage, usually microaneurysms.
  - *Subthreshold (micropulse) diode laser:* This modality uses very short (microsecond order) laser pulse duration combined with a relatively longer interval, allowing energy dissipation
  - *Intravitreal triamcinolone; in pseudophakic eyes intravitreal triamcinolone* steroid injection followed by prompt laser is comparable to ranibizumab with regard to visual improvement and reduced retinal thickening.
  - *Pars plana vitrectomy (PPV)* may be indicated when macular edema is associated with tangential traction from a thickened and taut posterior hyaloid.

Treatment for Proliferative Retinopathy

- *Laser photocoagulation*: Scatter laser treatment (panretinal photocoagulation) continues to be the mainstay of PDR treatment.
- *Laser parameters*:
  - *Spot size:* A retinal burn diameter of 400 μm is usually desired for PRP.
  - *Spacing:* Burns should be separated by 1-1.5 burn widths.

Extent of treated area: The initial treatment session should consist of 1,500 burns in most cases, though more may be applied if there is a risk of imminent sight loss from vitreous hemorrhage. 2,500–3,500 burns are likely to be required for regression of mild PDR, 4,000 for moderate PDR, and 7,000 for severe PDR.

Pattern of treatment: Treatment is generally restricted to the area outside the temporal macular vascular arcades. In very severe PDR it is advisable to treat the inferior fundus first, since any vitreous hemorrhage will gravitate inferiorly and obscure this area, precluding further treatment. Areas of vitreoretinal traction should be avoided.

Indicators of regression include blunting of vessel tips, shrinking and disappearance of NV, often leaving "ghost" vessels or fibrosis, regression of IRMA, decreased venous changes, absorption of retinal hemorrhages, disc pallor.

VEGF inhibition for proliferative retinopathy: PRCR.net Protocol S concludes that intravitreal ranibizumab treatment is as effective as PRP in patients at high risk of PDR for up to 5 years. The macular edema rate is reduced and the visual field is slightly better maintained with anti-VEGF treatment

Pars plana vitrectomy: Vitrectomy in DR is typically combined with extensive endolaser PRP.

Indications

- Severe persistent vitreous hemorrhage that precludes adequate PRP is the most common indication
- Progressive tractional RD threatening or involving the macula must be treated without delay. However, extramacular tractional detachments may be observed, since they often remain stationary for prolonged periods.

- Combined tractional and rhegmatogenous RD should be treated urgently.
- Premacular retrohyaloid hemorrhage, if dense and persistent should be considered for early vitrectomy because, if untreated, the internal limiting membrane or posterior hyaloid face may serve as a scaffold for subsequent fibrovascular proliferation and consequent tractional macular detachment or macular epiretinal membrane formation.
- Anterior segment neovascularization and media opacities.

4. How will you evaluate and manage a case of central retinal vein occlusion in a 45Y male? (10) (WBUHS MS 2023/DNB 2022)

Central retinal vein occlusion is the occlusion at or proximal to the lamina cribrosa of the optic nerve, where the central retinal vein exits the eye. The pathogenesis of CRVO is believed to follow the principles of Virchow's triad for thrombogenesis, involving vessel damage, stasis, and hypercoagulability.

The central retinal vein and artery share a common adventitial sheath at arteriovenous crossings posterior to the lamina cribrosa so that atherosclerotic changes of the artery may compress the vein and precipitate CRVO.

Risk Factors

- Age
- Hypertension
- Hyperlipidemia
- Diabetes
- Oral contraceptive pills
- Raised intraocular pressure
- Smoking

Other uncommon predisposing risks factors like myeloproliferative disorders, acquired and inherited hypercoagulable states and some inflammatory conditions.

Symptoms

Presentation is with sudden, unilateral blurred vision. In nonischemic CRVO, the blurring is mild and may be worse on waking and improves during the day. In ischemic CRVO, visual impairment is sudden and severe.

Classification of CRVO

CRVO can be classified as nonischemic CRVO (perfused) and ischemic CRVO (nonperfused) **(Table 3)**.

TABLE 3: Difference between nonischemic and ischemic CRVO.

	Nonischemic CRVO	*Ischemic CRVO*
Visual acuity	>20/200	<20/200
RAPD (relative afferent papillary defect)	Mild or absent	Present (>0, 7 log units of neutral density filter)
Visual field defect	Rare	Common (use of Goldmann perimeter is suggested, as 30 degree field misses peripheral changes)
Fundus appearance	• Less disc/macular edema, hemorrhage, cotton-wool spots • Mild venous tortuosity and dilation	• More disc/macular edema, hemorrhage, cotton-wool spots • Severe venous tortuosity and dilation
Fundus fluorescein angiogram	Less area of nonperfusion	Retinal capillary nonperfusion more than 10 disc areas
ERG/electroretinogram	Normal	Reduced b wave amplitude (≤60% of the normal mean value of both photopic and scotopic ERG), and reduced b/a
Prognosis	Good, less chance of anterior segment neovascularization/ neovascular glaucoma	• Poor, high chance of anterior segment/neovascularization/ neovascular glaucoma • The visual prognosis may be worse than central retinal arterial occlusion

Diagnosis

Fundus Fluorescein Angiography

- In nonischemic CRVO, FA shows marked delay in arteriovenous transit time, which is longer than 20 seconds, masking by retinal hemorrhages, and vessel wall staining.
- Late staining along the large retinal veins is a characteristic finding in moderate and severe degrees of central retinal vein obstruction.
- The ischemic form has extensive areas of capillary nonperfusion.
- Greater than 10 disc areas of retinal capillary nonperfusion is associated with an increased risk of neovascularization

Optical Coherence Tomography

- OCT is useful in the assessment of macular edema, and particularly in monitoring its course, especially with treatment of the edema.
- The OCT shows cystoid macular edema with or without subfoveal fluid. Epiretinal membrane or vitreomacular traction may also be evident.

Systemic Investigations

- Blood pressure
- Erythrocyte sedimentation rate (ESR)
- Complete blood count (CBC)
- Random blood glucose
- Random total and HDL cholesterol
- Plasma protein electrophoresis (dysproteinemias such as multiple myeloma)
- Urea, electrolytes and creatinine (renal disease in association with hypertension)
- Thyroid function tests (associated with dyslipidemia)
- ECG (left ventricular hypertrophy secondary to hypertension)

Management

- In a non-ischemic CRVO without macular edema, initial follow-up should take place after 4-6 weeks to monitor for development of edema or worsening ischemia.
- In a clearly nonischemic CRVO without macular edema, initial follow-up should take place after 4–6 weeks to monitor for development of edema or worsening ischemia.
- Patients with ischemic CRVO should be seen monthly for 6 months to detect the onset of anterior segment neovascularization. Routine gonioscopy of eyes at risk should therefore be performed and the pupillary margin should be examined prior to mydriasis.
- Macular grid laser is not recommended, since it may reduce angiographically the macular leakage but without benefit on the visual acuity. The CVOS showed no benefit in terms of visual acuity in older patients, although a trend towards better acuity was seen in younger patients
- *Intravitreal therapy used:*
  - Intravitreal steroids
  - Ranibizumab
  - Aflibercept
  - Intravitreal dexamethasone implant
  - Brolucizumab
  - Faricimab
- *Neovascularization:* According to CRVO study there is no apparent benefit in performing panretinal photocoagulation (PRP) before development of iris and angle neovascularization, provided frequent follow-up examinations can be performed, since prophylactic treatment does not totally prevent iris and angle neovascularization.

Prognosis: In cases that do not subsequently become ischemic, the prognosis is reasonably good with return of vision to normal or near normal in about 50%. The main cause for poor vision is chronic macular edema, which may lead to secondary RPE changes. To a certain extent the prognosis is related to initial visual acuity as follows:

- 20/60 or better, it is likely to remain so
- 20/80–20/200, the clinical course is variable, and vision may subsequently improve, remain the same, or worsen
- Worse than 20/200, improvement is unlikely

The prognosis of ischemic CRVO is extremely poor due to macular ischemia. Rubeosis iridis develops in about 50% of eyes, usually between 2 and 4 months (100-day glaucoma), and there is a high risk of neovascular glaucoma. The development of opticociliary shunts may protect the eye from anterior segment neovascularization and probably indicates a dramatic reduction in risk. Retinal neovascularization occurs in about 5% of eyes

5. Enumerate the risk factors, clinical features, classification and management of Retinopathy of prematurity. (2 + 4 + 4) (WBUHS MS 2023)

Risk Factors

- Low birthweight < 1,500 g
- Young gestational age (GA) < 30 weeks of gestation
- High, unregulated oxygen at birth, fluctuations in oxygenation
- Poor postnatal growth

Other Risk Factors

- Respiratory distress syndrome, duration of mechanical ventilation, and steroid use for bronchopulmonary dysplasia—considered risk factors for the *development* of ROP
- Bronchopulmonary dysplasia—considered risk factor for the *progression* of ROP
- *CNS injuries:* Intraventricular hemorrhage, periventricular leukomalacia—considered risk factors for *progression* of ROP
- Low plasma IGF-1 levels—IGF-1 is thought to mediate VEGF. Hence, low plasma IGF-1 levels may be a potential risk factor for the *development* of ROP
- Hyperglycemia
- Sepsis, white race, blood transfusion, and multiple births
- Proteinuria—due to shared embryogenesis between retinal vascularity and renal function

Classifications

To define the location, three concentric zones were established. Zone is based on the most posterior zone as the retina may be vascularized to different extents in different regions of the retina (i.e., nasal vs. temporal vs. superior vs. inferior). Since retinal vascular development proceeds from the optic nerve to the ora serrata, the zones are centered on the optic disc rather than the macula.

Zone I: The area defined by a circle centered on optic nerve, the radius of which extends from the center of the optic disc to twice the distance from the center of the optic disc to the center of the macula.

Zone II: The area extending centrifugally from the edge of zone I to a circle with a radius equal to the distance from the center of the optic disc to the nasal ora serrata.

- *Posterior Zone II:* A region of 2 disc diameters peripheral to the zone I border. This was an addition in ICROP3 to allow for nuance in characterizing more posterior disease, which is often more aggressive.

Zone III: The residual temporal crescent of retina anterior to zone II. By convention, zones II and III are considered to be mutually exclusive.

ICROP3 also added the notion of a "notch" in describing the location of ROP.

Notch: An incursion by the ROP lesion of 1 to 2 clock hours from one zone into another." If present, it should be documented by the most posterior zone with the qualifier "secondary to notch". For example, if most of the vascularization in zone 2 with a notch that extends into zone 1, the location would be "zone 1 secondary to notch".

Disease Severity (Stage)

Stage 1: Demarcation line—This line is thin and flat (in the retina plane) and separates the avascular retina anteriorly from the vascularized retina posteriorly.

Stage 2: Ridge—The ridge arises from the demarcation line and has height and width, which extends above the plane of the retina. Small isolated tufts of neovascular tissue lying on the surface of the retina, commonly called "popcorn" may be seen posterior to this ridge structure but do not constitute the degree of fibrovascular growth that is a necessary condition for stage 3.

Stage 3: Extraretinal fibrovascular proliferation—Intravitreal neovascularization or that which extends from the ridge into the vitreous.

Stage 4: Partial retinal detachment—Stage 4, in the initial classification was the final stage and initially known as the cicatricial phase. It was later divided into extrafoveal (stage 4A) and foveal (stage 4B) partial retinal detachments.

Stage 5: Total retinal detachment—retinal detachments are generally tractional and usually funnel shaped.

Stage 5A: The optic disc is visible by ophthalmoscopy.

Stage 5B: The optic disc is not visible secondary to retrolental fibrovascular tissue or closed-funnel detachment.

Stage 5C: Findings of stage 5B + accompanied by anterior segment abnormalities (e.g., anterior lens displacement, marked anterior chamber shallowing, iridocapsular adhesions, capsule-endothelial adhesion with central corneal opacification. Ultrasonography (B-scan) can be useful, but is not necessary, for the classification of stage 5B and 5C ROP.

Aggressive ROP: Aggressive ROP (A-ROP) is a new category presented in ICROP3. A-ROP includes aggressive posterior ROP (AP-ROP), which was first recognized in the international classification in 2005 to indicate a rapidly progressing, posterior form of ROP that can bypass the typical progression of stages.

Plus disease: Plus disease was characterized by additional signs of increased venous dilatation and arteriolar tortuosity of the posterior retinal vessels which can increase in severity to include iris vascular engorgement, poor pupillary dilatation, and vitreous haze was referred to as plus disease in the original classification

Preplus disease: Preplus disease was later described as vascular abnormalities of the posterior pole that are insufficient for the diagnosis of plus disease but that demonstrate more arterial tortuosity *and* more venous dilatation than normal

Management

Screening

- *First screening examination:* At 32 weeks of post menstrual age or 4 weeks of postnatal age whichever is later
- Infants <28 weeks or <1,200 g should be screened as early as 2–3 weeks of age to enable early identification of APROP

Follow-ups: The timing of follow-up examinations are based on retinal exam findings as classified by the International Classification of Retinopathy of Prematurity revisited.

- *Recommended follow up in 1 week or less:*
    - *Zone I:* Immature vascularization, stage 1 or 2 ROP
    - *Posterior zone II:* Immature vascularization
    - Suspected presence of A-ROP
- *Recommended follow up in 1–2 weeks:*
    - *Zone I:* Unequivocally regressing ROP
    - *Posterior zone II:* Immature vascularization
    - *Zone II:* Stage 2 ROP
- *Recommended follow up in 2 weeks:*
    - *Zone II:* Immature vascularization, stage 1 ROP, or unequivocally regressing ROP
- *Recommended follow up in 2–3 weeks:*
    - *Zone II:* Regressing ROP
    - *Zone III:* Stage 1 or 2 ROP

Termination of acute retinal screening examinations is based on age and retinal findings. Examinations can be stopped when:

- Retina is fully vascularized.
- Zone III retinal vascularization without previous ROP in zone I or II (may need a confirmatory examination if PMA < 35 weeks)
- PMA = 45 weeks and no type 1 ROP (i.e., "pre-threshold disease" (defined as stage 3 ROP in zone II, any ROP in zone I) or worse ROP)
- If previously treated with anti-VEGF (vascular endothelial growth factor) injection, follow until at least PMA = 65 weeks (FYI: Infant needs close follow-up during time of highest risk for disease reactivation PMA: 45–55 weeks)
- ROP has fully regressed (ensure there is no abnormal vascular tissue present that can reactivate and progress)

Long-term follow-up:

- After termination of acute retinal screening, preterm infants should be seen within 4–6 months after discharge from the NICU for vision development. Preterm infants are at increased risk for developing strabismus, amblyopia, high refractive error, cataract, and glaucoma.

Treatment

Currently ROP treatment guidelines are based on the Early Treatment of Retinopathy of Prematurity Study

Laser treatment is currently recommended for the following (defined as "type 1" ROP):

- *Zone I:* Any stage ROP with plus disease
- *Zone I:* Stage 3 ROP without plus disease
- *Zone II:* Stage 2 or 3 ROP with plus disease
- APROP

Follow-up is recommended in 3–7 days following either laser photocoagulation or anti-VEGF injection to monitor for reduction in retinal dilation, tortuosity and/or stage 3 ROP.

Eyes must be watched carefully for regression and reactivation. Very late recurrences of proliferative ROP have been reported following anti-VEGF therapy.

6. Discuss newer anti-VEGFs. (10) (DNB 2023)

Vascular Endothelial Growth Factor

The vascular endothelial growth factor (VEGF) family of cytokines plays a key role in vasculogenesis, angiogenesis, and lymphangiogenesis. This VEGF protein family comprises VEGF-A (main member), VEGF-B, VEGF-C, VEGF-D and placental growth factor (PlGF) in mammals.

Role in retinal diseases: Upregulation of VEGF and other proangiogenic factors results in neovascularization in DR **(Table 4)** and nAMD.

Anti-VEGFs: Anti-VEGFs are molecules that block the VEGF action in several ways thereby halting the disease process. Last two decades have seen a revolutionary growth in these molecules enlisted in **Table 5**.

TABLE 4: Different anti-VEGFs used in diabetic retinopathy.

FDA approval	*Anti-VEGFs*	*Blocks*	*Dosage (mg/0.05 mL)*	*Disease*
2004	Pegaptanib	VEGF-A165	0.3	nAMD
2005	Bevacizumab	All isoforms of VEGF-A	1.25	nAMD
2006	Ranibizumab	All isoforms of Pan VEGF-A	0.5	nAMD
2011	Aflibercept	VEGF-A, VEGF-B, PGF	2	nAMD
2012	Ranibizumab	All isoforms of pan VEGF-A	0.5	DME
2014	Aflibercept	VEGF-A, VEGF-B, and PGF	2	DME

TABLE 5: Next generation therapeutics.

Newer anti-VEGFs	*Dosage (mg/0.05 mL)*	*Molecule type and action*	*Trials*
Conbercept	0.5	Recombinant human fusion protein of extracellular domains of VEGFR1, VEGFR2, and IgG1Fc	PANDA-1, PANDA-2
Brolucizumab	6	Single-chain antibody fragment	HAWK and HARRIER
Abicipar pegol	–	Mono–designed ankyrin repeat protein	CEDAR and SEQUOIA, MAPLE
KSI–301	–	Anti-VEGF antibody-biopolymer conjugate	DAZZLE
Ranibizumab port delivery system	100 mg/mL	Permanent, surgically implanted intraocular device	LADDER, ARCHWAY
Faricimab	6	Bi-specific antibody targeting both VEGF-A and Ang-2	TENAYA and LUCERNE for w-AMD and YOSEMITE and RHINE for DME
EYLEA HD/8 mg aflibercept	8	4 times higher molar dose than 2 mg counterpart	PHOTON (for DME) and PULSAR (for nAMD)

Biosimilars: A biosimilar is defined as a "biologic that is highly similar to and has no clinically meaningful differences from an FDA-approved biologic". They should have similar pharmacokinetics, pharmacodynamics, safety profile, immunogenicity and clinical efficacy compared to the reference product **(Table 6)**. Biosimilars are manufactured in living cells rather than chemically synthesized. Their structure is reverse engineered and does not need to be identical to the original biologic, as long as other criteria are met.

TABLE 6: List of biosimilars.

Origin molecules	*Biosimilars*
Bevacizumab	• Mvasi • Zirabev • ONS-5010
Ranibizumab	• Ranibizumab-nuna (Sept 2021) • FYB201 (Cimerli, ranibizumab-eqrn) • Razumab • R-TPR-024 (RanizuRel) • Xlucane • LUBT010 • CKD-701 • SJP-0133 • PF582
Aflibercept	• SB 15 • MYL-1701P • FYB203 • CT-P42 • SOK583A1 • ABP-938 • ALT-L9 • OT-702/LY09004 • CHS2020

Others

- *OPT-302:* OPT-302 is a soluble form of vascular endothelial growth factor receptor 3 (VEGFR-3)or "Trap" molecule that blocks the activity of two proteins (VEGF-C and VEGF-D) that cause blood vessels to grow and leak, processes which contribute to the pathophysiology of retinal diseases. It is been developed to be used in combination with a VEGF-A inhibitor achieves more complete blockade of members of the VEGF family.

- *Gene therapy:* The biologic agent under study is a modified adenoviral vector containing a genetic package that, through the process of transfection, enables retinal pigment epithelial cells to produce a modified ranibizumab-like molecule that then dramatically reduces the number of intravitreal injections a patient requires. One injects the gene therapy underneath the retina in a surgical procedure; the other injects it into the eye just like a routine anti-VEGF treatment and is done in the ophthalmologist's office.
- *Drugs targeting immune system:* A part of the immune system called the "complement cascade" has long been identified as a culprit in AMD. Two new drugs that target the complement cascade and stop it from attacking the retina have recently been approved by the FDA—pegcetacoplan and avacincaptad pegol.
- *Stem cell*: Stem cells may be able to replace the retinal cells that are killed off by this disease. One strategy is to layer the stem cells on thin scaffolds. Another tactic is to put the cells into a fluid suspension that can be injected under the retina.

SUGGESTED READING

1. American Academy of Ophthalmology. EyeWiki. [online] Available from https://eyewiki.org/Main_Page [Last accessed March 2025].
2. McCannel CA. 2023–2024 Basic and Clinical Science Course™, Section 12: Retina and Vitreous. San Francisco: American Academy of Ophthalmology; 2023.
3. Ryan SJ, Hinton DR, Schachat AP, Wilkinson CP. Ryan Retina, 4th edition. 2009. Madrid: Marbán Books; 2009.
4. Salmon JF. Retinal vascular disease. Kanski's Clinical Ophthalmology: A Systematic Approach, 9th edition. Philadelphia: Elsevier; 2019.
5. Sihota R, Tandon R. Parsons' Diseases of the Eye, 23rd edition. New Delhi: Elsevier; 2019.
6. Venkatesh R, Joshi A, Acharya I. (2023). Optical Coherence Tomography Biomarkers in Diabetic Macular Edema. [online] Available from https://www.eophtha.com/posts/optical-coherence-tomography-biomarkers-in-diabetic-macular-edema [Last accessed March 2025].

CHAPTER

Retinal Detachment

Soumava Mandal, Rupak Roy, Sangeeta Roy, Debleena Mitra

QUESTIONS

1. **Describe in brief the mechanism of normal retinal adhesion between RPE and NSR. (10) (WBUHS MS 2019)**
2. **Peripheral Retinal Degenerations—difference between benign and not-so-benign peripheral degenerations. (10) (WBUHS MS 2019, 2020)**
3. **Clinical features and differential diagnosis of various types of retinal detachment. Management of giant retinal tear. (10) (DNB 2019)**
4. **Management of post-traumatic retinal detachment. (5) (DNB 2023)**
5. **Enumerate the indications of pars plana vitrectomy. (5) (DNB 2020)**
6. **Describe the properties of various intraocular gases used in VR surgery. What are the indications and complications? (5+3+2) (DNB 2021)**
7. **Principles, uses, and complications of silicone oil and their management. (2+2+2+4) (DNB 2020)**
8. **What are the various intravitreal implants available? Name a few intraocular steroid implants approved by the FDA and their indications, contraindications, and side effects. (10) (DNB 2020)**
9. **Pars plana vitrectomy-indications and technique. (10) (WBUHS MS 2019, 2020)**
10. **Sutureless PPV. (10) (WBUHS MS 2019, 2020)**

1. Describe in brief the mechanism of normal retinal adhesion between RPE and NSR. (10) (WBUHS MS 2019)

Physiologic Adhesion between the Retina and RPE

1. The viscous mucopolysaccharide substance between the villous processes of the RPE interdigitating with the photoreceptors.
2. There is an oncotic pressure difference between the choroid and subretinal space because proteins in the choroid cannot easily pass through the RPE and Bruch's membrane into the subretinal space.
3. The hydraulic forces because of intravitreal fluid pushing against the retina at a physiologic intraocular pressure. The hydraulic forces are produced by a more rapid passage of fluid from the subretinal space through the sclera than from the vitreous through the retina **(Fig. 1)**.

   Hydraulic forces are independent of the RPE pump and explain why the retina can remain attached after removal of the choroid and RPE in an eye wall resection, such as is sometimes used for removal of a choroidal melanoma.
4. The most important factor is - RPE pump, which actively removes fluid from the subretinal space, promoting adhesion of the RPE to the photoreceptors.

   These four types of force maintain the apposition of the retina and the RPE under normal physiologic conditions. The presence of vitreous traction, retinal breaks, and fluid currents in the eye may overcome these adhesive forces.

Clinical Application

1. Vitreoretinal traction forces play an important role in the pathogenesis of
   - Retinal tears,
   - Rhegmatogenous retinal detachments
   - Traction retinal detachments.

   Forces that act on the retina have both magnitude and direction **(Fig. 2)**. The equilibrium of the vector forces on the retinal surface is the pathogenesis of retinal detachment.

If the force of vitreous traction on the retina at the edge of a PVD is counterbalanced by retinal adherence to the eye wall, no tear will develop. If vitreous traction on the retina exceeds photoreceptor adherence to the RPE and retinal tensile strength, a retinal tear will develop to re-establish equilibrium.

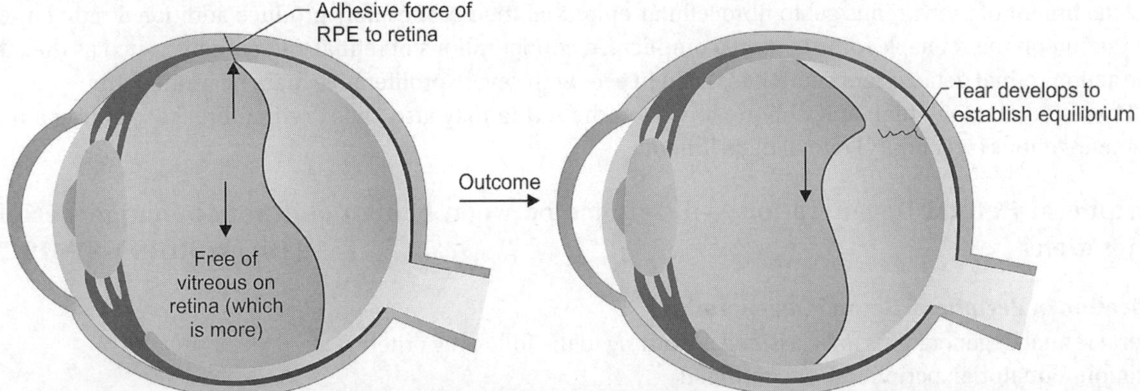

Fig. 1: Schematic diagram showing the mechanism of retinal detachment.

Most retinal breaks are caused by a combination of forces,

A. Vitreous traction
B. Fluid movement during rotary ocular movements
C. Traction associated with epiretinal membranes.

A. *Vitreous traction* may be exerted in many different directions with respect to the curved surface of the retina
   - Perpendicular
   - Tangential
   - Oblique

   The force exerted by the vitreous is primarily perpendicular or oblique to the surface of the retina. As the posterior hyaloid detaches, gravity causes the vitreous gel to pull away from the superior retina. A focal adhesion of the vitreous to the retina may cause a tear to develop if the force exerted by the vitreous on the retina exceeds the adherence of the photoreceptors to the RPE and the tensile strength of the retina.

   Most of the traction from an epiretinal membrane occurs tangentially on the surface of the retina, although there is a small inward radial component to this traction because of the concave shape of the eye wall.

   Radial/oblique traction on the retina is more likely to produce retinal breaks than is tangential traction.

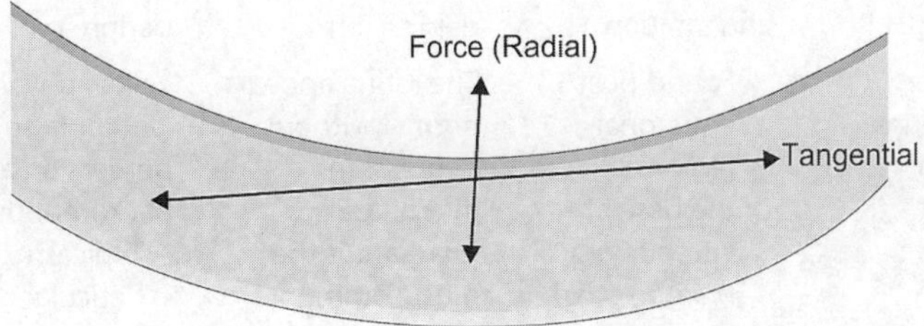

Fig. 2: Schematic diagram showing the direction of forces causing detachment.

B. Fluid movement and retinal breaks

Fluid currents: Rotational eye movements force fluid through a retinal tear, leading to retinal detachment. Fluid movement associated with rotational eye movements appears more likely to cause a retinal detachment when vitreous traction elevates the flap of a retinal tear than when a retinal hole is present without vitreous traction. The elevated retinal flap with vitreous traction may trap vitreous fluid and funnel it into the tear.

A retinal hole in the absence of vitreous traction does not catch the vitreous fluid from rotational eye movements as easily and thus is less likely to lead to retinal detachment.

C. Epiretinal membranes, cellular proliferation, and retinal breaks

1. The epiretinal membrane that initially conforms to the concave inner surface of the retina can cause a traction detachment of the retina in the configuration of a plane. The planar configuration occurs because this will minimize the tangential tension within the epiretinal membrane.
2. Attachment of the vitreous gel to fibrocellular epiretinal membranes may produce additional radial or oblique traction on the retina, leading to more complicated configurations of retinal detachments, such as the table-top traction retinal detachment sometimes seen in eyes with severe proliferative diabetic retinopathy

These radial, tangential, and oblique forces on the retina may also cause retinal breaks, creating a traction-rhegmatogenous (secondary) retinal detachment.

2. Peripheral Retinal Degenerations—difference between benign and not-so-benign peripheral degenerations. (10) (WBUHS MS 2019, 2020)

Classification of Peripheral Retinal Degenerations

Peripheral retinal degenerations are classified according to the following criteria:

- Location- equatorial, peripheral, or combined
- Pathomorphology- trophic, tractional, atrophic, or combined
- Depth of retinal changes- intraretinal, retinal, vitreoretinal, or chorioretinal
- Risk for retinal detachment
- Prognosis - progressive or stationary

The following are the commonly used classifications of peripheral retinal degenerations based upon the depth of retinal changes observed on optical coherence tomography (OCT):

- *Intraretinal degenerations:* Senile retinoschisis, white-without-pressure, white-with-pressure, dark-without-pressure, peripheral cystoid degeneration, snowflake degeneration **(Table 1)**.
- *Vitreoretinal degenerations:* Lattice degeneration, snail-track degeneration, retinal tufts, and peripheral retinal breaks **(Table 2)**.
- *Chorioretinal degenerations:* Paving stone degeneration and peripheral retinal drusen **(Table 3)**.

TABLE 1: Intraretinal degenerations.

	Senile retinoschisis	*White-without-pressure*	*White-with-pressure*	*Peripheral cystoid degeneration*	*Snowflake degeneration*
Definition	Splitting of layers of the neurosensory retina by thick fluid	Distinctive white appearance of the peripheral retina without indentation	Distinctive white appearance of the peripheral retina with scleral depression	Multiple small intraretinal microcystoid cavities; temporal periphery	Small yellowish dots in the peripheral retina appear white due to light reflection
Characteristics	Bullous elevation of peripheral retina (inferotemporal quadrant- most common)	• Found-post equatorial region at the base of vitreous/ora • Margins sharply demarcated	The retina appears normal without depression; inferonasal quadrant is the most common; myopic	Yellow tiny vesicles with blurred borders on a gray background; Types: • Typical • Reticular	May span wide band in more than one retinal quadrant, superotemporal most common may be combined with other degenerations

Contd...

Contd...

	Senile retinoschisis	*White-without-pressure*	*White-with-pressure*	*Peripheral cystoid degeneration*	*Snowflake degeneration*
Chances of RD	0.5-2.5%	Low risk	No	No	Very low
Treatment	Barrage laser • If symptomatic • Progressive detachment extending to macula	Observation	Observation	Observation	Barrage, if associated with hole/tear

TABLE 2: Vitreoretinal degenerations.

	Lattice degeneration	*Snail track degeneration*	*Retinal tufts*	*Peripheral retinal tears*
Definition	Retinal thinning with loss of neurosensory layer, vitreoretinal adhesions at margin of lesion	Groups of glistening white dots may be an early stage of lattice degeneration	Area of retinal degeneration caused by attachment to and pulling of the vitreous	Isolated tear due to defect in sensory retina from traction of vitreous after acute posterior vitreous detachment
Characteristics	Spindle-shaped areas of retinal thinning, with/without pigmentation, arborizing white lines, frost-like areas, between equator and the posterior border of the vitreous base; vitreous liquefaction over the lesion	Retinal thinning with vitreous liquefaction above the lesion, associated vitreoretinal tractions; superotemporal and superonasal quadrants	Types • Cystic, • Noncystic • Zonular traction tufts	Either retinal tear or retinal hole, retinal holes due to atrophic changes in neurosensory retina
Chances of RD	14–35%	In 54% chances of tear	If vitreous traction-tear/RD	3–18%
Treatment	Prophylactic barrage laser	Prophylactic barrage laser	Observation	Prophylactic barrage laser

TABLE 3: Chorioretinal degenerations.

	Paving Stone degeneration	*Peripheral retinal drusen*
Definition	Multiple rounded punched-out areas of choroidal and retinal atrophy	Extracellular protein and fat deposits between the RPE and Bruch's membrane due to the degeneration of RPE cells
Characteristics	Lesions are yellow-white in color and may reveal underlying choroidal vessels due to sclera being partly visible through the atrophic choroid, discrete margins that may be pigmented, may become confluent.	Small, round-shaped, clearly outlined, looks like crystals
Chances of RD	Benign lesion	Benign lesion
Treatment	Observation	Observation

Peripheral retinal degenerations that can predispose to develop RD

1. Lattice degeneration
2. Snailtrack degeneration
3. Degenerative retinoschisis
4. Cystic and zonular tractional retinal tuft
5. Retinal tear
6. Retinal hole

Lesions that do not Predispose to Retinal Detachment

1. Paving-stone degeneration,
2. Retinal pigment epithelial hyperplasia,
3. Retinal pigment epithelial hypertrophy
4. Peripheral cystoid degenerations

3. Clinical features and differential diagnosis of various types of retinal detachment. Management of giant retinal tear. (10) (DNB 2019)

Differentiating features and the differential diagnosis of the various types of retinal detachment are mentioned in **Tables 4 and 5**.

TABLE 4: Differentiating features of Various types of RD.

Clinical features	*Rhegmatogenous*	*Tractional*	*Exudative*
Symptom	Floaters and flashes, DOV sudden onset progressive	Gradual onset progressive DOV	Gradual onset progressive DOV
Laterality	U/L other eye may be involved later	U/L or B/L	Can involve both eyes simultaneously depending on the cause
PVD	Usually follows PVD	Not associated with PVD	Not associated with PVD
Break	Always present	Absent	Absent
Configuration of retina	Convex, bullous, corrugated folds	Concave	Covex with smooth surface, no folds
Mobility of retina	Mobile in fresh case, restricted in old case	Restricted	Mobile
Extent	Extends to ora	Seldom extends, localized in areas of FVP	Extends to ora
PVR	Present in due course of time	Absent	Absent
SRF shift	No shift	No shift	Shift with posture
RPE pump	Intact	Not affected	Occurs to RPE pump failure
Visual field defect	Develops fast	Develops slowly, may remain static for months	Develops fast
Treatment	Surgical	Surgical	No surgery, treat the underlying cause

TABLE 5: Differential diagnosis of various types of RD.

	Rhegmatogenous	*Tractional*	*Exudative*
Differential diagnosis	• Retinoschisis • TRD • Ex RD • CD	• TPH • VMTS • Combined RD	Etiologies • Uveitic: (a) inflammatory- VH, SO, post scleritis (b) Infectious – TB, syphilis • Non uveitic – (a) choroidal – ch melanoma, hemangioma, mets (b) Retinal – coat's, FEVR, vasoproliferative tumors (c) misc – CSCR, uveal effusion syndrome

Management of GRT

Definition

A giant retinal tear (GRT) is a full-thickness retinal break, which extends circumferentially for more than or equal to 3 clock hours (>/=90 degrees) in the presence of a posteriorly detached vitreous.

Giant Retinal Tears Need Special Consideration because (2)

1. They rapidly lead to extensive retinal detachment
2. Posterior flap has a tendency to roll over, fold, or invert
3. They have an increased risk of proliferative vitreoretinopathy
4. The chances of developing hypotony is high due to bare choroid, and so is the chance of CD

5. They require meticulous surgery to prevent complications
6. They have several ocular and systemic associations
7. Fellow eye involvement occurs frequently
8. Redetachments occur frequently in these cases

Clinical Features

Symptoms – presents with dimness of vision

Signs - Tobacco dusting in vitreous cavity,

Vitreous hemorrhage may result if a tear involves the retinal vessels.

Configuration: (1) GRT without detachment; (2) GRT with detachment with (a) flat posterior flap, (b) rolled posterior flap, and (c) inverted posterior flap; and (3) GRT with detachment with associated posterior extensions (radial rips) at or within the tear margin.

The chances of developing PVR are higher as a large area of RPE being exposed and increased liberation of RPE cells into the vitreous.

The fundus of the fellow eye should be examined to look for any predisposing lesion, including WWOP areas.

Investigations

USG - classical "double linear echo" sign is seen in GRT with two high-amplitude linear echoes, one extending from the optic disc and the other usually lying almost parallel to it (inverted posterior flap).

Treatment – is surgical.

The surgical principle- complete vitrectomy, unfolding of the retinal flap, sealing the tear with laser or cryo, and providing long-term intraocular tamponade.

Steps – pars plana vitrectomy with meticulous base shaving and proliferative tissue or epiretimal membrane removal are to be done. PFCL injection helps in the unrolling and repositioning of the inverted GRT. Endolaser is to be done along the break. Cryo can also be done at the edges of the break if the break is very anterior. PFCL – air exchange followed by gas or silicon oil exchange can be performed, or direct PFCL- gas/silicon oil exchange can be done. In this step, we need to be careful of retinal slippage.

Role of encircling element - the use of an encircling scleral band in GRT is controversial. Some studies have reported higher redetachment rates with encirclage due to redundant retinal folds, fish-mouthing, and increased posterior retinal slippage. While others report a lack of encircling elements to be associated with a higher rate of redetachment.

Role of lensectomy: With advancement of better visualization till ora with wide angle viewing system indications for lensectomy are cataract, subluxated lens or presence of anterior PVR.

Complication

a. Posterior slippage of GRT
b. Retention of PFCL bubble
c. PVR leads to formation of a new tear, extension of the existing tear, and redetachment.

Prophylaxis of fellow eye - Fellow eyes of nontraumatic GRT cases often show vitreoretinal pathology with risks as high as GRT occurring in these fellow eyes. However, there exists no evidence to support or refute the use of 360 prophylactic treatment in the fellow eyes.

Freeman noted several high-risk characteristics in fellow eyes of GRTs -high myopia (>10 diopters), increasing WWOP areas, and increasing condensation of the vitreous base. The objective in the management of such high-risk fellow eyes is to relieve the vitreous traction. A prophylactic scleral buckle in a phakic eye with an attached retina may be required in high-risk individuals. 360° retinopexy, either in the form of cryopexy or laser photocoagulation, may also be considered.

4. Management of post-traumatic retinal detachment. (5) (DNB 2023)

Ocular trauma is a major cause of monocular blindness and visual impairment throughout the world. Traumatic retinal detachment (TrRD) accounts for 10–40% of all detachments. In the absence of an established definition, the diagnosis of traumatic retinal detachment depends on the elicitation of a relevant history. Hoogewoud and coworkers proposed to define traumatic retinal detachments (TrRD) as rhegmatogenous retinal detachments (RRDs) caused by open or closed globe injuries due to direct or indirect mechanisms resulting in retinal breaks. RRD is the most common type of TrRD.

Management

Management consists of proper diagnosis, investigations, and treatment.

Diagnosis

1. Clinical

   A detailed history and comprehensive ophthalmic examination at the presentation play a key role in the diagnosis of TrRD. A comprehensive ophthalmic examination includes an external examination of the injury and its surroundings for obvious foreign bodies and lacerations. This should be followed by assessments of visual acuity, pupillary function, external slit lamp examination, and fundus examinations. All contact procedures (applanation tonometry, gonioscopy, and scleral depression) are not advised in case of suspected globe rupture until the entry site has been repaired. In clear media, Indirect ophthalmoscopy aids in the diagnosis, but as scleral indentation is not advisable, peripheral retinal examination is difficult.
2. Investigation

   A. *Ultrasonography:* In cases of poor visibility, ultrasonography (US) plays a vital role. It should be done with a closed lid and soft hands to minimize trauma to the already compromised globe. The US can help to distinguish RD from PVD. US can also be utilized when an IOFB (such as glass or plastic) cannot be seen directly or with a CT scan.
      - Ultrasound biomicroscopy (UBM) provides detailed imaging of the anterior segment up to a depth of 5 mm. It excels in detecting small foreign bodies of diverse compositions, even in opaque media, often overlooked by computed tomography (CT) or B-scan.

   B. *CT scan:* Though it does not have any critical role in detecting RD, but it has a paramount role in detecting metallic and paramagnetic IOFBs. 1–1.5 mm thin cuts in sagittal and coronal scans through the orbit should be done.

Treatment

1. *Laser retinopexy:* Laser burns form scar tissue around the tears, causing adhesion of the retina to underlying tissue. It is indicated in closed-globe injury and tears with or without minimal SRF. Non-contact Laser Indirect Ophthalmoscopy is the preferred choice for this.
2. *Scleral buckling:* Scleral buckling alone or combined with vitrectomy plays a crucial role in ocular trauma. In closed-globe injury, is typically indicated in cases of retinal dialysis. It is more preferred over vitrectomy in young patients with attached hyaloid due to the low risk of cataract.
3. *Vitrectomy:* It is the preferred choice of surgery in TrRD. It helps in PVR management (5FU and LMWH have also been tried to reduce the incidence of PVR), good anatomical and visual outcome. Silicon oil is the ideal tamponading agent after a vitrectomy.

5. Enumerate the indications of pars plana vitrectomy. (5) (DNB 2020)

1. Rhegmatogenous retinal detachment
2. Macular diseases: Full-thickness macular hole, Epiretinal membrane, Vitreomacular traction
3. Tractional myopic maculopathy
4. Vitreous hemorrhage
5. Tractional retinal detachment
6. Retained intraocular foreign body
7. Endophthalmitis – could be postoperative or post-traumatic or endogenous
8. Retained lens fragment after cataract surgery
9. Posteriorly dislocated IOL
10. Diagnostic vitrectomy is done in case of vitritis and infection
11. Rare indications such as malignant glaucoma, optic disc pit with maculopathy, Coat's disease, and intraocular malignancies for retinal and choroidal biopsies.

6. Describe the properties of various intraocular gases used in VR surgery. What are the indications and complications? (5+3+2) (DNB 2021)

Three different intraocular gases are commonly used in vitreoretinal surgery: air, sulfur hexafluoride (SF6), and perfluoropropane (C3F8). In the vitreous cavity, these gases are colorless, odorless, and inert.

Properties

Buoyancy and surface tension are the characteristics of intraocular gas that help in retinal reattachment after surgery. The high surface tension of gas enables the formation of an effective seal around a retinal break, thus allowing the retinal pigment epithelium (RPE) to absorb any remaining subretinal fluid to facilitate reattachment of the retina. Because the specific gravity of any gas is lower than that of water, the intraocular gas bubble has buoyancy that keeps the retina against the RPE, and this effect is greatest at the apex of the bubble.

An intraocular gas bubble has the following dynamics: expansion, equilibration, and dissolution **(Figs. 3A to C)**. The initial expansion is a result of the absorption into the bubble of nitrogen, oxygen, and carbon dioxide from the surrounding tissue fluid. Therefore, it is very important to turn off a nitrogen infusion during general anesthesia, if used, while performing a vitrectomy with gas tamponade. The most rapid rate of expansion occurs within the first 6 to 8 hours after gas injection. During the equilibrium phase, the partial pressures in the 2 compartments equilibrate as diffusion of nitrogen into the bubble is balanced by the diffusion of gas into the surrounding fluid. Finally, during dissolution, there is a net exit of gases as they are ultimately absorbed into the bloodstream.

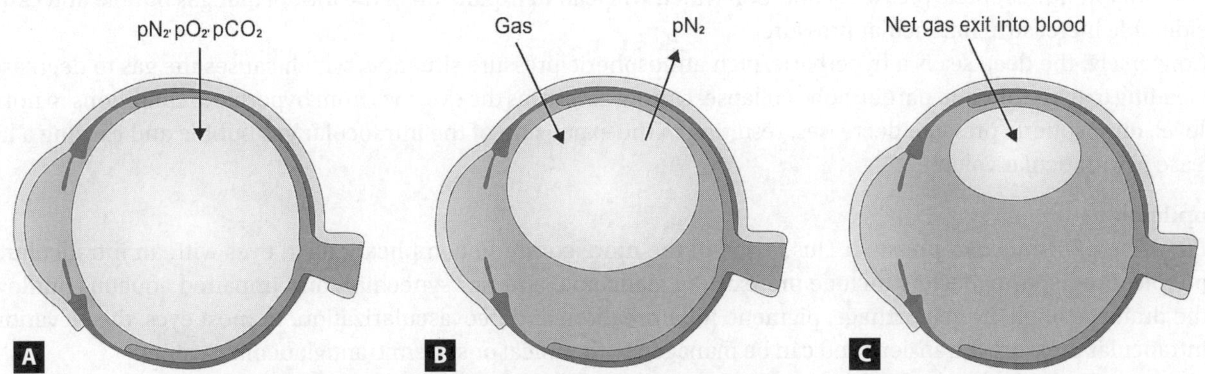

Figs. 3A to C: Different stages of gas tamponade in vitreoretinal surgeries. (A) Expansion of gas; (B) Equilibrium phase; and (C) Dissolution phase.

Choosing appropriate air/gas depends on the indications summarized in **Table 6**.

TABLE 6: Air/Gas properties.

	Molecular weight	*Physical properties*	*Duration*	*Maximal expansion (hours)*	*Largest size*	*Expansion (Pure)*	*Indications*
AIR	29	Floats	5–7 days	N/A	Immediate	No expansion	Tamponade of sclerostomies in routine cases (Epiretinal membrane surgeries)
SF6	146	• Floats • 20 %-non expansile • 26%-If some expansion is desired	1–2 weeks	24–48 hours	36 hours	2 X	• Non PVR, Primary RRD with superior tears • Routine macular hole surgery
C3F8	188	• Floats • 10–14%-non expansile • 16–18%-If some expansion is desired	6–8 weeks	72–96 hours	3 days	4X	• Inferior breaks RRD • Mild to moderate PVR retinal detachment • Giant retinal tear • Some chronic macular hole surgery

Indications of intraocular gases in vitreoretinal surgery

- *Pneumatic retinopexy in retinal detachment:* Pneumatic retinopexy is primarily indicated for uncomplicated retinal detachment with retinal breaks involving the superior 8 clock hours of the fundus. The desired volume of gas (usually 0.3 to 0.5 mL) is injected rapidly into the vitreous cavity in order to minimize the formation of small 'fish-egg' bubbles.
- *Macular hole surgery:* The presence of intraocular gas provides isolation of the macular hole from the vitreous cavity by surface tension at the gas-liquid interface. It may also mechanically tamponade the hole and provide a template over which a nascent bridging membrane forms.
- *Pneumatic displacement of submacular hemorrhage*: Submacular hemorrhage can result in sudden, dramatic visual loss and has many causes, such as choroidal neovascularization, polypoidal choroidal vasculopathy, trauma, and retinal artery macroaneurysm. The technique of pneumatic displacement involves the injection of an expansile pure C3F8 gas (about 0.3 mL) via the pars plana at 3.5 mm from the limbus with a 30-gauge needle, followed by strict prone positioning for 5–7 days.
- *Unrolling giant retinal tear:* A giant retinal tear may be unrolled using an intraocular gas bubble by placing the patient in a prone position and injecting gas via the infusion cannula while removing fluid from the anterior vitreous cavity at the same time (upside down fluid-gas exchange). Use of this technique is mostly historical now, since the availability of perfluorocarbon liquids.

Contraindications: Post gas injection, the patient is advised against high altitude/flight travel or deep-sea diving. High altitude is a low atmospheric pressure condition which will lead to expansion of the intraocular gas bubble and cause a considerable increase in intraocular pressure.

Conversely, the deep sea is a hyperbaric/high atmospheric pressure situation, which causes the gas to decrease in size, leading to hypotony and partial globe collapse. During ascent, as the eye goes from hyperbaric conditions to normal sea level, atmospheric pressure decreases, resulting in the expansion of the intraocular gas bubble and causing a large increase in intraocular volume.

Complications

- *Elevation of intraocular pressure:* This is one of the more common complications in eyes with an intraocular gas bubble. Predisposing factors include pre-existing glaucoma, anterior synechiae, and impaired aqueous outflow at the drainage angle by hemorrhage, pigment, inflammation, and neovascularization. In most eyes, the elevation in intraocular pressure is transient and can be managed with topical or systemic antiglaucoma agents.
- *Cataract:* Prolonged contact of intraocular gas with the posterior lens surface can lead to gas-induced cataract, presenting typically as "lens feathering."
- *Migration of intraocular gas bubble:* Migration of intraocular gas bubble into the subretinal space can rarely occur as a result of pneumatic retinopexy, and thus re-detachment can occur. In phakic or pseudophakic patients, an intraocular gas bubble may also migrate into the anterior chamber via weakened zonules or a larger posterior capsulotomy.
- *Inadequate gas bubble size:* An Inadequate gas bubble may ensue if the surgery is completed with a smaller-than-desired intraocular gas or if the gas escapes through a sclerotomy during the perioperative period, leading to hypotony. Inadequate gas bubble size may also be caused by premature absorption of the gas due to errors in reconstituting the gas mixture.

7. Principles, uses, and complications of silicone oil and their management. (2+2+2+4) (DNB 2020)

Principles

Silicone oil is used to tamponade the retina for anatomical successes in cases with proliferative vitreoretinopathy. It is made of repeating units of siloxane, and it can be combined with many inorganic and organic components to change its properties.

Physical Properties of Silicone Oil

1. *Specific gravity:* Usually, it is lighter than water so that it floats. In a few cases with inferior old retinal detachment or in patients who cannot maintain prone positioning, heavy silicone oil is used, which is heavier than water.

2. *Buoyancy:* Since the buoyancy of silicone oil is less, we have to fill up the vitreous cavity nearly 100% to get a good tamponade effect on the retina.
3. Surface tension and interfacial tension.
4. *Viscosity:* The lower the viscosity, the higher are the chances of emulsification.

Indications of Silicone Oil Use

1. Retinal detachment with severe proliferative vitreoretinopathy
2. Giant retinal tears
3. Severe proliferative diabetic retinopathy
4. Viral retinitis
5. Complicated pediatric retinal detachments
6. Trauma
7. Endophthalmitis
8. Macular hole surgeries are when the patient has to travel by air after the surgery or if the patient is unable to maintain a face-down position or to ensure prolonged tamponade after a failed surgery.
9. RIOFB

Complications of Silicone Oil

1. *Anterior chamber silicone oil:*
   a. This can happen during surgery in aphakia, loose zonular support, blockage of inferior PI, or rupture of the posterior capsule.
   b. AC completely filled with silicone oil is very difficult to diagnose. It can be diagnosed by the shimmering reflex on the iris and posterior bulging of the iris. Usually, the cornea is clear as there is no fluid in the AC, and corneal edema usually ensues after the removal of the oil.
   c. The silicone oil can be displaced with the help of air or viscoelastic agents, and inferior PI needs to be done to prevent pupillary block.
   d. If left untreated, then it might cause visual disturbances, corneal endothelial loss, and trabecular meshwork damage.
   e. Late migration of silicone oil in AC is caused by recurrent detachment and hypotony.
2. *Glaucoma:*
   a. *Pupillary block glaucoma:* It happens in aphakic patients when the peripheral iridectomy becomes nonfunctional or due to blockage by inflammatory products. It can be treated by reopening the inferior PI with a laser or surgically.
   b. *Overfill of silicone oil:* It has to be treated surgically to remove the excess oil. To avoid overfill pressure at the end of surgery, it should be normal.
   c. *Secondary open angle glaucoma:* It is caused by mechanical blockage of the trabecular meshwork by silicone oil or trabeculitis by emulsified silicone oil. It can be treated initially with topical medications. For intractable cases, glaucoma surgery with drainage devices is to be done.
   d. Migration of silicone oil in AC
   e. *Secondary angle closure glaucoma:* This is a diagnosis of exclusion after ensuring that the peripheral iridectomy is patent and there is no silicone oil in AC and no oil is trapped between the iris or crystalline lens and iris.
3. *Chronic hypotony:* It is defined as IOP</= 5 mm of Hg according to silicone oil study. It happens in the late postoperative period. It may be caused by a combination of increased uveal-scleral outflow and reduced production caused by ciliary body membrane formation. The treatment for his condition is not very rewarding. Reoperation with ciliary body membrane dissection and removal with reinjection of silicone oil can be done.
4. *Cataract formation:* Cataract formation in the postoperative period is inevitable in cases of silicone oil injection. Early silicone oil-induced cataract starts as lens vacuole formation leading to posterior subcapsular cataract. Rapid progression to hypermaturity can occur. Lens power calculation is a challenge in silicone oil-filled eyes.

5. *Recurrent retinal detachment:* This can happen due to a missed break or proliferative vitreoretinopathy, even under the presence of silicone oil.
6. *Emulsification:* It is the breaking up of large silicone oil bubbles into smaller droplets. It can lead to glaucoma, inflammation, and PVR formation. If there is emulsification, then the silicone oil has to be removed with multiple air-fluid exchanges.
7. *Keratopathy:* Prolonged use of silicone oil is associated with keratopathy. Band-shaped keratopathy is more common in early stages, and bullous keratopathy in later stages. Silicone oil migration in the anterior chamber has to be prevented as it causes endothelial damage.
8. Unusual vision loss following silicone oil tamponade.

8. What are the various intravitreal implants available? Name a few intraocular steroid implants approved by the FDA and their indications, contraindications, and side effects. (10) (DNB 2020)

Various intravitreal implants (Table 7)

Intravitreal implants are a specially designed drug delivery system to release drugs in a controlled manner over a longer duration, helping in its direct delivery into the vitreous, thus overcoming systemic pathways and obtaining a high drug concentration in the vitreous chamber.

TABLE 7: Various intravitreal implants.

Types	*Characteristics*	*Composition*	*Example*
(1) Non-biodegradable(NBI)	Requires surgical removal or replacement. Larger in size; hence, a larger incision is required for implantation	Ethylene vinyl acetate (EVA), polyvinyl alcohol (PVA), or polysulfone capillary fiber (PCF)	Vitrasert and Retisert.
(2) Biodegradable (BI)	Degrades and disintegrates overtime, thus eliminating all components from the body	Polylactic acid (PLA), polyglycolic acid (PGA), PLGA, or polycaprolactones	DEX Implant (Ozurdex)

Some intravitreal implants areas follows (steroids are enlisted in the next part):

	Composition	*Releaserate*	*Indication*	*C/I*	*S/E*
Vitrasert (NBI)	Active agent- 4.5 mg ganciclovir and inactive agent- 0.25% magnesium stearate	1μg/hour for a period of 5–8 months	AIDS associated CMV retinitis	Ocular surface infection, in combination with intravenous cidofovir, presence of retinal tear or detachment, and allergic reactions to acyclovir or ganciclovir	ERM
Ranibizumab Port delivery system(NBI)	20 μL ranibizumab	2.3μg/day for 6 months	nAMD-previously respon ded to at least two anti-VEGF injections	Ocularor periocular infections, active IOI, hypersensitive Reactions to ranibizumab, Recent history of stroke or myocardial infarction, and pregnancy, cautiously used in Patients with end-stage kidney disease or those on dialysis	Endophthal mitis, RD, implant dislocation, septum dislodgement, VH, conjunctival erosion, retraction, and bleb formation
Verisome (BI)	Verisome with ranibizumab	1.1 μg/mL and lasts up to 1 year	nAMD		

Some investigational implants are -

a. Cyclosporine-chronicuveitis.
b. Indomethacine-7 mg over 3 weeks.

c. Dendrimers
d. Hydrogels
e. Particulated drug delivery systems–Liposomes-neovascularization due to AMD, pathologic myopia, or presumed ocular histoplasmosis.
f. Liposomal amphotericin or AmBisome-leishmaniasis and various fungal infections in immunocompromised individuals and patients with renal impairment. It is also used off label for fungal endophthalmitis. Liposomal formulation has few toxic effects.
g. Microparticles-3-6 months
h. Nanoparticles.

TABLE 8: Intraocular steroid implants.

	Name		***Indication***
Fluocinolone acetonide (NBI)	Retisert (2005)	0.6 µg of drug per day Into the vitreous cavity. It lasts up to 3 years	Chronic noninfectious posterior uveitis, DME and ME In CRVO, persistent or Recurrent DME
	Iluvien	0.2 µg (low dose insert) or 0.5 µg/day (high dose insert) and lasts up to 3 years	DME Underevaluation for Dry AMD, RVO, and noninfectious uveitis
	Yutiq (2018)	0.25 µg/day for three years	Chronic NIPU
Triamcinolone acetonide (NBI)	I-vation	0.925 µg of triamcinolone Acetonide (TA), 2 years	DME
Dexamathasone (BI)	Ozurdex (2009)	0.7 mg dexamethasone, Which is released sustain ablyin the Vitreous for 6 months	Main-RVO with ME, DME, and NIPU. Off-label use in Irvine–Gass syndrome, nAMD, vasoproliferative retinal tumors, retinal telangiectasia, Coats' disease, radiation maculopathy, retinitis pigmentosa, macular Edema secondary to scleral Buckle and parsplana vitrectomy. As adjunct to ranibizumab
	Surodex	0.6 mg, Sustained release for 7–10 days following insertion in AC	Postopinflammation
Verisome(BI)		1.1 µg/mL and lasts up to 1 year	Verisome with TA: CME due to RVO

Steroid implants are contraindicated: In patients with hypersensitivity or active ocular or periocular infections (viral, mycobacterial, fungal) and glaucoma patients with a cup disk ratio > 0.8. Additionally, dexamethasone is contraindicated into torn posterior capsules, in a phakic eyes, or those with anterior chamber or scleral fixated intraocular lenses due to the risk of migration of the implant into the anterior chamber **(Table 8)**.

General side effects of steroids are: Increase in IOP causing glaucoma, cataract formation, migration into anterior chamber, corneal endothelial compromise. Apart from this, Retisert may cause ERM formation, and its components may dissociate, causing visual problems.

Biodegradable implants may cause uncontrolled drug release, leading to drug toxicity, cloudy vision, and their movement in front of the retina or anterior chamber.

9. Pars plana vitrectomy-indications and technique. (10) (WBUHS MS 2019, 2020)

Pars plana vitrectomy was introduced in 1970 by Robert Machemer, who first introduced pars plana vitrectomy (PPV) using a 17-gauge (17-G) cutter. PPV allows access to the posterior segment to treat vitreoretinal diseases. With recent advances, it is doing a great job in retaining, restoring of sight and prevention of blindness for patients of posterior segment diseases.

Indications

- *Nonclearing vitreous hemorrhage:* May be seen in proliferative diabetic retinopathy, trauma, posterior vitreous detachment, retinal detachment, intraocular tumors, or retinal vascular diseases.
- Rhegmatogenous retinal detachment
- Tractional retinal detachment
- Combined retinal detachment (Tractional +Rhegmatogenous Retinal Detachment)
- *Epiretinal membranes:* These can be idiopathic in origin or occur secondarily to a variety of conditions such as retinal vascular disease, uveitis, laser therapy, or retinal breaks
- Macular holes
- Vitreomacular traction (VMT)—can occur spontaneously, in sickle cell disease or diabetic retinopathy.
- Submacular hemorrhage secondary to choroidal neovascularization
- Intraocular foreign body
- Endophthalmitis -PPV can be both diagnostic and therapeutic.
- Retrieval of retained lens fragments after phacoemulsification
- Dropped intraocular lens (IOL)
- *Intraocular tumors*: Endoresection and tumor biopsies.
- Placement of intraocular implants: Ganciclovir implants have been used in cases of cytomegalovirus infection in HIV patients. Fluocinolone implants are used for idiopathic posterior uveitis or some refractory uveitis following the exclusion of infections.

Technique

The basic components of a vitrectomy setup include the following elements:

- Vitrectomy machine
- Surgical microscope and wide-angle viewing system (e.g., Zeiss RESIGHT, Oculus BIOM, AVI)
- Trocar-cannula system: for placing ports available in 20, 23, 25, and 27-gauge
- Infusion cannula
- Endoillumination light source
- Vitrectomy cutter
- Other instruments used depending on pathology are scissors, forceps, diathermy, endo-laser, extrusion cannula, or Fragmatome.

Steps

1. It can be done under general anesthesia or local anesthesia. Clean and drape the involved eye in an aseptic manner.
2. Trocar and cannulas are introduced through conjunctiva and sclera at the 2 o'clock, 10 o'clock, and inferotemporal regions, around 3-4 mm from the corneal limbus.
   - Inferotemporal port-for infusion cannula
   - 2 o'clock port- for endoillumination pipe
   - 10 o'clock port for vitrectomy cutter
3. Core vitrectomy is done
4. Induce posterior vitreous detachment (PVD) from the posterior pole by using high suction with the vitrector over the optic nerve. Triamcinolone acetonide can help with visualization if this is difficult.
5. Remove peripheral vitreous- Scleral indentation is a technique used to help with visualization of the peripheral retina. The entire retina should be visualized to find any breaks, holes, tears, or detachments.
6. After the initial few steps, depending on the pathology, the procedure can be:
   For retinal detachment:
   - Drain subretinal fluid to flatten the retina through the existing break/new break, using a soft-tipped cannula during fluid-air exchange.
   - Endolaser to seal all breaks
   - Intraocular tamponade-silicone oil/SF_6/C_3F_8

For membrane peeling:

- *For better visualization*: A higher magnification and resolution lens is used, which may be the 68-degree AVI lens or the green macular lens with the Zeiss RESIGHT. Also, a vital dye can be instilled to improve tissue visualization.
- The initial flap can be created with ILM forceps, an MVR blade, a Tano scraper, a Finesse Flex loop, or a pick. Then, the membrane peel can be completed.

Lens removal:

- For pars plana lensectomy, soft lenses can be removed using the vitrectomy cutter, but denser lenses may require the use of the Fragmatome. Use of the conventional fragmatome requires enlarging sclerotomies, often using an MVR blade.

Complications

- Cataract
- Glaucoma
- Endophthalmitis
- Retinal tear
- Retinal detachment
- Hypotony
- Suprachoroidal effusion
- Suprachoroidal hemorrhage
- Vitreous hemorrhage
- Cystoid macular edema
- Optic neuropathy
- Phototoxicity

10. Sutureless PPV. (10) (WBUHS MS 2019, 2020)

The original PPV used a single port, 17-gauge vitrectome that Machemer called the vitreous infusion suction vitrectome that required a 2.3 mm scleral incision.

In 1974, O'Malley and Heintz introduced a smaller 20-gauge, three port procedure that became the standard until the early 2000s, when 23-gauge and 25-gauge PPV systems were introduced and widely adopted. Most recently, there has been a shift toward smaller gauge vitrectomy with the introduction of the 27-gauge PPV by Oshima et al. in 2010.

Advantages of Small-Gauge Sutureless Pars Plana Vitrectomy

1. *Less traumatic wound construction and closure:* Initially, 25G vitrectomy was attempted with straight incisions as better self-sealing was expected with the smaller gauge. However, studies showed better wound closure and reduced hypotony with beveled incisions for 25 G.

   With smaller 27-gauge cannulas, the surgeon can perform a perpendicular trans-scleral, one-step entry into the vitreous cavity with minimal need for sutures. As a result, there is reduced tissue trauma, a faster start to the procedure, and lower hypotony rates. For 23- and 25-gauge PPV, postoperative hypotony rates have been reported to be 0–10.5% and 0–25.6%, respectively.
2. *Less perioperative and postoperative patient discomfort:* With smaller gauge PPV, anesthesia has transitioned from general endotracheal intubation to local retrobulbar or peribulbar anesthesia, thus decreasing the risks and the costs of general anesthesia. Decreased post-op inflammation and pain have been reported comparing 25-gauge systems to 20- and 23-gauge systems. Studies comparing 27-gauge PPV to 25-gauge PPV have also shown no instances of significant inflammation postoperatively.
3. *Comparable risk of endophthalmitis to large-gauge vitrectomy:* Studies indicate that small gauge sutureless PPV produces similar postoperative endophthalmitis rates compared to larger gauges that were sutured. The risk of endophthalmitis is directly related to communication between the sterile cavity and the environment. Therefore, there may be a concern that a sutureless wound may increase the risk of endophthalmitis. However, this has not been found to be the case, with several studies showing postoperative endophthalmitis rates of zero and none above 0.3%.

Disadvantages of Small-Gauge Sutureless Pars Plana Vitrectomy

1. *Infusion and aspiration flow rate limitation on effective vitreous removal:* Smaller gauze vitrectomy systems have a smaller radius of the lumen of the cannulas (r), infusion, and vitrectome, which increases the resistance (R) in them with a subsequent decrease in flow rates (F) in them, as understood by the equations below. This decreases effective vitreous removal.
   - $R = 8\,\eta L/(\pi r^4)$

   where, R = resistance, η = viscosity of fluid, L = length of tube, r = radius of tube.
   - $F = (\Delta P)/R$

   where, F = flow rate, P = pressure (infusion/aspiration), R = resistance.
2. *Longer operating time:* Average operating times for 27-gauge PPV are similar to or approaching operating times for 23- and 25-gauge. Studies have not shown a consensus but lean slightly toward a longer, but not significant, operating time for 27 gauge.
3. *Flexible instruments limiting small-gauge ppv in complex cases:* Smaller gauge instruments have decreased tensile strength of the shaft, which could lead to damage to the vitrectome, poor tissue handling during membrane dissection, and iatrogenic foreign body introduction. Within the cannula, forceful manipulation of small-gauge instruments can lead to bending and damage to the operating mechanism while performing peripheral vitrectomy. If the shaft of a forceps is bent during operation, then the surgeon may experience decreased control of the forceps while manipulating delicate tissue, such as during a membrane peel. With improvements in instrument designs, increased cut rates, and duty cycles of small gauze vitrectomy machines, these limitations have been addressed to a great extent.

SUGGESTED READING

1. Chang S, Lincoff H, Zimmermann NJ, Fuchs W. Giant retinal tears. Surgical techniques and results using perfluorocarbon liquids. Arch Ophthalmol. 1989;107(5):761-6.
2. Cheung R, Ly A, Katalinic P, Coroneo MT, Chang A, Kalloniatis M, et al. Visualisation of peripheral retinal degenerations and anomalies with ocular imaging. Semin Ophthalmol. 2022;37(5):554-82.
3. Engstrom RE, Glasgow BJ, Foos RY, Straatsma BR. Degenerative Diseases of the Peripheral Retina. Duane's Ophthalmology. Philadelphia: Lippincott Williams and Wilkins; 2006.
4. Freeman HM. Fellow eyes of giant retinal breaks. Trans Am Ophthalmol Soc. 1978;76:343-82.
5. Freeman HM. Giant retinal tears: 207 cases from the perfluorom study (Abstract). Am Acad Ophthalmol Vitreoretinal up data. 1997;168-71.
6. Kertes Pl, Wafapoor H, Peyman GA, Calixto N Jr, Thompson H. The management of giant retinal tears using perfluoroperhydrophenanthrene. A multicenter case series. Vitreon Collaborative Study Group. Ophthalmol. 1997;104(7): 1159-65.
7. Khurana AK, Sood S, Kumar A. Disorders of retina and vitreous. New Delhi: CBS Publishers & Distributors Pvt Ltd; 2014.
8. Kumar A, Agarwal D. Retina: Medical and surgical management. New Delhi: Jaypee Brothers Medical Publishers Pvt Ltd; 2022.
9. Mandura RA. Acquired Senile Retinoschisis of the Peripheral Retina Imaged by Spectral Domain Optical Coherent Tomography. Cureus. 2021;13(4):e14540.
10. McCannel CA. 2019-2020 Basic and Clinical Course: Retina and Vitreous. San Francisco, California: American Academy of Ophthalmology; 2019-2020. pp. 357-66
11. Nishitsuka K, Nishi K, Namba H, Kaneko Y, Yamashita H. Peripheral Cystoid Degeneration Finding Using Intraoperative Optical Coherence Tomography in Rhegmatogenous Retinal Detachment. Clin Ophthalmol. 2021;15:1183-7.
12. Schepens LL, Dobbie JG, McMeel JW. Retinal detachments with giant retinal breaks: pre- liminary report. Trans Am Acad Ophthalmol Otolarynogol 1962;66:471-68.
13. Shukla M, Ahuja OP. White with pressure (WWP) and white without pressure (WWOP) lesions. Indian J Ophthalmol. 1982;30(3):129-32.

CHAPTER

Vitreous Disorders

Soumava Mandal, Rupak Roy, Ekta Bharti, Ayantika Das

QUESTIONS

1. **Describe vitreous humor. Discuss its clinical importance. Draw the Amsler Dubois Chart with appropriate color coding for abnormal retinal findings. (10) (DNB 2023)**
2. **Surgical anatomy of vitreous and its role in retinal detachment. (10) (DNB 2021)**
3. **Advances in management of vitreous floaters. (5) (DNB 2023)**
4. **Discuss investigation and management of recurrent vitreous hemorrhage in a 30-year-old male. (3+4) (DNB 2023)**
5. **Write a short note on Asteroid Hyalosis. (5) (TNMGRMU MS 2023)**
6. **Write a short note on Vitreous degeneration. (5) (TNMGRMU MS 2022)**

1. Describe vitreous humor. Discuss its clinical importance. Draw the Amsler Dubois Chart with appropriate color coding for abnormal retinal findings. (10) (DNB 2023)

Vitreous Humor

The vitreous is a transparent extracellular gel consisting of collagen, soluble proteins, hyaluronic acid, and water. Its total volume is approximately 4.0 mL. The few cells normally present in the gel are located predominantly in the cortex and include hyalocytes, astrocytes, and glial cells. The vitreous provides structural support to the globe while allowing a clear and optically uniform path to the retina. Once liquefied or surgically removed, it does not reform. Vitreous opacities can be caused by a variety of pathological processes primarily involving other ocular sites; apart from vitreous hemorrhage, the conditions discussed below are those in which the vitreous gel is the primary site of pathology.

Development: The vitreous fluid is not present at birth (the eye being filled with only the gel-like vitreous body), but found after age 4-5, and increases in size thereafter. Produced by cells in the non-pigmented portion of the ciliary body, the vitreous humor is derived from embryonic mesenchymal cells, which degenerate after birth.

Biochemical properties*:* Its composition is similar to that of the cornea, but the vitreous contains very few cells. It is composed mostly of phagocytes, which remove unwanted cellular debris in the visual field, and hyalocytes, which turn over the hyaluronan. The vitreous humor contains no blood vessels, and 98–99% of its volume is water. In addition to water, the vitreous consists of salts, sugars, vitrosin (a type of collagen), a network of collagen type II fibrils with glycosaminoglycan, hyaluronan, opticin, and a wide array of proteins. Despite having little solid matter, the fluid is substantial enough to fill the eye and give it its spherical shape. This contrasts with the aqueous humor, which is more fluid, and the lens, on the other hand, which is elastic in nature and is tightly packed with cells. The vitreous humor has a viscosity two to four times that of water, giving it a gelatinous consistency. It has a refractive index of 1.336.

Surface features*:* The vitreous has many anatomical landmarks

Patella fossa: Shallow saucer-like concavity anteriorly, in which the lens rests, separated by Berger's space

Ligamentum hyaloideocapsular (Wieger's ligament): Circular thickening of vitreous 8–9 mm in diameter, delineates the patella fossa

Anterior hyaloid: Vitreous surface anterior to ora serrata. Continuous with and invests in the zonular fibers and extends forward between the ciliary processes

Vitreous base: Denser cortical area of vitreous. Firmly attached to the posterior 2 mm of the pars plana and the anterior 2–4 mm of the retina

Posterior hyaloid surface: Closely applied to the retinal internal limiting membrane. Firm attachment sites: Along blood vessels and at sites of retinal degeneration

Space of Martegiani: A funnel-shaped space overlying the optic disc with condensed edge

Cloquet's canal: A 1–2 mm wide canal within the vitreous, from the space of Martegiani to the space of Berger, along an S-shaped course mainly below the horizontal. It is labelled "hyaloid canal" in the above diagram.

Mittendorf's dot: A small circular opacity on the posterior lens capsule, which represents the site of attachment of the hyaloid artery before it subsequently regressed.

Bergmeister's papilla: A tuft of fibrous tissue at the optic disc, which represents a remnant of the sheath associated with the hyaloid artery before it subsequently regressed.

Clinical Significance

1. *Injury:* If the vitreous pulls away from the retina, it is known as a vitreous detachment. As the human body ages, the vitreous often liquefies and may collapse. It can also occur after injuries to the eye or inflammation in the eye (uveitis). The gel may liquefy, a condition known as synaeresis, allowing cells and other organic clusters to float freely within the vitreous humor. These allow floaters, which are perceived in the visual field as spots or fibrous strands. Floaters are generally harmless, but the sudden onset of recurring floaters may signify a posterior vitreous detachment or other diseases of the eye.
2. *Ageing effects:* Age-related vitreous degeneration such as vitreous liquefaction and posterior vitreous detachment (Once liquid vitreous enters the sub-hyaloid space between the vitreous cortex and the retina, it may strip the vitreous cortex off the retina with each eye movement).
3. *Different pathology:*
   a. Developmental anomalies: There can be various abnormalities in fetal vitreous vessel regression, such as persistent fetal vasculature syndrome
   b. Diabetic vitreopathy: It plays an important role in the progression of diabetic retinopathy.
   c. Myopic Vtreopathy
4. *Postmortem and forensic:* After death, the vitreous resists putrefaction longer than other body fluids. Within the hours, days, and weeks after death, the vitreous potassium concentration rises at such a predictable speed that vitreous potassium levels are frequently used to estimate the time since death (post-mortem interval) of a corpse.

2. Surgical anatomy of vitreous and its role in retinal detachment. (10) (DNB 2021)

Vitreous Body

- Patellar fossa - depression just posterior to the lens **(Fig. 1)**
- Hyaloideocapsular ligament of Weigert - annular region 1–2 mm in width and 8–9 mm in diameter where vitreous is attached to the posterior lens.
- Erggelet's or Berger's space - at the center of the hyaloideocapsular ligament.
- Cloquet's canal - Arising from Berger's space and coursing posteriorly through the central vitreous, the former site of the hyaloid artery in the primary vitreous.
- Area Martegiani - Posteriorly, Cloquet's canal opens into a funnel-shaped region anterior to the optic disc.

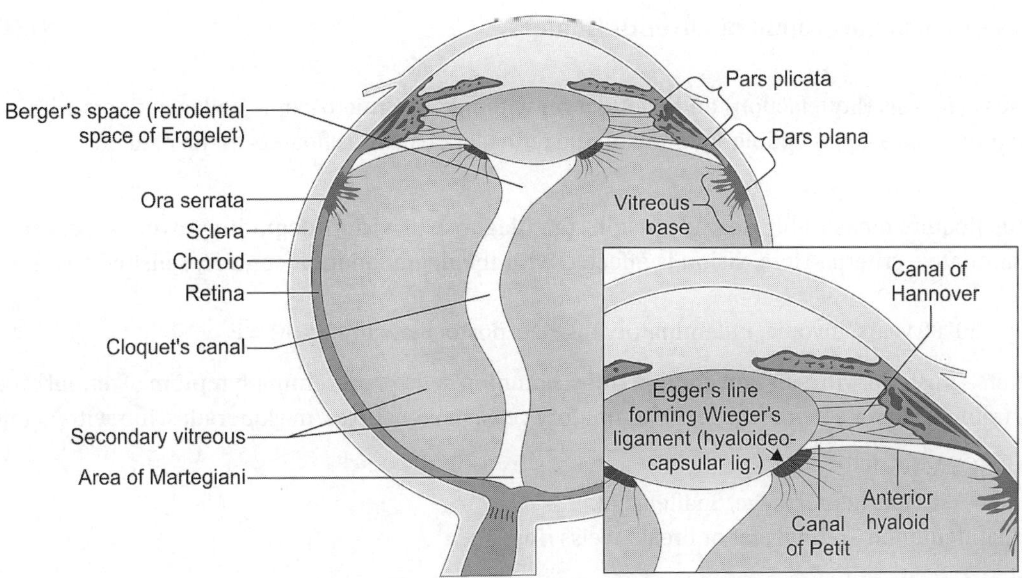

Fig. 1: Schematic diagram of vitreous anatomy.

- Vitreous fibers- bundles of fine, parallel fibers (collagen fibrils) coursing in an anteroposterior direction attach into the vitreous base where they splay out anterior and posterior to the oraserrata. Peripheral fibers are circumferential with the vitreous cortex, while central fibers undulate in a configuration parallel with Cloquet's canal. Posteriorly, these fibers attach in to the posterior vitreous cortex, but not the retina.

Vitreous Base

A three-dimensional zone that extends 1.5–2 mm anterior to the ora serrata, 1–3 mm posterior to the ora serrata, and several millimeters into the vitreous body itself. It is the strongest attachment of vitreous.

Vitreous Cortex

The peripheral shell of the vitreous body that courses forward and inward from the anterior vitreous base to form the anterior vitreous cortex, and posteriorly from the posterior border of the vitreous base to form the posterior vitreous cortex.

Vitreoretinal Interface

There is a basal lamina on the inner surface of the retina to which the cortical and basal vitreous are attached. The basal lamina posterior to the ora serrata is known as the internal limiting lamina (ILL) of the retina.

The vitreous is known to be most firmly attached at the vitreous base, at the disk and macula, and over retinal blood vessels.

Role of the vitreous in rhegmatogenous retinal detachment (RRD): Retinal detachment represents the presence of liquid between the retinal pigment epithelium layer and the neurosensory retina. In rhegmatogenous detachment, the fluid reaches the subretinal space through a retinal hole or tear. The origin of the subretinal fluid is the liquefied fraction of the vitreous body, so it depends on synchysis, while the retinal tear is most often associated with the phenomenon of PVD. An abnormally tight focal adhesion associated with consecutive vitreous syneresis traction causes these retinal tears. They are most often found along the posterior margin of the vitreous and in regions of degenerative retinal thinning called lattice degeneration.

To cause a rhegmatogenous retinal detachment, three factors must be present:

1. Liquefied vitreous gel
2. Abnormal traction forces that can cause a retinal tear
3. A retinal tear that allows liquefied vitreous to pass into the subretinal space.

3. Advances in the management of vitreous floaters. (5) (DNB 2023)

Floaters?

Due to vitreous syneresis (liquefaction) and contraction with age, are microscopic collagen fibers within the vitreous that tend to clump and cast perceptible shadows on the retina, appearing as floaters to the patient.

VDM?

When vitreous floaters measurably degrade vision, the diagnosis is vision-degrading myodesopsia based on some objective, quantitative criteria. Here, vision is affected with the degradation of contrast sensitivity while visual acuity remains intact.

Epidemiology – 50–80 years, myopia, inflammatory disease, postocular surgery, M = F.

Cause of floaters – Posterior vitreous detachment (most common cause), presenting symptom of retinal breaks or retinal detachment, trauma, vitreous hemorrhage, inflammatory cells, malignancies/masquerades, intravitreal injections.

Examination - BCVA, CS, IOP.
SL examination – Vitreous hemorrhage, Shaffer sign.
IO with scleral indentation - retinal tear or break, Weiss ring.

Management:

- Investigation – B-scan
- Treatment –
  a. Observation -as spontaneous resolution – 3 months – 1 year.
  b. Retinal break/tear – laser photocoagulation
  c. Persistent floater with Vision degrading myodesopsia (VDM) –
    - Nd: Yag laser vitreolysis – best option for Weiss ring but less amenable for a larger numbers of floaters (>3) or more peripheral lesions. Power required 3–10 mJ.
    - PPV ± cryoablation or laser photocoagulation retinopexy ± tamponading agent
    - Limited vitrectomy – preserving 3–4 mm of retrolental gel vitreous and avoid surgical PVD induction reducing the incidence of cataract, retinal tear or RD, especially in patients unhappy with MFIOL.
    - Combined cataract extraction + anterior vitrectomy
    - Nanoparticles to enhance laser ablation of vitreous opacities - capacity to absorb YLV to about 1000 times- still in research stage
    - Pharmacologic vitreolysis – Enzymatic/nonenzymatic

Liquefactants (agents that liquefy the gel vitreous)	tPA, plasmin, microplasmin, nattokinase, vitreosolve	Chondroitinase, hyaluronidase
Interfactants (agents that alter the vitreoretinal interface)-		Dispase, chondroitinase

  d. Organic causes – VH, uveitis, masquerades should be treated according to their respective line of management protocols.

4. Discuss investigation and management of recurrent vitreous hemorrhage in a 30-year-old male. (3+4) (DNB 2023)

Recurrent vitreous hemorrhage is the repeated presence of blood in the vitreous cavity, which is the space between the posterior lens capsule, the internal limiting membrane (ILM), and the non-pigmented epithelium of the ciliary body. The frequency of the etiologies of vitreous hemorrhage is variable according to the characteristics of the study population. In our case, in a 30-year-old male:

The most common causes include-

- Proliferative diabetic retinopathy (PDR),
- Posterior vitreous detachment (PVD) with or without retinal tear

- Ocular trauma
- Retinal vasculitis and Eales disease

Less common causes include-

- Polypoidal choroidal vasculopathy
- Retinal vein occlusion
- Proliferative sickle cell retinopathy
- Retinal arterial macro aneurysm
- Subarachnoid hemorrhage (Terson syndrome)
- Valsalva retinopathy
- Blood dyscrasias/coagulation disorders
- Retinal vessel avulsion

Investigation

History

A history of diabetes, hypertension, sickle cell disease, trauma, previous retinal conditions, or ocular surgery may give us some leading evidences.

Ocular Examination

NVI/NVA and IOP should be noted. A dilated fundus exam is needed to detect the distribution of hemorrhage and the possible etiology. Retinal tear or detachment should be ruled out using scleral depression. Examination of the fellow eye will give us important clues.

Diagnostic Modalities

- *USG-B scan*: If the fundal view is completely obscured. It is used to detect retinal detachment, posterior vitreous detachment, retinal tears, tractional membranes, intraocular tumors, and intraocular foreign bodies.
- *Fundus fluorescein angiography*- mild to moderate vitreous hemorrhage to help identify neovascularization and associated pathology.
- *Optical coherence tomography*—to detect associated macular edema or bleeding in the macular region (subhyaloid/sub-ILM/subretinal)
- *Orbital CT scan*- in open globe injury to assess orbital bony structures and integrity of eyeball.
- MRI- in suspected iron foreign body

Laboratory Tests

Complete hemogram, Hb electrophoresis, blood sugar, HbA1c, blood pressure, lipid profile, Mantoux test - are used according to clinical suspicion.

Treatment

Medical Management

1. General measures:
   - To avoid strenuous activity
   - Bilateral patching and bedrest to limit eye movement
   - Head end elevation to allow settling of the blood, permitting more complete fundoscopic examination -
   - To control blood pressure
2. Treatment of etiology:
   - If there is adequate visibility of the fundus and the etiology can be determined, treatment of the underlying cause should be attempted first.
   - Panretinal photocoagulation- neovascularization from proliferative retinopathy (diabetes, sickle cell, vasculitis, vessel occlusions) is treated, often guided by FFA. This causes the regression of NVEs and prevents further bleeding
   - Laser retinopexy—should be attempted if the VH is mild or the tear is superior. Red laser and Cryotherapy are alternate options in poor visibility.

- Laser Augmentation- if the eye was previously treated with laser, but NVE has recurred, dense laser augmentation is done in visible bare retina.

Surgical Management

- In an open globe injury, the eyeball should be repaired at the earliest time, and surgery of the posterior segment is followed after a few days.
- A short period of cautious observation for clearing of VH is reasonable. The duration of observation depends on the surgeon, severity of the disease, systemic status, and the condition of the other eye of the patient.
  - Anti-VEGF- Intravitreal anti-VEGF acts as a temporary measure to regress the neovascularization. It is supplemented by laser or is used pre-operatively to decrease intra-op bleeding. Intracameral anti-VEGF is seldom used in NVG before surgical intervention.
  - Pars plana vitrectomy is indicated in-
    1. Nonresolving VH
    2. Associated retinal detachment/ break seen on B-scan
    3. Intraocular foreign body
    4. Neovascular glaucoma
  - After thorough vitrectomy, endo laser is applied according to the etiology. Endodiathermy is also used to prevent rebleeding. Often, it is supplemented by intravitreal steroids or anti-VEGF. Silicone oil or gas tamponade is needed for retinal detachments. Peeling of the Internal limiting membrane may be needed in Valsalva retinopathy/ Terson syndrome.
- *Prevention of rebleed after vitrectomy*: Peripheral retinal ablation with cryotherapy or laser has been proven to be effective in proliferative retinal vascular diseases. Control of systemic co-morbidities is also a pre-requisite. Other factors that decrease the risk are- complete separation of vitreous from retina, pre-op laser, use of diathermy, and absence of tractional detachment.

5. Write a short note on Asteroid Hyalosis. (5) (TNMGRMU MS 2023)

Asteroid hyalosis is a condition in which there are minute white opacities in the vitreous composed of calcium-containing phospholipids. It is usually seen above 50 years and has a strong association with diabetes and hypertension.

Etiology- The asteroid bodies are round structures that stain positively for neutral fats, phospholipids, and calcium.

Risk factors- usually seen unilaterally in those above 50 years. It was positively correlated with age and inversely correlated with posterior vitreous detachment.

Pathology- the asteroid bodies exhibit structural and elementary similarity to hydroxyapatite and proteoglycans. These are composed of carbohydrates in the inner matrix and chondroitin-6-sulfate in the periphery.

Three studies conclude that asteroid hyalosis is mostly associated with aging.

1. Beaver Dam study
2. Australian Blue Mountain Eye Study
3. UCLA

Diagnosis: Funduscopic examination is the mainstay. Other investigations which can be done include- fluorescein angiography, USG b scan, OCT and slit lamp biomicroscopy.

Treatment: As the condition is rarely associated with vision loss, initial management is observation. If the patient complains of floaters with vision loss, a standard 3 port vitrectomy is needed to remove the vitreous opacities.

6. Write a short note of Vitreous degeneration. (5) (TNMGRMU MS 2022)

Vitreous is a transparent gel composed of water, collagen, and hyaluronic acid and occupies 80% of the volume of the eye. The vitreous body is divided into 2 areas- the central/ core area and the peripheral/cortical area. With age, the vitreous gel undergoes liquefaction, which is called synchysis, followed by collapse of the vitreous called syneresis.

Causes of vitreous degeneration:
- Advancing age
- Eye trauma/inflammation
- Myopia
- Previous history of any eye surgery.

Types of vitreous degeneration:
- Benign vitreous floaters
- Symptomatic vitreous floaters
- Degenerative vitreous syndrome
- Posterior vitreous detachment

Benign vitreous floaters:
- It is the starting phase associated with aging.
- The vitreous becomes stringy and shrinks.
- Appears as spots, strands, cobwebs or dark shadows
- Does not affect vision
- Particles and fibers moving in vitreous emit its shadow on the retinal wall

Symptomatic vitreous floaters or vitreous opacities:
- Floaters present with symptoms
- Multiple dark colored floaters present in vitreous gel
- Flashes of lights present
- Further progress to retinal detachment

Degenerative vitreous syndrome/DVS:
- Mostly seen in elders of 50 years or above
- A persistent form of the disorder that severely affects the vision
- Patient complaint about routine work like reading, driving, and other skills required to see

Treatment:
- For floaters only, no treatment is needed.
- Sudden increase in floaters: need full ophthalmoscopically examination
- Floaters with flashes of light- fundoscopy should be done, followed by appropriate treatment.
- If there is any detachment, vitreoretinal surgery is needed.

SUGGESTED READING

1. Bergstrom R, Czyz CN. Vitreous Floaters. In: StatPearls [Internet]. Treasure Island (FL): StatPearls Publishing; 2024.
2. In: Standring S, Gray NR, Hnery (Eds). Gray's anatomy: the anatomical basis of clinical practice, 40th edition. London: Churchill Livingstone; 2008.
3. McCannel CA. American Academy of Ophthalmology: 2019-2020 BCSC Section 12: Retina and Vitreous. 307-8, 331-40.
4. Sebag J. Vitreous Anatomy, Aging, and Anomalous Posterior Vitreous Detachment. In: Dartt DA (Ed). Encyclopedia of the Eye. Oxford: Academic Press; 2010. pp. 307-15.
5. Sultan ZN, Agoro Giannis EI, Iannetta D, Steel D, Sandinha T. Rhegmatogenous retinal detachment: a review of current practice in diagnosis and management. BMJ Open Ophthalmology. 2020;5(1):e000474.
6. www.sas.upenn.edu. (2007). Anatomy of the Eye. [Online] Available from https://www.sas.upenn.edu/~scottds/vision/visanat.htm [Last accessed March, 2025].

CHAPTER

Diseases of Macula

Rupak Roy, Kshitiz Kumar, Soumava Mandal, Sangeeta Roy, Ekta Bharti, Bratatee Roy

QUESTIONS

1. **Investigations for evaluation of Macular Diseases.** **(10) (WBUHS MS 2022)**
2. **Write briefly on Macular function tests (MFT).** **(10) (MS, DNB)**
3. **What is ICGA angiography? Differentiate between FFA and ICG angiography. What are the indications.** **(10) (WBUHS MS 2022)**
4. **Discuss ARMD.** **(10) (WBUHS MS 2021)**
5. **Discuss results of AREDS 2 trial on vitamins for AMD. How does it differ from AREDS 1 trial?** **(DNB 2020)**
6. **Diabetic macular edema—OCT findings and its management.** **(10) (WBUHS MS 2019, 2020)**
7. **Explain management of subretinal fluid and its complications.** **(10) (DNB 2019)**
8. **Pathology, evaluation, and management of full thickness macular hole.** **(10) (DNB 2019/DNB 2022)**
9. **Mention clinical features of retinitis pigmentosa.** **(5) (DNB 2023)**
10. **Define Pachychoroid spectrum and its clinical features.** **(10) (DNB 2021)**
11. **Optic disc pit maculopathy- clinical features, evaluation and management.** **(3 + 2 + 5) (DNB 2023)**
12. **Describe causes, diagnosis, management, and prognostic features of submacular hemorrhage.** **(WBUHS MS 2023)**

1. Investigations for evaluation of Macular Diseases. (10) (WBUHS MS 2022)

The various investigations that can be used to evaluate macular diseases are:

- *Fundus fluorescein angiography:* Fluorescence is the property of certain molecules to emit light of a longer wavelength when stimulated by an incident light of shorter wavelength (excitation is at 480 nm, stimulated molecules emit yellow green light of about 530 nm **(Fig. 1)**.
  - Sodium Fluorescein is a water-soluble dye (>70% bound to proteins) which is excreted over 24–36 hours. Fluorescein angiography involves surveillance of dye passage through retinal and choroidal circulation and its imaging
  - Contraindications—people with allergy to fluorescein, renal failure patients, pregnancy, mod-severe asthma, significant cardiac disease.
  - Technique **(Flowchart 1)**
  - *Phases of FFA:*
    - *Choroidal phase (Prearterial):* 9–15 seconds after dye injection, patchy lobular filling of choroid
    - *Arterial phase:* 1 second after choroidal phase, Retinal Arteriolar filling, and continued choroidal filling.
    - *Arteriovenous phase:* Complete artery and capillary filling with Laminar filling in veins
    - *Venous phase:* Laminar flow progress to complete filling, Late arterial reduced fluorescence
    - *Late recirculation phase:* Continued Recirculation, dilution and elimination of dye, gets weaker and vanishes from circulation after 10 minutes.

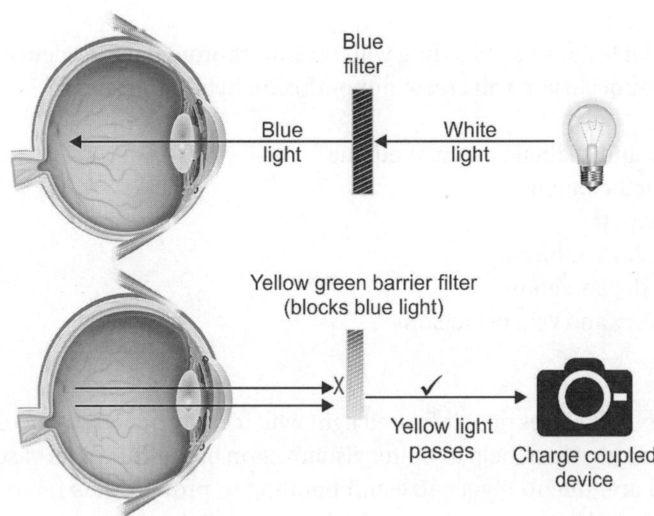

Fig. 1: Schematic diagram showing the principle of fundus fluorescein angiography (FFA). *(For Color version, See Color Plate 8)*

Flowchart 1: Techniques.

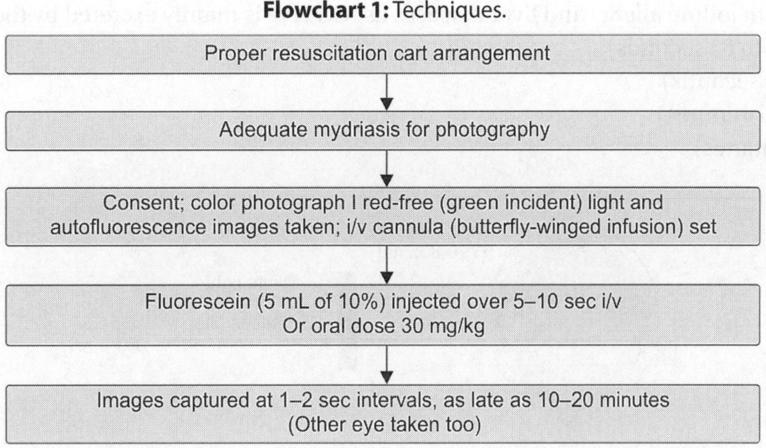

- *Dark appearance of fovea is due to:*
  - Absence of blood vessels in the foveal avascular zone
  - Blockage of background choroidal fluorescence due to xanthophyll pigment
  - Blockage of background choroidal fluorescence due to RPE cells at fovea
- *Causes of hyperfluorescence:*
  - *Autofluorescence:* Lipofuscin in RPE weakly absorbs blue light and emits weak yellow-green light (lesions—optic disc drusen and astrocytic hamartoma)
  - *Pseudofluorescence:* Nonfluorescent light visible prior to injection of sodium fluorescein passes filters due to overlapping wavelengths.
  - *Leakage:* With time intensity, size and fluorescence increases (DR, RVO, CME) occurs due to breakdown of inner retinal barrier
  - *Pooling:* Intensity increases with time but the size of defect remains constant, e.g., pigment epithelial detachment (sub-RPE) and CSR (sub-retinal).
  - *Staining:* Late phenomenon along with prolonged retention of dye, e.g., drusen, scar, fibrous tissue
  - *Window defect:* Atrophy/absence of RPE allows unmasking of background choroidal fluorescence, very early seen, increases in intensity and fades away without changing shape or size.

- *Causes of hypofluorescence:*
  - *Obstruction:* Preretinal lesions like bleeding will mask all choroidal fluorescence
  - *Filling defect:* Vascular occlusion will create nonperfusion hypofluorescence
- *Indications:*
  - Diabetic retinopathy and Diabetic macular edema
  - Pigment Epithelial Detachment
  - Central serous Retinopathy
  - Choroidal neovascular membrane
  - Age related macular degeneration
  - Branched Retinal artery and vein occlusions
  - Retinal vasculitis
  - Coat's disease

- *Indo-Cyanine Green Angiography:* Uses near infra-red light which easily penetrates ocular pigments like xanthophyll and melanin as well as exudates which help in better visualization of the choroidal vasculature.
  - 98% bound to albumin and due to bigger size and bonding to protein, gets retained in choroidal vessels for a longer time and also infrared light causes less scattering so imaging is better.
  - Uses high sensitivity cameras as the fluorescence is 1/25th of that of FFA.
  - Technique is similar; however, greater emphasis is given on the later phases of the ICGA images. (at 45 minutes)
  - C/I in patients with iodine allergy and liver diseases as ICG Dye is mainly excreted by the liver.
  - *Phases:* Early (up to 60 seconds)
    - Early mid (1–3 seconds)
    - Late mid (3–15 minutes)
    - Late (15–45 minutes)
  - *Filters* **(Fig. 2)**:

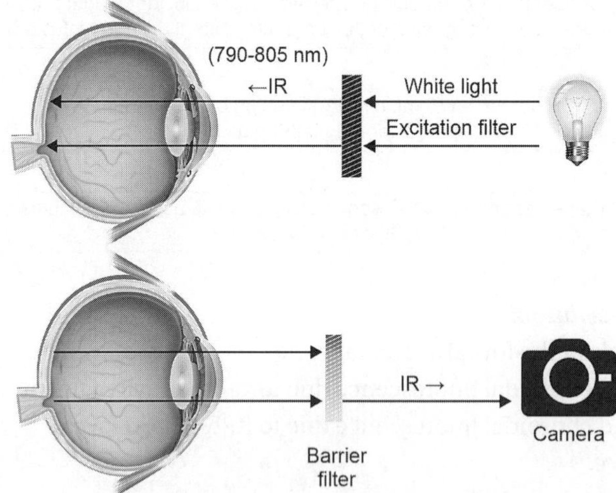

Fig. 2: Filters. *(For Color version, See Color Plate 8)*

- *Diagnosis*:
  - Hypercyanosence
    - Window defect
    - Leakage from retinal vessels
    - Abnormal vessels
  - Hypocyanosence:
    - Blocked (e.g., PED) (pigment, hemorrhage, exudation, and scar)
    - Filling defect
- *Indications*:
  - PCV

- ARMD
- Retinal Angiomatous Proliferation
- Chronic CSCR
- Posterior Uveitis
- Choroidal Tumors
- Breaks in Bruch's Membrane
- If Fluorescein Angiography is C/I

- *Optical Coherence Tomography:* Noninvasive and noncontact imaging system that uses a super-luminescent diode light source to create high resolution real time, cross-sectional tomographic images of retina. Recent third generation of OCT can image retinal Ganglion cell layer with an improved resolution of 2–3 μ.

  *Principle of OCT (**Flowchart 2**):*

Flowchart 2: Principle of optical coherence tomography (OCT).

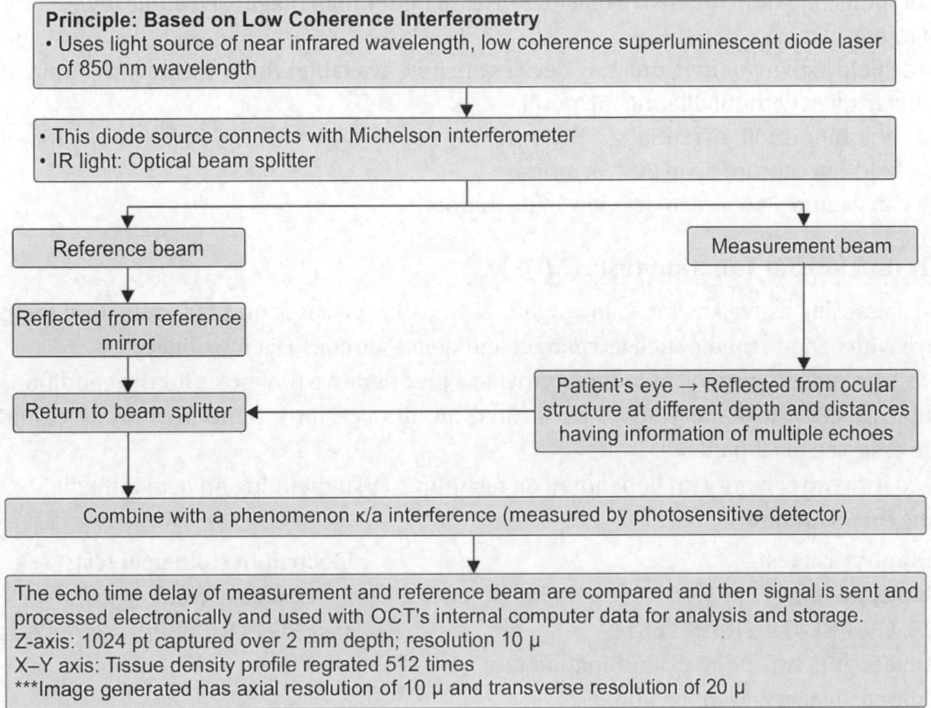

- *Applications of OCT:*
  - Follow-up and understanding pathology
  - Access response to medication, surgery, and laser treatment
  - Documentation and explaining prognosis of disease
  - Evaluation of OCT in glaucoma for evaluation of ONH, RNFL for progression of disease.
  - OCT for macular diseases like macular hole, ERM, Diabetic Retinopathy, CME, CSCR, ARMD, retinal vein occlusion
  - Limitations of OCT
  - Asteroid hyalosis
  - Cloudy media
  - High astigmatism
  - Dense cataract

- *Optical Coherence Tomography Angiography:*
  - New noninvasive technique that allows blood flow in retina and choroid to be visualized without the need for an injection of contrast media.

- *But,* leaking, staining, pooling (the three classic abnormalities) cannot be noted in this technique.
- Images are based on detection of RBC movement within microvasculature of the back of the eye using a series of OCT-B scans.
- *Applications:*
  - CNVM (visualize blood flow and abnormal vasculature)
  - Dry ARMD (to diagnose non-exudative CNVM)
  - Visualization of Abnormal choroidal vessels particularly after treatment
  - Diabetic Retinopathy (IRMA vs new vessel diagnosis, detect microvascular changes)
  - Macular telangiectasias, PCV, CSCR

- *Fundus Autofluorescence:*
  - Imaging using an enhanced fundus camera or scanning laser ophthalmoscopy permits visualization of accumulated lipofuscin in retinal pigment epithelium.
  - Useful to demonstrate more extensive macular disease better than diagnosed clinically.
- *Wide Field Imaging:*
  - Several wide field high resolution imaging devices are now available which are able to capture up to 80% of retina in single image often without dilating the pupil.
  - Wide field can capture 100° of retina.
  - Ultra-wide field can capture up to 200° of retina.
  - Pan retina can capture 360° ora to ora view of the retina.

2. Write briefly on Macular function tests (MFT). (10) MS, DNB

- Required for diagnosing as well as for following up of macular diseases and for evaluating the potential macular function in eye with opaque media such as cataract and dense vitreous Haemorrhage.
- Indicated in as a prelude to surgery, in order to provide a preoperative prognosis for the condition.
- Not all macular function tests need to be performed on all occasions. Some like VA assessment and papillary evaluation are assessed in all patients.
- **MFT**: Classified into two category (a) depending on technique (b) depending on ocular media.
  a. **Depending on technique:**
     1. **Psychophysical test**
        - Subjective test
        - VA, CV, PHOTOSTRESS TEST
        - Amsler grid, two-point discrimination test
        - Entopic imagery, Maddox Rod test
     2. **Electrophysiological test**
        - Objective test
        - ERG,EOG, VEP

  b. **Depending on ocular media**:
     1. **With clear media**
        - VA, CV, Photo stress test, Amsler grid
        - Two-point discrimination test,
        - Micro perimetry, FFA, OCT
     2. **With opaque media**
        - Laser interferometry
        - PAM, ERG, EOG, VEP
        - Entopic phenomenon

Psychological Tests: It is subjective test

A *Visual acuity test (VA)*
- *Distant VA:* By Snellen VA chart, LOGMAR CHARTS (Baily lovie charts), the ETDRS chart (Calibrated for 4 m), COMPUTER CHART
  - Distant VA is directly related to minimum angle of separations between 2 objects that allow them to be perceived as distinct.
- *Near VA:* It can be sensitive indicator of the presence of macular disease.
  - Done by near vision charts (including LOGMAR and ETDRS vision), test type book.
  - In patient with macular disease VA is frequently worse when the patient looks through a pin hole.

B. *Color vision testing:* Color vision depends on three populations of retinal cones, each with a specific peak sensitivity: blue (titan), green (deuteron), and red (protan). Normal color perception requires all these primary colors to match those within the spectrum.

- Acquired macular disease tends to produce blue-yellow defects, and optic nerve lesions
- Produce red-green defects.
- CV done by the ISHIHARA test, The CITY UNIVERSITY test, The HARDY-RAND-RITTLER test, The FRANSWORTH-MUNSEKK 100 hue test.

C. *Photostress rest:* It can differentiate visual loss caused by macular disease from that caused by an optic nerve lesion.

- Similar to dark adaptation test.
- BCVA distant is determined and ask to fixate on light of a Pen torch or an IDO held about 3 cm away for about 10 seconds, then photo stress recovery time (PSRT) is measured by time taken to read any three letters of pre-test acuity line. the test is performed on the other, presumably normal eye and results are compared.
- In a patient with macular lesion, the PSRT will be longer (50 seconds or more)as compared with the normal eye. whereas in a patient with an optic nerve lesion there will be no difference.

D. *Amsler grid:* Developed by Marc Amsler—

- Is a grid of horizontal and vertical lines used to monitor a person's central visual field.
- There are 7 charts, each consisting of a 10 cm outer square.
- *Techniques:* Pupils should not be dilated, and in order to avoid a photo stress effect, eye should not yet have examined on the slit lamp.
- The chart should be well illuminated and held at a comfortable reading distance, optimally around 33 cm.
- The patient may be provided with a recording sheet and pen and asked to draw any anomalies **(Fig. 3)**.
  - *Chart 1:* Standard grid.
    - White lines on a black background and a central white dot on which the patient fixate.
    - 400 small squares, each square measures 5 mm.
    - Held 30 cm from the patient, each squares subtends 1° on retina.
    - When patient cannot seen the central white spot this indicates a scotoma.
  - *Chart 2:* Has diagonal lines which help maintain central fixation. This helps then point out the limits of scotoma.
  - *Chart 3:* Has red lines on black background.
    - Helpful in detecting color scotoma.
  - *Chart 4:* This chart comprises random dots only.
    - Used to differentiate scotoma from metamorphopsia.
  - *Chart 5:* Has horizontal lines.
    - Helps to detect metamorphopsia along specific meridian.
  - *Chart 6:* Similar to chart 5, but has white background and central lines are oriented closer for detailed evaluation.
  - *Chart 7:* Has fine central grid.
    - Each square subtends on angle of half a degree when the chart is held at 30 cm from patient.

E. *Contrast sensitivity:* Measure of minimum amount of contrast needed to distinguish a test object.

- Indirectly assesses the quality of vision,
- Can detect early/subtle visual loss when VA is normal,
- Spatial frequency is the number of dark light cycles per visual angle,
- In macular disease there is a marked impairment for intermediate and higher spatial frequencies.

F. *Two-point discrimination test:* The ability to distinguish two illuminated point of light 2 mm diameter in size and 2 inches apart placed 2 feet away from patient's eye suggests good retinal function.

- Excellent method for testing macular functions in children and uncooperative adults in OPD clinic.

G. *Entopic Imaging:* Visual perceptions that are produced or influenced by native structures of one's own eye.

- If a focal source of light is pressed firmly against the exterior of eye through closed lids, the arborizing pattern of retinal blood vessels can be briefly made visible.

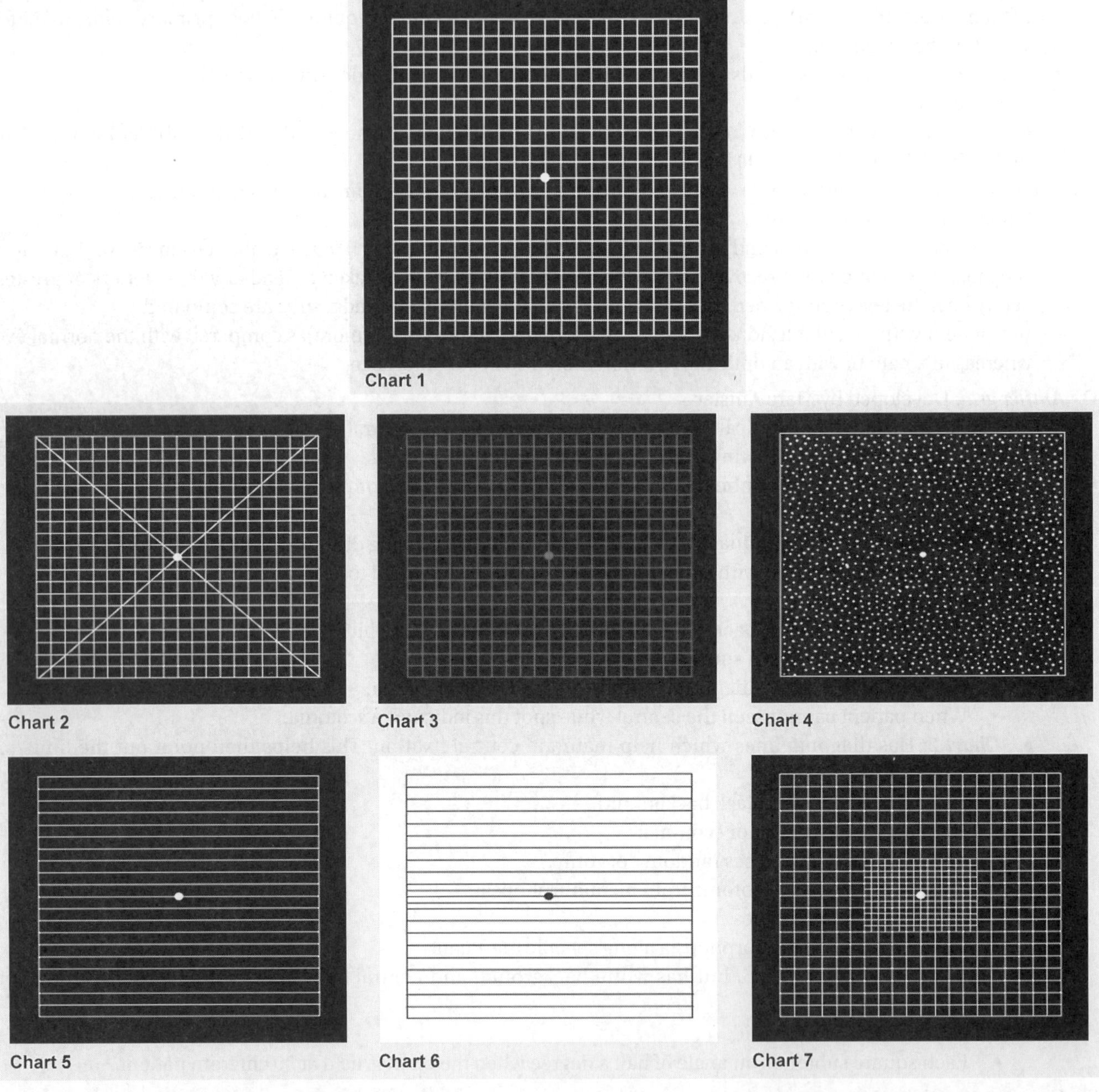

Fig. 3: Amsler grid. *(For Color version, See Color Plate 9)*

- Normal corpuscles is more than 15 corpuscles in one field,
- Abnormal finding are failure to see any corpuscles or partial less of corpuscles in one part of the field, visibility of less number of corpuscles and slow corpuscular movement.

H. *Maddox rod test:* When a patient sees a point source of light through the Maddox rod, a line perpendicular to axis of the parallel cylinders is perceived. Any break in this line in the centre is indicative of a central/macular lesion.
- Very sensitive test that can be performed in outpatient clinic without requirement of any specific equipment.
- Maddox rod is used to assess the macular functions; the light source should be placed between 33 cm and 40 cm in front of eye and each should be tested uniocularly.

I. *Laser interferometry:* Resolving power of macula is tested by using 2 coherent beams of light, which create a 3 D fringe pattern of retina,
   - Pupils are widely dilated and light beam is directed in to centre of pupil,
   - Pupil is scanned until the fringe pattern is seen and patient indicates the orientation of bands of light,
   - Laser interferometry can thus be used in eyes with immature cataracts.

J. *Micro perimetry:* Also known as fundus perimetry,
   - Allows for exact topographic correlation between fundus details and its light sensitivity,
   - Micro perimetry is a visual field test that incorporates perimetry and retinal imaging.

K. *Potential visual acuity meter (PAM):* Main components of PAM are a bright light source miniature Trans illuminator Snellen chart and +12 D lens.

L. *OCT:* Noninvasive noncontact imaging that produce high resolution cross-sectional image, useful in diagnosing macular disorders and to delineate retinal layers and detect subtle anatomical changes.

Test dependent on macular pigment

- These tests require the presence of macular pigment for perception (outer plexiform layer) .
  1. *Haidinger's Brushes:* Commonly used as a screening test for retinal pathology in strabismus patients with amblyopia.
     - Entopic phenomena,
     - In this test diffusely illuminated source of plane polarized white or blue light is used,
     - Brushes radiating from point of fixation to Maltese cross,
     - Contrasting yellow or blue hues,
     - Darker portion of Maltese pattern - yellow
     - Brighter pattern of Maltese pattern - blue,
     - Variation in absorption of plane polarized light by oriented molecules of xanthophylls in fovea,
     - Yellow pigment disrupted -> pathology in inner layer -> Brushes not seen.
  2. *Maxwell's spot:* A subject with normal macula will see a 3-degree dark ring surrounding fixation upon looking through a blue filter at a brightly illuminated white surface. Usually, a smaller dark spot is seen at a fixation point itself. The dark ring and spot will fade as the eye adapts to blue light.
     - Some physiologists believe that perception of Maxwell's spot depends on the screening of photoreceptors by macular pigment.

Other tests are: Foveal flicker sensitivity, grating psychophysics, dark adaptometry, visual cycle, electophysiologic test.

3. What is ICGA angiography? Differentiate between FFA and ICG angiography. What are the indications. (10) (WBUHS MS 2022)

The choroid plays an important role in the pathophysiology of the eye. Multimodal imaging offers different techniques to examine the choroid. Fundus fluorescein angiography offers limited visualization of the deep layers of the fundus due to the barrier property of the retinal pigment epithelium. Therefore, indocyanine green angiography (ICGA) is widely used in the angiographic examination of the choroidal structure.

Procedure

The standard dosing for ICG with confocal scanning laser ophthalmoscopy (CSLO) camera systems is 25 mg of ICG dissolved in 3 mL of saline and 1 mL of the solution is injected. For combined FA and ICGA images, saline is replaced with fluorescein sodium solution at 10, 20, or 25% concentrations. There are three phases for ICGA imaging:

- Early phase (<1 min)—Choroidal vessels start to fill from larger outer Haller's layer vessels followed by intermediate Sattler's layer. The choriocapillaris layer fills last but camera resolutions are not high enough to identify individual choriocapillaris. Thus, filling of choriocapillaris is usually seen as indistinct general haze, more evident in the posterior pole.

- *Middle phase:*
  - Early mid-phase (1-3 mins)—shows greater prominence of choroidal veins as well as retinal vessels.
  - Late mid-phase (3-15 mins)—shows fading of choroidal vessels but retinal vessels are still visible. Diffuse tissue staining is also present.
- Late or recirculation phase (15-45 mins)—Choroidal vortex veins are visible during this phase.

Difference between fundus fluorescein angiography (FFA) and indocyanine green angiography (ICGA) (Table 1)

TABLE 1: Difference between fundus fluorescein angiography (FFA) and indocyanine green angiography (ICGA).

Parameters	*FFA*	*ICGA*
Dye used	Sodium fluorescein (orange water soluble dye)	Indocyanine green (tricarbocyanine water soluble dye)
Dosage	5 mL of a 10% solution	25 mg/2mL followed by 5 mL bolus of saline
Protein binding of dye	80%	95% (lesser leakage from vessels)
Vasculature seen more prominently	Retinal vessels	Choroidal vessels
Excitation peak	490 nm	805 nm
Emission peak	530 nm	835 nm
Filter used	Blue-green	Infra-red
Image capture	Digital imaging system with CCD (charge coupled device)	Video angiography and scanning laser ophthalmoscopy
Excretion	Liver and kidney	Liver
Side effects	• Mild—nausea, vomiting, pruritus • Moderate—Urticaria, syncope, local tissue necrosis • Severe—Anaphylaxis, myocardial infarction, death	Less toxic than FFA

Indications of ICGA:

1. *Exudative Age-Related Macular Degeneration:*
   Using ICGA, CNV has been reclassified into three different morphologic types: focal spot or "hot spot", plaques (well or poorly defined), and mixed (i.e., a combination of the previous two) **(Figs. 4A and B)**.

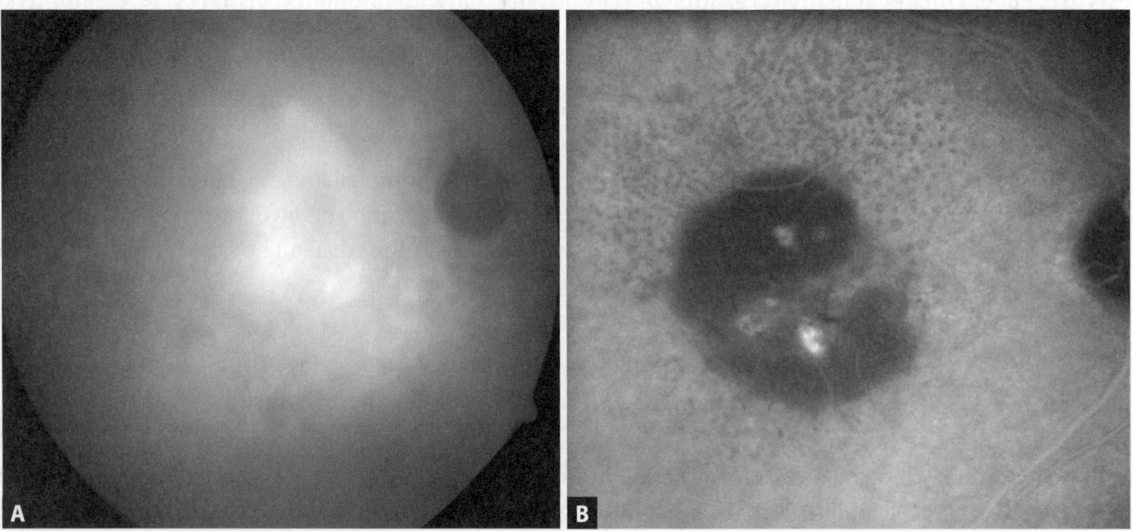

Figs. 4A and B: (A) A plaque with poorly defined margins, in the late phases of ICGA; (B) Two hot spots (the lower spot being more active).

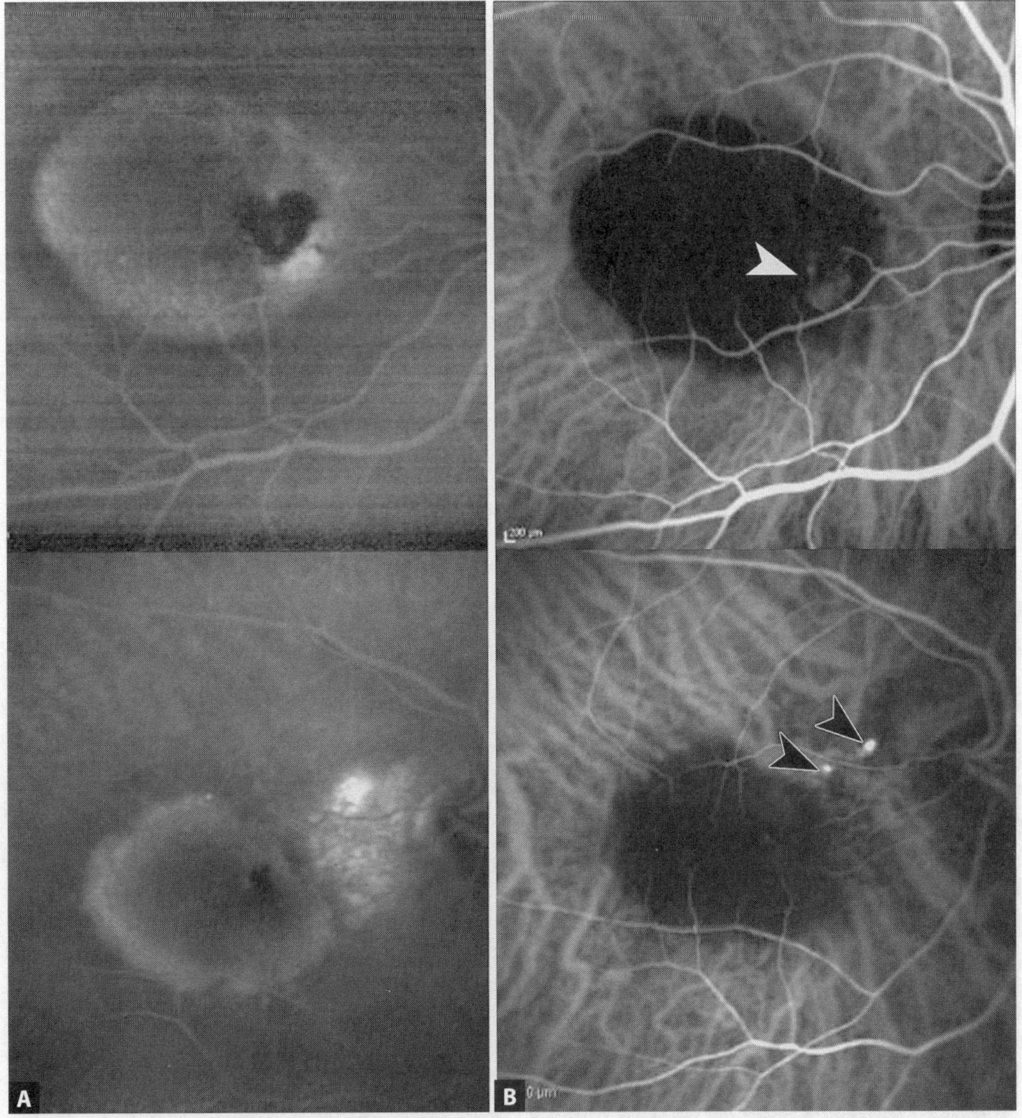

Figs. 5A and B: FA (A) and ICGA (B) images of serous PED with CNVM hot spots.

- In occult CNVM, 60% of eyes reveal plaques on ICGA, and approximately 30% of eyes show hot spots. The rest of the eyes have combined lesions. The visual prognosis of plaque may be worse compared to hot spots, and hot spots may be treated easily with PDT **(Figs. 5A and B)**.
- ICGA helps determine the presence of CNVM in a retinal pigment epithelial detachment (PED). In a PED without CNVM (nonvascularized PED), only hypocyanescence is noted throughout the phases of ICGA. In eyes with proven occult CNVM with serous PED (vascularized PED) on FFA, 62% showed plaque (size more than one disc area), 38% of eyes showed focal CNVM (with a maximum size of one optic disk area), and in 4% of eyes ICGA could not detect a CNVM **(Fig. 6)**.

2. *Retinal angiomatous proliferation (RAP) or Type 3 CNVM:* RAP may contribute to up to 20% of cases of wet AMD. The feeding retinal arteriole and the draining retinal venule in RAP can be visualized in ICGA. Typical features of RAP include intraretinal hemorrhage, retino-retinal anastomosis visible in the early phase of ICGA, high-flow vascular alterations, retino-choroidal anastomosis, and double retinal and choroidal circulation **(Fig. 6)**.

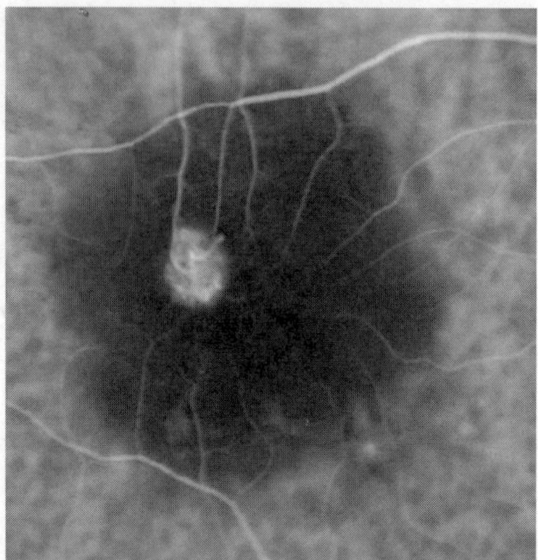

Fig. 6: ICGA image of RAP.

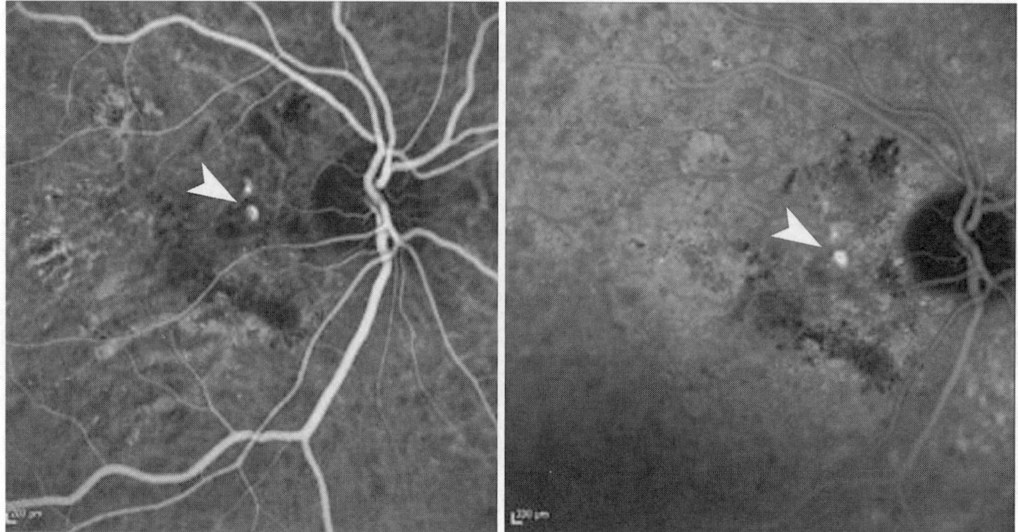

Fig. 7: ICGA image of PCV.

3. *Polypoidal Choroidal Vasculopathy:* ICGA is considered the gold standard for diagnosing PCV. ICGA should be advised to rule out PCV in the eyes with:
   - Massive spontaneous subretinal or submacular hemorrhage
   - Orange-red subretinal nodule
   - Notched or hemorrhagic PED, and
   - Poor response to anti-VEGF therapy.

In ICGA, even though the PCV network starts getting filled with the dye earlier than the retinal vessels, it gets filled slowly. Later the polyps become visible as hypercyanescent lesions **(Fig. 7)**.

4. *Central Serous Chorioretinopathy (CSCR):* ICGA may show an area of choroidal hypervascularity larger than the leakage spot seen in FA and is especially helpful in guiding photodynamic therapy to include entire hypervascular and leaking areas. ICGA also shows chronic CSCR complicated by CNVM changes.

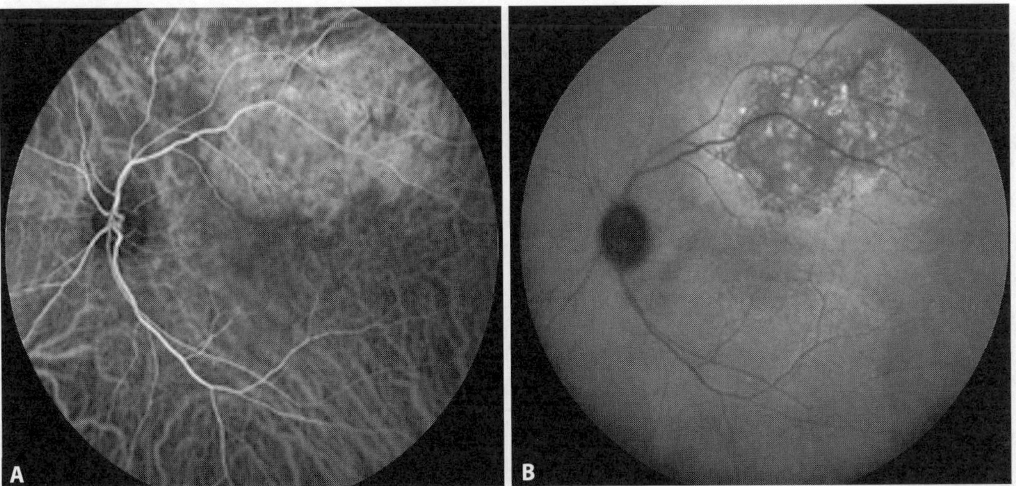

Figs. 8A and B: ICGA of circumscribed choroidal hemangioma (CCH). (A) Early phases; (B) Typical late dye wash-out of the CCH.

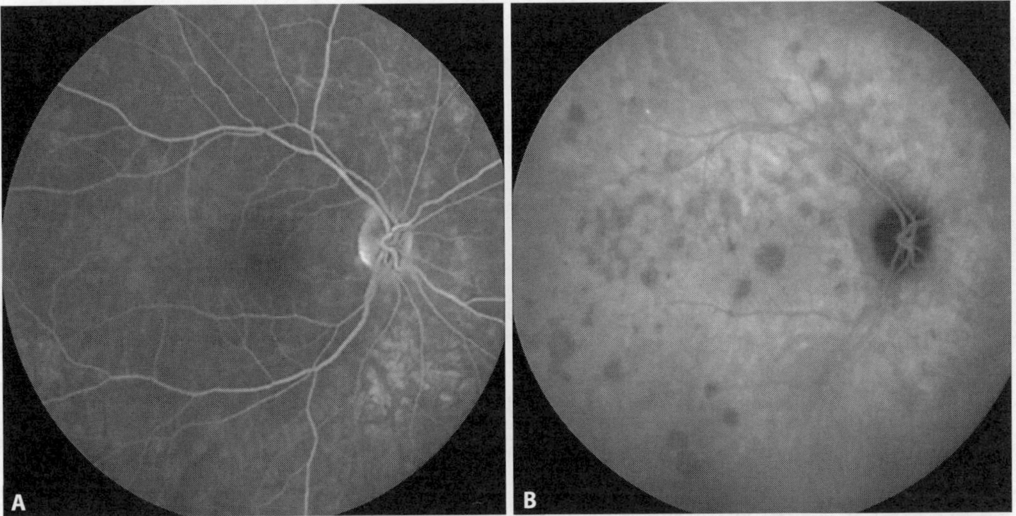

Figs. 9A and B: Multiple evanescent white dot syndrome (MEWDS). (A) FA spots are hyperfluorescent; (B) ICGA shows corresponding hypocyanescent patches.

5. *Choroidal Tumors:* ICGA and ultrasonography help identify choroidal hemangiomas and differentiate them from simulating tumors such as choroidal melanoma or metastasis. Choroidal hemangioma has a distinctive filling pattern on ICGA: progressive filling of abnormal choroidal vessels in the early phase, followed by an intense hypercyanescence at 2–4 minutes, with decreased cyanescence of the tumor at later frames compared to the rest of the choroid, known as the washout phenomenon **(Figs. 8A and B)**.
6. *Multiple evanescent white dot syndrome (MEWDS):* ICGA is helpful in the diagnosis of white dot syndromes, particularly if the fundus lesions are of an atypical appearance or have already faded away. In MEWDS, ICGA shows numerous hypocyanescent dots scattered throughout the posterior pole and a hypocyanescent area surrounding the optic nerve **(Figs. 9A and B)**. These hypocyanescent areas on ICGA disappear over time as the inflammation resolves.
7. *Acute Posterior Multifocal Placoid Pigment Epitheliopathy (APMPPE):* Acute posterior multifocal placoid pigment epitheliopathy is a multifocal inflammation involving the choriocapillaris, and the resulting delayed choroidal filling may manifest as a unique pattern of multifocal hypocyanescence in ICGA in areas seen in the retinal examination as yellow-white spots **(Figs. 10A and B)**.

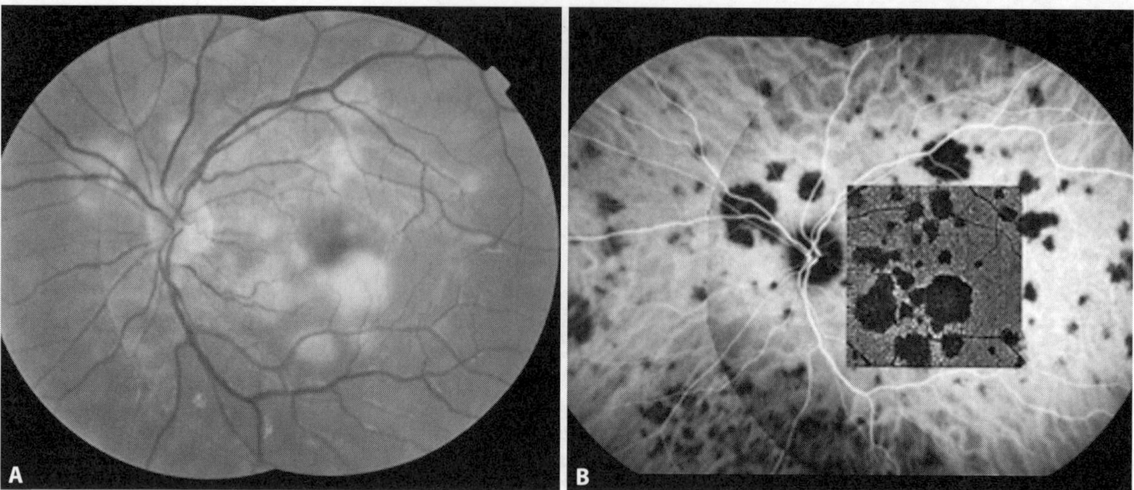

Figs. 10A and B: Acute posterior multifocal placoid pigment epitheliopathy (APMPPE). (A) Fundus photo shows multiple yellow placoid lesions in the posterior pole; (B) ICGA hypocyanescence is more numerous than clinically seen. *[For Color version (Fig. A), See Color Plate 10]*

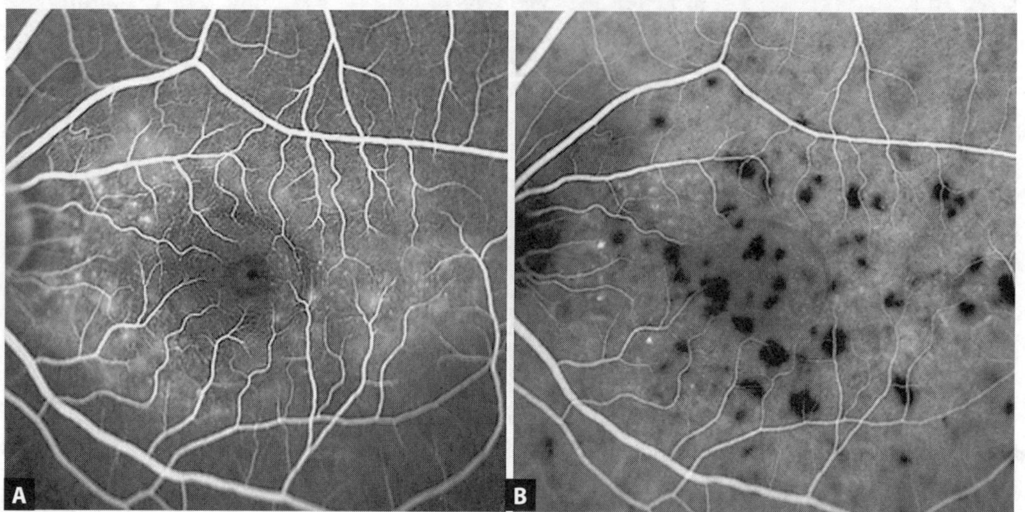

Figs. 11A and B: Vogt–Koyanagi–Harada disease. FA (A) and ICGA (B) showing hypocyanescent dark dots.

8. *Vogt–Koyanagi–Harada Disease:* Active disease can be differentiated from completely treated and inactive VKH by the ICGA pattern. ICGA signs of acute VKH include early choroidal vessel hypercyanescence, intermediate to late phase fuzziness of choroidal stromal vessels, disc hypercyanescence, and hypocyanescent dark dots (HDDs) **(Figs. 11A and B)**.

4. Discuss ARMD. (10) (WBUHS MS 2021)

ARMD

Definition: Age-related macular degeneration (AMD) is defined as a degenerative disorder that affect the macula which is characterized by the presence of specific clinical findings like drusen and RPE changes, in the absence of another disorder. Age related macular degeneration is mostly associated with impairment of vision in later stages of disease. (KANSKI PAGE – 598, 8TH EDI)

Etiology

Changes in the Bruch's membrane/choroid complex, the retinal pigment epithelium and photoreceptor cells play an important role. The disease may affect one, both, or all of these tissue components and the change in one of these tissue components influence the others that starts an 'intermediate disease mechanism" [Bird AC (2010)].

Prevalence

The prevalence of advanced ARMD was 1.6% in Beaver Dam Eye Study, with the exudative form being present in one eye 1.2% of the time, and geographic atrophy in one eye 0.6% of the time.[Klein R, Klein BEk, Linton KLP (1992). Prevalence of Age-related Maculopathy-The Beaver Dam Eye Study. Ophthalmology 99(6): 933-943.]

Classification (Table 2)

- *Conventional Classification:* There are two main types of AMD:
  1. Dry (non-exudative, non-neovascular) AMD—It is the most common type, consisting approx. 90% of diagnosed disease. Geographic atrophy (GA) is the advanced stage of dry AMD.
  2. Wet (exudative, neovascular) AMD though is less common than dry, but is associated with more chances of rapid progression to severe vision loss. The main manifestations are CNV and PED, but retinal angiomatous proliferation (RAP) and polypoidal choroidal vasculopathy (PCV), have been also included under neovascular AMD.

TABLE 2: Clinical classification of age-related macular degeneration (AMD).

Category	Definition, based on presence of lesions within two disk diameters of the fovea in either eye
No apparent ageing changes	• No drusen • No AMD pigmentary abnormalities
Normal ageing changes	• Only drupelets • No AMD pigmentary abnormalities
Early AMD	• Medium drusen (>63 µm but <125 µm) • No AMD pigmentary abnormalities
Intermediate AMD	• Large drusen(>125 µm) • Any AMD pigmentary abnormalities
Late AMD	• Neovascular AMD and/or any geographic atrophy

Non-neovascular AMD: In all stages of non-neovascular AMD, the defining lesion is the drusen. Drusen are typically round, yellow lesions located along the basal surface of the RPE, mostly in the postequatorial retina. This material corresponds to the abnormal thickening of the inner aspect of Bruch membrane.

Diagnosis

- Symptoms: Gradual impairment of vision over months or years.

Signs

- Presence of numerous intermediate to large soft drusen which may become confluent.
- Focal hyper- and/or hypopigmentation of the RPE.
- There may be variable loss of the retina and choriocapillaris associated with sharply circumscribed areas of RPE atrophy.
- Larger choroidal vessels may become visible and pre-existing drusen disappear with enlargement of atrophic areas.
- Rotenoid RPE detachment (see below).

OCT

- Drusen – Medium-sized and large drusens are seen as hyper-reflective irregular nodules beneath the RPE, located on or within the Bruch membrane.

- Increased hyper-reflectivity initially in the outer retinal layers and eventual photoreceptor loss are seen in GA.
- Outer retinal tubulations consist of degenerating photoreceptors aggregated into tubular structures that appear as roundish hyporeflective spaces, often around the margin of GA.
- Outer retinal corrugations. This recently described phenomenon is an undulating hyper-reflective layer on OCT thought to correspond to the histological finding of basal laminar deposit, a layer that accumulates between the RPE and the RPE basement membrane (the inner layer of the Bruch membrane) in AMD. Basal linear deposit is a distinct finding consisting of membranous debris laid down between the RPE basement membrane and the inner collagenous layer of the Bruch membrane that may progress focally to form drusen.

FA of atrophic areas shows a window defect due to unmasking of background choroidal fluorescence, if the underlying choriocapillaris is still intact. Exposed sclera may exhibit late staining.

Management

- Risk factors such as smoking, ocular sun protection, cardiovascular, and dietary should be addressed.
- Antioxidant supplementation if indicated.
- Amsler grid testing: patient may use this at home to monitor visual distortion. Any changes noted by patient should be evaluated promptly.

Neovascular AMD

The presence of macular neovascularization is the defining characteristics of neovascular AMD.

Symptoms: Sudden decrease in vision, metamorphopsia and/or paracentral scotoma.

Signs: Subretinal or intraretinal fluid (cystoid macular edema/CME), exudate and/or blood, a pigment ring or gray-green membrane, irregular elevation of the RPE or a PED, an RPE tear, and/or a sea fan pattern of subretinal vessels.

OCT: Shown as a thickening and fragmentation of the RPE and choriocapillaris. Subretinal and sub-RPE fluid, blood, and scarring are demonstrated. It is mainly useful in monitoring the response to the treatment.

FA: Indicated for diagnosis of neovascularization prior to commenting to anti-VEGF.CNV ca be classified on the basis of findings on FA

- *Classic CNV:* They show 'lacy' pattern (fills with dye in a well-defined pattern) during early transit subsequently leaking into the subretinal space over 1–2 minutes with late staining of fibrous tissue. Most CNV is subfoveal.
- Occult CNV (80%) is used to describe CNV when its limits cannot be fully defined on FA. Variants are fibrovascular PED and 'late leakage of an undetermined source' (LLUS).
- Predominantly or minimally classic CNV is present when the classic element is greater or less than 50% of the total lesion respectively.

ICG: CNV can be demonstrated as a focal hyperfluorescent "hot spot" or "plaque'; benefits adjunctive to FA include increased sensitivity in the detection of CNV. The distinction of CNV from other conditions that may have a similar presentation, particularly PCV, RAP and CSR.

Treatment

Antiangiogenic therapies: VEGF inhibitors block its interaction with receptors on the endothelial cell surface that retard or reverse vessel growth. Anti VEGF agents are Aflibercept (Eylea), Ranibizumab (Lucentis), Bevacizumab(Avastin), Pegaptanib.

Photodynamic therapy: Which uses Verteporfin, a light-activated compound preferentially taken up by dividing cells including neovascular tissue.

Laser: Thermal argon or diode laser ablation may be one of the treatment modalities.

5. Discuss results of AREDS 2 trial on vitamins for AMD. How does it differ from AREDS 1 trial? (DNB 2020)

The Age-Related Eye Disease Study (AREDS) was a clinical trial sponsored by the National Eye Institute that ran from 1992 to 2001. The study was designed to:

- Investigate the natural history and risk factors of age-related macular degeneration (AMD) and cataracts, and
- Evaluate the effects of high doses of antioxidants and zinc on the progression of the two conditions in those with AMD.

The original AREDS study was followed by AREDS2, a five-year study that started in 2006 to test whether the original AREDS formulation would be improved by adding omega-3 fatty acids; adding lutein and zeaxanthin; removing beta-carotene; or reducing zinc.

Results

- In the AREDS2 trial, adding omega-3 fatty acids or lutein + zeaxanthin to the AREDS formula had no additional overall effect on the risk of advanced AMD. However, AREDS2 participants who took antioxidants minus beta-carotene but with lutein + zeaxanthin (AREDS2 formula) had an incremental increase in benefit, compared to those who took the AREDS formula.
- AREDS2 participants who were former smokers who took a formulation with beta-carotene had a higher incidence of lung cancer. The investigators found no significant changes in the effectiveness of the formulation when they removed beta-carotene or reduced the zinc dose.
- Adding omega-3 fatty acids or lutein + zeaxanthin to antioxidants plus zinc (AREDS formula) had no overall effect on the need for cataract surgery

Comparing AREDS and AREDS2

The transition from the AREDS to AREDS2 study signifies an important evolution in the fight against age-related macular degeneration (AMD). While both studies shared the common goal of identifying effective nutritional strategies to slow the progression of AMD, there were notable differences in their formulations, findings, and subsequent recommendations for eye health.

AREDS focused on a formulation that included high doses of antioxidants and zinc. This combination was chosen based on the hypothesis that oxidative stress plays a key role in the development and progression of AMD. The significant finding from AREDS was that the formulation could reduce the risk of progression to advanced AMD by about 25% for individuals at high risk.

AREDS2 sought to build upon these findings by assessing the potential benefits of adding or modifying components in the original formula. Key changes included:

- *Introduction of Lutein and Zeaxanthin:* These carotenoids, found in high concentrations in the macula, were added due to their potential to protect against macular damage.
- *Exclusion of Beta-Carotene:* AREDS2 removed beta-carotene due to its association with increased risk of lung cancer in smokers. This change aimed to enhance the safety profile of the supplement.
- *Inclusion of Omega-3 Fatty Acids:* Although the addition of DHA and EPA omega-3 fatty acids did not show a significant benefit in the final analysis, their initial inclusion was based on promising preliminary research.
- *Adjustment of Zinc Dosage:* AREDS2 explored whether a lower dose of zinc would be as effective, aiming to reduce potential side effects without compromising benefits.

These modifications reflect a nuanced understanding of nutritional science and its application to eye health, particularly in the context of AMD management.

6. Diabetic macular edema—OCT findings and its management. (10) (WBUHS MS 2019, 2020)

Diabetic maculopathy is the most common cause of visual impairment in patients with diabetes mellitus.

Classification

Diabetic maculopathy is classified as -

- Exudative maculopathy
- Ischemic maculopathy
- Mixed maculopathy

Exudative maculopathy (Diabetic macular edema)

It is diagnosed stereoscopically as retinal thickening within 1 disc diameter of the center of the macula using fundus biomicroscopy. To characterize the severity of macular edema and for treatment guidelines, the term clinically significant macular edema (CSME) is used. Macular edema is clinically significant if one of the following conditions is present:

- Retinal thickening at or within 500 mm of the center of the macula; and/or
- Hard exudates at or within 500 mm of the center of the macula if associated with thickening of the adjacent retina; and/or
- A zone or zones of retinal thickening 1 disk area in size, at least part of which is within 1 disk diameter of the macular center.

It is more common in type 2 diabetes (Adult Onset). The incidence of macular edema increases significantly with increasing severity of diabetes in both younger onset and older onset diabetic patients as - IDDM - <5 yrs - 0% &> 20 yrs- 32%; and NIDDM - < 5 yrs - 3% &> 20 yrs - 28%.

Clinically significant macular edema is further classified into focal or diffuse, depending on the leakage pattern seen on the fluorescein angiogram (FA). In focal CSME, discrete points of retinal hyperfluorescence are present on the FA due to focal leakage of microaneurysms. In diffuse DME, areas of diffuse leakage are noted on the FA due to intraretinal leakage from a dilated retinal capillary bed and/or intraretinal microvascular abnormalities (IRMA), and/or (in severe cases) from arterioles and venules without discrete foci of leaking microaneurysms. There may be associated cystoid macular edema (CME). Cystoid macular edema results from a generalized breakdown of the inner BRB with fluid accumulation, primarily in the outer plexiform layer.

OCT finding

OCT studies of CSME, as defined by the ETDRS, have revealed three basic structural changes in the neurosensory retina: retinal swelling, CME, and serous retinal detachment

Kang et al. described four patterns of OCT findings associated with CSME (as defined by the ETDRS): foveal thickening with homogenous optical reflectivity throughout the entire thickness of retina (type 1); foveal thickening with decreased optical reflectivity in the outer layers of the retina (type 2); and foveal thickening with subretinal fluid accumulation with or without retinal traction (types 3A and 3B), respectively OCT pattern.

The following morphologic patterns on the basis of OCT examination has been proposed:

- Diffuse retinal thickening
- Cystoid macular edema
- Posterior hyaloidal traction
- Subretinal fluid
- Tractional retinal detachment

OCT has several advantages as a retinal imaging technique:

- It is noninvasive (no injected dye involved) and well tolerated (especially important in children).
- It provides quantitative information regarding retinal thickness with a high degree of accuracy and reproducibility.
- It clearly reveals the presence and extent of vitreomacular traction; and
- It serves as valuable teaching tool for fellows and residents and is easily understood by most patients. Moreover, OCT can be used to calculate the standardized change in macular thickness (SCMT).

Treatment

The treatment of various forms of maculopathy differs. Although there is no established treatment of diabetic macular ischemia, management decisions are complicated by its presence

- **Intravitreal anti-VEGF agents** - DRCR.net Protocol concludes that intravitreal ranibizumab more effectively improves visual acuity than focal/grid laser treatment for center-involved DMO. Laser treatment should be deferred for 6 months after commencement of anti-VEGF therapy.
- **Laser Photocoagulation**

Indications:

- Focal leaks > 500 u from the centre of macula.
- Focal leaks 300–500 from the centre of macula, if the treating ophthalmologist does not believe that the treatment is likely to destroy the remaining perifoveal capillary network.
- Areas of diffuse leakage that has not been treated previously.
- Avascular zones other than normal FAZ, not previously treated.
- Mechanism of action
- Reduces metabolic need.
- Direct diffusion of oxygen from choriocapillaries through scar to inner retina.
- Stimulates endothelial repair process.
- Types **(Table 3)**
- Focal
- Classic Grid
- Modified Grid

TABLE 3: Differences between focal, classic grid, and modified grid.

Parameters	*Focal*	*Classic grid*	*Modified grid*
Wavelength	Argon green, double frequency Nd:YAG, dye yellow		
Duration	100 ms		
Spot size	50 µ	50 µ	
Power	80 mw according (Titrated to requirement	50 mw (Titrated according to requirement)	
Inter burn distance	-	2 burns	
Burn type	Grade 23 (dirty white)/ Blanching or darkening of MA	Grade 12 (faint white)	
Remarks	Burns are given at 500 µ from the fovea to all MAs within 3,000 µ	Burns are given at 500 µ from the fovea in a pattern sparing papilla-macular bundle, can extend up to 2 disk diameters from the center of macula	Only thickened areas are treated and not the whole macula, can extend up to 2 disk diameters from the center of macula.
Follow-up	1 week, 1 m, 4 m FFA	1 week, 1 m, 4 m FFA	1 week, 1 m, 4 m FFA

Side effects:

- Paracentral scotomas
- Immediate risk of vision loss.

Poor prognostic factors:

- Hard exudates involving the fovea
- Mixed Maculopathy
- Severe retinopathy at presentation
    - *Subthreshold (micropulse) diode laser:* This modality uses very short (microsecond order) laser pulse duration combined with a relatively longer interval, allowing energy dissipation

- *Intravitreal triamcinolone:* In pseudophakic eyes intravitreal triamcinolone steroid injection followed by prompt laser is comparable to ranibizumab with regard to visual improvement and reduced retinal thickening.
- *Pars plana vitrectomy (PPV)* may be indicated when macular oedema is associated with tangential traction from a thickened and taut posterior hyaloid.
- *Intravitreal Dexamethasone Delivery System:* A sustained release drug delivery system for dexamethasone inserted transclerally into the vitreous produced statistically significant visual acuity improvement for 90 days after insertion and was well tolerated for 180 days.
- *Supplemental Oxygen and Hyperbaric Oxygenation:* Hyperbaric oxygenation reduced breakdown of the blood-retinal barrier in a rat model of diabetic retinopathy. In a small clinical series, 10-30 hyperbaric oxygen treatments resulted in no morphologic change in DME.

DME ***(Flowcharts 3 and 4)****:*

Flowchart 3: Diabetic macular edema (DME)

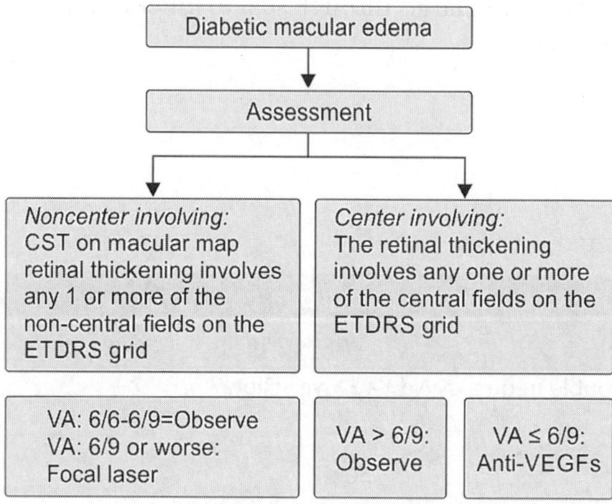

Flowchart 4: Diabetic Retinopathy clinical research (DRCR) network protocol.

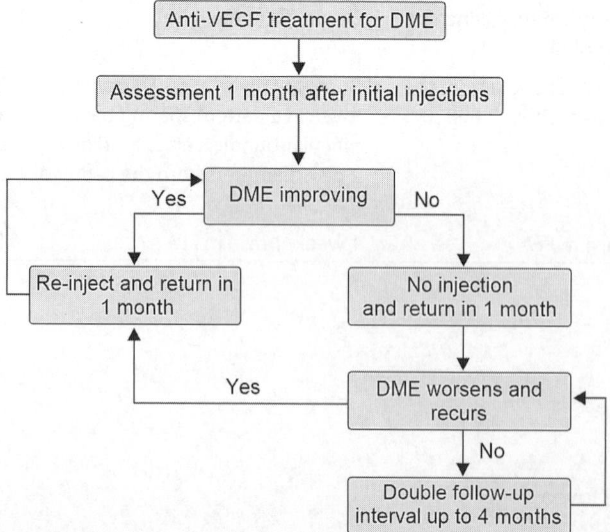

The Diabetic Retinopathy Clinical Research (DRCR) network protocol for CI-DME starts with:

- Initial injections are given monthly for 4–6 months and then allows for *holding on treatment*

- If there is no improvement in vision or central subfield thickness. No further improvement is defined as a <10% decrease in the central subfield thickness on OCT and a <1 line improvement in VA on the Snellen chart after the last injection, and in the opinion of the treating ophthalmologist, no further benefit can be expected with additional treatment.
- Or, if 6/6 Snellen vision and/or the resolution of DME has been achieved.

- Anti-VEGF treatment can be resumed if there is a worsening vision or CST on subsequent visits. If on consecutive visits, treatment is not required, the follow-up interval is doubled up to 4 months.
- Treatment is deferred when vision has improved to 6/6 and the OCT has become normal (normal foveal contour with reduction of retinal thickening at the macula, regression of the neurosensory detachment, and disappearance of cystic spaces in the neurosensory retina).

An alternative approach is a treat-and-extend regimen, wherein the interval between visits is adjusted based on the treatment response.

Patients may have persistent NCI-DME after treating CI-DME with anti-VEGFs or steroid therapy.

- BCVA of 6/9 or better, observe
- BCVA worse than 6/9—laser.
- *A plaque of hard exudates may deposit at the macula:* Steroids (triamcinolone acetonide or dexamethasone). In the absence of macular thickening, repeat injection of anti-VEGF for persistent exudates may resolve the exudates but chances of improvement would be less likely.

1. **Anti VEGFs (Table 4):**

TABLE 4: Anti-VEGF drugs and their mechanisms and doses.

Drug	*Mechanism*	*Dosage*	*Studies*
Ranibizumab	• Binds to the receptor-binding site on VEGF-A, which inhibits the binding of VEGF molecules to their receptors on the surface of endothelial cells • Each molecule of ranibizumab has only one binding site for VEGF, which implies that two molecules of ranibizumab are necessary to bind a VEGF dimer	0.3 mg	RIDE, RISE, RESOLVE
Bevacizumab	Binds to soluble VEGF and inhibits the binding of VEGF molecules to its receptors on the surface of endothelial cells. It has two binding site per molecule. Prevents all VEGF-A isoforms from binding to endothelial cell receptors	1.25 mg	BOLT
Aflibercept	• Soluble decoy receptor that binds vascular endothelial growth factor-A (VEGF-A), VEGF-B, and placental growth factor (PIGF) • It is called a decoy receptor since VEGF does not bind to its original receptors and mistakenly binds with aflibercept, thereby reducing VEGF activity. Inhibits neovascularization	2 mg	VISTA and VIVID,
Faricimab	• Inhibitory effect on both VEGF-A and Ang-2 • Anti-VEGF-A effect inhibits endothelial proliferation, reduces vascular permeability, and suppresses neovascularization. • Anti-Ang 2 effect improves vascular stability and desensitize the vessels to the actions of VEGF-A.	6 mg	BOULEVARD, STAIRWAY, YOSEMITE and RHINE

2. **Steroids:**

Switching to intravitreal steroids can be considered in the following situations:

- Responding to anti-VEGFs but difficult to maintain frequent follow-up visits
- Pseudophakic patients who have reached a plateau – persistent intraretinal fluid (IRF)/VA <6/12
- Persistent edema and needing cataract surgery
- Occurrence of systemic vascular event while on anti-VEGFs

- Associated features such as extensive hard exudates and presence of hyperreflective dots on OCT
- Eyes post vitrectomy **(Table 5)**

TABLE 5: Eyes postvitrectomy: drugs and doses.		
Dexamethasone	0.7 mg	MEAD
Fluocinolone acetonide	0.19 mg	FAME

3. **Laser therapy**

- In cases of focal edema with identifiable microaneurysms, the treatment is directed at the involved area. Done between 500-3000 micrometers from center of fovea. Spot size of 50-100 micrometer is chosen.
- Subthreshold laser using micropulse mode of laser delivery.
- Scatter laser for DME. Here exposure time would be less. But increased foveal thickness post treatment is an adverse event.

Additional laser photocoagulation to treat persistent edema

- Persistent CSME with visible microaneurysms
- If a switch to steroid is not possible.

4. **Vitrectomy:**

Indications

- DME with vitreomacular traction or tractional epiretinal membrane (ERM) or a taut posterior hyaloid.
  - The anteroposterior and tangential traction is released, resulting in better oxygenation to the inner retina, which may improve capillary blood flow in the perifoveal area and reduce hypoxia-induced VEGF drive.
  - Traction can be relieved through segmentation, delamination, en bloc dissection, bimanual dissection, shaving with cutter.
- The ILM contributes to tangential traction and helps prevent recurrences of ERM especially in cases of vitreoschisis.

Treatment of DME with associated conditions ***(Table 6):***

TABLE 6: Treatment of DME with associated conditions.	
PDR with DME	Panretinal photocoagulation (PRP). DME treated as per standard protocol. In the presence of vision-threatening traction, vitrectomy + PRP
DME in Pseudophakic eyes	• DME with no component of Irvine–Gass syndrome: anti-VEGFs for CI-DME • In the presence of both DME and Irvine–Gass syndrome: topical nonsteroidal anti-inflammatory drugs (NSAIDs) should be used followed by anti-VEGFs. • In nonresponders: Switch to steroids
DME in Pregnancy	*Close observation:* If progressive deterioration of vision, intravitreal steroids: dexamethasone implants.
DME in vitrectomized eyes	Intravitreal steroids+ Anti-VEGFs
DME in Macular ischemia	Anti-VEGFs or steroids
DME with glaucoma	Anti-VEGFs and laser
DME with cataract	Anti-VEGFs/Steroids with cataract surgery

7. Explain management of subretinal fluid and its complications. (10) (DNB 2019)

Subretinal fluid is collection of fluid between RPE and neurosensory retina.

Approach to management:

Detailed history:

- Including onset and duration of DOV
- Past, personal (smoking), family history (genetic retinal diseases) should be asked for.

Clinical examination:

- Reduced vision—can vary from mild to moderate DOV to profound loss of vision.
- Pupil can show RAPD (in RD involving >2 quadrants or RD with macula off)
- Fundoscopy will show elevated neurosensory retina.

Noninvasive investigation:

- Color fundus picture (widefield)—single or multiple areas of elevated retina.
- Associated features- vitreous hemorrhage, disk edema, sclerosed vessels, perivascular cuffing, retinal hemorrhage, retinal tears or breaks.
- Optical coherence tomography—separation of neurosensory retina from RPE with collection of fluid in sub retinal space.
- Optical coherence tomography angiography- newer, invasive imaging
- Allows visualization of retinal and choroidal circulation without any contrast medium.
- Fundus autofluorescence- with scanning laser ophthalmoscopy.
- SRF appears as area of hypo auto fluorescence.
- Collection of lipofuschin at the margin of SRF appears hyper auto fluorescent. This indicates active disease.
- Gravitational tract can be seen in chronic CSCR.

Invasive imaging technique:

- Fundus fluorescein angiography- shows pooling of dye in a defined anatomical space.
- Other associated features are staining, leaky vessels filling defects etc.
- Pattern of leak- starry sky appearance seen in VKH due to diffuse pinpoint leaks,
- Ink blot or smoke-stack pattern seen in CSCR.
- Window defect seen in atrophic ARMD, FTMH, and RPE tears.
- Indocyanine green angiography—delineates choroidal circulation.
- Better imaging modality than FFA in PCV, RAM, chronic CSCR, postuveitis, choroidal tumors, Break in Bruch's membrane.

Treatment modalities

I. Observation- minimal SRF without any break or tear, not affecting vision can be observed for up to 2 months.

II. *Medical:*
Indications—macular edema, ARMD, tumors, and proliferative retinopathy intravitreal anti-VEGF injections **(Tables 7 and 8)**.

III. *Laser:*
- Conventional laser—Suitable for extrafoveal leaky vessels or polyp or CNVM.
  - Uses argan green and diode lasers.
  - It is used during retinal detachment repair following PPV and extrusion of SRF or in surgical treatment of PDR.
- Subthreshold micropulse laser—For subfoveal collection of fluid in CSCR or DME.
- Significantly less damage on OCT.
- Focal laser—For clinically significant macular edema.
- Directed to microaneurysm 500 microns from fovea.
  - *Spot size:* 50–100 μ; pulse duration: 50–100 ms; power—enough to barely whiten the microaneurysm.
  - *Grid laser:* Also for clinically significant macular edema and persistent macular edema (>3 months), resulting from BRVO.
- *Verteporfin+ PDT:* Subfoveal predominantly classic CNVM with vision of ≤6/60
- Verteporfin is used as photosensitizing agent followed by application of 689 nm wavelength light.

IV. *Surgical treatment:*
- Pneumatic retinopexy
- Scleral buckling with or without drainage of subretinal fluid.

TABLE 7: Anti-VEGF doses.

Anti-VEGF	*Dose*	*Halflife (days)*
Ranibizumab (lucentis)	0.5 mg (0.05 mL)	9
Bevacizumab (Avastin)	1.125 mg (0.05 mL)	20
Aflibercept (Eylea)	2 mg (0.05 mL)	5–6
Brolucizumab (Pagenex)	6 mg (0.05 mL)	3
Pegaptanib (Macugen)	0.3 mg	6 (94 hours)
Faricimab (Vabysmo)	6 mg	7.5

TABLE 8: Trials related to anti-VEGF.

Disease	*Study name*
AMD	• MARINA • ANCHOR • PIER • PrONTO • CATT • HAWK and HARRIER
DME	• READ 2 • RISE AND RIDE • VIVID AND VISTA • YOSEMITE AND RHINE • DRCR NET PROTOCOL
PCV	• LAPTOP • EVEREST • EVEREST II
STAGE 3 + ROP	BEAT-ROP
Macular edema due to BRVO	BRAVO

- Cryotherapy
- Endolaser
- Pars plana vitrectomy with vitreous substitutes.

Complications

- Due to persistent subretinal fluid- can cause poor central vision and delayed recovery after treatment
  - Seen in cases resistant to medical/laser treatment.
  - Can be seen after scleral buckling for RRD
- Complications after anti-VEGF injection:
  - Increase in IOP
  - Cataract
  - Endophthalmitis
  - Risk of thromboembolic events
  - Rebound macular events
  - Immunoreactivity
  - Retinal detachment
- Complications after surgery-
  - Post surgical endophthalmitis
  - Choroidal hemorrhage
  - Scleral perforation
  - Raised IOP
  - Silicon oil-associated glaucoma
  - Cataract
  - Band keratopathy
  - Retinal breaks

8. Pathology, evaluation, and management of full thickness macular hole. (10) (DNB 2019/DNB 2022)

Pathology

Vitreomacular traction: Historically, vitreomacular traction has been suspected to cause macular hole which has been confirmed with the advent of newer OCTs'. Vitreomacular traction is caused by partial vitreous detachment around the fovea.

Foveal cyst: Fellow eye of many macular hole patients showed the presence of a foveal cyst. OCT showed the presence of vitreous cortex attachment at the roof of these cysts. Then it was hypothesized that foveal cysts are the initial changes in the structure of fovea that further progresses to a full thickness macular hole.

Contraction of the premacular cortex:

Gass in 1988 postulated that the tangential contraction of the remnants of posterior hyaloid membrane causes the detachment of the central photoreceptors leading to the separation of the fovea. Based on this theory Gass proposed the staging of macular hole and also the surgical technique of dissecting the posterior hyaloid and ILM peeling.

Evaluation: The patients of macular hole present with progressive loss of vision, central scotoma or metamorphopsia. On presentation, the initial clinical examinations should include visual acuity assessment, slit lamp examination and fundus examination with slit lamp biomicroscopy and indirect ophthalmoscopy.

After the initial clinical examination an optical coherence tomography (OCT) has to be done. Based on the clinical and OCT findings, the macular hole is classified into four stages.

Stages of macula hole: The staging of macular hole was described by Gass in 1988.

Stage 1—impending macular hole:

Stage 1A—loss of foveolar depression, central yellow spot and no vitreofoveal detachment

Stage 1B— loss of foveolar depression, yellow ring with bridging interface, no vitreofoveal detachment. The yellow ring is the edematous border of the disrupted outer retina.

Stage 2: Central round retinal defect with rim of elevated retina with or without prefoveal opacity

Stage 3: Central round defect >/= 400 um diameter retinal defect, no Wess ring, rim of elevated retina with or without prefoveolar opacity.

Stage 4: Central round defect, rim of elevated retina, Wess's ring with prefoveolar opacity

After the advent of OCT, Chan et al., in 2004, proposed a stage 0 macular hole when the posterior hyaloid is attached to the foveal center resulting in minor changes of the foveal pit.

Differential Diagnosis

- Lamellar macular hole
- Macular pseudoholes
- Foveal cysts of other origins
- Microholes

Management of Macular Holes

Macular holes can be treated surgically only although vitreolysis has been described as nonsurgical treatment of small stage 2 macular holes but not with great success. Stages 1A and B macular hole can be observed.

Macular Hole Surgery Principles

Pars plana vitrectomy is done to remove the posterior hyaloid attachment from the fovea. Extensive vitrectomy with vitreous base shaving is described to allow injection of more gas mixture and to prevent postoperative risks of retinal breaks and retinal detachment by preventing the gas bubble from exerting traction on the remaining vitreous fibers.

Epiretinal membrane peeling when present and internal membrane peeling is done with the help of brilliant blue dye (0.025%).

Other vital dyes that are rarely used for ILM peeling are indocyanine green (0.05%) and tryphan blue.

In patients with large macular holes special techniques like inverse peel is done where ILM flap is used to cover the macular hole. In failed macular holes retinal autografts, amniotic membrane grafts or anterior lens capsule is used to tuck inside the macular hole.

Gas Injection

Gas helps in dehydrating the edges of the macular hole and then by preventing fluid current from hampering the healing process. It also acts as a scaffold for the retinal tissue to bridge the gap. Various gas-like C_3F_8, C_2F_6, SF_6, and air. The rationale of using one gas over other is the size of the macular hole which will determine the expected duration of the gas bubble. Silicone oil is used as a tamponading agent only when the patient has to travel by air after the surgery or if the patient is unable to maintain facedown position or to ensure prolonged tamponade after a failed surgery.

Postoperative Positioning

Traditionally, Postoperative prone position is advised for 7 days after macular hole surgery to keep the macular hole edges insulated from fluid currents till the healing process starts. This positioning is not required if the gas mixture injected is able to cover the macula for one week.

Prognosis

Best corrected visual acuity on presentation: Visual acuity >6/60 is considered as better visual prognosis than visual acuity <6/60.

Duration: Less than 1 year of presentation has better visual prognosis.

Stage of hole: Stage 2 and 3 macular holes on presentation have better prognosis than stage 4 macular hole.

Size of macular hole: Large macular holes have poorer closure rates and they are more prone to secondary closure after the surgery.

9. Mention clinical features of retinitis pigmentosa. (5) (DNB 2023)

Symptoms

- It is usually a bilateral disease but can have asymmetrical presentation.
- Patients usually present with loss of night vision and loss of peripheral field of vision
- Tunnel vision in advanced cases
- Loss of depth perception
- Photopsia
- Photophobia
- Glare
- Poor dark adaptation

Signs

- The classic clinical triad of RP is arteriolar attenuation, retinal pigmentary changes (could be either hypopigmentation and/or hyperpigmentation in form of bone-spicule and pigment clumpings), and waxy disc pallor.
- Mottled appearance of the retina
- RP combined with deafness(congenital or progressive) is called Usher syndrome.

10. Define Pachychoroid spectrum and its clinical features. (10) (DNB 2021)

The Pachychoroid Spectrum refers to a group of retinal disorders characterized by increased choroidal thickness (**pachychoroid**), dilation and enlargement of large outer choroidal vessels (**pachyvessels**), and *attenuation* inner choroidal choriocapillaris layer (inner most choroid). They are often associated with **subretinal fluid** and **retinal pigment epithelial detachment** (**PED**).

Key diseases in this spectrum include:

1. **Pachychoroid pigment epitheliopathy (PPE)**
   - *Clinical Features:* PPE is considered a **precursor** to other pachychoroid disorders. It is characterized by abnormalities in the retinal pigment epithelium (RPE), such as *pigmentary changes* and or irregularities, **but without the presence of subretinal fluid**. Patients often remain asymptomatic or have mild visual disturbances.
   - *Management:* Since PPE is often asymptomatic, management involves regular monitoring with imaging techniques like OCT to detect any progression to more serious conditions like CSCR or pachychoroid neovasculopathy.
2. **Central serous chorioretinopathy (CSCR)**
   - *Clinical features:* CSCR typically affects young to middle-aged males, with stress, systemic corticosteroid use, and other factors such as hypertension or sleep disturbances as triggers.

     The condition results in serous detachment of the neurosensory retina (NSD) appearing as blister on biomicroscopy often leading to blurred vision, micropsia (perceiving objects smaller than they are), and relative scotomas (blind spots).
   - *Management: Observation* is the first line of treatment for *acute cases.*

     For *chronic or recurrent cases,* treatments include focal laser photocoagulation, photodynamic therapy (PDT), or anti-VEGF (vascular endothelial growth factor) injections.
3. **Pachychoroid Neovasculopathy (PNV)**
   - *Clinical features:* PNV involves the formation of **new** *abnormal blood vessels* beneath the RPE, similar to age-related macular degeneration (AMD).

     Patients may experience blurred vision, and there is often the presence of subretinal fluid (SRF)

     This condition can be distinguished from AMD by the absence of drusen (yellow deposits under the retina) and the presence of pachyvessels.
   - *Management:* PNV is managed primarily with anti-VEGF therapy to control neovascularization. PDT may also be considered for persistent cases.
4. **Polypoidal Choroidal Vasculopathy (PCV):** PCV is characterized by the presence of abnormal branching choroidal vessels with polyp-like structures.

   It predominantly affects individuals of Asian or African descent.
   - *Clinical features:* There are recurrent serosanguinous (serous and bloody) neurosensory detachments, and it often mimics other forms of choroidal neovascularization.

     Patients may present with visual disturbances, exudative fluid accumulation (SRF), and subretinal & choroidal hemorrhages.
   - *Management:* Management of PCV includes anti-VEGF injections and PDT. Some cases may require combination therapy to control the condition effectively.

Imaging Techniques for Diagnosis and Management

The diagnosis and management of pachychoroid diseases rely heavily on multimodal imaging techniques, including:

- **Optical coherence tomography (OCT)**: To assess choroidal thickness, subretinal fluid, and pigment epithelial detachment.
- **OCT angiography (OCTA)**: For detecting choroidal neovascularization.
- **Indocyanine green angiography (ICGA)**: For visualizing pachyvessels and other choroidal abnormalities

OCT scans play a critical role in diagnosing and distinguishing between the various disorders within the pachychoroid spectrum.

The OCT features specific to the pachychoroid spectrum include:

Key OCT Features:

- **Increased choroidal thickness**:
  - *Enhanced depth imaging-OCT (EDI-OCT)* reveals an increase subfoveal choroidal thickness (>350 microns),
  - This is a *hallmark feature across all pachychoroid diseases.*

- **Pachyvessels**:
  - *Dilated choroidal vessels (>200 microns)* in the outer choroidal layer are visible on EDI-OCT scans. Seen across all pachychoroid diseases.
- **Subretinal fluid (SRF)**:
  - SRF accumulation between the neurosensory retina and RPE layers is one of the defining features. Seen in CSCR, PNV & PCV.
- **Pigment epithelial detachment (PED)**:
  - *Pigment Epithelial Detachments (PEDs)* is the separation of RPE from the Bruch's membrane. It can be a serous PED or flat & irregular PED (FIPED) often accompanied by neovascularization beneath the RPE – "double-layer sign (DLS)".
  - PPE & CSCR: serous PED
  - PNV & PVV will have FIPED/DLS
- **Retinal pigment epithelium (RPE) Changes**:
  - In conditions like *Pachychoroid Pigment Epitheliopathy (PPE)*, subtle RPE changes such as *hyperreflective foci* and *irregularities* are observed without significant subretinal fluid.
- **Neovascularization**:
  - *Choroidal Neovascularization (CNV)* is prominent in pachychoroid neovasculopathy (PNV) and is visualized as a hyperreflective area beneath the RPE on OCT, often accompanied by fluid or hemorrhage.
- **Polypoidal Lesions**:
  - *Polypoidal Choroidal Vasculopathy (PCV)* presents with characteristic polyp-like ovoid structures beneath tall rising thumb like or notched PED seen on OCT, often associated with branching vascular networks (BVN) identified by FIPED/DLS just next to tall rising PED. These are best visualized with the help of additional imaging like indocyanine green angiography (ICGA).

Each condition's OCT appearance can overlap with others, making multimodal imaging important for accurate diagnosis.

Representative Images (Figs. 12 and 13)

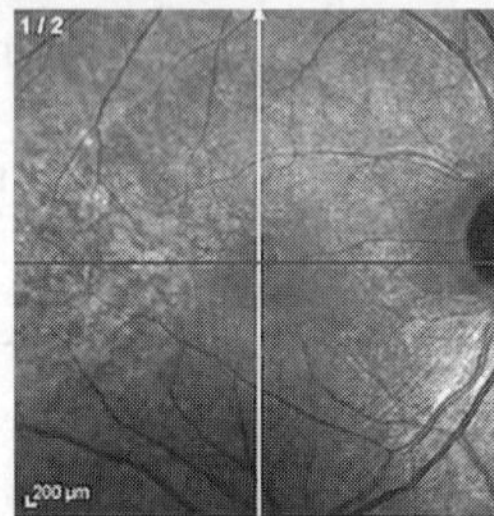

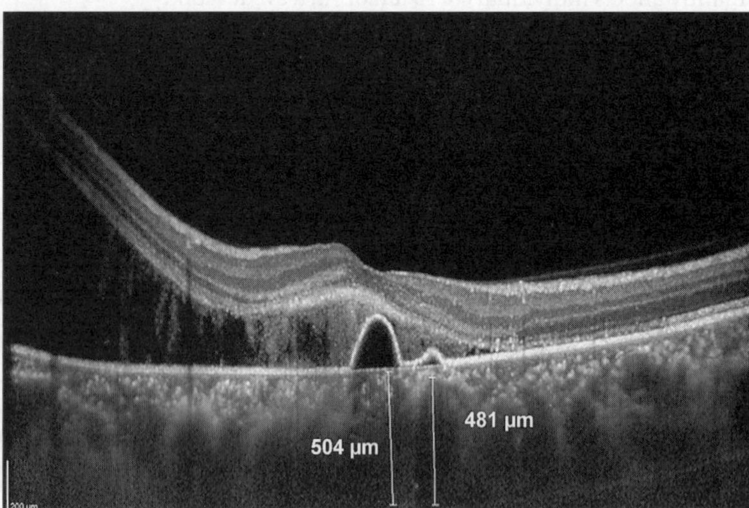

Fig. 12: Multimodal imaging.

One can see:

- NSD with fibrinous SRF
- PED with "Double—layer sign"/FIPED
- SFCT > 350 µm: Pachychoroid
- Dilated Large Choroidal Vessels (>200 µ)

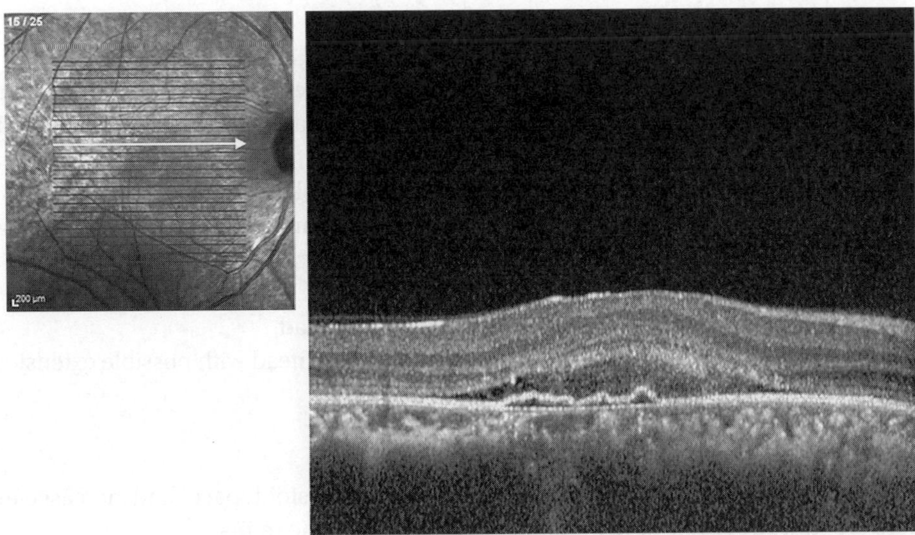

Fig. 13: Optical coherence tomography (OCT) multimodal imaging.

One can see:

- Fibrinous SRF with NSD
- "Double - layer sign"/FIPED

11. Optic disc pit maculopathy- clinical features, evaluation and management. (3+2+5) (DNB 2023)

Optic disk pit maculopathy (ODPM) is a rare eye condition associated with congenital optic disc pits, which are small, round, or oval depressions in the optic nerve head. This condition can lead to maculopathy due to the accumulation of fluid in the retina, potentially affecting vision. Below is a summary of the clinical features, evaluation, and management strategies for ODPM **(Figs. 14A to D)**.

Clinical features

- *Optic Disc Pit (ODP):*
  - *Location:* Typically located temporally on the optic disc.
  - *Appearance:* Greyish or whitish depression on the optic disk, often unilateral.
  - *Association with Maculopathy:* In approximately 40–50% of cases, optic disc pits are associated with maculopathy.
- *Maculopathy:*
  - *Serous Retinal Detachment (SRD):* The most common feature, characterized by fluid accumulation under the retina.
  - *Schisis-like cavity:* Splitting of the retinal layers, typically in the inner layers.
  - *Vitreomacular Traction (VMT):* May occur and contribute to maculopathy.
- *Symptoms:*
  - *Visual Loss:* Gradual, painless vision loss in the affected eye.
  - *Central Scotoma:* A central area of vision loss due to macular involvement.
  - *Metamorphopsia:* Distortion of vision.

Evaluation

- *Clinical examination:*
  - *Fundus examination:* Direct visualization of the optic disc pit and associated maculopathy.
- *Optical coherence tomography (OCT):* Optical Coherence Tomography (OCT) is a crucial imaging tool for evaluating optic disc maculopathy. It provides high-resolution cross-sectional images of the retina, allowing detailed assessment of retinal layers and associated abnormalities. Here are the key OCT features commonly observed in optic disk maculopathy:

1. *Serous retinal detachment (SRD)*
   - *Description:* Accumulation of fluid beneath the retina.
   - *OCT Appearance:* Hyperreflective fluid located between the retinal pigment epithelium (RPE) and the neurosensory retina. The detachment is typically seen in the macula but can also extend toward the periphery.
2. *Retinoschisis*
   - *Description:* Splitting of the retinal layers, often affecting the outer plexiform layer.
   - *OCT appearance:* Presence of two or more hyperreflective lines separated by a hyporeflective space, representing the split retinal layers. This can be seen as a "split" or "schisis" cavity.
3. *Optic Disc Pit*
   - *Description:* A congenital depression or defect in the optic nerve head.
   - *OCT appearance:* The pit is seen as a depression in the optic nerve head with possible extension into the retinal layers. Fluid may be seen extending from the pit into the macula.
4. *Macular Edema*
   - *Description:* Swelling of the macula due to fluid accumulation.
   - *OCT appearance:* Thickening of the macular area with intraretinal cystoid spaces and increased retinal reflectivity. Cystoid spaces are typically visible as hyperreflective areas within the retina.
5. *Vitreomacular traction (VMT)*
   - *Description:* Abnormal adhesion of the vitreous gel to the macula, causing traction.
   - *OCT appearance:* Presence of a hyperreflective line at the vitreomacular interface with possible distortion or wrinkling of the macular retina. This can lead to macular thickening or edema.
6. *Epiretinal membrane (ERM)*
   - *Description:* A thin layer of fibrous tissue on the retinal surface.
   - *OCT appearance:* Hyperreflective membrane on the surface of the retina, often associated with wrinkling or distortion of the retinal surface. This can cause macular distortion and edema.
7. *Internal limiting membrane (ILM) changes*
   - *Description:* Changes or damage to the innermost retinal layer.
   - *OCT appearance:* Alterations in the reflectivity or continuity of the ILM, especially in cases where ILM peeling has been performed as part of surgical intervention.

Management

The management of ODPM is challenging, and there is no standard treatment protocol. Options include:

- *Observation:*
  - *Indications:* For asymptomatic cases or those with minimal macular involvement and stable vision.
  - *Approach:* Regular monitoring with clinical examinations and OCT imaging to track any changes in the condition. If vision remains stable and macular involvement is minimal, intervention may not be necessary.
- *Pars plana vitrectomy (PPV)*
  - *Indications:* Often recommended for patients with significant macular involvement, such as extensive macular edema, serous retinal detachment, or retinoschisis.
  - *Procedure:*
    - *Vitrectomy*: Removal of the vitreous gel to relieve traction on the retina.
    - *Internal Limiting Membrane (ILM) Peeling:* Removal of the ILM to facilitate better retinal reattachment and fluid absorption.
    - *Gas tamponade:* Injection of a gas bubble (e.g., SF6 or C3F8) into the vitreous cavity to help flatten the retina and promote reattachment.
    - *Postoperative Positioning:* Patients may need to maintain a specific head position (prone positioning) to optimize the effect of the gas bubble and aid in retinal reattachment.
- *Endolaser or retinopexy:*
  - *Indications:* Often used when there is persistent fluid accumulation or when additional stabilization is needed after vitrectomy.

- *Procedure:* Application of laser treatment around the optic disc pit combined with gas tamponade. This approach aims to seal the pit and reduce fluid leakage into the macula.

- *Prognosis:*
  - Visual prognosis varies. While some patients regain good visual acuity after treatment, others may have permanent vision loss due to chronic maculopathy.
  - *Long-Term Follow-Up:* Regular follow-up is essential to monitor for any recurrence of fluid accumulation or other complications.

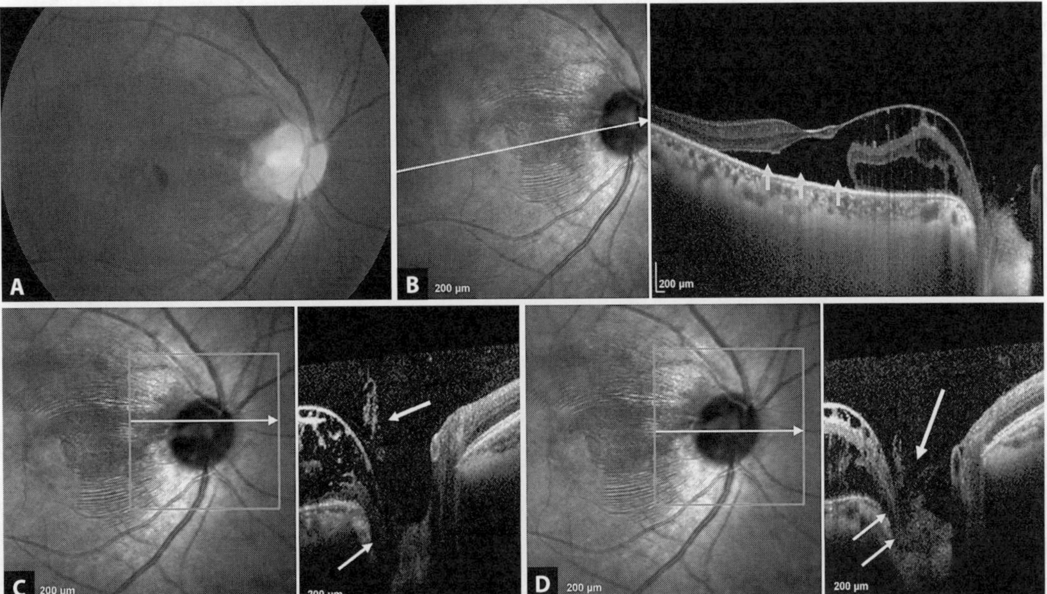

Figs. 14A to D: Preoperative images. (A) Digital fundus photograph of right eye showing macular neurosensory detachment with a pseudohole and greyish yellow double optic disc pits in the temporal segment; (B) Confocal scanning laser ophthalmoscope (cSLO) image of macula and optic disc showing the same; spectral domain optical coherence tomography (SD—OCT) along the green line shows schisis—detachment (yellow arrows), outer layer hole, retinoschisis of inner, middle and outer retina; (C) cSLO and SD—OCT images of superior pit show communication between perineural and intraretinal spaces (red arrows) and a hyperreflective membrane or glial tissue overlying the pit (blue arrow); (D) cSLO and SD—OCT images of inferior pit show communication between perineural and intraretinal spaces (red arrows) and a glial tissue overlying the pit (orange arrow). *(For Color version, See Color Plate 10)*

12. Describe causes, diagnosis, management, and prognostic features of submacular hemorrhage. (WBUHS MS 2023)

Definition

Submacular hemorrhage (SMH) is defined as the presence of blood in the space between the retinal pigment epithelium (RPE) and the neurosensory retina at the macular area arising from choroidal and retinal vessel abnormalities

Causes

There are several pathologies that can be associated with subretinal hemorrhage. The differential diagnosis for subretinal hemorrhage is listed below:

- Choroidal Neovascularization (CNV): The new vessels may rupture leading to SMH. CNV leading to SMH can be seen in following settings
  - Age related macular degeneration, AMD (CNV type 1, under the RPE); (CNV type 2, under the neurosensory retina); (CNV type 3, RAP lesion)
  - High myopia

  - Trauma (choroidal rupture leading to CNV)
  - Angioid streaks
  - Inflammation of the retina/choroid, including punctate inner choroidopathy (PIC).
  - Idiopathic
- Surgical trauma in the following settings can lead to SMH:
  - Drainage of subretinal fluid in scleral buckle procedures
  - Inadvertent scleral perforation (strabismus, AGV, and Baerveldt)
  - During radioactive plaque placement in melanomas
  - Laser photocoagulation with high power can lead to retinal/choroidal bleed.
- Penetrating and Blunt ocular trauma: Can lead to choroidal/retinal vessel rupture
- Other:
  - Ruptured retinal artery macroaneurysm (classically multi-layered hemorrhage including sub-ILM)
  - Sickle cell disease
  - Necrotic tumors
  - Coagulopathies
  - Central retinal vein occlusion rarely can have SMH
  - Diabetic retinopathy

Pathogenesis of Retinal Damage and Visual loss - experimental studies in animal models have shown visual damage happens due to:

- Stripping/shearing of photoreceptor outer segments due to clot contraction
- Toxic effect of iron (oxidative stress to the photoreceptors with subsequent photoreceptor apoptosis)
- Establishment of diffusion barrier between RPE and neurosensory retina (blocks the bidirectional nutrient exchange)

Diagnosis of Submacular Hemorrhage

A comprehensive ophthalmic examination is essential to diagnose submacular hemorrhage, and this often includes the following:

- *Clinical Examination:*
  - Fundus examination through direct ophthalmoscopy or slit-lamp biomicroscopy is used to visualize the macula and the extent of hemorrhage
  - The hemorrhage may appear as a red or dark patch under the macula, and it may be associated with retinal edema or exudates
- *Fluorescein Angiography (FA):*
  - FA can help identify the underlying cause of the hemorrhage, such as choroidal neovascularization or retinal vascular abnormalities. It also helps assess the leakage and the extent of vascular abnormalities
- *Optical Coherence Tomography (OCT):*
  - OCT can provide high-resolution images of the retina, allowing for visualization of the hemorrhage's depth, location, and effect on the macula. It can also help detect associated macular edema or retinal fluid
- *Indocyanine Green Angiography (ICGA):*
  - ICGA is especially useful for evaluating choroidal neovascularization (CNV), which may not always be well-demonstrated on fluorescein angiography
- *Fundus Autofluorescence:*
  - Can provide insight into the health of the retinal pigment epithelium (RPE) and help detect any macular atrophy or pigmentary changes that may have occurred as a result of the hemorrhage.

Prognosis

Natural history series of SMH show variable visual outcomes, largely dependent on etiology of SMH and its location with respect to the fovea.

Reported visual outcomes in eyes with SMH are variable.

Factors associated with a poorer visual prognosis may include:

- Presence of CNV
- Thicker SRH
- Larger hemorrhage
- Old SMH - >2 weeks old
- Untreated SMH

Good visual outcome is sometimes possible in select patients with small SMH, early intervention and mostly those managed without surgical intervention.

Treatment modalities:

- *Surgical removal of SMH without tPA*
  - Extraction of SMH may be traumatic when large retinotomies are created and shearing forces during mechanical extraction of the clot.
  - Major complications include disciform scarring and PVR with recurrent RD
- *Surgical removal of SMH with tPA*
  - *Tissue plasminogen activator (tPA)* is a serine protease with fibrin-specific thrombolytic activity that forms a complex with fibrin to activate plasminogen to plasmin which then cleaves fibrin and dissolves the clot.
  - Proposed but not proven benefit of intravitreal tPA to hasten clot lysis prior to surgical extraction of hemorrhage
  - Advantages may include smaller retinotomy and less traumatic surgery (less trauma by the photoreceptors by dissolving fibrin clot with tPA)
  - Potential toxic effect of tPA must be kept in mind (safe dose is about 25-50 ug per injection in humans); toxicity may result in RPE changes, exudative RDs, recurrent hemorrhages in vitreous cavity and hyphema.
- *Submacular surgery trials*
  - Group B: NEI sponsored, randomized clinical trial comparing submacular surgery versus observation for treatment of large submacular hemorrhage secondary to subfoveal CNV related to nAMD—No benefit of submacular surgery for CNV-associated submacular hemorrhage in nAMD patients over observation alone.
  - Complication rate (cataracts, rhegmatogenous retinal detachment, and proliferative vitreoretinopathy) much higher in surgery arm relative to observation.
- *Macular translocation*
  - PPV followed by circumferential peripheral retinotomy, evacuation of SMH and macular rotation +/- RPE patch grafting.
  - Results are variable with improvement in BCVA observed in patients with severe macular hemorrhage and vision loss
  - Proliferative vitreoretinopathy, recurrence of choroidal neovascularization, cataracts and recurrent retinal detachment are main complications
- *Pneumatic displacement:*
  - IV injection of expansile (SF6/C3f8) gas that requires prone positioning for several hours, followed by face down positioning for 3-4 days
  - Efficacy in improving BCVA with pneumatic displacement in combination with IV tPA and/or anti-VEGFs are encouraging; the positioning requirement limits usefulness in older patients
- *Use of anti-VEGF agents in SMH*
  - *Thin* and *extrafoveal SMH* is best treated with intravitreal anti-VEGF agents alone (*ranibizumab, aflibercept,* or *bevacizumab*)
  - Intravitreal anti-VEGF therapy alone or in combination with pneumatic displacement strategies can preserve and improve visual acuity in patients with SMH due to CNV related to nAMD.

SUGGESTED READING

1. Gass JD, Sever RJ, Sparks D, Goren J. A combined technique of fluorescein fundoscopy and angiography of the eye. Arch Ophthalmol. 1967;78(4):455-61.
2. Gologorsky D, Rosen R. Principles of Ocular Imaging. United States: CRC Press Ltd.; 2024.
3. Guyer DR, Yannuzzi LA, Slakter JS, Sorenson JA, Hanutsaha P, Spaide RF, et al. Classification of choroidal neovascularizaton by digital indocyanine green videoangiography. Ophthalmology. 1996;103:2054-60.
4. Owens SL. Indocyanine green angiography. Br J Ophthalmol. 1996;80(3):263.
5. Stanga PE, Lim JI, Hamilton P. Indocyanine green angiography in chorioretinal diseases: indications and interpretation: an evidence-based update. Ophthalmology. 2003;110(1):15-21.
6. Yannuzzi LA, Rohrer KT, Tindel LJ, Sobel RS, Costanza MA, Shields W, et al. Fluorescein angiography complication survey. Ophthalmology. 1986;93(5):611-7.

CHAPTER

Strabismus

Suman Mukherjee, Anchal Mitra, Erum Hayet

QUESTIONS

1. **Describe sensory and motor adaptations to strabismus.** **(10) (DNB 2020)**
2. **Define anomalous retinal correspondence (ARC). Explain its development and methods to evaluate ARC.** **(10) (DNB 2019)**
3. **Define Amblyopia. Briefly discuss the classification and management.** **(10) WBUHS MS 2023**
4. **Define and classify esotropia. Discuss clinical features and management of essential infantile esotropia.** **(10) (WBUHS MS 2018, 2023)**
5. **How will you manage a case of 5-year-old boy with esotropia?** **(WBUHS MS 2016, 2024)**
6. **A 7-year-old child presented with intermittent exotropia. Discuss the evaluation and management.** **(10) (WBUHS MS 2021)**
7. **What is intermittent exotropia? What are the indications for surgery? What are the available surgical options?** **(2 + 3 + 5) (DNB 2023)**
8. **Nystagmus short note.** **(5) (WBUHS MS 2019)**
9. **Briefly discuss about Duane retraction syndrome.** **(10) (WBUHS DO 2019)**
10. **Discuss the diagnosis and management of dissociated vertical divergence. How will you differentiate from inferior oblique overaction.** **(10) (DNB 2018)**
11. **Indication and principles of inferior oblique weakening procedure. Write a short note.** **(5) (DNB 2018)**
12. **Muscle transposition in paralytic strabismus. Write a short note.** **(5) (TNMGRMU MS 2022)**
13. **Discuss the complications of strabismus surgery.** **(10) (WBUHS MS 2015, 2023)**

1. Describe sensory and motor adaptations to strabismus. (10) (DNB 2020)

Sensory adaptations to strabismus

The ocular sensory system in children 6–8 years has the ability to adapt to anomalous states of confusion and diplopia. These occur in the age group 6–8 years because the plasticity of the developing visual system.

Binocular vision is embarrassed in two ways:

- Diplopia
- Confusion

The visual system copes in two ways:

- Suppression
- ARC

Suppression is a binocular sensory adaptation that occurs when the patient is using both eyes in the presence of strabismus. It is binocular innate and transient phenomenon.

Stimuli for suppression include Diplopia, confusion and burred image from one eye. Suppression can be categorized as

- Central or peripheral - In central suppression the image from fovea of the deviating eye is suppressed to avoid confusion. In peripheral suppression the image from peripheral retina of deviating eye is suppressed to avoid diplopia.

Monocular of alternating monocular suppression always develops in the deviating eye when image formation of deviating eye is constantly suppressed alternating suppression develops in alternating squints and in the cases, amblyopia is less likely to develop.

Facultative or obligatory facultative suppression happens when eyes are misaligned, and obligatory suppression happens at all times.

Suppression can be tested with the following methods.

- Worth 4-dot test
- Bagolini striate lenses
- Synaptophore
- Red filter test
- Four base-out prism test

Suppression should be appropriately treated with appropriate refraction and proper alignment of eyes, simultaneously with treatment of amblyopia.

Abnormal Retinal Correspondence

ARC is a condition in which non corresponding retinal element acquire a common subjecting visual direction, i.e., fusion occurs in the presence of small angle manifest squint.

There are three types of ARC

- Harmonious -Where the angle of anomaly = angle of strabismus
- Unharmonious–Where angle of anomaly is less than angle of strabismus
- Paradoxical - If angle of anomaly is in opposite direction .

Features of ARC

- Fovea of fixating aye is paired with non-foveal element
- It's a positive sensory adaptation
- Binocular responses in ARC are not as good as bifoveal BSV
- Usually happens in microtropia

Advantages of ARC

- Stabilizes the angle of strabismus
- Gives some level of BSV
- Gives some depth perception

ARC can be tested with

- Bagolini striate lenses
- Synaptophore
- Red filter test
- Worth 4 dot test

Motor Adaptations

- Motor adaptation to strabismus involves the adoption of a compensatory head posture (CHP) and occurs primarily in children to maintain BSV. In these children loss of a CHP may indicate loss of binocular function and the need for surgical intervention. Acquired paretic strabismus in adults may have a CHP to eliminate diplopia and helps to centralize the binocular visual field. The patient will turn the head into the direction of the field of action of the weak muscle, so that the eyes are then automatically turned the opposite direction.

- *A face turn* will be adopted to control a purely horizontal deviation. For example, if the left lateral rectus is paralyzed, diplopia will occur in the left gaze. The face will be turned to the left, which deviates the eyes to the right, away from the field of action of the weak muscle and area of diplopia. A face turn may also be adopted in a paresis of a vertically acting muscle to avoid the side where the vertical deviation is greatest (e.g. in a right superior oblique weakness the face is turned to the left).

  A head tilt is adopted to compensate for torsional and/or vertical diplopia. In a right superior oblique weakness, the right eye is relatively elevated, and the head is tilted to the left toward the hypotropic eye. This reduces the vertical separation of the diplopic images and permits fusion to be regained.
- *Chin elevation or depression* may be used to compensate for weakness of an elevator or depressor muscle or to minimize the horizontal deviation when an 'A' or 'V' pattern is present.

2. Define anomalous retinal correspondence (ARC). Explain its development and methods to evaluate ARC. (10) (DNB 2019)

ARC is a sensory adaptation that develops in strabismus patient where light from one point in space is being focused hits the fovea of one eye and hits an extra foveal retinal point in contralateral eye.

Development of ARC – The major cause of ARC is the foveal misalignment due to strabismus in most cases. The development of ARC depends upon the level of misalignment. Microtropia is a small angle strabismus (<10 PD) in which diplopia may not be present since ARC is able to occur. So horopter is an imaginary plane in an external space relative to both the observed eye for a given fixation target. All points on horopter stimulate corresponding retinal elements and are therefore seen singly in the same plane.

Pannum fusional space is a zone in front and behind the horopter in which objects stimulate slightly non corresponding retinal points. The objects in Pannum fusional space stimulate slightly dissimilar points on retina but still form a single image. In microtropia (<10 PD) the level of deviation due to strabismus is low enough and the motor misalignment is within the acceptable amount of error for each retinal point such that Diplopia is not found, and ARC takes place.

For ARC to take place, a neurological adaptation has to occur, and it has generally happened in childhood where the maturation of visual cortex has not yet occurred. It is thought that the adaptation that causes ARC occurs in the occipital cortex where image fusion happens, particularly in the primary visual cortex V1 where binocular neurons are found.

In terms of prevalence ARC is more common with micro strabismus (<10 PD) and in children with deviation of >40 PD. The prevalence of ARC is <16%. In addition, there is a higher chance of achieving ARC as an esotrope V/S and exotrope because anatomically there is greater input and territory in the visual cortex from the nasal retina compared to the temporal retina.

Types of ARC – ARC types depend upon objective and subjective angle.

- Harmonious ARC – the objective angle is equal to subjective angle.
- Unharmonic ARC – the subjective angle is less than objective angle
- Paradoxical ARC – if the localization of subjective and objective angles is crossed or uncrossed it is called paradoxical ARC. Objective angle is the motor deviation angle and subjective angle is the sensory deviation or how far the extrafoveal point is from the actual fovea.

Evaluation of ARC

Patients with ARC presents with strabismus and no diplopia. The severity of ARC can also differ depending on how strong the connection to the extrafoveal point is.

Diagnostic procedures for ARC

- Worth 4-dot test – If BSV is present all four dots are seen, if all four dots are seen with manifest deviation harmonious ARC is present.
- *Bagolini striated glass* – if the lines are seen intersecting at their centers to form an oblique cross with manifest deviation present then one can say that harmonious ARC is present.
- *Red filter test* – if a red is placed over the patient`s eye and an esotropic patient reports crossed diplopia or exotropic patient reports uncrossed diplopia then ARC may be present.

- *Synaptophore* – it can be used to assess the subjective and objective angle of deviation and any anomalies in binocular vision when an image is presented to each eye. A difference between the subjective and objective angle (the angle of anomaly) indicates that the patient has a form of ARC.

3. Define Amblyopia. Briefly discuss the classification and management. (10) (WBUHS MS 2023)

Definition: Amblyopia is clinically defined as reduction of visual acuity in one or both eyes, caused by abnormal binocular interaction during the critical period of visual development, that cannot be attributed to any ocular or visual system abnormality or to refractive error. Clinically amblyopia is present when an interocular difference of 2 lines or more in a visual acuity table (without specifying any), or visual acuity worse than or equal to 20/30 with the best optical correction.

Types of amblyopia

Amblyopia can be categorized based on its underlying causes, referred to as refractive, strabismic, visual deprivation, and occlusion (reverse).

Refractive amblyopia

Refractive amblyopia is caused by untreated refractive errors unilaterally or in both eyes.

This condition results from blurred visual input caused by hyperopia, astigmatism, or myopia, typically with a difference of refractive error exceeding 1 diopter (D) between the eyes.

Generally, eyes with hyperopia or astigmatism are more prone to developing amblyopia than myopia, as myopic eyes can still maintain a clear focus on nearby objects.

The first-line treatment for individuals with bilateral refractive amblyopia involves a thorough assessment of BCVA and the prescription of corrected lenses to fully correct the underlying refractive errors.

Strabismic amblyopia

This condition can develop when both eyes fail to align correctly. In pediatric cases, the brain employs a mechanism to prevent diplopia by suppressing the visual input from one eye, leading to impaired visual development in that eye. In these individuals, both retinas receive stimulation in noncorresponding areas, hindering the establishment of proper binocular vision and the fusion of images from both eyes.

In cases of amblyopia associated with strabismus, the tropia, or deviation of the eye from its normal position concerning the central line of vision, tends to be unequal and not alternating. Such conditions are usually observed in patients with esodeviations.

Visual deprivation amblyopia

Deprivation amblyopia occurs due to any pathology that obstructs the visual pathway, leading to partial or complete blockage and consequently causing blurred or degraded images to be projected onto the retina. Various factors, including early-onset or congenital cataracts, corneal opacity intraocular inflammation of either noninfectious or infectious origin, vitreous hemorrhage, retina damage, optic nerve pathologies, or ptosis.

Although deprivation is the least common form of amblyopia, it tends to be the most severe and challenging form to treat. The prognosis for patients with this condition is usually more favorable when early intervention (within the first 2 months of age) is undertaken, particularly in cases involving the removal of cataracts or the cause of the optical opacity.

Mixed amblyopia

Amblyopia is considered mixed when caused by two amblyogenic factors. Combination of anisometropic and strabismic amblyopia is common, especially in partially accommodative esotropia, microtropia, and monofixation syndrome.

Occlusion or reverse amblyopia

Occlusion amblyopia is uncommon, resulting from prolonged visual deprivation in the healthy eye, often induced by pharmaceutical cycloplegia or therapeutic patching. Visual acuity typically returns to normal once atropine or patching is discontinued, and optimal refractive correction spectacles are used for the healthy eye.

The severity of resulting amblyopia tends to be more pronounced when the degree of visual deprivation is greater. The critical period for visual development is primarily concentrated within the first 7 years of life, with the initial few years and even months being particularly critical. Delaying the start of amblyopia treatment makes it increasingly challenging to achieve clinical reversal of the condition.

Management

Examination

A comprehensive ocular eye examination should encompass the following:
- Binocular and stereoacuity testing
- Ocular alignment, fixation, and motility
- Cycloplegic Refraction and BCVA
- Anterior segment assessment
- Fundus examination

Treatment
- Cycloplegic refraction and full correction of error - Optical correction alone is successful in improving the amblyopia in nearly 1/3 of patients (anisometropic, strabismic, or mixed)
- Occlusion therapy for non-preferred eye
- For non-compliant children, penalization therapy (optical/pharmacological)
- Surgery for visual deprivation amblyopia

Patching
- The gold standard treatment for amblyopia is patching the better eye to force the brain to use the weaker eye. Depriving the fellow/fixating eye of vision forces the amblyopic eye to strike suppression and to use the visual cortex corresponding to the eye to recover connections for better vision.
- In 3–7 years children with severe amblyopia (vision 6/30–6/60) – full time patching has same result as 6 hrs of patching.
- In 3–7 years of children with moderate amblyopia (vision 6/12 or more) – patching for 2 hours has same result as 6 hours of patching.
- Patching hours should include at least 1 hour of near work.
- Amblyopia treatment in children of 7–12 years of age for 2–6 hours can be beneficial even if earlier treatment is taken.
- Treatment in children 13–17 years of age might be beneficial if not been treated earlier.

Penalization

A cycloplegic drug, typically atropine, can inhibit accommodation in the eye without amblyopia.

Neuropharmacological treatment- citicoline, levodopa. Carbidopa is found to be effective

- *Newer treatment*

  Perceptual learning: Perceptual learning (PL) is based on the principle that performance of sensory tasks can be improved with practice. Helps in facilitating the neural connections at the cortical level. Revital vision is non-invasive software using Gabor patches, *CAM Vision stimulator*- amblyopic eye is stimulated by slowly rotating high contrast, square wave grating of different spatial frequency for 7 minutes.

  Dichoptic therapy: The aim of binocular treatment is to not only improve visual acuity of the amblyopic eye but also restore binocular fusion and stereopsis. BYNOCS -Advanced AI Based Therapy for Amblyopia Through Digital Games & Activities, Dig Rush, games–anaglyph glasses are used.

End point of medical therapy
- Stabilization of vision
- Equalization of vision in both eyes.
- Freely alternating fixation with equal vision in strabismic amblyopia.
- With achievement of end point, patching is slowly withdrawn depending upon recurrence in the individual child.

4. Define and classify esotropia. Discuss clinical features and management of essential infantile esotropia. **(10) (WBUHS MS 2018, 2023)**

Definition

Esotropia is defined as misalignment of eyes in which one eye deviates toward the nose. The tern "esotropia" is derived from the Greek word where "eso" means within and tropia means "a turn".

Types of Esodeviations

Incomitant

Paralytic

- Neurogenic (e.g. abducens palsy, divergence palsy)
- Myogenic (e.g. myasthenia)

Restrictive

- Musculofascial (e.g. Duane's)
- Other restrictive conditions (tumor, postoperative, dysthyroid, strabismus fixus)

Spastic

Concomitant

- *Accommodative:* Esodeviations due to excessive convergence associated with accommodation are called accommodative esotropia
  - *Refractive (hypermetropic)*
    - Normo-accommodative (normal AC/A ratio)
    - Hyper-accommodative (high AC/A ratio)
  - *Nonrefractive, hyperaccommodative*
    - Hyper-accommodative (high AC/A ratio)
    - Hypo-accommodative (normal AC/A ratio, weak accommodative mechanism) hypoaccommodative
- *Partially accommodative-* with associated nonaccommodative esotropia with or without convergence excess
- *Nonaccommodative*
  - Essential infantile
  - Essential acquired or late-onset
    - Basic
    - Convergence excess
    - Divergence insufficiency
  - Acute concomitant
  - Microtropia
  - Cyclic esotropia
  - Sensory esotropia
  - Nystagmus blockage syndrome
  - Esophoria

Essential Infantile Esotropia

Definition: Infantile esotropia is esotropia with an onset before the age of six months, with a constant, large angle of strabismus (> 30 PD) in the absence of nervous system disorders.

Clinical features

- *Large angle esotropia,* usually >30 prism diopters.
- *Free alternation* or *cross fixation* in alternators, and fixation preference of the normal eye in amblyopes.
- No significant refractive error *(deviation not contributed by refractive error)*.
- *No neurological defect.*

- Confirmed by *4–6 months.*
- May be associated with *inferior oblique overactions, nystagmus, or dissociated vertical deviations.* Inferior oblique overactions are associated with V-phenomenon.
- *Asymmetric optokinetic nystagmus.* This is an asymmetry of smooth pursuit movements: tracking of objects temporal to nasal is smooth while tracking nasal to temporal is cogwheel

Differential Diagnosis
- Pseudoesotropia
- Congenital 6th nerve palsy
- Type 1 Duane retraction syndrome
- Mobius syndrome
- Congenital fibrosis of extraocular muscles.

Management
- *Correction of refractive error:* Corrective lenses are often prescribed if the hyperopia is greater than 2.50 diopters and/or when there are 1.50 diopters or more of anisometropia.
- *Amblyopia treatment:* Amblyopia treatment is often reserved for those patients with a strong fixation preference. Unilateral preference of fixation or resistance of the child to allow covering one eye indicates amblyopia.
- *Medical therapy options:* Botulinum toxin (Botox®) has been suggested as an alternative to surgery in patients with small to medium angle esotropia. Botox® may also be used to augment the effects of extraocular muscle surgery.
- *Surgical therapy options:* Frequently, bilateral medial rectus recession is the initial surgery for infantile esotropia. Alternatively, recession and resection of horizontal eye muscles of the same eye may be preferred if there is amblyopia or an anatomic defect of one eye.

Parents should be made aware that the goal of treatment is to get the eyes aligned and encourage the best sensory development possible which might take >1 surgical procedure.

If signs of inferior oblique overaction are noted, surgical weakening of the inferior oblique muscle is usually performed simultaneously.

The other associated conditions of DVD and latent nystagmus usually appear late later in life and may be addressed surgically at that point.

Timing of Surgery

Large angle esotropia (constant deviation) should be operated at the earliest, 4–6 months of age, or once the diagnosis and the deviation and associated overactions can be assessed properly. Small angle esotropias are to be carefully monitored with proper hyperopic correction till about 6 months or till the examination can be done satisfactorily. Surgery done before two years of age results in better binocular vision and stereopsis.

Prognosis

Patients with infantile esotropia frequently have good vision despite reduced binocularity. Earlier surgery is associated with improved binocularity. Treatment of amblyopia, along with multiple surgeries, may be required to achieve the best visual and binocular outcomes.

5. How will you manage a case of 5-year-old boy with esotropia? (WBUHS MS 2016, 2024)

The management of a case of a 5-year-old boy with esotropia starts with a good evaluation of the esotropia and completes with proper history taking, classification and ocular examination. Esotropia is characterized by inward deviation of one or both the eyes.

- The deviation can be comitant or non-comitant. In comitant esotropia the variation between the angle of deviation is within 5Δ in different gazes.
- Esotropia can be unilateral or alternating or bilateral.
- The deviation may be constant or intermittent.

- A proper history taking of the 5-year-old boy along with parents should be done to ascertain the type of esotropia and the associated ocular condition.

Chief complaints: Diminution of vision, AHP and asthenopic symptoms associated or not.

History of Present Illness, Onset, and Duration

Esotropia can give us a clue so as to which type of esotropia the child has. Infantile esotropia generally develops within 6 months of birth and accommodative esotropia develops usually between 6 months to 7 years of age.

- History of asthenopia can indicate toward accommodative squint.
- History of squint recurring at regular intervals can indicate toward cyclical esotropia.
- History of poor general health or head injury or meningitis preceding esotropia can indicate toward acute onset esotropia.
- Antenatal history of smoking, drug/alcohol/smoking addiction has high probability of being associated with infantile esotropia.
- Birth history of Prematurity, seizures, developmental delay, hydrocephalous are all risk factors for infantile esotropia.

Ocular Examination

- External examination – epicanthal fold and broad nasal base may mimic pseudo-esotropia. Nystagmus should be noted. AHP can be present in DRS, congenital 6th nerve palsy.
- Assessment of visual acuity of a 5-year-old should be through Snellen's chart.
- Assessment of stereoacuity should be done through Randot stereogram or Titmus test.
- Cycloplegic refraction preferably with atropine should be done for all 5-year-old presenting with esotropia.
- Dilated fundus examination to look for associated cataracts, optic atrophy or macular degeneration.
- Measurement of Deviation with Hirsberg, cover-uncover test, Prism cover test. The deviation is generally larger than 30 PD in infantile esotropia and is constant for both distant and near. In accommodative esotropia the deviation varies between 20 and 40 PD and near deviation is larger than distant. Accommodative convergence is normally 3–5 PD per 1D of accommodation but in accommodative esotropia (non-refractive) it is more than that.
- Ocular movement – full versions and ductions should be elicited. Look for classical triad of DVD/inferior oblique overaction (IOOA) and latent nystagmus in infantile esotropia.
- Sensory anomalies and binocular function should be tested with Worth four dot/ Maddox rod/ Diplopia charting/ Fusional amplitudes/Hess charting.

Treatment

The treatment of a 5-year-old boy with esotropia will depend upon the type of esotropia diagnosed.

- For infantile esotropia the amblyopia component should be managed first with patching and glasses, the ocular misalignment should be managed subsequently with surgical intervention. The procedure can either be recession of both medial rectus or unilateral R&R.
- Refractive accommodative esotropia can be managed with full cycloplegic correction.
- For non-accommodative refractive esotropias with high AC/At ratio bifocals may be required.
- Residual esotropias can be managed with surgery.
- Cyclical esotropias can be surgically managed for acute onset esotropia, root cause should be found and eliminated
- High myopia esotropia may require surgical correction.

6. A 7-year-old child presented with intermittent exotropia. Discuss the evaluation and management. (10) (WBUHS MS 2021)

Intermittent exotropia is the outward deviation of eyes which happen intermittently under condition of visual inattention, bright light, fatigue or ill health. The eyes are straight with BSV at times and manifest with suppression at other times. It can be presented by long duration of exophorias.

Intermittent exotropia has been divided into:

- *Basic exotropia/nonspecific exotropia:* Angle of deviation is same for distal and near or the difference is not more than 10PD.
- *Divergence excess:* Distance deviation is 10PD or more than near deviation.
- *Simulated or pseudo-divergence excess:* In this type of IDS, the distance deviation is greater than near but after 30–60 min of monocular occlusion the difference is not there. This happens because of high AC/A ratio, or tenacious proximal convergence.
- *Convergence insufficiency:* Where near deviation is 10PD greater than distance deviation.

Regarding the evaluation of a child with IDS, a thorough history taking should be done. Age of onset, frequency of deviation, birth history, family history should be noted.

Physical Examination

- Visual acuity – age-appropriate method or Snellen chart here should be need for visual acuity assessment.
- Test of stereopsis and binocular vision should be assessed with tests like TNO test and worth 4-dot test.
- Pupillary examination and anterior segment examination should be done.
- Ocular motility and strabismus should be examined with Hirschberg, Krimsky, alternate cover test, and prism cover test.
- Cycloplegic refraction should be carried out and any refractive error should be corrected.
- Assess control of IDS
- Fundus examination should be carried out to detect any retinal vitreous pathology.
- Patch test should be carried out to alternate between true and simulated distance exotropia.

Treatment opinion included Nonsurgical management and surgical management:

Nonsurgical Management

- Observation for well controlled asymptomatic patient
- Correction of refractive errors sometime just correction of refractive error can improve control of intermittent exotropia
- Amblyopia if any should be treated with PTO. Alternate occlusion may be needed in patient with equal fixation preferences.
- Orthoptics – convergence exercises may be helpful in patients with convergence insufficiency or in those who have a remote near pout of convergence.

Surgical Management

Indications of surgery include

- >20 PD difference in near and distance angle of deviation
- Deteriorating control of IDS
- Increase in magnitude of deviation
- Decreasing stereoacuity
- Amblyopia development
- Cosmesis

Types of surgery

- U/L or B/L lateral rectus recession can be planned on basis of angle of deviation
- Recession – Resection procedure – U/L R&R with MR resection and LR recession can be performed. Especially in cases of amblyopic eye U/L R&R is preferred.
- MR resection – Specially in case of convergence insufficiency.
- In case of A&V pattern associated with inf oblique muscle may be weakened along with Horizontal muscle surgery.

Reported prognosis and success rates are good with the above surgeries for IDS. Long time follow up of patients are needed.

7. What is intermittent exotropia? What are the indications for surgery? What are the available surgical options? (2 + 3 + 5) (DNB 2023)

It is characterized by occasional outward deviation of one or alternate eyes. Frequency, duration of deviation, and control vary from individual to individual. Exotropia can be manifest or latent, if manifest it can be intermittent or constant. Intermittent exotropia is the most common form of manifest exotropia and is usually noticed parents in early childhood (2–5) years of age.

In children, it tends to manifest under conditions of fatigue, illness, daydreaming or inattentive, while in adults it can manifest after taking sedatives or intoxication.

Examination

Patients with intermittent exotropia typically have equal visual acuity in both eyes, although a fixation preference can be associated with strabismic amblyopia.

Ocular motility is typically full, and the deviation is comitant.

A full sensorimotor evaluation should be completed with strabismus measurements taken at distance and near and in all directions of gaze. A far distance (>6 m) measurement should be done.

Lateral incomitance- presence of difference in size of deviation in primary position and lateral gaze. It can occur primarily or as a result of past surgeries.

The classification of exotropia and the new castle scores are mentioned in **Tables 1 and 2**.

TABLE 1: Classification of exotropia.

Basic exotropia	The angle of the exodeviation measures the same at distance and at near.
Convergence insufficiency	The angle of the exodeviation measures greater at near than distance by ≥ 10 prism diopters.
True divergence excess	The angle of the exodeviation measures greater at distance than nearby ≥10 prism diopters.
Pseudodivergence excess	The angle of the exodeviation measures greater at distance than nearby ≥ 10 prism diopters but this difference becomes minimal after 60 minutes of monocular occlusion (patch test) or measurement of near angle with +3.00 diopter lenses.

TABLE 2: The Newcastle Score—quantitative method of ability to control the deviation based on home and clinic control.

Home control *Exotropia seen:*	
• Never	0
• <50% of time fixating at distance	1
• >50% of time fixating at distance	2
• <50% of time fixating at distance, also seen at near	3
Clinic control *Exotropia seen at near:*	
• Immediate realignment after dissociation	0
• Realignment with aid of blink or re-fixation	1
• Remains manifest after dissociation/prolonged fixation	2
• Manifests spontaneously	3
Exotropia seen at distance:	
• Immediate realignment after dissociation	0
• Realignment with aid of blink or re-fixation	1
• Remains manifest after dissociation/prolonged fixation	2
• Manifests spontaneously	3
Total score (home + near + distance) =	

Management

Non-surgical Treatment

The aim is to encourage the use of both the eyes together by elimination of suppression), aiding recognition of double vision when eyes are misaligned, and building fusional reserves to control the exodeviation. This may be preferred in patients with small (<20 prism diopter) deviations, very young patients in whom accurate measurements cannot be made, or surgical overcorrection could lead to amblyopia or loss of fixation.

- *Correction of refractive error:* Uncorrected refractive errors can impair fusion and thus lead to manifest deviations. Cycloplegic refraction should be done in all patients, and a trial of corrective lenses advised.
- *Orthoptics:* These may be used to improve the control of the deviation. The aim is to make the patient aware of the manifest deviation. *Convergence exercises* are helpful in patients with a remote near the point of convergence or who demonstrate poor fusional convergence amplitudes.

Active anti-suppression and diplopia awareness techniques are useful in patients with suppression.

- *Overcorrecting minus lenses:* This is based on the principle of stimulating accommodative convergence and thus reducing an exodeviation.
- *Part-time occlusion:* This is a passive anti-suppression technique, particularly useful for very young children. Alternate eye occlusion should be advised in patients with equal fixation patterns. This may result in improved control of the deviation.
- *Prismotherapy:* The conventional approach includes the use of a base in prism to enhance bifoveal stimulation. Large amounts of prisms are often required, which might deteriorate vision quality and lead to low compliance.

Signs of Progression

- Gradual loss of fusional control - increased frequency of manifest phase of squint.
- Increase in size of deviation
- Decrease of stereoacuity
- Development of suppression

Indications of Surgery

- Large angle deviation (>20 PD)
- Signs of progression
- Failure of conservative therapy
- Poor control of squint.

Surgical Options

- Unilateral medial rectus muscle resection combined with a lateral rectus muscle recession
- Bilateral lateral rectus muscle recessions.
- Augmented lateral rectus recession - true divergence excess
- Bilateral medial rectus resection- convergence insufficiency
- A or V patterns - oblique muscle surgeries or vertical shift of recti muscle
- Lateral Incomitance - Patients with preoperative lateral incomitance are likely to be overcorrected with surgery. Thus, reducing the amount of recession is suggested if the deviation in lateral gaze is 50% less than the deviation in the primary position.

Residual Exotropia

- Small residual exotropia -be managed with non-conservative measures.
- Optical correction - a full correction should be given for any underlying myopic refraction.
- Orthoptic exercises - anti suppression exercises or fusional exercises should be continued till alignment is obtained.
- Prismotherapy - base-in-prisms equal to fully neutralize the deviation may be helpful to avoid diplopia and maintain bifoveal fusion.

- Large residual exotropia (15–18 prism diopters) - Patients with a large residual exotropia in the first postoperative week will probably require additional surgery. It is better to wait for 8–12 weeks before re-operating for the residual exotropia. If the primary surgery was bilateral lateral rectus recession of 6 mm or less, re-recession of the lateral rectus might be planned. If the primary recession was >6 mm, bilateral medial rectus resections with a conservative approach might be planned, as overcorrections are common after resecting against a large recession.

8. Nystagmus short note. (5) (WBUHS MS 2019)

Definition

Nystagmus is the involuntary, to and fro, rhythmic, repeated eye movement in which the first phase is the slow phase which drifts away from the fixation followed by a ref-fixation fast phase.

Types

- Horizontal jerk nystagmus – slow phase > fast phase
- Pendular nystagmus – slow phase = fast phase
- Torsional nystagmus – has a rotatory component

Classification (Old)

- *Physiologic nystagmus*
  - End-point nystagmus
  - Vestibular (caloric or rotational) nystagmus
  - Optokinetic nystagmus
  - Voluntary nystagmus

Pathologic Nystagmus

- Nystagmus associated with poor vision – retinal disease, ON hypoplasia, ant segment abnormality
- Nystagmus associated with neurologic diseases (motor)
- Nystagmus associated with strabismus -Latent/Manifest-latent nystagmus, Manifest nystagmus, Nystagmus blockage syndrome
- Miscellaneous – spasmus nutans, PAN

Nystagmoid Conditions

- Oculopalatal myoclonus
- Opsoclonus
- Ocular bobbing
- Heimann–Bielschowsky's unilateral vertical bobbing

CEMAS Classification

Classification of Eye Movement Abnormalities and Strabismus (CEMAS) Involuntary Ocular Oscillations

1. *Peripheral Vestibular Imbalance*
   Meniere, Drug toxicity
2. *Central Vestibular Imbalance*
   Downbeat, Upbeat, Drug toxicity
3. *Instability of Vestibular Mechanisms*
   Periodic Alternating Nystagmus
4. *Disorders of Visual Fixation*
   Vision Loss, See-Saw Nystagmus, Drug toxicity
5. *Disorders of Gaze Holding*
   Gaze Evoked, Acquired Pendular, Drug toxicity
6. *Acquired Pendular Nystagmus*
   Central myelin, Oculopalatal, Whipple, Drug toxicity
7. *Saccadic Intrusions and Oscillations*
   Square Wave Jerks, Macro-saccadic oscillations, opsoclonus, flutter, pulses

8. *Miscellaneous Eye Movements*
   Superior Oblique Myokymia, Ocular motor neuromyotonia
9. *Infantile Nystagmus Syndrome*
   Congenital, motor, sensory, idiopathic, nystagmus blockage
10. *Fusion Maldevelopment Nystagmus Syndrome*
    Old "Latent, manifest latent," nystagmus blockage
11. *Spasmus Nutans Syndrome*
    Without optic pathway glioma
    With optic pathway glioma

Approach to a Case of Nsytagmus

- *History*
  - Onset?
  - *Visual behavior:* Does the child hold objects very close?
    - Able to grasp toys/objects?
    - Behavior with familiar/unfamiliar faces
  - *Is there day-night disparity in vision?*
    - Difficulty in dim illumination- rod dystrophies
    - Difficulty in bright illumination- Cone dystrophies/achromatopsia
  - *AHP* (GOOD sign) – (indicates that the child has a null point, hence functional vision fixation)
  - *Oculodigital sign* (POOR vision)- LCA, advanced ROP
  - Oscillopsia? Head bobbing?
  - Birth history, Developmental history, neurological history
- *Assessment of visual acuity*
  - Monocular vision – with Spielmann occluder, fogging with +3.50 to +5.00 lens
  - Binocular vision
  - Near vision
- *Measurement of abnormal head posture by goniometer*
- *Examination - to rule out sensory cause*
  - *Anterior segment* -total cataract, corneal opacity, coloboma, aniridia
  - *Posterior segment* – retinal dystrophy, disc pallor, foveal hypoplasia, coloboma
- *Investigation* –
  - ERG-INS with poor vision, severe photophobia, bilateral high myopia, Oculodigital sign, Paradoxical pupil
  - MRI-ON atrophy, ON abnormality, Neurological sign, Spasmus nutans, See-saw nystagmus
- *Treatment*:
  - *Optical:*
    - Correction of refractive error with Glasses ± tints and Contact lens
    - Prisms- yoked prism places the eyes in null position abolishing the need of AHP. The base of prism is always toward the AHP.
    - For convergence null- B/L base out prisms with – 1.00 Ds lenses to stimulate convergence
  - *Medical:*
    - Gabapentin, memantine
    - Topical brinzolamide to improve foveation
    - Chemodenervation with Botulinum toxin in ocular muscles
  - *Surgical – to correct face turn; turns the eyes in the direction of face turn*
    - *Anderson's procedure* – B/L Recession of yolk muscle pair.
    - *Augmented Anderson procedure* – B/L Recession of yolk muscle pair (12 mm LR + 9 mm MR)
    - *Kestenbaum procedure* - B/L 5 mm Recession + 5 mm Resection (10 mm/eye). Recession of LR of the abducted eye and resection of MR of adducted eye.
    - *Park's modification of Kestenbaum (Classic Maximum)* – Rs and Rc of a total of 13 mm/eye (5, 6, 7, and 8)

9. Briefly discuss about Duane retraction syndrome. (10) (WBUHS DO 2019)

Duane Retraction syndrome (DRS) is a congenital motility disorder caused by the absence of partial development of the Abducent nerve and nucleus. There is aberrant innervation of the lateral rectus by the oculomotor nerve. Similar developmental anomalies of one or more cranial nerve have been grouped under congenital cranial dysinnervation disorder (CCDD).

Clinical Features

- Complete or less often partial absence of abduction
- Retraction of globe on adduction
- Narrowing of palpebral fissure during adduction (induced ptosis)
- Partial deficiency of adduction
- Upshoot or downshoot of globe with adduction (Leash Phenomenon)
- Widening of palpebral aperture with abduction
- Strabismus in primary gaze
- Compensatory head turn

Epidemiology

- More common in females than male
- 80% cases are unilateral, left more than right
- 70% cases are isolated
- 30% are associated with other congenital anomalies such as Okihiro syndrome, Wildervanck syndrome, Mobius syndrome, and Goldenhar syndrome

Types

- *Type 1*—abduction limitation, normal or minimally defective adduction, presents with an esotropia in primary gaze with a compensatory head turn to the involved side. This is the most common type.
- *Type 2*—adduction limitation, slight abduction limitation, presents with an exotropia in primary gaze with a compensatory head turn to the uninvolved side. Least common type.
- *Type 3*—limitation or complete absence of abduction or adduction. Can present with either esotropia or exotropia in primary gaze, and will have a compensatory head turn to the involved side.

Pathophysiology

A disturbance in the embryological development between 4 and 8 weeks of gestation results in an absent abducent nerve with anomalous innervation of the lateral rectus muscle by a division of oculomotor nerve.

Simultaneous co-contraction of the lateral rectus and medial rectus causes the globe contraction.

Management

- *Non-surgical management*
  - Spectacles/contact lenses to correct refractive error
  - Prism glasses to correct anomalous head posture
  - Botulinum toxin injection
- *Surgical management*

  The indications for surgical management are:
  - Abnormal head posture >15 degrees
  - Significant deviation in primary position
  - Significant upshoot or downshoot leading to palpebral fissure changes.
- Esotropic DRS
  - For small angles <20 PD
  - Single medial rectus recession
  - For large angles
  - B/L medial rectus recession

- Exotropic DRS
  - Small angles <20 PD
  - Single Lateral rectus recession
  - Large angles
  - B/L lateral rectus recession
- Upshoots/downshoots/globe retraction
  - Recession of Medial rectus and Lateral rectus
  - Y-split of Lateral rectus
  - Posterior fixation suture to LR
- Duction improvement- transposition of superior rectus/inferior rectus

10. Discuss the diagnosis and management of dissociated vertical divergence. How will you differentiate from inferior oblique overaction. (10) (DNB 2018)

DVD is an innervational disorder found in 50% patients with Infantile strabismus (Esotropia /Exotropia). It is typically associated nystagmus. It can happen several years after the initial strabismus surgery. DVD is characterized by updrift with Excyclotorsion of the eye when under cover or during periods of visual inattention. DVD is usually the most prominent component on Dissociated Strabismus complex.

Sometimes abduction is the most prominent and principal Dissociated movement, then it is called Dissociated horizontal Deviation (DHD). Sometimes, excyclotorsion is the most prominent Dissociated movement, then it is called as Dissociated torsional deviation.

The main characteristic of these dissociated vertical deviations is that these deviations violate Herring's law. No movement is seen in fixing eye when deviated eye returns to fixation.

DVDs are frequently Bilateral and asymmetric.

Signs and symptoms of DVD:

- No asthenopic and visual symptoms as eye is suppressed.
- Diplopia/confusion may occur
- Can be phoric or tropic
- On uncover the eye slowly drifts back
- Generally, bilateral and asymmetric
- Amblyopia can occur
- Cosmetic blemish
- Can be associated with long Eso, Intermittent Exo, Latent Nystagmus.

Measurement of DVD

- Hirsberg Test
- With Prism bars and translucent occludes. With occluded in place, base downward prism bar is introduced in increasing strength and the occlude is switched to other eye. This is repeated till the deviating Eye shows no vertical movement to refixate.
- Bielschowsky phenomenon – as intensity of light shown to the fixing eye is decreased the Dissociated eye comes down.
- Red glass test – If red glass is presented before any eye that eye dissociates.

Management of DVD

- *Non-surgical* –
  - Observation can be done in mild cases.
  - Refractive Error correction helps.
  - Encouraging fixation by DVD eye by occlusion of dominant eye can help.
- *Surgical* – Treatment is surgical if (>6–8 PD)

- The deviation is noticeable and occurs frequently during the day.
- If there is an increase in frequency of number of times DVD happens in a day.
- Increasing risk of Amblyopia with DVD.
- Poor control by AHD.

Surgical options available are:

- Unilateral DVDs can be treated with U/L vertical muscle surgeries.
- B/L asymmetric DVD should be treated by Bilateral vertical muscle surgeries. Superior rectus recession and Inferior rectus resections can be performed.

If inferior oblique overaction is present along with inferior oblique weakening. Procedures can be performed. Superior rectus (SR) recession can also be tried with Faden of SR.

The difference between IOOA and DVD are mentioned in **Table 3**.

TABLE 3: Difference between IOOA and DVD.

IOOA	*DVD*
• Happens in adduction and elevation	• Happens in primary position
• Associated V pattern in IOOA	• Nothing such
• Obeys Herring's Law	• Does not obey Herring' s law
• Rapid Refixation when cover is removed	• Slowly refixates
• Nothing such	• Red fitter glass test and Biclchowsky positive

11. Indication and principles of *inferior oblique* weakening procedure. Write a short note. (5) (DNB 2018)

Inferior oblique id a cyclo-vertical muscle originating from the orbital floor lateral to the nasolacrimal groove and inserting behind the equator under the lateral rectus insertion. It has close proximity to the inferior rectus and lateral rectus via the ligament of Lockwood. It is also closely related to the neuro-vascular bundle, optic nerve and the vortex vein.

Inferior oblique overaction manifests as over-elevation in adduction.

Indications for Inferior oblique weakening procedures are:

- Superior oblique paresis
- Inferior oblique over-action
- V-pattern horizontal strabismus with inferior oblique over-action
- Dissociated vertical deviation

Inferior oblique weakening procedures are:

- Recession
- Anterior- transposition
- Antero-nasal transposition
- Tenectomy
- Myotomy
- Disinsertion
- Extirpation

Steps of Isolating the inferior oblique muscle:

- Globe is retracted in superonasal quadrant
- Incision is made in inferotemporal quadrant 8 mm form limbus in bulbar conjunctiva and intermuscular septum.
- A perpendicular incision is made in the tenon's fascia to expose the bare sclera
- Under direct visualization, a muscle hook is placed under the belly of the muscle and the inferior oblique muscle is hooked and freed of all the attachment.

Myotomy –muscle is incised close to the insertion and allowed to retract without placing any sutures.

Myectomy – is a self-adjusting procedure in which 2 clamps are placed, one close to the insertion and the other 4–8 mm from the first clamp. The muscle is excised between the clamps and ends are cauterized to prevent bleeding.

Recession – the muscle is recessed and re-attached to the sclera along its course at a desired point. The basis is the more anterior the placement of IO, the more the muscle becomes a depressor.

- Park's point- the anterior end of IO is attached to 2 mm lateral and 3 mm posterior to the lateral end of inferior rectus muscle, and the posterior end is 5 mm posterior.
- Fink's recession – IO is inserted 8 m posterior and 2 mm inferior to the lateral rectus insertion.
- Elliot Nankin's recession – anterior end of IO is inserted at the lateral end of IR insertion and posterior end is 5 mm posterior.

Anterior transposition – IO is placed just below the anterior border of lateral rectus.

Total antero-positioning – IO is re-inserted anterior to the IR muscle. This weakens the elevator action and converts the muscle into a depressor.

Antero-nasal transposition – the new insertion is 2 mm nasal and 2 mm posterior to the nasal border of IR muscle insertion. This converts the IO muscle into an intorter and depressor and improves elevation in adduction.

Complications

- Anti-elevation syndrome – caused by misplacing of posterior fibers of inferior oblique too anteriorly and bunching of inferior oblique.
- Recurrent overaction–incomplete muscle capture, i.e., missed fibers of IO at insertion during hooking of the muscle. It is necessary to look for any missed muscle fibers along the bare sclera while hooking the muscle.
- Fat-adherence syndrome– excessive adipose tissue released by breach in tenon's capsule while exposing Inferior Oblique will lead to scarring and hemorrhage.
- Bleeding/hemorrhage– due to close proximity to vortex vein
- Injury to the macula – IO inserts close to the area of macula hence extreme caution should be taken to avoid perforation of sclera.

12. Muscle transposition in paralytic strabismus. Write a short note. (5) (TNMGRMU MS 2022)

Muscle transposition surgeries involve the redirection of the paths of extraocular muscle. Main indication of muscle transposition includes paralytic strabismus where force direction tests are free, and force regeneration reveals absence of any active force generation.

MOA: The main aim of transposition surgery is to realign eyes in primary position. It is believed that transposition causes a change in vector forces which aids in alignment of eyes in primary position.

Transposition procedures for 6th nerve palsy:

- *Full Tendon Transposition:* This involves dis insertion of full width tendons of vertical rectus muscles and transposition toward lateral rectus.
- *Crossed Adjustable Technique:* The transposed vertical rectus muscles are passed beneath the lateral rectus muscle and attached to respected opposite corners of lateral rectus muscle insertion.
- *Hummelsheim Procedure:* This involves the transposition of ½ tendon width of vertical rectus muscle reducing the risk of anterior segment ischemia by sparing half tendon width and its ciliary vessels.
- *Modified Hummelsheim:* When a simultaneous recession of MR muscle and or resection of transposed tendon is performed with Hummelsheim.
- *Jensen's procedure:* In this procedure muscle bellies of IR and SR are dissected and tied together with LR without being disinserted.
- *Nishida procedure:* In this technique vertical rectus muscles are hooked and split halfway till 15 mm. Following this the temporal half of muscle belly is secured 8 mm post to insertion. Following this the same sutures are then secured with sclera at a distance of 8 mm from origin of LR along the sup and inf edge.

- *Superior rectus transposition:* Transposing only SR muscle to LR
- *Inferior rectus transposition:* Only IR is transposed to insertion of LR

Transposition procedure for 3rd nerve palsy

- *Sup oblique tendon transposition:* The sup oblique tendon is exposed and disinserted and then sutured to the sclera at the sup border of medial rectus.
- *Lateral rectus to MR transposition:* The full tendon disinsertion and then attachment at MR origin can be done superior through SR muscle or inferiorly through IR muscle
- *Medial transposition with Y splitting:* The LR muscle is split halfway till 15 mm and disinserted upper half is passed through SR and lower half is passed through IR to get attached at MR insertion.

Transposition in vertical muscle palsy

- *Knapp's procedure:* Both MR and LR are disinserted and transposed superiorly
- *Modified Knapp:* Both horizontal recti are split halfway, and the sup halves are transposed to superior rectus.
- *Augmented Knapp's:* Along with post fixation suture.
- *Inverse Knapp's:* In case of double depressor palsy or absence of IR.

13. Discuss the complications of strabismus surgery. (10) (WBUHS MS 2015, 2023)

A perfect result from strabismus surgery includes minimum immediate postoperative discomfort, normal versions and ductions, no apparent conjunctival scars, orthotropia, and normal palpebral changes. Complications can occur during strabismus surgery which need to be diagnosed and treated early to optimize postoperative outcome.

Complications can be grouped as

1. Intraoperative anesthesia related complications
2. Intraopertaive surgical site complications
3. Postoperative surgical site complications
4. Postoperative strabismus complications

- *Intraoperative anesthesia related complications*
  - *Oculo-cardiac reflex*– reflex bradycardia due to compression of the extra-ocular muscle tendon stimulating the trigeminal nerve. The incidence of OCR is more with medial rectus muscle.
    It can be prevented by retro or peri- bulbar anesthetic block which blunts the afferent limb of the reflex arc. Intravenous anticholinergics like atropine or glycopyrrolate also decrease the incidence of oculo-cardiac reflex.
  - *Allergy*- hypersensitivity to anesthetic agents like suxamethonium.
  - *Cardiac arrest* - can occur due to underlying undetected cardiac disease.
- *Intraoperative surgical site related complications*
  - *Scleral perforation* –occurs passage of the suture needle through the sclera from an inadvertent deep pass
    Risk factors-thin sclera in high myopes with a staphyloma, very posterior suture placement, because it is more difficulty to visualize the suture and place at a proper depth.
    Good exposure of sclera and clear visibility of the needle tip all the time is required
    If perforation is suspected, a dilated fundus examination is required to identify potential retinal complications.
    Laser retinopexy should be performed at the time of surgery if a large retinal tear or small retinal tear in a patient with high risk of retinal detachment is noted
  - *Lost muscle* –occurs when the extra-ocular muscle slips free of the sutures or surgical instruments during surgery. There is no direct attachment between the muscle tendon and globe allowing the muscle and its capsule to retract posteriorly into the orbit.
  - *PITS*- (Pulled In two syndrome) –occurs when the muscle is torn at the junction of tendon and muscle belly resulting in loss of posterior muscle belly.
    More common in medial rectus muscle as it has no fascial attachments to the orbit.
    Attempts should be made to retrieve the muscle promptly, but in case it cannot be retrieved, a transposition surgery can be done.

- *Slipped muscle*– a slipped muscle occurs when less than full-thickness sutures are used to capture the muscle tendon, effectively only capturing the superficial muscular capsule instead of securing the muscle belly.

  More common in case where muscle is tight such as dysthyroid orbitopathy.

  A slipped muscle can be repaired during surgery by locating the muscle capsule attachment to the globe. The muscle can be traced in the muscle capsule posteriorly and attached to the globe.

- *Postoperative surgical site related complication* –
  - *Suture granuloma* – has become less common with better suture materials. Earlier silk sutures used to cause suture granulomas, but with vicryl sutures, the incidence has reduced. Topical corticosteroids for several weeks are used for treatment.
  - *Conjunctival incision*- when conjunctival epithelial cells are buried beneath the conjunctival surface during surgery.
  - *Dellen* – shallow, clearly defined excavations at the margins of the cornea or sclera. Any disruptions of the tear layer on the sclera or cornea can cause dehydration creating a dellen. Treated with lubricants.
  - *Conjunctival scarring* – the conjunctiva remains chronically hyperemic and pink. The risk is increased for a reoperation and after a surgical resection.
  - *Anterior segment ischemia*- occurs when blood supply to anterior segment is interrupted. Simultaneous surgery on three rectus muscles of the same eye can cause ASI. It presents with iritis, corneal edema and treated with topical and systemic corticosteroids to relieve inflammation.
  - *Palpebral fissure changes* – risk is more in subjects undergoing vertical rectus recessions or resections with high surgical doses, particularly inferior rectus.

    It can be minimized by limiting the surgical dosage of vertical rectus muscle and careful dissection of the lid retractors away from the extra-ocular muscles during surgery.

- *Postoperative surgical site related complication*
  - *Overcorrection and under corrections* – small residual under-corrections or consecutive exotropias can be managed by orthoptic fusional vergences or with prism glasses.

    A marked over correction after a recession may be due to slippage and managed without delay. The decision for re-surgery should be made after observing for a version for incomitance and FDT.
  - *Diplopia* – It happens in patients who can form vision with both eyes with imperfect vision alignment. Occurs more in over correction and complicated strabismus. Most of post op diplopia resolves with time but in 0.8% of patients it is intractable. Post op diplopia is more common in patients who complain of diplopia with preoperative prism testing. Diplopia can be prevented with careful assessment of binocular potential prior to surgery.

    Prism can be used in select cases to alleviate diplopia. Mono-ocular occlusion with a patch or occlusion foil may be used when prism is not effective.
  - *Iatrogenic brown syndrome:* Develops due to with excessive tightening of superior oblique (SO) muscle
  - *Anti elevation syndrome:* Restriction of elevation of eye in abduction with inferior oblique anteriorization

SUGGESTED READING

1. Hered RW. 2023-2024 Basic and Clinical Science Course™, Section 6: Pediatric Ophthalmology and Strabismus. American Academy of Ophthalmology; 2023.
2. Salmon JF. Kanski's Clinical ophthalmology, 9th edition. Elsevier; 2019. Chapter 18.
3. Sharma P. Strabismus Simplified. 2nd edition, 2019. New Delhi: CBS. Chapters 4-6.
4. Sharma P. Strabismus Simplified. 2nd edition, 2019. New Delhi: CBS. Chapters 7-12.
5. www.eyewiki.org. (2025). [online] Available from www.eyewiki.org [Last accessed March, 2025].

CHAPTER

Neuro-Ophthalmology

Suman Mukherjee, Soumyajit Guha, Rituparna Sarkar, Tiyasha Koner

QUESTIONS

1. **Describe the details of Anterior Ischemic Optic Neuropathy—Clinical features, evaluation, management, and differential diagnosis. (10) (WBUHS MS 2019)**
2. **Optic neuritis—causes, types, signs and symptoms, and treatment? (10) (TN MGRMU 2021)**
3. **What are the etiopathogenesis, management, differential diagnosis, and prognosis of a case of acute onset 3rd nerve palsy in a 56-year-old woman? (3 + 3 + 2 + 2) (DNB 2019, BHU MS 2020)**
4. **Horner's syndrome—cause, clinical features, and evaluation. (2 + 3 + 5) (WBUHS MS 2023)**
5. **Internuclear ophthalmoplegia. Discuss. (10) (DNB 2018, WBUHS MS 2022)**
6. **Clinical features, investigations, and treatments in case of neuromyelitis optica. (3 + 4 + 3) (DNB 2016)**
7. **Describe the causes and management of toxic optic neuropathy. (10) (MS WBUHS 2019, 2023)**
8. **Describe the clinical features and causes of papillitis. What are the differential diagnoses? (10) (MS 2021)**
9. **Describe the clinical features, evaluation, and management of Idiopathic intracranial hypertension. (3 + 3 + 4) (MS WBUHS 2021)**
10. **Describe the clinical features and management of ophthalmic migraine. (10) (MS WBUHS 2022)**
11. **Differential diagnosis of painful ophthalmoplegia in a 40-year-old woman. (10) (DNB 2022)**
12. **Discuss traumatic optic neuropathy. What is optic nerve fenestration surgery? (5 + 5) (DNB 2022)**
13. **Clinical features and management of superior oblique palsy. (10) (WBUHS MS 2019)**
14. **Optic atrophy—causes, classification, clinical features, and management. (10) (WBUHS DO 2018)**
15. **Enumerate the various ophthalmological causes of headache in an adult. How will you approach the patient? (10) (MS 2023)**
16. **What is disc edema? How is it different from papilledema? What are the common causes of optic disc edema? How do you differentiate papilledema from papillitis? (BHU MS 2021)**
17. **Discuss clinical features, field defects, and management of pituitary adenoma. (10) (DNB 2018)**
18. **Marcus Gunn Pupil-diagnosis, evaluation, management. (10) (TN MGRMU 2022)**
19. **Holmes Adie Pupil. (10) (DNB 2020)**
20. **Examination and management in a case of anisocoria. (10) (DNB 2021)**

1. Describe the details of Anterior Ischemic Optic Neuropathy—Clinical features, evaluation, management, and differential diagnosis. (10) (WBUHS MS 2019)

AION is the most common acute neuropathy in patients older than 50 years. Anterior Ischemic Optic Neuropathy may be due to arteritic (most common giant cell arteritis) or non-arteritic causes (e.g., hypertension, dyslipidemia, diabetes mellitus. Nocturnal hypotension etc.). Patients with AION experience monocular vision loss that develops over hours to days. Visual field loss always occurs. Inferior altitudinal visual field loss is the most common type. RAPD is present unless bilateral optic nerves are involved. Following features are helpful in distinguishing between them **(Table 1)**.

TABLE 1: Differentiating features between arteritic and non-arteritic AION.

Characteristic	***Arteritic features***	***Non-arteritic features***
Mean age	70 years	60 years
Sex	Female >> Male	Male and female equally affected
Associated symptoms	Headache, scalp tenderness, jaw claudication, and transient vision loss	Usually none, Painless vision loss
Visual acuity	<6/60 in >60% of cases	>6/60 in >60% of cases
ONH/Fundus findings	• Pallid ONH edema common • Cup normal or large • Cotton-wool spots • Choroidal or retinal ischemia	• Hyperemic ONH edema • Cup small
ESR	Elevated	Normal
CRP	Elevated	Normal
Platelet count	Elevated or normal	Normal
Fluorescein angiography findings	Delayed ONH and choroidal filling	Delayed ONH filling
Natural History	• Condition rarely improves, • Untreated fellow eye involved, 54–95% within 1–2 weeks	• 31% of cases improve • Fellow eye involved 15% at 5 years
Treatment	Systemic steroids	No definite treatment, control of hypertension, diabetes mellitus, dyslipidemia etc. improves prognosis

Treatment of AAION: When AAION due to GCA is suspected, immediate initiation of high dose corticosteroid therapy is crucial. Adjunctive daily Aspirin can also be prescribed. A temporal artery biopsy should be done to confirm the diagnosis as soon as possible. IV methylprednisolone (1g/day for the first 3-5 days) is usually recommended, followed by oral prednisolone (1 mg/kg/day) may be used, tapered slowly over 12 months or more, depending on response. Treatment should not be delayed to save the involvement of the fellow eye.

There is no proven prophylaxis for the fellow eye in case of non arteritic AION. Aspirin may be used to reduce the risk of secondary stroke. Systemic disease e.g., hypertension, dyslipidemia, diabetes mellitus, coagulopathy, sleep apnea must be treated if present.

Differential diagnosis:

- Arteritic AION
- Non-arteritic AION
- Idiopathic optic neuritis
- Optic nerve inflammation related to syphilis or sarcoidosis
- Infiltrative optic neuropathy
- Anterior orbital lesions with optic nerve compression
- Diabetic papillopathy

2. Optic neuritis—causes, types, signs and symptoms, and treatment? (10) (TN MGRMU 2021)

Causes of Optic Neuritis

Optic neuritis may be due to the following causes: Demyelinating, Parainfectious, Infectious, and Non-infectious inflammation.

Demyelinating optic neuritis: Myelinated optic nerve fibers lose their insulating myelin layer; hence nerve conduction is hampered. Demyelinating conditions that may involve the visual system include the following:

- Isolated optic neuritis (no clinical evidence of generalized demyelination)
- Multiple sclerosis (MS). Most common demyelinating disease.
- Devic disease (neuromyelitis optica). A rare autoimmune disease, autoantibodies form against aquaporin-4 protein in the cell membrane of astrocytes. It causes bilateral optic neuritis.
- Schilder disease. A very rare progressive generalized disease with early onset. It causes bilateral optic neuritis.

Parainfectious optic neuritis: Associated with viral infection such as measles, mumps, varicella zoster, whooping cough, may also occur following immunization. Children are commonly affected. Bilateral papillitis is the rule.

Infectious optic neuritis: Sinus-related optic neuritis is common. Sphenoethmoidal sinusitis may result into recurrent visual loss with severe headache. Infectious optic neuritis can also occur due to Cat-scratch disease (by Bartonella henselae), Syphilis (by Treponema pallidum), Lyme disease (by Borrelia burgdorferi), Cryptococcal meningitis, Varicella zoster virus infection.

Non-infectious optic neuritis: May be due to Neurosarcoidosis or autoimmune optic neuritis.

Neuroretinitis: Combination of optic neuritis and retinal, usually macular inflammation. May be due to cat-scratch disease (60%), idiopathic (25%), syphilis, Lyme disease, mumps etc.

Types of Optic Neuritis

According to ophthalmoscopic appearance, optic neuritis are of following types:

- *Retrobulbar neuritis:* Optic nerve head (ONH) is not involved. Most common type in adults and frequently associated with Multiple sclerosis (MS)
- *Papillitis:* Characterized by hyperemia and edema of the ONH, may be associated with peripapillary flame shaped hemorrhage. Most common type in children.
- *Neuroretinitis:* Characterized by papillitis in association with inflammation of the RNFL and macular star figure.

Sign and symptoms of optic neuritis

The clinical signs of optic neuritis are:

- Visual acuity (distance and near) impairment
- Dyschromatopsia
- Impaired contrast sensitivity
- Reduced stereoacuity
- Generalized depression of visual field, particularly pronounced centrally
- Relative afferent pupillary defect
- Optic disc hyperemia and edema.

Symptoms of optic neuritis: Patient generally presents with gradually progressing dimness of vision associated with pain (especially with upward and inward movement of eye). Other symptoms are impaired color vision, desaturated color vision, movement phosphene, visual obscuration in bright light, Uhthoff's phenomenon (episodic transient obscuration of vision with exertion) etc.

Treatment of Optic Neuritis

Demyelinating optic neuritis: Indications for steroid treatment are when visual acuity within the first week of onset is worse than 6/12, treatment may speed up recovery by 2-3 weeks and may delay the clinical onset of MS over short term.

Steroid regimen: Intravenous methylprednisolone sodium succinate 1 g daily for 3 days, followed by oral prednisolone (1 mg/kg daily) for 11 days, subsequently tapered over 3 days. Oral prednisolone may increase the risk of recurrence of optic neuritis if used without prior intravenous steroid.

Parainfectious optic neuritis: Prognosis for spontaneous visual recovery is very good and treatment is not required in the majority of cases. However, in case of severe visual loss or in bilateral involvement intravenous steroids should be considered with antiviral cover where appropriate.

Infectious optic neuritis: Associated sphenoethmoidal sinusitis is treated with systemic antibiotics, and surgical drainage if required.

Non-infectious optic neuritis: In case of neurosarcoidosis response to systemic steroid therapy is often rapid and patient requires long-term low dose therapy. Methotrexate may also be used as an adjunct or as monotherapy.

3. What are the etiopathogenesis, management, differential diagnosis, and prognosis of a case of acute onset 3rd nerve palsy in a 56-year-old woman? (3 + 3 + 2 + 2) (DNB 2019, BHU MS 2020)

An acute onset of oculomotor nerve palsy in a 56-year-old woman can present in different ways causing somatic extraocular muscle dysfunction (levator palpebrae superioris, superior, inferior and medial recti and inferior oblique) and autonomic muscles (Sphincter pupillae and ciliary). From its course from nucleus in the midbrain through basilar region, cavernous sinus and orbital cavity pathology to any segment can give rise to 3rd nerve palsy. Between the brain stem and the cavernous sinus, the pupillomotor parasympathetic fibers are located superficially in the superomedial part of the 3rd nerve. They derive their blood supply from the pial blood vessels (hence any surgical lesion, e.g., aneurysm, trauma, uncal herniation involve pupil), whereas the main interior trunk of the nerve is supplied by the vasa nervosum (Medical lesions, e.g., hypertension, diabetes usually spare pupil).

Etiology

Lesion of nucleus and fascicles: Ischemia, hemorrhage or metastatic infiltration.

In the basilar area

- Compression by any vascular aneurysm (posterior communicating artery at its junction with the ICA)
- Infiltrative (e.g., leukemia)
- Head trauma, resulting in extradural or subdural hematoma may cause a tentorial pressure cone with downward herniation of the temporal lobe. This compresses the 3rd nerve at the tentorial edge.

Intracavernous

- Diabetes
  - Pituitary apoplexy
- Pathology of cavernous sinus, like meningioma, carotid-cavernous fistula, granulomatous inflammation (Tolosa-Hunt syndrome). In this case due to their proximity 4th, 6th, and one division of Trigeminal nerve are often involved.

Intraorbital

- Any lesion at superficial orbital fissure (orbital apex syndrome)
  - Trauma

Differential diagnosis

- Myasthenia Gravis
- Thyroid associated orbitopathy
- Internuclear ophthalmoplegia
- Chronic progressive external ophthalmoplegia
- Orbital pseudotumor
- Giant cell arteritis

Management

Diagnosis is done clinically.

In a conscious patient presenting with ophthalmoplegia, ptosis and mydriasis a compressive etiology (intracranial aneurysm) must be ruled out. A computed tomography angiography (CTA) and/or magnetic resonance imaging (MRI and MRA) should be performed (90% sensitivity in aneurysms of 3 mm or greater diameter). Gold standard is digital subtraction angiography (DSA).

In case of pupil sparing 3rd nerve palsy ischemic causes are more likely. Inflammation and compression should also be considered. Following tests may be considered. Vital signs (e.g., blood pressure monitoring), complete blood count, ESR, CRP, FBS, PPBS. Brain and orbit imaging (CT or MRI).

Treatment: Treatment depends on the cause of the palsy. Ischemic disease that causes pupil sparing 3rd nerve palsy is generally improved within 4 to 12 weeks if hypertension and diabetes are well controlled. Residual deficit can be corrected with prisms or strabismus surgery after 6 months of stability.

Those with compressive causes are often diagnosed with aneurysm, tumor, trauma may require neurosurgical intervention.

4. Horner's syndrome—cause, clinical features, and evaluation. (2 + 3 + 5) (WBUHS MS 2023)

Clinical features of Horner syndrome

The majority of cases are unilateral, spine injury or autonomic diabetic neuropathy may give rise to bilateral involvement. Painful Horner syndrome of acute onset may be due to carotid dissection.

- Mild ptosis (1-2 mm) due to Muller muscle inaction and miosis due to unopposed action of sphincter pupillae resulting anisocoria.
- Anisocoria is accentuated in dim light. Pupillary constriction to light and near stimulus is normal.
- Hypochromic heterochromia (irides of different color, the Horner being lighter), seen in congenital or longstanding cases.
- Slight elevation of the inferior eyelid (inferior ptosis)
- Reduced ipsilateral sweating.

Clinical features if Horner's Syndrome are tabulated in **Table 2**.

TABLE 2: Clinical features associated with Horner Syndrome based on lesion location and cause.

Location in the sympathetic pathway and etiology of lesion	*Common symptoms or specific features*
Central (first order)	
• Lateral medullary syndrome (Wallenberg syndrome)	• Anhidrosis of ipsilateral face. • Ipsilateral impairment of pain and temperature sensation over the face, contralateral pain and temperature impairment over the trunk and limbs, limb ataxia, bulbar disturbance (e.g., dysarthria, dysphagia, nystagmus)
• Trochlear nucleus/fascicle in brainstem	• Contralateral CN IV palsy.
• Pontine lesion	• Ipsilateral CN VI palsy.
• Spinal cord lesion	• Quadriparesis or paraparesis, sensory deficit, bladder or bowel difficulty, hyperreflexia.
• Diabetic autonomic neuropathy	
Preganglionic (second order)	
• Superior sulcus of lung (Pancoast syndrome), mediastinum, C8-T1 nerve roots	• Anhidrosis of ipsilateral face • Cough, hemoptysis and swelling in the neck, ipsilateral shoulder pain, pain and paresthesia along medial arm, forearm, and 4th, 5th digits.
• Neck lesion (thyroid tumor, enlarged lymph nodes, trauma, post-surgical)	• Arm pain, hand weakness.
• Rowland-Payne syndrome (C6 nerve roots)	• Paralysis of the phrenic, vagus, and recurrent laryngeal nerves
Postganglionic (third order)	
• Internal carotid artery dissection	• Acute pain in temple, orbit, throat, neck, arm or behind ear, amaurosis fugax, dysgeusia, diplopia, tongue, or facial numbness.
• Cavernous sinus lesion	• Ipsilateral CN VI palsy, trigeminal neuropathy
• Superior cervical ganglion lesion	• Anhidrosis of forehead
• Trigeminal autonomic cephalgias (e.g., cluster headache)	• Headache, periocular pain, rhinorrhea, conjunctival hyperemia
• Intraoral trauma or tumor	• Ear pain, vertigo, hearing loss.

Evaluation

Pharmacological Tests:

Apraclonidine is used to confirm the diagnosis, hydroxyamphetamine, and adrenaline may be used to differentiate a preganglionic (1st or 2nd order neuron) from a postganglionic lesion (3rd order neuron).

Apraclonidine 0.5% or 1%: One drop is instilled into both eyes to confirm or refute Horner syndrome. The pupils are checked at 30 minutes and if negative rechecked at 45 minutes. A Horner pupil will dilate due to alpha-1 receptor upregulation in denervated dilator pupillae, but a normal pupil will not be affected. The ptosis also improved. Sensitivity is around 90%.

Phenylephrine 1%: In an established postganglionic lesion, the Horner pupil will dilate and ptosis may be temporarily relieved. A central or preganglionic Horner pupil and normal pupil will not dilate because in postganglionic Horner syndrome the dilator pupillae muscle develops denervation hypersensitivity to adrenergic neurotransmitter.

Hydroxyamphetamine 1%: Two drops are instilled into each eye. A normal or preganglionic Horner pupil will dilate but a postganglionic Horner will not, because it potentiates the release of noradrenaline from functioning postganglionic nerve endings only.

The mainstay of investigation is neuroimaging. CT or MR angiography examining the region from the aortic arch to the circle of Willis will facilitate exclusion of neck, apical lung, thyroid, and skull base lesion. MRI to exclude brain stem stroke.

5. Internuclear ophthalmoplegia. Discuss. (10) (DNB 2018, WBUHS MS 2022)

Internuclear ophthalmoplegia (INO) is an ocular movement disorder that presents as an inability to perform to conjugate lateral gaze and ophthalmoplegia due to damage to the interneuron between two nuclei of cranial nerves VI (Abducens) and CN III (Oculomotor). This interneuron is called the medial longitudinal fasciculus (MLF). INO can be unilateral or bilateral.

Anatomy

The MLF is a heavily myelinated nerve tract connecting the oculomotor nucleus (CN III) of the ipsilateral side with the paramedian pontine reticular formation (PPRF) and CN VI in the contralateral pons. The PPRF or para-abducens nucleus is the key structure in conjugate horizontal gaze and horizontal saccades. Damage to the PPRF results in impaired horizontal saccade in the same direction. PPRF sends a signal to the CN VI. Some axons from the CN VI innervate the ipsilateral lateral rectus resulting in the abduction of the ipsilateral eye. The signal for contraction of the contralateral medial rectus for adduction of the contralateral eye is sent from the CN VI to the contralateral medial rectus subnucleus of CN III via the internuclear pathway called MLF. The activation of the contralateral medial rectus and ipsilateral lateral rectus muscle produces horizontal conjugate eye movement. The side of the INO is named by the side of the adduction deficit, which is ipsilateral to the MLF lesion **(Fig. 1)**.

Etiology

- Demyelination (common cause in young patients)
- Stroke (common cause in aged patients)
- Other causes include infection, neoplasm, trauma, and progressive supranuclear palsy.

Clinical Features

Symptoms

- Horizontal diplopia which becomes more prominent on looking at objects on the opposite side of the lesion. No diplopia on primary gaze.
- Difficulty in tracking high-speed objects.
- Headache and vertigo
- Vertical oblique diplopia

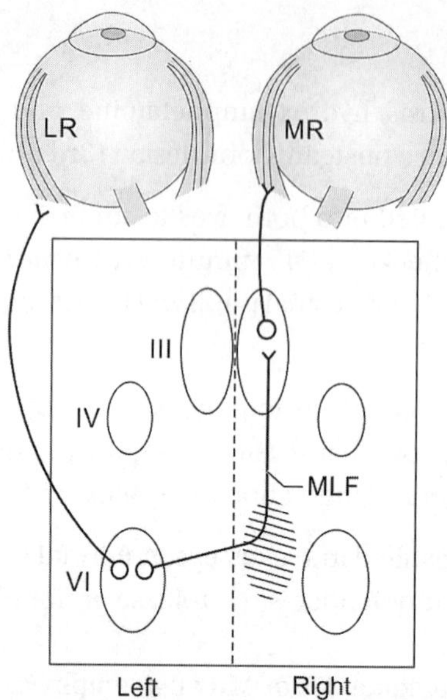

Fig. 1: Diagram showing the pathway involving horizontal gaze centers.
Courtesy: Eyewiki.

Signs

- Ipsilateral partial or complete adduction deficit with contralateral, dissociated, horizontal abducting saccade/nystagmus on attempted gaze to the contralateral side.
- A skew deviation with the ipsilateral hypertropic eye may be noted. Vertical gaze nystagmus may be noted on upgazed.
- Convergence is not affected.

Associated Syndromes

"Wall-eyed" bilateral INO or WEBINO syndrome: A large-angle exotropia occurs with bilateral INO due to midbrain lesion near the CN III nuclei.

One- and- a- half syndrome: Combination of horizontal gaze palsy and ipsilateral INO. It is caused by a pontine pathology that is large enough to involve the MLF and the PPRF or the CN VI nucleus on the same side of the brainstem. Abduction of the eye contralateral to the lesion remains unaffected. Vertical gaze is also preserved.

Diagnosis

- Diagnosis is done clinically.
- Quantitative infrared oculography may increase the precision for the diagnosis of subtle INO cases.
- MRI of brain (especially FLAIR image) or CT scan of brain.

Differential diagnosis

- *Pseudo-INO:* This is usually seen in established cases of myasthenia gravis and Guillain-Barré syndrome.
- Third nerve palsy.
- Progressive supranuclear palsy (PSP).
- Chiari malformation.

Management

Dalfampridine, a potassium channel blocker, showed improvement in saccades, binocular conjugacy, and ocular motility in patients with INO secondary to demyelination in Multiple sclerosis.

If the etiology of INO is inflammation or infection, high-dose corticosteroids can help.

Patients with WEBINO may get benefit from patching, prism, or strabismus surgery to correct any residual primary position symptomatic deviation that does not recover. Injection of botulinum toxin in one or two extraocular muscles may temporarily reduce the diplopia and improve binocular function in INO.

6. Clinical features, investigations, and treatments in case of neuromyelitis optica.

(3 + 4 + 3) (DNB 2016)

Neuromyelitis optica previously called Devic's disease is an immunological and inflammatory disease of the central nervous system causing demyelination of optic nerve and spinal cord.

It is now a part of the neuromyelitis optica spectrum disorder (NMOSD).

Epidemiology: It is the 2nd most common type of demyelinating disease. Women are more affected, usually in the childbearing age group (15-40 years). Seen in African and Asian descent.

Pathophysiology

- The humoral immune system is mainly involved in the pathogenesis.
- It is characterized by the presence of a disease specific IgG antibody against the aquaporin 4 (AQP4) water channel. These channels are mostly present in the optic nerve and spinal cord and other areas of CNS.
- The mechanism involves production of these aquaporin autoantibodies peripherally which then enter the CNS and bind astrocyte foot processes. This causes complement mediated cell damage, granulocytic infiltration, and astrocyte death.
- Death of astrocytes further causes death of oligodendrocytes, resulting in demyelination and neuronal cell death.

Clinical Features

- Flu like symptoms like fever, malaise, headache.
- Reduced visual acuity optic disc swelling, later on optic atrophy
- Reduced visual field
- Reduced color vision
- RAPD in unilateral/bilateral cases.
- Optic disc swelling progressing to optic atrophy
- Features of myelitis include paraparesis and tetraparesis, sphincter dysfunction.
- Transverse myelitis can occur presenting as complete spinal cord syndrome involving motor, sensory and autonomic pathways.
- Involvement of area postrema leads to hiccups and nausea.

Diagnosis

Diagnostic criteria are divided into those with Serum positive AQP4-IgG and those without AQP4-IgG or NMOSD.

NMOSD with positive AQP4-IgG

- At least one core clinical feature
- AQP4-IgG positive
- Exclusion of alternative diagnoses.

NMOSD without AQP4-IgG/unknown AQP4-IgG status

- At least two core clinical features due to one or more clinical attacks and meeting the following criteria.
  - At least one core clinical feature must be optic neuritis, acute myelitis with longitudinally extensive transverse myelitis lesions (LETM) or area postrema syndrome.
  - Dissemination in space
  - Fulfilment of MRI requirements.
- AQP4-IgG negative
- Exclusion of alternative diagnoses.

Core clinical features are:

- Optic neuritis
- Acute myelitis
- Area postrema syndrome

- Acute brainstem syndrome
- Symptomatic narcolepsy
- Symptomatic cerebral syndrome with NMOSD typical brain lesions.

MRI requirements
- Acute optic neuritis—brain MRI showing normal finding or nonspecific white matter lesions OR optic nerve MRI with T2 hyperintense lesion/T1 weighted gadolinium extending over >1/2 optic nerve length or involving optic chiasm.
- Acute myelitis—intramedullary MRI lesion extending >3 contiguous segments OR >3 contiguous segments of focal spinal cord atrophy.

Tests
- Serum AQP4 antibody
- Neuroimaging-MRI

Treatment
- For acute episodes intravenous glucocorticoids are given. (IVMP 500-1000 mg daily for 5-10 days) followed by IV immunoglobulin or plasmapheresis.
- Eculizumab and inebilizumab—both humanized antibodies have shown to be effective in trials.
- Other immunosuppressive used—methotrexate, azathioprine, and mmf.

7. Describe the causes and management of toxic optic neuropathy. (10) (MS WBUHS 2019, 2023)

Toxic optic neuropathy is the damage to the optic nerve due to toxins. It is characterized by bilateral symmetrical vision loss, papillomacular bundle damage, central scotoma, and reduced color vision.

Etiology
- Alcohols—methanol, ethylene glycol
- Antibiotics—chloramphenicol, sulfonamides
- Antimalarials—quinine, HCQs, chloroquine
- Antitubercular—ethambutol, isoniazid, streptomycin
- Antiarrhythmic—amiodarone
- Anticancer—vincristine, methotrexate
- PDE inhibitors
- Heavy metals—lead, mercury
- Others—carbon monoxide, tobacco

Risk factors
- Nutritional deficiency—thiamine, riboflavin, niacin, pyridoxine, cobalamin, folic acid
- Using systemic medications in high doses
- Exposure to toxic substances in the environment

Pathophysiology

The proposed mechanism of toxic insult is the impairment of vascular supply of the tissue or its metabolism. Another mechanism could be mitochondrial injury and imbalance of intracellular and extracellular free radical homeostasis.

Clinical Features

Symptoms
- History of drug use, medications, and alcohol
- Painless, bilateral symmetrical loss of vision
- Color vision reduced-usually red
- Central scotoma

- Reduced contrast perception
- Photophobia
- Poor dark adaptation

Signs
- Decreased visual acuity
- Normal, swollen/hyperemic optic disc early in course of disease
- Temporal disc pallor in later stages
- Central field loss with preserved peripheral vision
- Abnormal ERG and VEP

Examination
- Snellen visual acuity
- HFA for field evaluation
- Slit lamp examination—vortex keratopathy in amiodarone toxicity
- Swinging flashlight test—RAPD
- Direct ophthalmoscopy for optic nerve and retina

Laboratory tests
- Routine blood investigations and urinalysis
- Heavy metal screening
- Serum vitamin B_{12} and folate levels

Diagnostic procedure
- Ishihara tests/Panel D15 test
- OCT helps detect early sign of toxicity even before fundus changes appear and also helps in monitoring those at risk.
- ERG and VEP—useful in early subclinical toxic neuropathy
- MRI of optic nerves and chiasma with/without gadolinium is done to rule out compressive lesions in cases of doubtful etiology.

Treatment
- Removal of the offending agent
- Medical therapy includes vitamin supplementation.

8. Describe the clinical features and causes of papillitis. What are the differential diagnoses? (10) (MS 2021)

Papillitis is defined as the inflammation of the optic nerve head also called papilla. It is characterized by swelling and hyperemia of the optic nerve head.

It can be unilateral or bilateral.

Causes
- Idiopathic
- Infectious
- Ischemic-AION
- Tumor-glioma, sphenoid wing meningioma

Clinical Features

Symptoms
- Loss of vision in one eye
- Headache
- Decreased color sense

- Central field defect
- Pain with eye movement

Signs
- Visual acuity is reduced.
- Color vision defective
- Pupillary light reflex may be depressed.
- Central/paracentral scotoma
- Disc swollen with blurred margins
- Disc hyperemic
- Vessels in the retina appear engorged.
- Hemorrhages on the disc or near the disc.

Diagnosis
- Clinical diagnosis
- Serological testing
- Visual field testing
- Oct of the optic nerve

Management
- I.V. corticosteroids are usually given at a dose of 1 mg/kg body weight and tapered slowly over 6 months.
- Treatment depends on the cause.

Differential diagnosis
- Optic neuritis
- Papilledema
- Malignant hypertension
- Diabetic papillopathy
- Papillophlebitis
- Neuroretinitis

9. Describe the clinical features, evaluation, and management of Idiopathic intracranial hypertension. (3 + 3 + 4) (MS WBUHS 2021)

Idiopathic intracranial hypertension (IIH) also called pseudotumor cerebri is a disorder characterized by increased intracranial tension due to an unknown cause.

Risk factors
- Women of childbearing age group though it can occur in any age group.
- Systemic conditions such as anemia and coagulation disorders
- Hypothyroidism
- Addison's disease
- SLE
- Obstructive sleep apnea
- Behcet's syndrome
- Uremia

Pathology

The pathophysiology includes multiple hypotheses:
- The earliest proposed theory for IIH was cerebral edema but this criticized as this was not associated features of neurological involvement.
- The theory of stenosis of distal part of the transverse venous sinuses. This resulted in cerebral venous hypertension and impaired CSF absorption.

- Another theory was -increase in intra-abdominal pressure causing increased cardiac filling pressure with will reduce the venous return from the brain leading to increased intracranial venous pressure and IIH.
- The presence of microthrombus in the venous sinus is proposed to block CSF absorption in the arachnoid granulations.
- Some studies have suggested the role of Vitamin A in the pathogenesis of IIH.

Clinical features are typically bilateral and symmetric

- Headache—diffuse, associated with retro-ocular pain and vomiting
- Transient vision loss
- Pulsatile tinnitus which worsens with posture
- Visual disturbance—involves the peripheral field with inferonasal defect/arcuate defect.
- Horizontal diplopia is mostly seen associated with 6th Cranial nerve palsy.
- Papilledema is the hallmark of IIH
- Funduscopically—choroidal changes across macula, choroidal neovascularization
- Pediatric patients may have associated ocular dysmotility, 3rd and 4th nerve palsies.

Diagnosis

- Complete ocular examination
- Visual field examination
- Optic nerve imaging
- Neuroimaging to rule out other causes of raised intracranial tension
  - MRI
  - MRV

Lumbar puncture should be done in all patients suspected of IIH. An opening CSF pressure >= 25 cm of water with patient in lateral position is diagnostic.

Values between 20 and 25 cm of water are taken equivocal.

Values = 28 cm of water can be considered in obsessed patients.

MRI findings include

- Empty sella
- Enhancement of optic nerve
- Flat posterior pole
- Distension of subarachnoid space
- Tortuous intraorbital optic nerve
- Stenosis of cerebral venous sinuses

Treatment

General measures are aimed at-

- Reduce the symptoms and preserve vision
- Weight reduction in obese patients

Medical treatment

- First-line drug is Acetazolamide, a CA inhibitor for reducing CSF production.
- If intolerant then, drugs like TOPIRAMATE can be used. It is a weak CA inhibitor which helps improve headaches and lowers body weight.
- Furosemide can also be used.

Surgical treatment is useful for those with:

- Recent onset visual field defect
- Worsening existing visual field
- Severe vision loss

- Refractory headache
- Non-compliance with medical therapy

The choice of procedures is based on patients clinical presentations.

- Optic nerve sheath fenestration
- CSF shunting
- Venous sinus stenting

10. Describe the clinical features and management of ophthalmic migraine. (10) (MS WBUHS 2022)

Migraine is a headache disorder characterized by profound unilateral headache associated with other symptoms. The symptoms differ from person to person and include—

- Nausea
- Vomiting
- Changes in mood
- Extreme fatigue
- Sensitivity to light/noise/smell.

These symptoms can occur during the attack or in between migraine attacks. These symptoms can last from hours to days.

Phases of migraine attack

- Prodrome—beginning of the migrainous attack
- Aura- these appear 10 minutes to an hour before the start of actual headache. Classical aura includes vision changes, confusion, tingling of hands or face and difficulty in speaking.
- Headache—throbbing type pain which is unilateral.
- Postdrome may last up to 2 days where the patients suffer from confusion and are exhausted.

Types of migraine

- *Migraine with aura*
  - Migraine with typical aura
  - Migraine with brainstem aura
  - Hemiplegic migraine
  - Retinal migraine—affects one eye and includes temporary loss of vision and changes in eyesight.
- *Other types*
  - Chronic migraine

The commonest neuro-ophthalmic symptoms include

- *Photophobia*
  - Increased sensitivity to light
  - Bilateral
  - Induces visual and color perception and visual perceptual distortions
  - Worsening of headache with exposure to light.
- Visual aura-bilateral, with scintillating scotomas which expand in the visual hemifield.

Signs and symptoms

- Visual aura without migraine has features similar to transient ischemia attack or occipital lobe seizures.
- Atypical duration of Aura with hemianopia.
- Bilateral visual impairment
- Retinal migraine- monocular loss of vision with c-shaped, colored, scintillating scotomas.

Visual hallucination

- Floaters

- Palinopsia—visualization of the image even after the stimulus has been removed.

  Diagnosis of Retinal Migraine from International Classification of Headache disorders.

Criteria—at least two attacks of migraine and fulfil criteria from column A and column B. causes of Amaurosis fugax should be eliminated.

Column A: Aura with fully reversible monocular positive and/or negative visual phenomena confirmed during attack by at least one of the following—

- Clinical visual field examination
- Patient's drawing of a monocular field defect.

Column B: Two or more of the following—

- Gradual aura over 5/more minutes
- Aura symptoms lasting for 5-60 minutes
- Headache during or within 60 minutes of aura.

Management

- *Primary prevention*
  - Lifestyle modification- diet and physical activity
  - Avoidance of triggers
  - Medications like tricyclic anti-depressants, anti-epileptics, beta blockers and calcium channel blockers.
  - In cases of chronic migraine, botulinum toxin helps reduce headache.
  - Randomized control trials showed the efficacy of using magnesium for prophylaxis.
  - Prophylaxis is dependent on the specific patient's comorbidities.
- *Medical therapy*
  - Use of analgesics, like NSAIDS in acute cases.
  - Triptans – are a group of drugs which are agonists to 5-HT-1B/1D receptors, causing vasoconstriction of the intracranial blood vessels. They also cause inhibition of the pain pathways.
  - Triptans are contraindicated in coronary artery disease and stroke.
  - Ergotamines are group of drugs which stimulate serotonergic receptors, are less frequently given.

11. Differential diagnosis of painful ophthalmoplegia in a 40-year-old woman. (10) (DNB 2022)

Painful ophthalmoplegia is a condition where there is pain with eye movement along with weakness in the extraocular muscles. The etiologies are extensive:

- Trauma
  - Orbital fracture
- Vascular
  - Aneurysm- posterior communicating artery
  - Carotid cavernous fistula
- Ischemic
  - Diabetic
  - Hypertension
- Tumors
  - Intracranial,
  - Orbital
  - Metastasis
- Infectious
  - Orbital cellulitis
  - Cavernous sinus thrombosis
  - Herpes zoster ophthalmicus

- Inflammation
  - Sarcoid
  - GCA
  - Tolosa Hunt Syndrome
- Miscellaneous
  - Ophthalmoplegic migraine

Approach to the patient

- Clinical history
  - Onset and progression- acute, subacute, chronic
  - Nature of pain- sharp, throbbing, dull.
  - Associated symptoms
    - Visual disturbance- vision loss, diplopia
    - Systemic features of fever and weight loss
    - Neurological features
  - Medical history
    - Comorbidities- Diabetes, hypertension, thyroid dysfunction
    - Autoimmune disorders
    - Malignancy
    - Medications or previous surgeries
- Clinical examination
  - External examination- swelling, redness, proptosis, lid, and adnexal abnormalities
  - Pupillary reflexes
    - Anisocoria
    - Afferent pupillary defects
  - Fundoscopy- for optic nerve head swelling and retinal changes.
  - Extraocular movement
  - Cranial nerve examination
    - CN 3/4/6- extraocular movements
    - CN 5- corneal sensation, facial pain
    - CN 2-visual acuity
- Investigations
  - Blood examination
    - Inflammatory markers- ESR, CRP
    - Autoimmune markers- ANA, ANCA
    - Infectious markers- blood cultures, serologies (e.g., syphilis and tuberculosis)
  - Imaging
    - CT brain and orbit- for bony trauma, orbital mass, and sinusitis
    - MRI brain and orbit- superior for soft tissue.
    - MRA/MRV- assess for aneurysms or vascular occlusions.
  - Lumbar puncture- if CNS infection/inflammation is suspected.
  - Histopathological examination for suspected orbital tumors and sarcoidosis.

Management

- Immediate measure
  - For emergency cases like aneurysms
- Symptomatic therapy
  - Pain management with analgesics

- Targeted therapy
  - Infections- antibiotics, antivirals
  - Inflammatory- steroids or immunosuppressants
  - Vascular causes- surgery (aneurysm) or endovascular treatment for fistulas
  - Neoplasm- surgery, radiation, or chemotherapy.

12. Discuss traumatic optic neuropathy. What is optic nerve fenestration surgery? (5 + 5) (DNB 2022)

Traumatic optic neuropathy is an acute injury of the optic nerve secondary to trauma. The injury can be direct or indirect, direct injury results from anatomical disruption of the nerve fibers by penetrating orbital trauma, bone fragments within the orbital canal. Indirect injury results from transmission of forces to the optic nerve.

The visual loss can be complete or partial.

Causes of traumatic optic neuropathy

- Road traffic accidents
- Penetrating orbital trauma
- Falls
- Assault
- Sports

Classification of traumatic optic neuropathy

- Direct
- Indirect
- Based on the site of injury
  - Orbital
  - Intracanalicular
  - Intracranial
- Based on structure affected
  - Optic disc avulsion
  - Anterior optic neuropathy- anterior 10 mm of optic nerve, pt presents with CRAO, BRAO, CRVO, AION
  - Posterior optic neuropathy- involves the posterior part of optic nerve with no ophthalmological evidence of trauma, optic nerve head appearing normal. These cases present with disc pallor 5-6 weeks later.

Clinical Features

Symptoms

- Loss of vision
- Visual field defects
- Decreased color vision

Signs

- Reduced visual acuity
- Reduced color vision
- Afferent pupillary defect
- Visual field defect
- Optic disc edema may be normal in cases of retrobulbar optic neuropathy, disc edema may be present followed later by optic atrophy (after 3-4 weeks)

Diagnosis

- Full ophthalmological examination
- Visual field testing in cases of adequate vision
- Visual evoked potential (VEP)- to assess the electrical activity of the optic nerve

- Neuroimaging – CT scan of orbit with axial and coronal thin sections of 1 mm through the optic canal. This helps visualize-
  - Optic nerve
  - Optic canal
  - Detection of fracture
  - Evaluation of the surrounding sinuses.

Management

Spontaneous recovery has been seen in 15-30% of patients. There are two treatment options-

1. High dose corticosteroids
2. Surgical decompression

Medical therapy

- High dose corticosteroids minimize inflammation and swelling by their antioxidant properties and inhibition of free radical induced damage. These agents used after trauma were seen to have a neuroprotective effect.
- CRASH trial evaluated the efficacy of steroids.
- Erythropoietin (EPO) has shown neuroprotective effect on the injured retinal ganglion cells by inhibiting the activity of caspase three through the PI-3-kinase/Akt pathway.

Surgical

- Surgical decompression is performed in cases of optic nerve compression
  - Bony fragments compressing the optic nerve
  - Compressive retro-orbital hemorrhage
  - Hematoma near the optic nerve

Contraindications of surgery

- Optic nerve avulsion
- Traumatic CCF

Optic nerve fenestration surgery

De Wecker was the first person to describe optic nerve sheath decompression (ONSD) in 1872. It is also called optic nerve sheath fenestration (ONSF).

- In this procedure the pressure around the optic nerve is relieved in case of raised intracranial tension.
- The pressure is relieved by creating a slit in the dura mater of the optic nerve with subsequent CSF release.

Indications

- Pseudotumor cerebri/IIH
- CVST
- Intracranial lesion causing impairment of CSF outflow

Contraindications

- Raised ICT without visual loss
- Raised ICT with headache
- Active infections of CNS

Surgical techniques

- Medial orbitotomy with transconjunctival approach
- Superomedial lid crease incision approach
- Lateral orbitotomy approach

Complications

- Ocular motility dysfunction

- Binocular diplopia
- Pupillary dysfunction/anisocoria
- Failure of ONSD
- Cranial nerve palsy
- Permanent vision loss from vascular causes
- Orbital hematoma
- Subconjunctival hemorrhage

13. Clinical features and management of superior oblique palsy. (10) (WBUHS MS 2019)

Superior oblique palsy occurs due to dysfunction of the trochlear nerve, cranial nerve four. The actions of the superior oblique muscle:

- Primary action-intorsion
- Secondary action-depression in adduction
- Tertiary action-abduction

Causes of 4th cranial nerve palsy

- Isolated 4th nerve palsy
    - Congenital
    - Trauma
    - Microvascular
    - Idiopathic
- non-isolated –
    - Neoplasm,
    - Trauma,
    - Infection
    - Inflammation

Clinical Features

Symptoms

- Diplopia
- Asthenopia

Signs

- Compensatory head tilt to opposite site
- Chin down position
- Facial symmetry

Diagnostic tests

- Park's 3-step test
- Torsion assessment
    - Subjective- synoptophore, double Maddox rod
    - Objective- indirect ophthalmoscopy
- Diplopia charting
- Hess chart/Lees'
- Imaging in case of neurological involvement

Management

- Non-surgical – using prisms in cases of small comitant hypertropia.
- Surgical
    - Levoelevation- Right IO recession

- Levodepression- right SO tucking left IR recession/modified Harada Ito procedure.
- All levoversions- hypertropia < 25pd- Right IO recession
- Hypertropia >25pd right IO recession + right SO tuck.

14. Optic atrophy—causes, classification, clinical features, and management. (10) (WBUHS DO 2018)

Optic atrophy is the condition where the retinal ganglion cell axons which make up the optic nerve undergo apoptosis and die. It is an irreversible process of vision loss occurring due to multiple causes of optic nerve damage anywhere along its path from retina up to lateral geniculate body.

Etiology

- Congenital- LHON, Autosomal dominant optic atrophy
- Post-traumatic
- Post neuritic- optic neuritis
- Ischemic- GCA
- Toxic- tobacco, ethambutol
- Metabolic- diabetes, nutritional
- Pressure/traction- glaucoma, papilledema
- Consecutive

Pathophysiology

- Optic nerve is a myelinated structure made of millions of axons from the retinal ganglion cells.
- It transmits the visual information from the retina to the brain.
- The myelination is by oligodendrocytes which do not regenerate after damage, hence in optic atrophy, loss of ganglion cell axons and reduction of myelin causes gliosis of the optic nerve.

Classification

- Pathological
  - Ascending optic atrophy- here the primary lesion is in the retina/optic nerve. E.g., RP, CRAO, glaucoma
  - Descending optic atrophy- the primary lesion is in the brain/optic nerve. E.g., tumors/trauma.
- Ophthalmoscopic
  - Primary-orderly degeneration of optic nerve fibers with minimum alteration of ONH morphology. E.g., CRAO, AION
  - Secondary- optic atrophy secondary to disc edema, papillitis.
  - Consecutive- following disease of retinal vasculature, e.g., Retinitis pigmentosa.
- Etiological

Clinical features

Symptoms

- Vision loss

Signs

- Optic nerve pallor
- Distinct disc margins
- Absence of neural rim

Diagnosis

- History is important for identifying the etiology
- Complete physical examination
- Screen for vitamin B_{12}, folate, heavy metals, TORCH panel, VDRL, FTA-ABS, ANA, ACE, homocysteine.
- Check for RAPD
- Visual field examination- 30-2 to localize the lesion

- Color vision examination
- OCT RNFL- for thickness of peripapillary RNFL and GCL
- ERG/mERG- to rule out retinal disease
- CT scan with contrast to look for bony pathologies
- MRI of brain and orbit with contrast.

Management

- Primary prevention- as optic atrophy is an end stage condition, every effort should be made to remove the process causing the damage. This is the goal of primary prevention.
- The management depends on the etiology.

15. Enumerate the various ophthalmological causes of headache in an adult. How will you approach the patient? (10) (MS 2023)

Ophthalmological causes of headache

- Giant cell arteritis
- Acute angle closure glaucoma
- Ocular ischemic syndrome
- Increased intracranial tension
- Malignant hypertension
- Ophthalmic Migraine
- Tolosa hunt syndrome
- Anterior uveitis
- Herpes zoster ophthalmicus
- Convergence insufficiency
- Accommodative spasm
- Refractive error

Approach to headache

A detailed history taking will allow proper classification of some cases of headache. It should consist of:

1. Duration of headache
2. Duration of episode
3. Frequency
4. Location
5. Intensity
6. Course
7. Triggering factors
8. Family history

- Duration of episode- in unilateral neuralgic headache it lasts for seconds. Cluster headache lasts from 20 minutes to 2 hours. Typical migraine headache lasts from 4 to 72 hours. Chronic persisting headache is seen in GCA or IIH.
- Frequency- migraine is associated with throbbing type headache once/twice a year or many times in a month.
- Location- headaches can be unilateral or bilateral, retrobulbar.
- Intensity- most intense pain is seen in migraine and paroxysmal headaches. GCA causes intermediate pain. Venous thrombosis causes alternating phases of mild to intermediate pain.
- Course- in CST, the pain has a diurnal course with morning and nocturnal pain.
- Triggering factors- from migraine triggers include- alcohol, change in sleep-wake cycle, stress, and agitation.

Full ophthalmological examination

- Visual acuity- lower acuity can be managed by refractive correction.
- Presence of vesicles in the forehead and around the eyes of one half of face is suggestive of herpes zoster ophthalmicus.
- Presence of acutely raised intraocular pressure can cause headache and pain round the eyes in glaucoma.
- Fundoscopy to look for papillitis or papilledema.
- Jaw claudication is seen in GCA.

Treatment

- It depends on the diagnosis.

16. What is disc edema? How is it different from papilledema? What are the common causes of optic disc edema? How do you differentiate papilledema from papillitis? (BHU MS 2021)

Optic disc edema refers to the swelling of the optic disc with a concurrent increase in fluid within or surrounding the axons. Papilledema implies optic disc edema due to increased intracranial pressure (ICP). Papilledema is used to describe optic disc edema resulting from increased intracranial pressure while disc edema could be due to any cause. While disc edema can be unilateral or bilateral, papilledema is usually bilateral, however, it can be asymmetric, to begin with.

Signs of disc edema Mechanical signs

- Elevation of the optic disc
- Blurring of the optic disc peripapillary margins
- Filling in of optic cup
- Exudates in disc or
- Edema of peripapillary nerve fiber
- Retinal or choroidal folds

Vascular signs

Hyperemia of disc

- Venous congestion Peripapillary hemorrhage
- Exudates in disc or
- Edema of peripapillary area
- Nerve fiber layer infarcts

Causes of true disc edema

- Inflammatory-papillitis, neuroretinitis, papillophlebitis, and uveitis
- Ocular hypotony due to any cause
- Vascular-CRVO, diabetic papillopathy, uremia, AION
- Orbital causes-tumors, Graves orbitopathy, orbital cellulitis
- Infiltrative conditions-leukemias, lymphomas

Causes for pseudo disc edema

1. Optic nerve head drusen
2. Myelinated nerve fibers
3. Morning glory syndrome
4. Tilted disc
5. Small hypermetropic disc
6. Optic disc hypoplasia
7. Bergmeister's papilla

Table 3 highlights the differences between papilledema and papillitis.

TABLE 3: Difference between papilledema and papillitis.

	Papilledema	*Papillitis*
Laterality	Bilateral	Unilateral
Symptoms	Transient loss of vision	Sudden diminution of vision
	No pain	Pain on extra ocular movement
Pupillary reaction	Normal	RAPD
Media	Clear	Posterior vitreous cells
Disc elevation	2-6 D	Does not exceed 2-3 D
Venous engorgement, peripapillary hemorrhages	More frequent	Less frequent

17. Discuss clinical features, field defects, and management of pituitary adenoma. (10) (DNB 2018)

Pituitary Adenomas

Classification

Pituitary adenomas are classified based on the type of hormone secreted. Approximately 25% of primary pituitary tumors do not secrete hormones.

- Prolactin secreting adenoma
- Corticotropic adenoma
- Somatotrophic adenoma

Ophthalmic features

Patients with large pituitary lesions may present with:

- *Headache:* Due to local effects, without typical raised intracranial pressure (ICP) features.
- *Visual symptoms:* Gradual onset, often unnoticed by the patient until well established.
- *Color desaturation:* An early sign of chiasmal compression.
- Optic atrophy is present in approximately 50% of cases with field defects. When optic atrophy is present the prognosis for visual recovery after treatment is guarded.
- Papilledema is rare.

Visual field defects

These depend on the location and direction of enlargement of the compressive lesion:

- *Bitemporal Superior Quadrantanopia:* Typically, the first visual field defect.
- *Bitemporal Hemianopia:* Classic chiasmal visual field lesion.
- *Junctional Scotoma:* Central or paracentral defect on the side of optic nerve involvement.

Investigation

- *MRI with gadolinium contrast:* Demonstrates the relationship between the mass lesion and the chiasm.
- *CT:* Shows enlargement or erosion of the sella.
- *Endocrinological evaluation:* Complex, requiring assessment by an endocrinologist.

Types of pituitary adenomas

- *Prolactin-secreting (Lactotrophic) adenoma:* Most common type, causing infertility, amenorrhea, and galactorrhea in women.
- *Corticotropic adenoma:* Causes Cushing's disease, characterized by central obesity and moon face.
- *Somatotrophic adenoma:* Secretes excessive growth hormone, causing acromegaly in adults and gigantism in children.

Treatment

- *Observation:* For incidentally discovered, clinically silent tumors.

- *Medical therapy:* Reduction in tumor size and secretion using agents like dopamine agonists and somatostatin analogues.
- *Surgery:* Tumor debulking via a trans-sphenoidal approach.
- *Radiotherapy:* Rarely employed due to complications.

18. Marcus Gunn Pupil-diagnosis, evaluation, management. (10) (TN MGRMU 2022)

Unilateral Ptosis with Jaw-Winking Phenomenon

Definition

Unilateral ptosis with jaw-winking phenomenon, also known as Marcus Gunn jaw-winking ptosis, is a rare congenital condition characterized by ptosis (drooping eyelid) associated with abnormal eyelid elevation during jaw movements.

Pathophysiology

This condition results from abnormal innervation of the levator muscle (cranial nerve III) and the external pterygoid muscle (cranial nerve V), leading to synkinetic movement of the eyelid and jaw.

Genetics

Unilateral ptosis with jaw-winking phenomenon typically occurs sporadically.

Clinical Features

- Laterality
- Usually, unilateral but can be bilateral in some cases.

Severity

- Mild to moderate ptosis.

Constant

- Ptosis may vary in severity during rest and primary position.

Time of onset

- Typically diagnosed after birth, often during feeding.

Jaw-wink

- Elevation of the ptotic eyelid with oral or jaw movements.

Classification of Jaw-Wink

- *Mild:* Elevation of ptotic eyelid ≤2 mm.
- *Moderate:* Elevation of ptotic eyelid between 3 and 6 mm.
- Severe: Elevation of ptotic eyelid ≥7 mm.

Associated conditions

- *Strabismus:* Seen in over half of patients.
- *Superior Rectus Palsy:* May occur.
- *Anisometropia:* May occur.
- *Amblyopia:* May occur.

Diagnosis

Retraction of the ptotic lid in conjunction with stimulation of the ipsilateral pterygoid muscles by chewing, sucking, opening of mouth or controlateral jaw movement.

Less common stimuli to winking include jaw protrusion, smiling, and clenching teeth. Jaw winking does not improve with age.

Management

Refractive Errors

Correct refractive errors and manage amblyopia if necessary.

Strabismus

Address squint correction before ptosis surgery.

Ptosis Surgery

- *Mild-to-moderate jaw-wink:* Correct ptosis similarly to simple congenital ptosis, considering ptosis severity and levator function.
- *Severe jaw-wink:* Levator disinsertion followed by unilateral or bilateral frontalis suspension.

Alternative surgical techniques

- Levator muscle excision
- Partial levator myectomy
- Fixation of transected levator to the superior orbital rim
- Bilateral levator excision and frontalis suspension
- Ipsilateral levator excision and frontalis suspension
- Levator extirpation followed by frontalis flap suspension
- Levator transection followed by brow suspension

19. Holmes Adie Pupil. (10) (DNB 2020)

An Adie pupil, also known as tonic pupil or Adie syndrome, results from damage to the parasympathetic nerve supply controlling the sphincter pupillae and ciliary muscle. This condition often follows a viral infection and may be inherited in an autosomal dominant pattern. The ciliary ganglion and dorsal root ganglion are presumed sites of dysfunction. Typically affecting young women, Adie pupil usually presents unilaterally (80% of cases) before potentially progressing to the second eye within months or years. Common symptoms include anisocoria (unequal pupil size) and impaired near vision due to reduced accommodation.

Signs of Adie Pupil

- *Pupil appearance:* A large, regular (or sometimes irregular) pupil is characteristic.
- *Light reflex:* The direct light reflex is absent or sluggish.
- *Pupillary border movements:* Vermiform movements of the pupillary border are typically observed on slit lamp examination.
- *Consensual light reflex:* Constriction is also absent or sluggish in response to light stimulation of the fellow eye.
- *Near response:* The pupil responds slowly to near stimuli, with slow redilation afterwards. Accommodation may be impaired, with slowed and impaired focusing for near and prolonged focusing in the distance.
- In longstanding cases the pupil may become small.

Associations and complications

- *Holmes-adie syndrome:* Diminished lower limb deep tendon reflexes and other features of autonomic nerve dysfunction may be present.
- *Autonomic nerve dysfunction:* Excessive sweating (Ross syndrome), orthostatic hypotension, bowel obstruction, or urinary retention may occur.
- *Generalized dysautonomia:* Adie-type pupils can be present in generalized dysautonomia, with various underlying causes.

Pharmacological testing

- *Pilocarpine test:* Instillation of 0.1-0.125% pilocarpine into both eyes leads to constriction of the abnormal pupil due to denervation hypersensitivity.
- *Syphilis serology:* Checking syphilis serology is recommended in patients with bilateral tonic pupils.

Treatment

- *Supportive care:* Treatment is usually not required, but reading glasses can help with near vision difficulties.

- *Cosmetic measures:* Sunglasses or low-concentration pilocarpine drops can be used for cosmetic purposes and to reduce photophobia.
- *Thoracic sympathectomy:* This procedure can be considered for excessive sweating.

20. Examination and management in a case of anisocoria. (10) (DNB 2021)

Definition

Anisocoria refers to the condition of having pupils of unequal sizes.

Physiological Anisocoria

Present in 10% of the population in room light and 20% in dim light, with a difference of 0.4 mm pupil diameter.

Causes of Anisocoria

- *Structural Defects:* Congenital or acquired defects of the iris.
- *Horner's Syndrome:* Interruption of sympathetic innervation to the eye.
- *Third Cranial Nerve Palsy:* Damage to the oculomotor nerve.
- *Adie's Tonic Pupil:* Damage to the ciliary ganglion or short ciliary nerves.

Horner's syndrome (More anisocoria in dim light)

Causes

- *Central Horner's Syndrome:* Lesions in the hypothalamus or brainstem.
- *Preganglionic Horner's Syndrome:* Lesions in the cervical spine or sympathetic chain.

Postganglionic Horner's Syndrome: Lesions in the superior cervical ganglion or along the internal carotid artery.

Symptoms

- *Miosis:* Constricted pupil.
- *Ptosis:* Drooping eyelid.
- *Anhidrosis:* Reduced sweating.

Investigation

- *Cocaine Test:* Blocks reuptake of norepinephrine.
- *Apraclonidine Test:* Direct alpha receptor agonist.
- *Hydroxyamphetamine Test:* Promotes release of noradrenaline.

More anisocoria in light

- *Damage to parasympathetic outflow to the iris sphincter:* The parasympathetic pathway is responsible for the constrict constriction in bright light, thus increasing anisocoria in bright light.

Lesions anywhere in the common pathway for the pupillary reaction to light can cause absolute paralysis of pupillary constrictor

EW nucleus damage

- Damage to pupillomotor fibers in the subarachnoid portion of the oculomotor nerve and nerve fascicle
- Damage to ciliary ganglion and iris

Etiologies of Tonic Pupil

- *Local causes*

  Inflammation, tumors, infiltrative disorders, and infections such as herpes zoster, measles, syphilis, diphtheria, influenza, and rheumatoid arthritis can lead to damage to the ciliary ganglion.
- Neuropathic Tonic Pupil
- *Adie's Tonic Pupil*

  The etiology of Adie's tonic pupil is obscured in many cases but can be associated with secondary viral or bacterial infection causing inflammation and damage to neurons in the ciliary ganglion

In Adie's syndrome, deep tendon reflexes may be reduced.

Clinical Features
Patients with Adie's tonic pupil are usually asymptomatic, but can also present with the following:

- Mydriasis
- Difficult in near vision and glare

Initially, the patients may have only loss of deep tendon reflexes.

With time, resting pupil size may be smaller; however, the normal tone of the pupil never returns. The tonic pupil may become smaller over time, known as "Little old Adie's pupil

On examination, the anisocoria increases in bright light. Direct light reflex is absent, but the near reflex is present or tonic due to aberrant reinnervation of the sphincter. Instillation of 0.125% pilocarpine constricts the pupil due to cholinergic denervation supersensitivity. A normal pupil does not respond to this diluted concentration of pilocarpine.

Management

- *Adie's tonic pupil:* 0.125% pilocarpine three times a day.
- *Horner's syndrome:* Treatment of underlying cause.
- *Third cranial nerve palsy:* Treatment of underlying cause.

SUGGESTED READING

1. Bhatti MT. 2023-2024 Basic and Clinical Science Course™, Section 5: Neuro-Ophthalmology. American Academy of Ophthalmology; 2023.
2. Gervasio KA, Peck TJ, Fathy CA, Sivalingam MD, Friedberg MA (Eds). The Will's Eye Manual: Office and Emergency Room Diagnosis and Treatment of Eye Disease, 8th edition. Lippincott Williams & Wilkins; 2021. Chapter 10.
3. Salmon JF. Kanski's Clinical Ophthalmology, 9th edition. Elsevier Health Sciences; 2019. Chapter 19.
4. Sihota R, Tandon R. Parsons' Diseases of Eye, 23rd edition. Elsevier India; 2019.f
5. www.eyewiki.org. (2025). [online] Available from www.eyewiki.org.

CHAPTER

Ocular Injuries

Rajkumari Bigyabati

QUESTIONS

1. **Classify ocular trauma. Describe the effects of blunt trauma on posterior segment of eye. (10) (WBUHS MS 2021)**
2. **Briefly discuss Zones of globe injury. Write a note on Ocular trauma score. (5 + 5) (RGUHS MS 2020)**
3. **Discuss the ocular injuries in RTA. (10) (BHU MS 2018, WBUHS MS 2023)**
4. **Describe briefly on Traumatic Hyphema. (10) (WBUHS MS 2019)**
5. **Discuss etiopathogenesis and management of post-traumatic hyphema. (5 + 5) (WBUHS DO 2018)**
6. **An 8-year-old female child had accidental blunt trauma to the eye with a tennis ball and presented to the emergency with total hyphema. Outline the steps of evaluation and management. (6 + 4) (DNB 2018)**
7. **What is pure and impure blow out fracture? Describe mechanism, clinical features, investigations, and management of blow-out fracture. (1 + 2 + 2 + 2 + 3) (DNB 2021)**
8. **What are the types of Blow out fracture? Describe mechanism, clinical features, investigations, and management of blow out fractures. (2 + 2 + 2 + 2 + 2) (DNB 2020, WBUHS MS 2021)**
9. **A 10-year-old boy suffered injury to orbit with a tennis ball. His complaints are diplopia in up gaze and associated giddiness and nausea on looking up. What is the probable diagnosis and why? What investigation will you order and likely results of those investigations? How will you treat this patient? (3 + 3 + 4) (DNB 2020)**
10. **Siderosis oculi. (10) (TN MGRMU MS 2018)**
11. **Siderosis bulbi: causes, evaluation, and management. (2 + 5 + 3) (TN MGRMU 2020)**
12. **Chalcosis. (10) (RGUHS MS 2018)**
13. **Describe chemical injury of eye, clinical features, and management. (4 + 3 + 3) MS WBUHS 2018**
14. **How will you manage a case of chemical injury? (10) (WBUHS DO 2020)**
15. **What is Dua's classification of chemical injuries? How is it better than Rooper-Hall classification? Management strategies of grade III and grade IV chemical injuries. (3 + 2 + 5) DNB 2019**
16. **A 28-year-old male comes to the emergency room with history of accidental instillation of activated lime. How will you manage this patient? What is the difference in presentation and management of acid burns from alkali burns? (7 + 3) (DNB 2019)**
17. **Principle of suturing of corneal laceration. (5) (BHU MS 2020)**
18. **Management of retained intraocular foreign body. (5) (TNMGRMU MS 2018)**
19. **A 12-year-old child sustained injury to right eye while playing with bow and arrow. Discuss the management of corneoscleral perforation with iris prolapse in this patient. (DNB 2020)**
20. **How will you manage a patient with cracker injury? (10) (DNB 2021)**

1. Classify ocular trauma. Describe the effects of blunt trauma on posterior segment of eye. (10) (WBUHS MS 2021)

Classification of Ocular Trauma

Ocular trauma can be classified into the following types:

- Mechanical globe injury
- Non-globe injury
  - Orbital injury
  - Adnexal injury
- Non-mechanical injury
  - Chemical injury
    - Alkali injury
    - Acid injury
  - Thermal injury

The Birmingham Eye Trauma Terminology System (BETTS) of Mechanical globe injury **(Flowchart 1)** was created by Kuhn to provide a standardized classification of eye injury based on the amount of injury sustained on the eyewall into Open and Closed globe injuries.

Flowchart 1: BETTS classification of ocular injury.

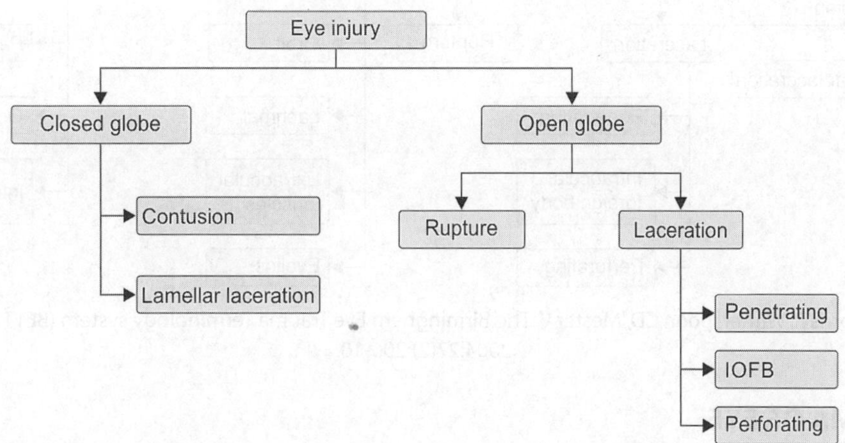

According to ocular trauma terminologies proposed by Bermingham Eye Trauma Terminology (BETT) for mechanical trauma, the terminologies mentioned above are defined as follows:

- *Closed globe injury* is one in which the eyewall does not have full thickness damage but shows intraocular damage and includes contusion and lamellar laceration.
  - *Contusion* is a closed-globe injury resulting from blunt trauma and damage may occur at the site of impact or at a distant site.
  - *Lamellar laceration* is a closed-globe injury in which there is partial thickness wound of the eyewall caused by a sharp object or blunt trauma.
- *Open globe injury* refers to full-thickness wound of cornea or sclera or both and include rupture and laceration
  - *Rupture* refers to full-thickness wound of eyewall caused by impact of large blunt trauma due to markedly raised intraocular pressure by an inside-out mechanism.
  - *Laceration* refers to a full-thickness wound of eyewall at the site of impact caused by a sharp object by an outside-in mechanism and includes penetrating and perforating injuries.
    - *Penetrating injury* refers to a single lacerating injury caused by a sharp object which traverse the eyewall only once and has only wound of entry.

- *Perforating injury* refers to two full thickness lacerations (wound of entry and exit) of the eyewall caused by a sharp object or missile and these two wounds are caused by the same object.
- *Intraocular foreign body (IOFB) injury* is a penetrating injury has only entrance wound with retained foreign body.

Modified Birmingham Eye Trauma Terminology Classification **(Flowchart 2)** was developed to address the shortcoming of BETT that did not include the wide range of ocular trauma. In this classification Periocular injury was added to Mechanical globe injury as follows:

Flowchart 2: Modified Birmingham Eye Trauma Terminology classification.

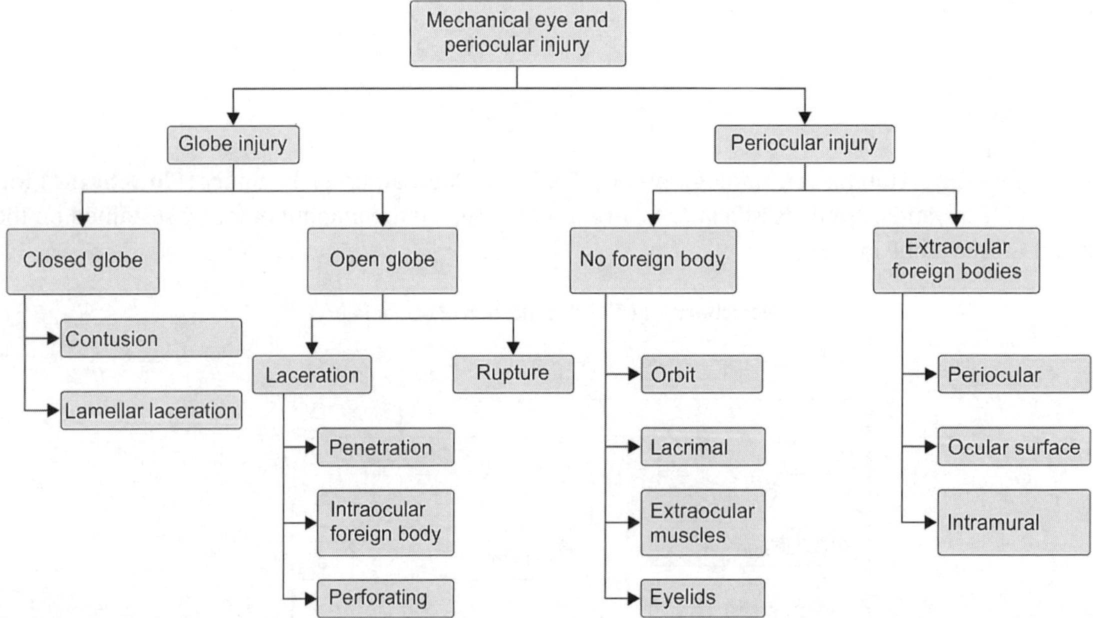

Source: Kuhn F, Morris R, Witherspoon CD, Mester V. The Birmingham Eye Trauma Terminology system (BETT). J Fr Ophthalmol. 2004;27(2):206-10.

BLUNT TRAUMA OF EYE

Blunt trauma is the most common cause of various intrinsic eye injuries resulting in open and closed globe injuries. Closed globe injuries are a more common pediatric age group. They can be caused by a variety of activities causing blunt trauma to the eye like while playing with sport items, wooden stick, toy gun pellets, firecrackers, road traffic accident, assault and occupational injuries. Closed globe Injury can cause hematoma or black eye, corneal scratches, damage to sphincter pupillae muscle causing traumatic mydriasis. Lens, ciliary body, choroid, vitreous, retina and optic nerve can also be damaged causing visual impairment and blindness.

Blunt trauma can lead to retrobulbar hemorrhage, orbital fracture, eyelid laceration and canalicular involvement. Blunt trauma can cause injury to the eye by Direct blow to eyeball by big blunt object like fist, stick, big stone, cricket or tennis ball and by accidental blunt trauma to eye may occur in road traffic accident, sport injuries, injuries by agriculture and industrial instruments.

The grade of injury depends upon the size and velocity of the object and site of impact. The mechanism leading to consequences of the blunt trauma can be one of the following:

- Direct blow on the globe (coup injury) with maximum damage at the point of impact
- Compression wave force (counter coup) which is transmitted through fluid contents to all directions, including the angle of anterior chamber, pushes the iris-lens diaphragm posteriorly, and also strikes the choroid and retina causing maximum damage at a point distant from actual point of impact.

- Reflected compression wave force which reflects towards the posterior pole after striking the outer coats, causing maximum damage to the fovea.
- Rebound compression wave force which rebounds back anteriorly after striking the posterior wall of the globe, damaging retina and choroid by forward pull and lens-iris diaphragm by forward thrust from the back.
- Anteroposterior compression and horizontal expansion which leads to globe rupture.
- Indirect force from bony wall and elastic contents of orbit may cause ocular damage when globe suddenly strikes against these structures.

Blunt trauma may damage the ocular structures by one or more of the following mechanisms:
- Mechanical tearing of ocular tissues.
- Damage to ocular tissue cells leading to disruption of their physiological activity.
- Vascular damage of ocular structures resulting in ischemia, edema and hemorrhages.
- Trophic changes due to disruption of nerve supply
- Delayed complications can occur as a result of long-term sequelae of trauma.

Types of lesions caused by blunt trauma are:
- Closed globe injury
- Globe rupture (open globe injury)
- Extraocular lesions

Effect of Blunt Trauma on Posterior Segment

Vitreous

- *Vitreous hemorrhage:* Vitreous hemorrhage occurs in blunt trauma in association with posterior vitreous detachment.
- *Tobacco dusting:* Liquefaction and appearance of clouds of pigment cells is seen as tobacco dusting is seen floating in the vitreous and they may not be associated with retinal tear.
- *Vitreous detachment:* It can be anterior causing Vitreous base avulsion or posterior leading to posterior vitreous detachment.
- *Vitreous prolapse:* Vitreous can prolapse into the anterior chamber following dislocation or subluxation of lens.

Choroid

- *Choroidal rupture:* Rupture involves choroid, Bruch membrane and RPE and may be direct or indirect. Direct ruptures occur anteriorly at the site of impact and are located anteriorly running parallel to the ora serrata while indirect ruptures occur at the site of impact. Rupture of choroid may be single or multiple and located temporal to optic disc. A fresh rupture may be obscured by subretinal, subhyaloid or vitreous hemorrhage. Weeks to months later, choroidal rupture appears as a whitish, crescent-shaped, vertical streaks of exposed underlying sclera concentric to the optic disc with fine pigments at its margin and retinal vessels pass over it.
- *Choroidal hemorrhage:* Subretinal hemorrhage may occur which may break through the internal limiting membrane resulting in subhyaloid or vitreous hemorrhage.
- *Choroidal detachment:* Blunt trauma can lead to choroidal detachment.
- *Traumatic choroiditis:* It can occur following trauma seen as patches of pigmentation and discoloration in the fundus.
- *Secondary choroidal neovascularization:* This is a late complication which may result in hemorrhage, scarring and visual deterioration.

Retina

- *Commotio retinae (Berlin's edema):* Commotio retinae is caused by concussion of sensory retina following a blow to the eye resulting in cloudy swelling. The involved area appears as grey or milky white cloudiness. Commotio most frequently involves the temporal fundus and occasionally the macula with a "cherry red spot" seen at the fovea. Spontaneous resolution occurs without sequelae within 6 weeks in mild cases and prognosis is good. Severe involvement of macula may be associated with intraretinal hemorrhage leading to sequelae like progressive RPE degeneration and macular hole.

- *Chorioretinitis sclopetaria:* This is a term that describes a closed globe injury following a high-velocity projectile passing into the orbit very near the globe. The sudden force cause deformation of the globe leading to splitting of the chorioretinal layers, which retracts, leaving the intact sclera exposed. This is the result of difference in elasticity of various parts of eyeball. Bruch's membrane and retinal pigment epithelium are inelastic and rupture easily with compressive forces. Retina and sclera are elastic, requiring very high energy impact with high velocity projectile objects to disrupt. Such force can create significant shock waves with enough force to disrupt and retract the choroid and retina, with bare sclera at the site of injury.
- *Retinal tears:* Retina tears may occur more commonly in the periphery following a contusion.
- *Traumatic proliferative retinopathy (Retinitis proliferans):* Proliferative retinopathy may develop secondary to vitreous hemorrhage, forming tractional bands.
- *Retinal detachment:* Detachment of retina may follow retinal tears or vitreoretinal traction bands.

Optic Nerve

- *Optic neuropathy:* Optic neuropathy can develop following blunt or penetrating trauma to the orbit. Optic nerve damage is either direct by compression or hemorrhage, shearing by acceleration of the nerve at the optic canal sheath where it is tethered to the dural or by transmission of shock wave through the orbit. Relative afferent pupillary defect may be the only objective finding in optic nerve damage. Papilledema and hemorrhage near the disc margin are found in more severe cases.
- *Optic nerve avulsion:* This is a rare complication which occurs when an object intrudes between the globe and orbital wall, displacing the eye. Mechanism of injury may be by sudden extreme rotation or anterior displacement of globe. Avulsion of optic nerve may occur as an isolated injury or may occur in association with other injuries of the globe or orbit. The lesion appears on fundoscopy as a striking cavity where the optic nerve head has retracted from its dural sheath. There is no treatment for optic nerve avulsion and visual prognosis is poor.

2. Briefly discuss Zones of globe injury. Write a note on Ocular trauma score. (5 + 5) (RGUHS MS 2020)

Zone of Globe Injury

Zones of globe injury are used to classify open and closed globe injuries which are useful for documentation as well as for prognosis of the injury. The highest zone injury is used when classifying an injury.

Open Globe Injury

- Zone 1 - Cornea and Limbus
- Zone 2 - Posterior to limbus to 5 mm posterior to sclera
- Zone 3 - Posterior to 5 mm from limbus
  - 5 to 8 mm posterior to limbus
  - >8 mm posterior to limbus

Closed Globe Injury

- Zone 1 - External anterior segment including conjunctiva, sclera and cornea
- Zone 2 - Internal anterior segment including lens, zonules and pars plicata
- Zone 3 - Posterior segment including vitreous, retina, optic nerve, choroid and ciliary body

Ocular Trauma Score

The Ocular Trauma Classification Group analyzed >100 variables from records of over 2500 eye injuries and developed the Ocular Trauma Score (OTS) depending upon presenting vision and score deducted according to clinical conditions. OTS is used to prognosticate visual outcome after an open-globe injury. OTS scores range from 1 (most severe injury with worst prognosis at 6 months) to 5 (least severe injury and least poor prognosis at 6 months) and has a predictive accuracy of 80%.

TABLE 1: Computational method for deriving OTS score.		
Initial visual factor	***Raw points***	
A. Initial raw score based on initial visual acuity	NPL=	60
	PL or HM =	70
	1/200 to 19/200 =	80
	20/200 to 20/50 =	90
	≥ 20/40 =	100
B. Globe rupture		-23
C. Endophthalmitis		-17
D. Perforating injury		-14
E. Retinal detachment		-11
F. Relative afferent pupillary defect (RAPD)		-10
Raw score sum = sum of raw points		

How to Calculate OTS Score (Tables 1 and 2)?

- *Step 1:* Assign initial raw score based on visual acuity (A)
- *Step 2:* Take raw points associated ocular injuries (from B to F)
- *Step 3:* Add raw points in step 1 and 2 and obtain a raw score sum and derive OTS score from it.

TABLE 2: Estimated probability of follow-up visual acuity category at 6 months.

Raw score sum	*OTS score*	*NPL (nil perception of light)*	*PL/HM (perception of light/ hand movement)*	*1/200 -19/200*	*20/200 – 20/50*	*≥20/40*
0-44	1	73%	17%	7%	2%	1%
45-65	2	28%	26%	18%	13%	15%
66-80	3	2%	11%	15%	28%	44%
81-91	4	1%	2%	2%	21%	74%
92-100	5	0%	1%	2%	5%	92%

3. Discuss the ocular injuries in RTA. (10) (BHU MS 2018, WBUHS MS 2023)

Road traffic accident is one of the most common causes of ocular trauma, often resulting in some degree of visual loss. Ocular injuries in road traffic accident may involve the eyelids, lacrimal system, orbital wall, conjunctiva, cornea, sclera and extraocular muscles and cause a variety of symptoms like prolapse of uveal tissue, vitreous loss, traumatic cataract, vitreous hemorrhage, choroidal rupture or globe rupture and optic nerve avulsion. Injuries seen in RTA are:

Hematoma

Road traffic accident can cause hematoma of eyelid or black eye, which is a collection of blood in the soft tissue around the eye. It is due to blunt injury to the eyelid or forehead following RTA leading to rupture of blood vessels beneath the skin.

Symptoms

- Bruising and swelling around eyes
- Pain
- Headache
- Temporary blurring of vision

Serious Conditions Associated with Hematoma

- *Trauma to globe or orbit*
  - *Orbital roof fracture:* This should be ruled out when black eye is associated with subconjunctival hemorrhage without a visible posterior limit.
  - *Basal skull fracture:* This may give rise to bilateral ring hematomas or panda eyes.

Eyelid Laceration

RTA can cause eyelid laceration which refers to partial or full thickness defects in the eyelid. As lid damage may be associated with serious ocular injuries, presence of lid laceration mandates careful exploration of the wound and examination of globe.

Lid lacerations result from contact with sharp objects causing partial or full thickness defect of lid. Blunt trauma from road traffic accidents frequently causes lid laceration in adolescents and young adults.

Clinical Features

Symptoms

- Pain emanating from eye or surrounding facial structures
- Bleeding
- Supraorbital anesthesia
- Blurring of vision

Signs

Tissue disruption, erythema or edema of the eyelid or surrounding structures are seen in eyelid laceration. Medial canthal tendo avulsion causes displacement or abnormal laxity of medial canthus and this can occur with concomitant disruption of canalicular system. Punctum can be displaced. Horizontal lid laceration with protrusion of preseptal fat with or without ptosis indicate perforation of orbital septum and damage to levator aponeurosis.

Systemic antibiotics should be administered for contaminated wounds.

Extraocular Foreign Bodies

An extraocular foreign body or adnexal foreign body is the entry of an object on the ocular surface or periocular region. They are quite common among industrial workers, builders and agriculture workers but can occur following RTA. Common foreign bodies such as particles of dust, sand, glass, dried leaves and small insects or wings of insects and particles of iron, coal and stone can be found.

Types of Extraocular Foreign Bodies

Depending upon the site of impaction, they can be of the following types:

- Lid or palpebral foreign body
- Conjunctival foreign body
- Corneal foreign body
- Lacrimal foreign body: Foreign body can lodge in the lacrimal gland or any part of the lacrimal drainage system
- Orbital foreign body within the muscle cone or in peripheral space

Clinical Features

Symptoms

- Discomfort in eye or foreign body sensation
- Profuse watering
- Redness of the eye
- Defective vision if foreign body is lodged in visual axis.
- Pain and photophobia which is more in corneal foreign body.

Signs

- There is marked blepharospasm and conjunctival congestion.
- The foreign body located in the external surface can be seen by external examination or under slit lamp.

Blunt Trauma of Eye

Blunt trauma is the most common cause of various intrinsic eye injuries resulting in open and closed globe injuries. Road traffic accident can cause closed globe injuries which can lead to hematoma or black eye, corneal scratches, damage to sphincter pupillae muscle causing traumatic mydriasis. Lens, ciliary body, choroid, vitreous, retina and optic nerve can also be damaged causing visual impairment and blindness. Blunt trauma can lead to retrobulbar hemorrhage, orbital fracture, eyelid laceration and canalicular involvement. Mode of injury in road traffic accident is accidental blunt trauma to eye.

The mechanism of injury leading to consequences of the blunt trauma can be one of the following:

- *Direct blow on the globe (coup injury)* with maximum damage at the point of impact
- *Compression wave force (counter coup)* which is transmitted through fluid contents to all directions, including the angle of anterior chamber, pushes the iris-lens diaphragm posteriorly, and also strikes the choroid and retina causing maximum damage at a point distant from actual point of impact.
- *Reflected compression wave force* which reflects towards the posterior pole after striking the outer coats, causing maximum damage to the fovea.
- *Rebound compression wave force* which rebounds back anteriorly after striking the posterior wall of the globe, damaging retina and choroid by forward pull and lens-iris diaphragm by forward thrust from the back.
- *Anteroposterior compression and horizontal expansion* which leads to globe rupture.
- *Indirect force* from bony walls and elastic contents of orbit may cause ocular damage when globe suddenly strikes against these structures.

Mechanism of Damage

Blunt trauma may damage the ocular structures by one or more of the following mechanisms:

- Mechanical tearing of ocular tissues.
- Damage to ocular tissue cells leading to disruption of their physiological activity.
- Vascular damage of ocular structures resulting in ischemia, edema, and hemorrhages.
- Trophic changes due to disruption of nerve supply
- Delayed complications can occur as a result of long-term sequelae of trauma.

Effect of Blunt Trauma

Blunt trauma may present with one or more of the following features:

Eyelids

Periocular hematoma (black eye), orbital floor fracture, basal skull fracture can occur in closed globe injury which may give rise to characteristic appearance of bilateral ring hematoma or panda eyes.

Conjunctiva

Subconjunctival hemorrhage, conjunctival congestion, conjunctival tears, foreign body in conjunctiva are some of the manifestations in ocular injuries.

Cornea

- *Epithelial damage:* There can be corneal abrasion or breach in the epithelium that is painful and stains with fluorescein and punctate epithelial erosion. Vision is grossly impaired if the defect involves the pupillary area.
- *Corneal edema:* Corneal edema can develop due to endothelial dysfunction. It is usually associated with stromal edema and Descemet membrane folds.
- *Descemet membrane tear:* They are usually vertical tears associated with birth trauma.
- *Recurrent corneal erosion:* They present with pain, redness, watering and photophobia due to loose attachment of epithelium to underlying Bowman's membrane.
- *Corneal endothelial blood staining:* This may be secondary to hyphema and may clear in about two years starting from periphery to center.
- *Corneal tear:* Partial or lamellar tear which may be self-sealing or full thickness tear may occur.
- *Corneal scar:* Corneal scar may develop after a long time following corneal injury, usually in 2 to 3 months.

Sclera

- Partial or full thickness scleral tear can occur with or without vitreous prolapse.
- Occult scleral tear can commonly occur at the equator where sclera is thinnest.

Hyphema

Accumulation of red blood cells in the anterior chamber is due to disruption of vessels of iris and ciliary body, usually due to trauma or underlying medical conditions.

Pupil

- *Traumatic mydriasis (Iridoplegia):* Iridoplegia is due to sphincter muscle spasm and may be associated with traumatic cycloplegia.
- *Traumatic miosis:* Occurs due to irritation of ciliary nerves and may be associated with spasm of accommodation.
- *Pupillary margin rupture:* Multiple tears can occur at the pupillary in blunt trauma.

Iris

- *Iridodialysis:* Separation of iris root from ciliary body results in a D-shaped pupil with biconvex black area in the periphery. It can cause glare, photophobia and monocular diplopia if it occurs in the other quadrants than superiorly which are covered by upper eyelid.
- *Sphincter tears:* Multiple tears in pupillary margin are a common occurrence in closed globe injury.
- *Iris stromal tear:* Radial tear in iris stroma may occur sometimes that can extend up to ciliary body.
- *Traumatic aniridia:* Blunt trauma can result in 360-degree iridodialysis, and the torn iris sinks to the bottom of anterior chamber resulting in traumatic aniridia.
- *Anteflexion of iris:* Rotation of detached portion of iris in which its posterior surface faces anteriorly occur following extensive iridodialysis.
- *Retroflexion of iris:* Retroflexion of iris occurs when the whole iris doubled back into the ciliary region and becomes invisible.
- *Inflammatory changes:* Traumatic iridocyclitis and post traumatic iris atrophy can occur following ocular trauma.

Ciliary Body

- Ciliary shock may develop as a reaction of severe trauma resulting in temporary cessation of aqueous secretion resulting in hypotony.
- Angle recession is caused by trauma where tear occurs between longitudinal and circular muscle fibers of ciliary body which has increased risk of development of late glaucoma.

Lens

- *Vossius ring:* It occurs due to striking of contracted pupil against crystalline lens seen as a circular ring of brown pigment on an anterior lens capsule which is always smaller than size of pupil.
- *Traumatic cataract:* Concussional cataract occurs due to traumatic damage to lens itself and minute rupture in lens capsule with influx of aqueous humor, hydration of lens fibers and consequent opacification. This leads to opacification along the posterior suture leading to rosette or flower-shaped posterior subcapsular cataract. A ring-shaped anterior subcapsular opacity may underline the Vossius ring.
- *Zonular dialysis:* Tearing of the suspensory ligaments may occur partially or completely following ocular trauma.
- *Subluxation:* Subluxation of lens occurs due to partial zonular dialysis which tends to deviate towards the meridian of intact zonules. The anterior chamber may deepen over the area of zonular tear if the lens tilts posteriorly. Uniocular diplopia may occur if subluxation renders the pupil partly aphakic. Subluxation may cause iridodonesis, phacodonesis and lenticular astigmatism due to lens tilt.
- *Dislocation of lens:* Dislocation is a rare complication and occurs due to 360-degree rupture of zonules. It may be commonly intraocular or sometimes extraocular. Intraocular dislocation may be posterior dislocation into vitreous, or less commonly anterior dislocation into anterior chamber. Extraocular dislocation may be phacocele in the subconjunctival space or it may fall outside the eye.
- *Traumatic absorption of lens:* Absorption of lens may sometimes occur following trauma in young children them aphakic.

  For Clinical features of posterior segment, please refer text of **Question 1**.

Open Globe Injury

RTA can cause open globe injury which is defined as a full-thickness wound of eyewall. It includes:

- Globe rupture
- Globe laceration
  - Penetrating injury
  - Perforating injury
  - Intraocular foreign bodies

Globe Rupture

Globe rupture refers to full-thickness wound of eyewall caused by blunt injury leading to sudden increase in intraocular pressure resulting in dehiscence of eye wall and collapse of globe.

Pathophysiology

When a blunt object hits the eye which is filled with an incompressible liquid with sufficient momentum, this creates energy transfer energy transfer over a large. This causes great increase in intraocular pressure, leading to rupture of the eyewall at its weakest point, which may or may not be at the site of impact. This wound is produced by an inside -out injury force and frequently leads to tissue herniation. Rupture occurs where the sclera is thinnest and weakest which is near the equator just behind the insertion of the rectus muscles. Other regions prone to rupture include the limbus, insertion of optic nerve and previous surgery sites. Ruptured globe result in diffuse injury leading to further damage like choroidal rupture and vitreous hemorrhage.

Risk Factor

There is an increased chance of blunt globe rupture in post-surgical cases of cataract surgery by large incision, LASIK, glaucoma filtering surgery and corneal transplant. Globe rupture is more common than globe laceration in elderly persons and females more than males.

Clinical Features

Signs

- Dense subconjunctival hemorrhage
- Presence of scleral step sign
- Prolapse of uveal tissue, lens dislocation, vitreous loss and intraocular hemorrhage
- Irregular or peaked pupil with angle pointing toward the site of scleral wound
- Hyphema
- Intraocular pressure may rise during the initial period following injury, but decrease ultimately
- Retinal injury may lead to commotio retinae, retinal breaks and detachment
- Choroidal rupture
- Optic neuropathy
- Optic nerve avulsion
- *Occult globe rupture:* This may be present without a visible scleral defect and may be suspected when there is extensive chemosis which may be hemorrhagic, relative hypotony, and vitreous hemorrhage.
- *Posterior globe dehiscence:* Pathognomonic signs of this are presence of a deeper than normal anterior chamber with posteriorly retracted plateau iris following acute ocular trauma.

Globe Laceration

RTA can cause globe laceration which refers to full-thickness wound of eyewall caused by sharp objects. It includes:

- Penetrating injury
- Perforating injury
- Intraocular foreign bodies

Penetrating and Perforating Injuries

RTA can cause ocular penetrating and perforating injuries which are open globe injuries that can result in severe loss of vision or even loss of eye.

Penetrating injury is defined as a single full-thickness wound of the eyewall caused by a sharp object and has only simple entrance wound with no exit wound. They are caused by a sharp object that penetrates into the eye but does not go through and through.

Perforating injury refers to two full thickness wounds, one entry and one exit caused by a sharp object or missile. These types of injuries go through the eye and therefore have an entrance and exit wound.

Sharp objects cause well-defined laceration of the globe. The extent of damage caused by flying objects is determined by their kinetic energy. Objects having high kinetic energy can cause considerable ocular damage.

Introduction of infection to the eye can occur during penetrating or perforating injuries. Depending upon the virulence of the organism and host defense mechanism, this can lead to a variety of infections like endophthalmitis and panophthalmitis.

Ocular penetrating and perforating injuries can be due to injury from any sharp or high velocity object and are frequently caused by accidents.

Risk Factors

Penetrating and perforating injuries are three times more common in males than females and occur mostly in younger age group. Failure to wear adequate eye protection while performing high risk activities contributes to risk of these type of injuries.

Symptoms

- Pain, loss of vision or double vision are the main complaints of patients sustaining penetrating and perforating injuries.
- Other symptoms are severe redness, sensitivity to light and foreign body sensation.
- Foreign body sensation and blurred vision are the symptoms encountered in more subtle injuries.

Signs

These are due to mechanical effects of penetrating or perforating trauma on different ocular structures enumerated below:

- *Conjunctival wounds:* These are quite common and usually associated with conjunctival laceration and subconjunctival hemorrhage.
- *Corneal wounds:* Corneal wounds can be uncomplicated and complicated with
  - *Uncomplicated corneal wound:* These wounds are not associated with prolapse of intraocular contents. The margins of such wound swell up leading to automatic sealing of the wound and restoration of anterior chamber.
  - *Complicated corneal wound:* These wounds are associated with prolapse of iris, and even lens matter and vitreous.
- *Scleral wound:* Anterior scleral lacerations may be complicated with iridociliary prolapse and vitreous incarceration, which may result in fibrous proliferation along the plane of incarcerated vitreous and tractional retinal detachment. Retinal breaks are frequently associated with posterior scleral lacerations.
- *Wound of lens:* Small wound in the anterior capsule may seal and lead to formation of traumatic cataract. Extensive lens rupture can occur with vitreous loss in severe damage.
- *Severely wounded eye:* This refers to a badly damaged eye in which there is extensive corneoscleral tears associated with prolapse of uveal tissue, lens rupture, vitreous loss along with injury to retina and choroid with no chance of getting useful vision.
- *Other signs:*
  - Shallow or flat anterior chamber
  - Very deep anterior chamber
  - Peaked pupil
  - Hyphema
  - Vitreous hemorrhage
  - Retinal tear
  - Retinal hemorrhage

Intraocular Foreign Bodies

RTA can lead to retention of foreign bodies like iron, glass, wood, stone, copper inside the eye. Ocular siderosis or siderosis bulbi is chronic pigmentary degenerative process of the eye following retention of intraocular foreign body containing iron. Siderosis may develop within days to as long as years after injury. It can also occur due to iron derived from blood. Iron has affinity for ocular structures of epithelial origin such as cornea, iris, trabecular meshwork, lens and retina leading to iron deposition and causing altered morphology of these tissues. The course of the disease is variable depending upon the iron content, size and location of the foreign body.

Pathophysiology

Ocular damage by siderosis can occur by two mechanisms, direct and indirect siderosis.

Direct siderosis refers to direct cellular damage caused by elemental iron ions producing hydroxyl radical formation following through Haber-Weiss ($O_2^{\cdot}- + Fe^{3+} \rightarrow Fe^{2+} + O_2$) and Fenton reaction ($Fe^{2+} + H_2O_2 \rightarrow Fe^{3+} + OH^- + OH^{\cdot}$) where ferric iron ($Fe^{3+}$) and molecular oxygen radical ($O_2^{\cdot}-$) produce Fe^{2+}, which reacts with hydrogen peroxide to produce hydroxyl radical ($OH^{\cdot}$). Hydroxyl radical, being a strong oxidizing agent, can lead to release of glutamate, which causes calcium ion (Ca^{2+}) influx, which trigger excitotoxity and apoptosis. Ultimately, this leads to pyknosis and irreversible retinal damage involving degeneration of retinal pigment epithelium and photoreceptors.

Indirect siderosis or vascular siderosis, refers to damage to vascular tissue causing ocular tissue damage distal to the location of intraocular foreign body. Iron associates with acid mucopolysaccharide, which is the main component of vascular adventitia, leading to its accumulation leading to microvasculopathy of the retinal vasculature and subsequent degeneration of inner retinal layers supplied by capillaries of central retinal artery.

Clinical Manifestations

The initial presenting symptoms of siderosis bulbi include a gradual progressive dimness of vision. Dyschromatopsia and positive scotomas are other presenting symptoms. Late-stage symptoms are progressive loss of visual field and nyctalopia.

The earliest signs of siderosis bulbi are mydriasis and heterochromia.

- *Cornea:* Iron granules may deposit in any layer of cornea but more prominent in deeper layers. A slit lamp examination may reveal rust-colored or yellowish pigment deposits within corneal stroma or endothelium.
- *Trabecular meshwork:* Iron deposition in the trabecular meshwork produces increase in intraocular pressure that may lead to fibrosclerosis due to iron toxicity, resulting in medically uncontrollable secondary open angle glaucoma.
- *Iris:* Iron can deposit in the stroma resulting in acquired hyperchromic heterochromia of iris. Iris is first stained greenish and turns brown or rusty later on.
- *Pupil:* Pupillary examination may reveal an anisocoria and a fixed, dilated pupil. Abnormal pupillary reactions like Tonic or Adie's pupil may be present. Iron mydriasis or light-near dissociation may be observed which is due to parasympathetic neuropathy resulting from iron deposition in sphincter and dilator pupillae muscles. An exaggerated pupillary constriction to diluted pilocarpine is seen due to denervation hypersensitivity.
- *Lens:* The lens epithelium appears yellow-brown or rusty from minute dots of intracellular iron. Rusty dark-brown anterior subcapsular deposits may develop. Eventually, the lens becomes cataractous, with diffusion of ionizable iron throughout the lens fibers.
- *Retina:* Accumulation of iron in the RPE and inner limiting membrane of neurosensory retina leads to degeneration of these parts, followed by full-thickness retinal degeneration and secondary gliosis. Rhegmatogenous retinal detachment may result from vitreous degeneration in association with retinal degeneration. Retinal pigmentary degeneration results from narrowing of arterioles and sheathing which resembles retinitis pigmentosa. Long standing disruption of retinal function leads to optic atrophy. Cystoid macular edema can develop, and optic disc swelling can be observed.

Orbital Blowout Fracture

RTA can cause blowout fracture of orbit which is isolated comminuted fractures that occur when the orbital wall is pressed indirectly. These fractures mainly involve the orbital floor and medial wall.

Classification

- *Pure blowout fracture:* This type of fracture does not involve the orbital rim.
- *Impure blowout fracture:* This fracture type involves the orbital rim and adjacent facial bones.

Etiology

Blowout fracture of orbit is generally results from trauma to the orbit by a relatively large striking object which is greater than 5 centimeters, such as part of an automobile in RTA.

The orbital floor is mostly predisposed to blowout fracture because of its anatomy. The inferior orbital nerve and artery courses within the bony floor of the orbit and the roof of this bony canal is only 0.23 mm thick, making it the thinnest and weakest and most prone to blowout fracture. The medial wall is the thinnest, posterior medial orbital wall is only 0.37 millimeters thick and may also be fractured. Since the bones of the orbital roof and lateral wall are thick, they are able to withstand the trauma and isolated blowout fracture does not occur in these walls.

Pathophysiology

Orbital blowout fracture can be explained by two theories.

In the hydraulic theory, when the eyeball is struck directly, the eyeball is thrust posteriorly and there is sudden transient rise in intraocular pressure. The increased in intraocular pressure leads to fracture of the weakest wall, usually the floor, and pushes the bone fragments into maxillary sinus, along with soft tissue from orbit. The medial wall may be fractured by the same mechanism.

In the buckling theory, blunt trauma to the face by a blow to the cheek transmits a pressure wave posteriorly, which compresses the bones of the orbit acutely ii an antero-posterior direction causing the weakest point in the orbit to buckle and fracture.

Clinical Features

Symptoms

Patient with blowout fracture may complain of pain or diplopia or both.

- *Periorbital edema and extravasation of blood:* This cause variable ecchymosis of the subconjunctival and periocular region and hematoma.
- *Emphysema of eyelid:* Subcutaneous emphysema occurs more frequently in medial wall fracture, which typically develops and makes it worse on blowing the nose.
- *Infraorbital nerve anesthesia:* This occurs in the distribution of infraorbital nerve involving the lower lid, cheek, side of nose, upper lip, upper teeth and gums.
- *Diplopia:* Mechanisms leading to diplopia may be either by hemorrhage and edema in the orbit may make the septa which connect the inferior rectus and inferior oblique muscles to become taut and restrict movement of the globe or by mechanical entrapment within the fracture of structures such as inferior rectus, inferior oblique, adjacent connective tissue and fat. Forced duction test is positive in these cases. Diplopia caused by entrapment of connective tissue and fat may subsequently improve but persist if there is significant muscle involvement.
- *Ipsilateral epistaxis:* This may result from bleeding maxillary sinus into the nose.
- *Enophthalmos:* Enophthalmos may be present from the onset of blowout fracture if the fracture is severe but usually tends to manifest after a few days as edema resolves. Factors responsible for enophthalmos escape of fat into maxillary sinus, backward traction of globe by entrapped inferior rectus muscle and enlargement of orbital cavity by displacement of fragments.
- *Defective ocular motility:* In medial wall fracture, defective ocular motility involving adduction and adductions seen if the medial rectus is caught in the fracture.
- *Ocular damage:* Ocular damage may be associated with blowout fracture, but they are uncommon as a blowout fracture is nature's way of protecting the globe during injury.

4. Describe briefly on Traumatic Hyphema. (10) (WBUHS MS 2019)

5. Discuss etiopathogenesis and management of post-traumatic hyphema. (5 + 5) (WBUHS DO 2018)

6. An 8-year-old female child had accidental blunt trauma to the eye with a tennis ball and presented to the emergency with total hyphema. Outline the steps of evaluation and management.

(6 + 4) (DNB 2018)

Hyphema is accumulation of red blood cell in the anterior chamber. Microhyphema is collection of a small amount of blood that is evident only after microscopic examination. Blood accumulates due to disruption of vessels of iris and ciliary body, usually due to trauma or underlying medical conditions. Most common cause of hyphema is blunt trauma.

Etiopathogenesis

Traumatic Hyphema can occur after blunting or lacerating or penetrating ocular trauma and sometimes following intraocular surgeries.

Compressive force to the globe can result in injury to intraocular structures like iris, ciliary body, trabecular meshwork and their vasculature. Shearing force from the injury can tear these vessels resulting in bleeding and accumulation of blood in the anterior chamber. Penetrating trauma causes direct injury to these vessels.

Evaluation of Hyphema

- A detailed history leading to hyphema should be elicited such as recent ocular trauma or surgery, past history of bleeding diathesis or anticoagulation therapy, clotting disorders or sickle cell disease.
- Symptoms associated with hyphema range from blurry vision, ocular distortion to pain, headache and photophobia depending upon the etiology.
- A routine ophthalmic work-up is mandatory for examination of hyphema such as visual acuity, pupillary examination, intraocular pressure measurement, slit-lamp examination and gonioscopy.
- A large hyphema can be visible on gross examination, but detailed examination should be done under the slit-lamp. The height of the hyphema can be measured from the inferior corneal limbus in millimeters and documented. Color of hyphema can vary from red to black where fresh hyphema will appear red and blood that has clotted will appear darker or black.

Grading of Hyphema

- *Grade O:* No visible layering, but red blood cells within the anterior chamber (microhyphema)
- *Grade I:* Layered blood occupying less than one third of anterior chamber
- *Grade II:* Blood filling one third to one half of anterior chamber
- *Grade III:* Layered blood filling one half to less than total of anterior chamber
- *Grade IV:* Total filling of anterior chamber with blood. Complete filling anterior chamber with bright red blood is called total hyphema. If the anterior chamber is filled with dark red blood is called blackball or 8-ball hyphema which is suggestive of impaired aqueous circulation and decreased oxygen concentration.

Complications

- Corneal blood staining
- Obstruction of trabecular meshwork leading to raised intraocular pressure
- Pupillary block mainly by blackball hyphema
- Peripheral anterior synechiae
- Posterior synechiae
- Amblyopia may develop in pediatric population in longstanding cases
- *Rebleeding:* Typically, rebleeding occurs within the first five days when the initial clot lyses leading to breakdown of the fragile damaged vessel wall and second episode of bleeding. Risk of rebleeding is higher in patients with raised intraocular pressure, large hyphemas, hypertensives, sickle cell trait and those using anticoagulants. Rebleeding carries a higher risk of associated complications.

Management

Uncomplicated hyphemas should be managed conservatively with and eye shield, limited activity and head elevation. The head of the bed should be elevated to at least 45 degrees to allow hyphema to settle inferiorly out of the visual axis and limit corneal endothelial and trabecular meshwork exposure to red blood cells.

Activities are limited including reading which increase the chance of rebleeding by causing pupillary constriction and dilatation.

Topical cycloplegics are useful for patients with significant ciliary spasm. This limits pupillary play and thus prevent rebleeding.

Topical steroids may reduce associated inflammation and decrease the risk of rebleeding.

In cases of elevated intraocular pressure, topical aqueous suppressants are given (beta-blockers and alpha-agonists) as first line therapy. If topical management fails to control raised IOP, systemic carbonic anhydrase inhibitors (acetazolamide) and hyperosmotic agents (mannitol) may be required. But these agents are avoided in sickle cell disease as they promote sickling.

Antifibrinolytics such as aminocaproic acid (ACA) and tranexamic acid (TA) are used on patients with higher chance of rebleeding or other complications.

Surgery is indicated if intraocular pressure is not controlled with medical therapy or when complications like corneal bloodstaining, persistent large hyphema and rebleeding develop. Anterior chamber washout can be done by anterior chamber irrigation and aspiration through a small incision. Oter interventions for hyphema include hyphema evacuation with closed vitrectomy or clot irrigation with filtering procedures.

Prognosis

Most patients recover fully without any deficit. Complications occur when hyphema is associated with comorbidities such as sickle cell trait or in cases of increasing size of hyphema. Prognosis also depends upon the grade of hyphema. Elevated intraocular pressure is seen in 13.5% of grade I to II hyphemas, but risk increase to about 52% in grade IV hyphemas. Grade I hyphemas have about 90% chance of recovering normal vision whereas grade IV has only 50% to 75% prognosis for normal vision mostly due to corneal blood staining.

7. What is pure and impure blow out fracture? Describe mechanism, clinical features, investigations, and management of blow-out fracture. (1 + 2 + 2 + 2 + 3) (DNB 2021)

8. What are the types of Blow out fracture? Describe mechanism, clinical features, investigations, and management of blow out fractures. (2 + 2 + 2 + 2 + 2) (DNB 2020, WBUHS MS 2021)

Blowout fractures of orbit are isolated comminuted fractures which occur when the orbital wall is pressed indirectly. These fractures mainly involve the orbital floor and medial wall.

Types of Blow Out Fracture

- *Pure blowout fracture:* This type of fracture does not involve the orbital rim.
- *Impure blowout fracture:* This fracture type involves the orbital rim and adjacent facial bones.

Mechanism of Blow-out Fracture

Blowout fracture of orbit generally results from trauma to the orbit by a relatively large striking object which is greater than 5 centimeters, such as a fist, cricket or tennis ball or part of an automobile.

The orbital floor is mostly predisposed to blowout fracture because of its anatomy. The inferior orbital nerve and artery courses within the bony floor of the orbit and the roof of this bony canal is only 0.23 millimeters thick, making it the thinnest and weakest and most prone to blowout fracture. The medial wall is the thinnest, posterior medial orbital wall is only 0.37 millimeters thick and may also be fractured. Since the bones of the orbital roof and lateral wall are thick, they are able to withstand the trauma and isolated blowout fracture does not occur in these walls.

Orbital blowout fracture can be explained by two theories.

In the hydraulic theory, when the eyeball is struck directly, the eyeball is thrust posteriorly and there is sudden transient rise in intraocular pressure. The increased in intraocular pressure leads to fracture of the weakest wall, usually the floor, and pushes the bone fragments into maxillary sinus, along with soft tissue from orbit. The medial wall may be fractured by the same mechanism

In the buckling theory, blunt trauma to the face by a blow to the cheek transmits a pressure wave posteriorly, which compresses the bones of the orbit acutely ii an antero-posterior direction causing the weakest point in the orbit to buckle and fracture.

Clinical Features

Patient with blowout fracture may complain of pain or diplopia or both.

- *Periorbital edema and extravasation of blood:* This cause variable ecchymosis of the subconjunctival and periocular region and hematoma.
- *Emphysema of eyelid:* Subcutaneous emphysema occurs more frequently in medial wall fracture, which typically develops and makes it worse on blowing the nose.
- *Infraorbital nerve anesthesia:* This occurs in the distribution of infraorbital nerve involving the lower lid, cheek, side of nose, upper lip, upper teeth and gums.
- *Diplopia:* Mechanisms leading to diplopia may be either by hemorrhage and edema in the orbit may make the septa which connect the inferior rectus and inferior oblique muscles to become taut and restrict movement of the globe or by mechanical entrapment within the fracture of structures such as inferior rectus, inferior oblique, adjacent connective tissue and fat. Forced duction test is positive in these cases. Diplopia caused by entrapment of connective tissue and fat may subsequently improve but persist if there is significant muscle involvement.
- *Ipsilateral epistaxis:* This may result from bleeding maxillary sinus into nose.
- *Enophthalmos:* Enophthalmos may be present from onset of blowout fracture if the fracture is severe but usually tends to manifest after a few days as edema resolves. Factors responsible for enophthalmos escape of fat into maxillary sinus, backward traction of globe by entrapped inferior rectus muscle and enlargement of orbital cavity by displacement of fragments.
- *Defective ocular motility:* In medial wall fracture, defective ocular motility involving adduction and adductions seen if the medial rectus is caught in the fracture.
- *Ocular damage:* Ocular damage may be associated with blowout fracture, but they are uncommon as a blowout fracture is nature's way of protecting the globe during injury.

Investigations of Blow-out Fracture

- *History:* A history of recent trauma to the eye or midface prior to occurrence of fracture can be elicited from almost all patients of blowout fracture.
- *Plain X-ray:* Water's view or nose-chin view is most useful in diagnosis of fracture of orbital floor. The common findings on X-ray are—irregularity and fragmentation of orbital floor, depression of bony fragments and hanging drop opacity of superior maxillary antrum from herniation of orbital contents through the nose.
- *CT scan:* Axial CT scans of orbit with coronal sections in thin cut of 1.0 to 1.5 millimeters is particularly useful in evaluating the extent of fracture. The nature of density of maxillary antral soft tissue may be helpful in diagnosing prolapsed orbital fat, extraocular muscle hematoma or antral polyps. Herniation of contents into maxillary antrum is seen as hanging drop or tear drop sign.
- *Hess test:* This test is useful in assessing and monitoring diplopia.

Management

Initial Management

Initial treatment of blowout fracture is conservative by general and medical measures.

- *Avoid blowing nose:* The patient is instructed not to blow the nose as this may lead to surgical emphysema and herniation of soft tissue.
- *Cold compress:* This may be helpful immediately following trauma by causing vasoconstriction and decreasing swelling.
- *Systemic antibiotics:* Antibiotics should be given to prevent secondary infection from maxillary sinus.
- *Analgesics and anti-inflammatory drugs:* These are given to control pain and reduce swelling.

Subsequent Management

The aim of subsequent management of blowout fracture is to prevent permanent diplopia and cosmetically unacceptable enophthalmos which depend on fracture size, herniation of orbital contents into maxillary sinus and muscle entrapment. Management depends on one of the following categories:

- *Small cracks not associated with herniation:* This does not require treatment as it rarely leads to permanent complications.
- *Fracture involving less than half of the orbital floor:* No treatment is required if there is little, or no herniation and diplopia is improving. But this requires treatment if the enophthalmos is >2 mm.
- *Fracture involving more than half or more of orbital floor:* This is usually associated with entrapment of orbital contents and persistent diplopia in primary position and should be repaired within 2 weeks. When surgery is delayed, the result of surgery is unsatisfactory due to secondary fibrotic changes in the orbit.

Surgical Management

Surgical repair of blowout fracture is done to restore the continuity of the fractured wall and may be done with or without implants.

Indications for Surgery

- Diplopia not resolving significantly
- Fracture with large herniation of tissues into maxillary antrum.
- Incarceration of tissues in the fracture resulting in globe retraction
- Enophthalmos >3 mm.

Technique of Surgical Repair of Orbital Floor Fracture

- A transconjunctival incision is made across the length of the eyelid just below the base of the tarsus.
- Blunt dissection is performed in the eyelid in the plane between orbital septum and orbicularis muscle down to the orbital rim.
- The periosteum is opened and lifted off from the orbital floor.
- The herniated orbital contents are repositioned back into the orbit.
- An orbital implant is fashioned in the shape of a guitar pick with the narrow portion placed posteriorly.
- The implant may be fixed by a variety of methods such as using synthetic material like Supramid, silicone, Teflon or fixing with cyanoacrylate
- The periosteum is sutured
- Intraoperative steroids should be given for 3 to 5 days to limit orbital swelling.

Technique of Surgical Repair of Medial Wall Fracture

- Fracture of medial wall can be done either by an open or endoscopic approach.
- In open approach, the medial orbital wall is assessed by a transconjunctival or subciliary or a transcaruncular incision.
- In endoscopic approach, after cutting the uncinate process ethmoidectomy is performed to delineate the fracture site.
- Reduction of herniated orbital tissue is done and an implant such as silastic which is made slightly larger than the defect is inserted.
- Forced duction test and pulse test in which the globe is gently pushed externally, and pulsation is observed through endoscope, are performed to confirm whether full ocular motility is achieved, and implant is placed properly.
- Nasal packing is done postoperatively.

9. A 10-year-old boy suffered injury to orbit with a tennis ball. His complaints are diplopia in up gaze and associated giddiness and nausea on looking up. What is the probable diagnosis and why? What investigation will you order and likely results of those investigations? How will you treat this patient? (3 + 3 + 4) (DNB 2020)

The probable diagnosis is blow out fracture of inferior wall of orbit with entrapment of orbital muscles especially inferior rectus muscle with orbital fat. This causes ophthalmoparesis through restriction of orbital muscles that worsens on up gaze on the affected eye while the normal eye elevates without restriction. This leads to diplopia in up gaze associated with oculocardiac reflex like giddiness and nausea on looking up and arrhythmia.

Worsening of diplopia on up gaze will occur in complete third nerve palsies since there is weakness of both superior rectus and inferior oblique muscles and is a differential diagnosis, but mode of injury goes more in favor of inferior wall blow out fracture with inferior muscle and fat entrapment.

Worsening in up gaze also occurs in inferior oblique overaction, since the affected eye will elevate more than normal in up gaze, but the mode of injury does not go in favor of this disease.

Investigation

- *Forced duction test*
  - This test is necessary to evaluate extraocular muscle entrapment.
  - The test is performed by grasping the conjunctiva near the attachment of inferior rectus muscle with a forceps and attempting to move the globe through superiorly.
  - A positive forced duction test is inferred when the eye cannot be placed in supraduction and indicates a mechanical restriction of inferior rectus muscle.
- *Orbital Computed Tomography (CT)*
  - The patient with suspect of orbital floor blow-out fracture will be advised to undergo Axial CT scans of orbit with coronal reconstruction preferably with thin cut of 1.0 to 1.5 mm to avoid artefact.
  - This scan can show the fracture as a trap-door displacement of the orbital floor or completely displaced bony fragment if a second fracture is present at the junction of floor and medial wall, with herniation of inferior rectus muscle and orbital fat.
- *Plain X-ray:*
  - Water's view or nose-chin view is most useful in diagnosis of fracture of orbital floor.
  - The common findings on X-ray are irregularity and fragmentation of orbital floor, depression of bony fragments and hanging drop opacity of superior maxillary antrum from herniation of orbital contents through the nose.

Treatment

This case needs early surgical repair of the orbital wall with relaxation of the entrapped muscles.

Initial Management

Initial treatment of blowout fracture is conservative by general and medical measures.

- *Avoid blowing nose:* The patient is instructed not to blow the nose as this may lead to surgical emphysema and herniation of soft tissue.
- *Cold compress:* This may be helpful immediately following trauma by causing vasoconstriction and decreasing swelling.
- *Systemic antibiotics:* Antibiotics should be given to prevent secondary infection from maxillary sinus.
- *Analgesics and anti-inflammatory drugs:* These are given to control pain and reduce swelling.

Subsequent Management

The aim of subsequent management of blowout fracture is to prevent permanent diplopia and cosmetically unacceptable enophthalmos which depend on fracture size, herniation of orbital contents into maxillary sinus and muscle entrapment.

Fracture associated with entrapment of orbital contents and persistent diplopia in primary position involve more than half or more of orbital floor and should be repaired within 2 weeks. When surgery is delayed, the result of surgery is unsatisfactory due to secondary fibrotic changes in the orbit.

Surgical Management

Surgical repair of blowout fracture is done to restore the continuity of the fractured wall and may be done with or without implants.

Technique of Surgical Repair of Orbital Floor Fracture

- A transconjunctival incision is made across the length of the eyelid just below the base of the tarsus.
- Blunt dissection is performed in the eyelid in the plane between orbital septum and orbicularis muscle down to the orbital rim.

- The periosteum is opened and lifted off from the orbital floor.
- The herniated orbital contents are repositioned back into the orbit.
- An orbital implant is fashioned in the shape of a guitar pick with the narrow portion placed posteriorly.
- The implant may be fixed by a variety of methods such as using synthetic material like Supramid, silicone, Teflon or fixing with cyanoacrylate
- The periosteum is sutured
- Intraoperative steroids should be given for 3 to 5 days to limit orbital swelling

10. Siderosis oculi. **(10) (TN MGRMU MS 2018)**

11. Siderosis bulbi: causes, evaluation, and management. **(2 + 5 + 3) (TN MGRMU 2020)**

Siderosis oculi or ocular siderosis or siderosis bulbi is chronic pigmentary degenerative process of the eye following retention of intraocular foreign body containing iron. Siderosis may develop within days to as long as years after injury. It can also occur due to iron derived from blood. Iron has affinity for ocular structures of epithelial origin such as cornea, iris, trabecular meshwork, lens and retina leading to iron deposition and causing altered morphology of these tissues. The course of the disease is variable depending upon the iron content, size and location of the foreign body.

Causes

Siderosis bulbi is caused by intraocular foreign body containing metallic iron. Most common cause is injury during hammering. Chiseling and lathe turning are other common causes. Other causes include welding, road traffic accidents, injury from nail gun, gunshot, or explosion injuries.

Ocular damage by siderosis can occur by two mechanisms, direct and indirect siderosis.

Direct siderosis refers to direct cellular damage caused by elemental iron ions producing hydroxyl radical formation following through Haber-Weiss ($O_2^{\cdot}- + Fe^{3+} \rightarrow Fe^{2+} + O_2$) and Fenton reaction ($Fe^{2+} + H_2O_2 \rightarrow Fe^{3+} + OH^- + OH^{\cdot}$) where ferric iron ($Fe^{3+}$) and molecular oxygen radical ($O_2^{\cdot}-$) produce Fe^{2+}, which reacts with hydrogen peroxide to produce hydroxyl radical ($OH^{\cdot}$). Hydroxyl radical, being a strong oxidizing agent, can lead to release of glutamate, which causes calcium ion (Ca^{2+}) influx, which trigger excitotoxity and apoptosis. Ultimately, this leads to pyknosis and irreversible retinal damage involving degeneration of retinal pigment epithelium and photoreceptors.

Indirect siderosis or vascular siderosis, refers to damage to vascular tissue causing ocular tissue damage distal to the location of intraocular foreign body. Iron associates with acid mucopolysaccharide, which is the main component of vascular adventitia, leading to its accumulation leading to microvasculopathy of the retinal vasculature and subsequent degeneration of inner retinal layers supplied by capillaries of central retinal artery.

Evaluation

History: To avoid siderosis, a detailed history of the injury must be elicited, and thorough evaluation of anterior and posterior segments are necessary. Slit lamp examination along with Seidel's test, gonioscopy and retinal examination should be performed to rule out intraocular foreign body.

Clinical Manifestations

Symptoms: The initial presenting symptoms of siderosis bulbi include:

- Gradual progressive dimness of vision
- Dyschromatopsia and positive scotomas are other presenting symptoms.
- Late-stage symptoms are progressive loss of visual field and nyctalopia.

Signs: The earliest signs of siderosis bulbi are mydriasis and heterochromia.

Cornea: Iron granules may deposit in any layer of cornea but more prominent in deeper layers. A slit lamp examination may reveal rust-colored or yellowish pigment deposits within corneal stroma or endothelium.

Trabecular meshwork: Iron deposition in the trabecular meshwork produces increase in intraocular pressure that may lead to fibrosclerosis due to iron toxicity, resulting in medically uncontrollable secondary open angle glaucoma.

Iris: Iron can deposit in the stroma resulting in acquired hyperchromic heterochromia of iris. Iris is first stained greenish and turns brown or rusty later on.

Pupil: Pupillary examination may reveal an anisocoria and a fixed, dilated pupil. Abnormal pupillary reaction like Tonic or Adie's pupil may be present. Iron mydriasis or light-near dissociation may be observed which is due to parasympathetic neuropathy resulting from iron deposition in sphincter and dilator pupillae muscles. An exaggerated pupillary constriction to diluted pilocarpine is seen due to denervation hypersensitivity.

Lens: The lens epithelium appears yellow-brown or rusty from minute dots of intracellular iron. Rusty dark-brown anterior subcapsular deposits may develop. Eventually, the lens becomes cataractous, with diffusion of ionizable iron throughout the lens fibers.

Retina: Accumulation of iron in the RPE and inner limiting membrane of neurosensory retina leads to degeneration of these parts, followed by full-thickness retinal degeneration and secondary gliosis. Rhegmatogenous retinal detachment may result from vitreous degeneration in association with retinal degeneration. Retinal pigmentary degeneration results from narrowing of arterioles and sheathing which resembles retinitis pigmentosa. Long standing disruption of retinal function leads to optic atrophy. Cystoid macular edema can develop, and optic disc swelling can be observed.

Diagnostic Tests

Radiological evaluation: They play a key role to detect IOFB as well as assess damage in ocular siderosis. Imaging modalities that can be used include X-ray, ultrasonography (USG), computed tomography (CT), magnetic resonance imaging (MRI, ultrasound biomicroscopy (UBM) and optical coherence tomography (OCT). Electrophysiological tests like electroretinography (ERG) can be used to assess retinal damage. Other tests like fluorescein angiography (FA), electrooculogram and visual field assessment can be used to assess further damage.

On *plain X-ray,* metallic foreign bodies are seen as radio-opaque foreign bodies but have limitations in localizing and predicting nature of foreign body.

USG can detect both metallic and non-metallic intraocular foreign bodies, which appear as hyperechoic lesion with acoustic black shadowing on B-scan. USG can identify associated ocular injuries such as lens dislocation, vitreous hemorrhage, retinal detachment and choroidal detachment even in the presence of media opacity. Limitations of USG are that it does not provide accurate size of foreign body, may miss foreign bodies lying in the posterior one-third of orbit or within orbital soft tissues, is operator dependent and caution must be exerted in suspected open globe injury.

Non-contrast CT is the gold-standard for identifying IOFBs, providing high accuracy in predicting the nature, location and size of foreign body. Thin scans (1-3 mm) have higher resolutions and are preferred.

MRI has better sensitivity (95%) than CT scan for non-metallic IOFB and visualize soft tissues, optic nerve and orbital apex without radiation exposure but contraindicated on ferromagnetic IOFB due to possible movement within the electromagnetic field.

UBM is useful for imaging foreign bodies located anteriorly like those lodged in the subconjunctival space, cornea, angle, iris, ciliary body but avoided in suspected open globe injury due to increased risk of infection.

OCT is a non-contact, non-invasive ocular imaging investigation tool. Anterior segment OCT can visualize IOFB in the anterior segment, but not beyond the iris due to poor penetrance.

Posterior segment OCT is a useful tool for accurate localization of IOFB in the posterior segment and for quantifying the amount of cystoid macular edema.

ERG is the gold standard electrophysiological test for diagnostic test for subclinical siderosis bulbi. Early phase of the disease shows supernormal response with increase in amplitude of both a and b waves. Subsequently, the amplitude of b-wave decreases with reduction of b/a ratio to <1. An extinguished response is seen in ERG in advanced cases with absent a and b waves.

Fluorescein angiography in ocular siderosis may show hyperfluorescent window defects due to capillary non-perfusion, RPE changes and ischemic maculopathy.

Visual field assessment: This may show progressive visual field constriction in ocular siderosis.

Management

Prompt removal of IOFB is advocated to avoid the development of endophthalmitis and siderosis. Antibiotics are given both by topical and systemic route to combat common pathogen and booster dose of tetanus vaccine administered.

Anterior segment IOFB should be removed promptly with forceps or intraocular magnet through limbal paracentesis.

Posterior segment IOFB can be removed with the help of intraocular magnet or forceps after performing pars plana vitrectomy.

Deferoxamine, a free iron chelating agent, has been shown to prevent development of damage due to ocular siderosis when used subconjunctivally in the dose of 10-100mg. In advanced case of siderosis, iron is already bound to tissues, damaging them which cannot be reversed. Deferoxamine has many side effects such as color vision impairment, nyctalopia, RPE alterations, reduction in ERG amplitudes, bone dysplasia and sensorineural hearing loss and so, not recommended in ocular siderosis.

12. Chalcosis. (10) (RGUHS MS 2018)

Chalcosis or chalcosis bulbi, is a chronic reaction to a copper containing intraocular foreign body. The condition may manifest within days, or the patient may remain asymptomatic for years. The course of the disease is variable depending on the copper content, size and location of the foreign body and the patient's healing response to the foreign material. Copper alloy may affect ocular structures like the cornea, iris, lens, vitreous and retina and timely intervention is necessary to prevent long-term damage.

Pathophysiology

When an IOFB containing copper enters the eye, uncharged elemental copper is oxidized to Cu^+ ions which have an affinity to deposit in intraocular basement membranes like internal limiting membrane and Desmet's membrane.

Copper content of foreign bodies is important in development of chalcosis. Typical causes of chalcosis are foreign bodies containing less copper (<85%) such as brass which incites a localized inflammatory response. Foreign bodies containing less than 70% copper are relatively inert, causing low grade chronic inflammation or no discernable symptoms. Foreign bodies with higher concentration of copper (85%) cause generalized deposition of copper with serious outcomes.

Histopathologic changes due to copper exposure are of four patterns. The first pattern is suppuration, which is an acute inflammatory reaction with accumulation of neutrophils and few macrophages and intensity of inflammation depends on proximity to the copper containing foreign body. The second pattern is chronic granulomatous inflammation, with accumulation of plasma cells, lymphocytes and macrophages which stain positive for copper. The third pattern is reactive fibrosis around the foreign body, resulting in a fibrous capsule composed of dense hyalinized connective tissue, with copper in the inner portion of the capsule. This dense fibrous capsule surrounding the foreign body may protect the eye from further damaging effects of copper. The fourth pattern is disseminated deposition of copper in various ocular structures like cornea and iris, leading to visible changes in these structures.

Clinical Manifestations

Earliest symptoms of pain and intraocular hemorrhage may be associated with penetrating ocular injury by copper containing foreign body. Staining of intraocular structures may occur in late stage.

Sclera: Copper inside the sclera may lead to tissue softening and abscess formation.

Cornea: Kayser-Fleischer ring is due to deposition of copper in Descemet's membrane seen as a 1 to 2 mm wide, green-brown ring (golden-brown metallic sheen) in the periphery of cornea which may extend superiorly, inferiorly or circumferentially.

Anterior chamber: Copper concentrations in the aqueous may be elevated in chalcosis with presence of cell and copper-colored metallic particles.

Iris: Iris may have a greenish tinge due to deposition of copper.

Lens: Sunflower cataract may form in the lens which appear as a metallic, green-grey or golden-yellow disciform opacity which has serrated edges and lateral radiations.

Vitreous: Vitreous may show green, red or brown granular deposits of copper, vitreous strands, haze, degeneration and liquefaction.

Retina: Copper granules may deposit in the internal limiting membrane of retina as hyperreflective deposits within inner retinal layers and circinate, fleck-like deposits surrounding the fovea and mid-peripheral retina. Retinal gliosis may occur in vicinity of copper containing intraocular foreign body and copper deposits may occur in the walls of retinal capillaries.

Diagnosis

X-ray of anteroposterior and lateral view of orbit is necessary in the diagnosis intraocular foreign body.

Computed tomography (CT) in the setting of trauma is the first line imaging modality for detection of metallic IOFB.

Ophthalmic B-scan ultrasonography is avoided in cases of suspected globe rupture, but useful for follow-up visits of occult metallic foreign bodies not detected on initial examination. Optical coherence tomography (OCT), ultrasound biomicroscopy and electrorenogram (ERG) are also useful in such situations.

ERG is useful in progressive retinal toxicity due to chalcosis to detect decreased photopic and scotopic response amplitudes and increased implicit time which can be reversed when intraocular copper concentration returns to normal.

Anterior segment OCT may show copper deposits forming a characteristic linear pattern of hyper-reflective dots along Descemet's membrane.

Histological examination: Copper deposits can be demonstrated in histopathological specimens after staining with certain dyes such as rhodamine and alizarin blue in fibrous capsule around copper containing IOFB, Descemet's membrane, internal limiting membrane and vitreous.

Differential Diagnosis

Wilson disease should be differentiated from chalcosis as both presents with Kayser-Fleicher ring and sunflower cataract. But Wilson disease may reveal low ceruloplasmin and high urinary copper level with liver dysfunction and presents with neurological symptoms.

Management

The copper containing IOFB should be removed urgently with meticulous wound closure to restore the integrity of globe. Broad spectrum antibiotics and anti-inflammatory like oral or peribulbar steroids are administered after ensuring tetanus immunization status.

After accurate identification of the non-metallic copper containing IOFB, removal may be done by performing a vitrectomy with or without lensectomy and scleral buckle placement. Internal limiting membrane peeling may be performed simultaneously if copper deposition is found on superficial retina.

13. Describe chemical injury of eye, clinical features, and management. (4 + 3 + 3) (MS WBUHS 2018)

14. How will you manage a case of chemical injury? (10) (WBUHS DO 2020)

Chemical Injury of Eye

Chemical ocular injuries are non-mechanical injuries inducing chemical changes in the eye. They include acid and alkali injury of conjunctiva and cornea which can vary from trivial to severe leading to visual impairment and disfigurement. The severity of ocular chemical injury depends on the causative agent, the duration of contact, time from injury to initiation of treatment and the treatment given as these factors influence the depth of penetration of the chemical agent, the ocular structures affected, wound healing, repair and regeneration process. Following chemical injuries, repair and regeneration response takes place slowly extending over 12 to 18 months with chronic inflammation, scarring and fibrosis leading to further damage. Early recognition and timely intervention give the best possible outcome of this potentially blinding condition.

Epidemiology

Chemical injury represents 10 to 22% of all ocular trauma and majority of these injuries result from industrial accidents. A minority of chemical injuries result from domestic accidents and hate crime like acid attack may be an uncommon cause of ocular chemical injury.

Etiology

The main causative agents of ocular chemical injuries are acids and alkalis, the latter being responsible for 50% of cases.

Common causes of ocular chemical injuries are:

Acid

- *Sulphuric acid (H_2SO_4):* Found in car and inverter batteries
- *Sulphurous acid (H_2SO_3):* Found in bleach and refrigerants
- *Acetic acid (CH_3COOH):* Found in vinegar and glacial acetic acid
- *Hydrochloric acid (HCL):* Ingredient of household cleaners and found in swimming pool disinfectants
- *Hydrofluoric acid (HF):* Found in rust removers, metal cleaners, glass polishing and mineral refining agents
- *Nitric acid (HNO_3):* Found in dyes, common laboratory reagent, fertilizer and explosives

Alkali

- *Lime [$Ca(OH)_2$]:* Most common cause of alkali injury and found in plaster, cement, mortar, whitewash
- *Ammonia (NH_3):* Found in cleaning agents, fertilizers, refrigerants
- *Potassium hydroxide (KOH):* Constituent of caustic potash
- *Magnesium hydroxide [$Mg(OH)_2$]:* Found in firework sparklers, flares
- *Lye (NaOH):* Ingredient of drain cleaners, airbags

Mode of Chemical Injury

Chemical injury occurs due to contact with chemical under circumstances such as:

- *Domestic accidents:* With detergents, cosmetics, ammonia and solvents.
- *Agricultural accidents:* Due to fertilizers, pesticides, insecticides, weedicides.
- *Workplace accidents:* With lime, mortar, cement, paint.
- *Chemical laboratory accidents:* With reagents containing acids and alkalis.
- *Deliberate chemical attacks:* As in hate crime with acids.
- Chemical warfare injuries.
- *Self-inflicted chemical injuries:* Seen in malingering and in psychopaths.

Pathophysiology

Acid

Acids interact with water contents of tear film and tissue to produce heat that cause charring of conjunctival and corneal epithelium and also cause tissue coagulation and collagen shrinkage. Acids bind to the ocular surface epithelium, which acts as buffer and prevents further penetration of acids. Strong acids cause instant coagulation of all proteins which act as barrier and prevent deeper penetration of acid into tissues and lesions become sharply demarcated. Thus, acid burns are less serious than alkali burns. The exception is Trifluoracetic acid and Hydrofluoric acid which have low molecular weight and dilute solutions of these acids penetrate deeply before dissociating. With calcium and magnesium, they form insoluble salts but form soluble salts with other cations, which release more fluoride after dissociation causing further tissue damage.

Alkali

Alkalis are hydrophilic and lipophilic and cause dissociation of tissues by release of hydroxyl ions that saponify fatty acids in cell membrane. They cause hydrolysis of interfibrillar glycosaminoglycans rendering tissues more susceptible to enzymatic degradation and disruption of extracellular matrix and collagen shrinkage, leading to deeper penetration of the alkali. Alkalis are hygroscopic and extract water from cells, leading to total necrosis. They combine with lipids of cells to form soluble compound, which produce softening and gelatinization of cells.

Magnesium hydroxide causes serious injuries due to thermal as well as chemical effects.

Lime forms calcium salts as soon as it penetrates the cell membrane, which prevents further penetration and damage. But lime particles retained in the fornices can act as reservoir of alkali and cause severe damage if not removed in time.

Alkali burns spread widely, their action continues for some and effects difficult to circumscribe and thus have guarded prognosis.

Duration of contact and surface area affected determine the depth of penetration and severity of damage in ocular chemical injuries. Depending on the degree of penetration, cornea, conjunctiva, tenon's capsule, episcleral, sclera, iris and lens can be affected. Damage to blood vessels at limbus leads to limbal ischemia with loss of limbal stem cells. Damage to ciliary body by ischemia or distortion of trabecular meshwork by collagen shrinkage leads to low or high intraocular pressure. All chemicals cause marked reduction in glucose and ascorbate in aqueous due to damage to ciliary body, leading to retarded collagen synthesis and hypotony.

Clinical Features

Symptoms

- Severe pain
- Blepharospasm
- Epiphora
- Reduced visual acuity

Signs

- *Cornea:* Mild superficial chemical burns cause de-epithelization of central corneal epithelium, leaving a rim of intact peripheral epithelium adjacent to limbus. This epithelial defect heals rapidly by migration from intact epithelium.

  More severe superficial chemical injuries affect the corneal, limbal and conjunctival epithelium resulting in sectorial limbal involvement. The central cornea is affected along with the inferior limbus and adjacent conjunctiva because of gravitation of chemical liquid to lower fornix and reflex rolling up of eye due to Bell's phenomenon at the time of injury, covering upper ocular surface. The denuded epithelium heals by migration of tongue-shaped projection of epithelium from remaining intact epithelium.

  More severe injuries result in total loss of corneal and limbal epithelium associated with partial or total loss of conjunctival epithelium. In cases of partial loss of conjunctival epithelium, surviving conjunctival epithelium migrates to reach centripetally to reach the limbus and cover the cornea. During migration, they bring along blood vessels, lymphatics and fibrovascular tissue and cover the cornea with a fibrovascular pannus of variable thickness. Cornea can be covered entirely or there can be a central epithelial defect.

  Corneal nerves may be damaged leading to corneal hypoesthesia or anesthesia. Hyperesthesia or photophobia may occur after wound healing due to aberrant nerve regeneration. Severe neurotrophic keratopathy may result from melting of stroma not covered with epithelium associated with nerve damage.
- *Conjunctiva:* Following chemical injury, surviving conjunctival epithelium covers the corneal defect and undergoes conjunctival transdifferentiation where there is transformation of conjunctival epithelial cells on the corneal epithelial phenotype.
- *Eyelids:* Lids may become swollen, contracted, and rigid leading to exposure. Lagophthalmos can result from lid margin burn. Lid margin can become distorted with inadequate lid movements causing tear film abnormalities and dry eye.
- *Iris:* Iris may show engorged vessels, hemorrhage, atrophy or necrosis and *anterior* and posterior synechiae can develop.
- *Pupil:* Pupil may be constricted or dilated with limited or absent pupillary response.
- *Intraocular pressure:* The intraocular pressure may be raised, low or normal. The intraocular pressure is raised due to distortion of the drainage angle as a consequence of sudden corneal and scleral collagen shrinkage and clogging of trabecular meshwork with inflammatory debris and release of prostaglandin. Hypotony is due to extensive scarring and fibrosis of the ciliary body. Sometimes, low aqueous due to ciliary body damage may be compensated by defective drainage due to trabecular damage, giving a normal pressure.
- *Lens:* The lens can swell a few days after chemical eye injury leading to phacomorphic glaucoma.

Stages of Ocular Chemical Injury

It can be divided into three stages as follows:

- *Stage of acute ischemic necrosis*
  - Conjunctiva is markedly edematous, congested, necrosed with copious purulent discharge.
  - Cornea develops corneal edema with widespread sloughing of epithelium and opalescence of stroma resulting in varying degree of corneal opacity and sloughing of whole cornea in severe cases.
  - Iris is severely inflamed, and granulation tissue may replace iris and ciliary body in severe cases.
- *Stage of reparation*
  - Conjunctival and corneal epithelium regenerate
  - Corneal vascularization occurs
  - Inflammation of iris subsides
- *Stage of complications:* Characterized by development of complications such as
  - Symblepharon
  - Recurrent corneal ulceration
  - Complicated cataract
  - Secondary glaucoma
  - Dry eye
  - Neurotrophic keratopathy

Phases of Ocular Recovery

According to McCulley, the phase of ocular recovery following chemical injury can be divided into phases as given in the **Table 3** below.

TABLE 3: Phases of ocular recovery following chemical injury.

Phase	*Day*	*Recovery*
Initial	0	Clinical manifestations relate to severity of injury and can be graded according to degree of involvement of cornea, conjunctiva and limbus
Acute	0-7	Epithelial regrowth begins to occur from the undamaged limbal stem cells. Treatment should be directed at encouraging growth while controlling inflammation
Early repair	7-21	Corneal/conjunctival epithelium and keratocytes proliferate during this stage. Mild injuries re-epithelize completely, more severe injuries can have persistent epithelial defects. Collagen synthesis continues while activity of collagenases peaks by 14-21 days. Treatment should be attempted to maximize collagen synthesis and minimize collagenase activity
Late repair	>21	• In mild injuries, repair is complete when limbal stem cell population is intact • In grade II injuries where there is focal stem cell loss, focal conjunctivalization of cornea may occur • In more severe injuries, there is delayed re-epithelization of cornea, leading to either repopulation by conjunctival epithelium or stromal ulceration and permanent scarring • In case of severe limbal damage, the eye cannot be salvaged despite optimal management

Management

Diagnosis

History: A meticulous history should be taken to document time of injury, the type of chemical, the mechanism of injury, whether eye was rinsed following injury and for how long, and whether eye protection was worn at the time of injury.

Physical examination: A complete ophthalmic examination should be performed after irrigation of the eye to assess the extent and depth of injury after normalizing the pH of the eye by irrigation and the degree of involvement of cornea, conjunctiva, limbus and any other structures should be assessed and documented. The palpebral fissures and fornices are checked for any retained chemical foreign bodies.

Fluorescein staining: Fluorescein staining and examination under cobalt blue light are useful in assessing degree of involvement of conjunctiva and cornea.

Intraocular pressure measurement: IOP measurement is important as elevation of IOP may be seen in acute and chronic alkali injuries.

Treatment

Eye Irrigation

Immediate and thorough copious irrigation with any clean water or saline is the cornerstone in management of ocular chemical injury. The pH of both eyes should be checked before conducting a full ophthalmic examination and irrigated if found to be not in the normal range. Irrigation removes the offending substance, limiting the duration of chemical exposure and restore the physiologic pH. Irrigation can be done with readily available solutions like tap water at the spot of injury or other readily available solutions like normal saline, ringer lactate, or balanced saline solution. Other useful solutions for eye irrigation are the phosphate buffer solution, hypertonic saline, and Diphoterine, which is a hypertonic amphoteric solution that can be used for both acid and alkali burns.

The patient should be seated upright with head supported and tilted towards the affected side. Topical anesthesia can be administered, and eyelids are kept open. Irrigating fluid should be administered from nasal to temporal side and away from non-infected eye to avoid injury to that eye. Irrigation should be done for at least 30 minutes using 1 to 3 L of fluid or continued until the physiological pH is reached (by monitoring with pH paper). During irrigation, the patient is instructed to blink and to look in all directions, thus ensuring that the conjunctival sacs are well irrigated.

Mechanical Removal of Contaminants

Contact lenses should be removed as their presence can lead to persistence of chemical burn despite irrigation.

The fornices should be swept with sterile cotton tipped applicators to remove any retained caustic foreign body as they cause continued chemical exposure. Retained particles can also be removed with the help of forceps under topical anesthesia.

Medical Management

The aim of medical management is to minimize collagen breakdown and control inflammation, prevent corneal melting, promote re-epithelization and enhance rapid and uncomplicated healing.

- *Antibiotics:* Topical antibiotic ointment like Erythromycin eye ointment four times daily is used to prevent superinfection and provide lubrication. For severe injuries, stronger antibiotics like topical fluoroquinolone (Moxifloxacin) are used 4-6 times daily to prevent infection.
- *Steroid eye drops:* Topical steroids are the mainstay of treatment of chemical eye injury to reduce inflammation and prevent further corneal breakdown. Topical steroids like dexamethasone 0.1% or prednisolone 1% can be used four times daily in mild injuries and hourly in severe injuries in the first week following injury. After about one week of intensive steroid therapy, tapering is required as steroids may interfere with corneal wound healing and collagen synthesis. After three weeks, there is no fibroblast migration and steroids can be readministered if required.
- *Cycloplegics:* Mydriatics and cycloplegics like Atropine or Cyclopentolate are used to treat iridocyclitis, prevent or break posterior synechiae and improve comfort.
- *Artificial tears:* preservative free lubricating eye drops should be used generously for comfort and to promote healing.
- *Ascorbic acid:* Ascorbic acid, a cofactor in collagen synthesis, may be depleted following chemical eye injury. Ascorbic acid can be used topically as a 10% sodium ascorbate eye drop every hour or orally in the dose of 1 to 2 g/day. It restores the aqueous level of ascorbic acid, reduces collagen degradation, corneal ulceration and perforation.
- *Autologous serum:* Autologous serum eyedrops is a useful adjunct therapy for promoting corneal wound healing as they provide growth factors, collagenase inhibitors, retinoic acid and fibrinogen activator.
- *Sodium citrate:* Citrate drops used as 10% topical eye drops, stabilizes polymorphonuclear cells from releasing proteolytic enzymes which can dissolve the cornea by chelating calcium and also inhibiting collagenases.
- *Doxycycline:* Doxycycline, 100mg twice daily, acts to reduce the effect of matrix metalloproteinases which can degrade type I collagen. They chelate zinc which is necessary for collagenase.
- *1% Medroxyprogesterone:* It is a progestational steroid which is less potent than corticosteroid. It can be used as a substitute for corticosteroid after 10 to 14 days therapy.

Surgical Treatment

- *Debridement of necrotic and contaminated tissue:* Contaminated and necrotic epithelium should be removed as early as possible because necrotic tissue serves as source of inflammation and inhibit epithelization. Removal can be done with a cotton bud to promote re-epithelization.
- *Conjunctival/Tenon's transposition (Tenoplasty):* Tenoplasty is a procedure of advancement of Tenon's to the limbus. In grade IV burns, anterior segment necrosis can result from loss of limbal blood supply which can lead to sterile corneal ulceration. Tenoplasty is performed by exploring the fornix closest to the ischemic area to identify viable, perfused tissue that is pink or red in color and bleeds on manipulation and mobilized and advanced to cover the ischemic area. This is done to re-establish limbal vascularity and facilitate re-epithelization.

  Free conjunctival autografts can be used in unilateral burns to treat corneal melting unresponsive to other mode of treatment.
- *Amniotic membrane transplantation (AMT):* Amniotic membrane transplantation is done to restore the conjunctival surface rapidly and to reduce limbal and stromal inflammation. AMT hastens healing of damaged cornea, reduce pain and in moderate chemical eye injuries. The benefit of AMT is both physical and biological. Physically, AMT improves patient comfort by reducing eyelid friction and also prevents symblepharon formation. Biologic effects of amniotic membrane are due to its expression of TGFB1 and epidermal growth factors, which have roles in wound healing.
- *Limbal stem cell transplantation (LSCT):* Limbal stem transplantation has been employed to replace loss of limbal stem cells which occur due to limbal ischemia following chemical eye injury. Limbal stem cells are responsible for repopulation of corneal epithelial cells and inhibition of conjunctival growth over cornea. In unilateral injury, limbal autografts can be taken from contralateral eye after acute phase of injury. in bilateral cases, limbal grafts can be taken from living related donors after HLA matching or from cadaveric donors which require aggressive immunosuppression therapy.
- *Cultivated oral mucosal epithelium transplantation:* This procedure can be used to reduce inflammation and promote re-epithelization in corneal burns. The cells are harvested from the patient's buccal mucosa which does not require immunosuppressive therapy.
- *Keratoprosthesis:* Keratoprosthesis can be used in severe chemical injury leading to chronic inflammation and scarring where visual recovery becomes challenging. In severely damaged eyes, limbal stem cell transplants and corneal transplants do not survive, and Boston Keratoprosthesis can be used in these cases. Immunosuppression therapy is not necessary for keratoprosthesis as it is independent of stem cell function.

Treatment of Complications

- *Secondary glaucoma:* Anti-glaucoma medication is often required to treat glaucoma. Oral acetazolamide is preferred, as with damage and distortion of trabecular meshwork and uveoscleral pathway, mechanism of action of drugs acting on these pathways may be ineffective. In severe cases of glaucoma, a tube shunt is preferred depending upon the conjunctival health. Phacomorphic glaucoma may need urgent removal of lens with secondary implant later.
- *Dry eye:* The treatment options for dry eye include instillation of artificial tears frequently, punctal occlusion, correction of lid malposition, oral mucous membrane grafts and salivary transplantation.
- *Conjunctival adhesions:* Symblepharon may be released and repaired, and fornix reconstruction can be done with amniotic membrane graft or oral mucous grafts.
- *Lid repair:* Lid repair should be performed early in eyelid tissue loss to prevent exposure with skin grafts or oral mucous membrane grafts. Tarsorrhaphy may be required to prevent exposure and promote healing.
- *Persistent epithelial defect:* Recombinant human nerve growth factor promotes healing of persistent epithelial defects. Nerve growth factor drops can promote corneal nerve regeneration if conjunctival sensation around cornea is preserved. Substrate regenerating eyedrops promote substrate regeneration and coenzyme Q10 promote epithelial healing. Recalcitrant cases may be treated by tarsorrhaphy, amniotic membrane grafts and conjunctival flaps. Limbal stem cell transplantation may be required to treat persistent epithelial defects with total limbal stem cell deficiency.

15. What is Dua's classification of chemical injuries? How is it better than Rooper-Hall classification? Management strategies of grade III and grade IV chemical injuries. (3 + 2 + 5) (DNB 2019)

Two classifications are currently used for grading chemical eye injury, namely Rooper-Hall classification and Dua's classification.

Dua's classification is based on limbal involvement in clock hours and percentage of conjunctival involvement for grading the severity and predicting the prognosis of chemical eye injury. The conjunctival involvement should be calculated only for bulbar conjunctiva up to the conjunctival fornices. Here, analogue scale is used which records the amount of limbal involvement in clock hours of affected limbus/percentage of conjunctival involvement **(Table 4)**.

TABLE 4: DUA'S classification of ocular chemical injury.

Grade	*Limbal involvement (clock hours)*	*Conjunctival involvement (%)*	*Analogue scale*	*Prognosis*
I	0 clock hours	0%	0/0%	Very good
II	≤3 clock hours	≤30%	0.1-3/1-30%	Good
III	>3-6 clock hours	>30-50%	3.1-6/31-50%	Good
IV	>6-9 clock hours	>50-75%	6.1-9/51-75%	Good to guarded
V	>9-<12 clock hours	>75-<100%	9.1-11.9/75.1-99.9%	Guarded to poor
VI	12 (total limbus) involved	Total conjunctiva (100%) involved	12/100%	Very poor

Source: Dua HS, King AJ, Joseph A. A new classification of ocular surface burns. Br J Ophthalmol. 2001;85(11):1379-83.

Rooper-Hall classification is based on the extent of limbal ischemia and degree of corneal involvement **(Table 5)**.

TABLE 5: Roper-Hall classification of ocular chemical injury.

Grade	*Cornea*	*Limbal ischemia*	*Prognosis*
I	Corneal epithelial damage	No limbal ischemia	Good
II	Cornea hazy but iris details visible	< 1/3 limbal ischemia	Good
III	Total epithelial loss, stromal haze, iris details obscured	1/3 to 1/2 limbal ischemia	Guarded
IV	Cornea opaque, iris and pupil obscured	>1/2 limbal ischemia	Poor

Source: Roper-Hall MJ. Thermal and chemical burns. Trans Ophthalmol Soc U K (1962). 1965;85:631-53.

The limitation of Rooper-Hall classification is that as it was introduced before the concept of limbal stem cell, conjunctival involvement is not taken into account nor any allowance made for overlap between grades. Dua's classification provides further subclassification of grade IV ocular burns by Rooper-Hall into three separate grades. Thus, Dua's classification is superior to Rooper-Hall classification in predicting outcome of severe ocular chemical injuries.

16. A 28-year-old male comes to the emergency room with history of accidental instillation of activated lime. How will you manage this patient? What is the difference in presentation and management of acid burns from alkali burns? (7 + 3) (DNB 2019)

Activated lime is alkali which is hydrophilic and lipophilic and causes dissociation of tissues by release of hydroxyl ions that saponify fatty acids in cell membrane. Alkali causes hydrolysis of interfibrillar glycosaminoglycans rendering tissues more susceptible to enzymatic degradation and disruption of extracellular matrix and collagen shrinkage, leading to deeper penetration of the alkali. It is hygroscopic and extract water from cells, leading to total necrosis. Alkali combines with lipids of cells to form soluble compound, which produce softening and gelatinization of cells.

Lime forms calcium salts as soon as it penetrates the cell membrane, which prevents further penetration and damage. But lime particles retained in the fornices can act as reservoir of alkali and cause severe damage if not removed in time.

Management of Accidental Instillation of Activated Lime

Eye Irrigation

Immediate and thorough copious irrigation with any clean water or saline is the cornerstone in management of ocular chemical injury. The pH of both eyes should be checked before conducting a full ophthalmic examination and irrigated if found to be not in the normal range. Irrigation removes the offending substance, limiting the duration of chemical exposure and restore the physiologic pH. Irrigation can be done with readily available solutions like tap water at the spot of injury or other readily available solutions like normal saline, ringer lactate, or balanced saline solution. Other useful solutions for eye irrigation are phosphate buffer solution, hypertonic saline, and Diphoterine, which is a hypertonic amphoteric solution that can be used for both acid and alkali burns.

The patient should be seated upright with head supported and tilted towards the affected side. Topical anesthesia can be administered, and eyelids are kept open. Irrigating fluid should be administered from nasal to temporal side and away from non-infected eye to avoid injury to that eye. Irrigation should be done for at least 30 minutes using 1 to 3 L of fluid or continued until the physiological pH is reached (by monitoring with pH paper). During irrigation, the patient is instructed to blink and to look in all directions, thus ensuring that the conjunctival sacs are well irrigated.

Mechanical Removal of Contaminants

Contact lenses should be removed as their presence can lead to persistence of chemical burn despite irrigation.

The fornices should be swept with sterile cotton tipped applicators to remove any retained caustic foreign body as they cause continued chemical exposure. Retained particles can also be removed with the help of forceps under topical anesthesia.

Medical Management

The aim of medical management is to minimize collagen breakdown and control inflammation, prevent corneal melting, promote re-epithelization and enhance rapid and uncomplicated healing.

- *Antibiotics:* Topical antibiotic ointment like Erythromycin eye ointment four times daily is used to prevent superinfection and provide lubrication. For severe injuries, stronger antibiotics like topical fluoroquinolone (Moxifloxacin) are used 4-6 times daily to prevent infection.
- *Steroid eye drops:* Topical steroids are the mainstay of treatment of chemical eye injury to reduce inflammation and prevent further corneal breakdown. Topical steroids like dexamethasone 0.1% or prednisolone 1% can be used four times daily in mild injuries and hourly in severe injuries in the first week following injury. After about one week of intensive steroid therapy, tapering is required as steroids may interfere with corneal wound healing and collagen synthesis. After three weeks, there is no fibroblast migration and steroids can be readministered if required.
- *Cycloplegics:* Mydriatics and cycloplegics like Atropine or Cyclopentolate are used to treat iridocyclitis, prevent or break posterior synechiae and improve comfort.
- *Artificial tears:* preservative free lubricating eye drops should be used generously for comfort and to promote healing.
- *Ascorbic acid:* Ascorbic acid, a cofactor in collagen synthesis, may be depleted following chemical eye injury. Ascorbic acid can be used topically as a 10% sodium ascorbate eye drop every hour or orally in the dose of 1 to 2 g/day. It restores the aqueous level of ascorbic acid, reduces collagen degradation, corneal ulceration and perforation.
- *Autologous serum:* Autologous serum eyedrops is a useful adjunct therapy for promoting corneal wound healing as they provide growth factors, collagenase inhibitors, retinoic acid and fibrinogen activator.
- *Sodium citrate:* Citrate drops used as 10% topical eye drops, stabilizes polymorphonuclear cells from releasing proteolytic enzymes which can dissolve the cornea by chelating calcium and also inhibiting collagenases.
- *Doxycycline:* Doxycycline, 100mg twice daily, acts to reduce the effect of matrix metalloproteinases which can degrade type I collagen. They chelate zinc which is necessary for collagenase.
- *1% Medroxyprogesterone:* It is a progestational steroid which is less potent than corticosteroid. It can be used as a substitute for corticosteroid after 10 to 14 days therapy.

Surgical Treatment

- *Debridement of necrotic and contaminated tissue:* Contaminated and necrotic epithelium should be removed as early as possible because necrotic tissue serves as source of inflammation and inhibit epithelization. Removal can be done with a cotton bud to promote re-epithelization.

- *Conjunctival/Tenon's transposition (Tenoplasty):* Tenoplasty is a procedure of advancement of Tenon's to the limbus. In grade IV burns, anterior segment necrosis can result from loss of limbal blood supply which can lead to sterile corneal ulceration. Tenoplasty is performed by exploring the fornix closest to the ischemic area to identify viable, perfused tissue that is pink or red in color and bleeds on manipulation and mobilized and advanced to cover the ischemic area. This is done to re-establish limbal vascularity and facilitate re-epithelization.

  Free conjunctival autografts can be used in unilateral burns to treat corneal melting unresponsive to other mode of treatment.
- *Amniotic membrane transplantation (AMT):* Amniotic membrane transplantation is done to restore the conjunctival surface rapidly and to reduce limbal and stromal inflammation. AMT hastens healing of damaged cornea, reduce pain and in moderate chemical eye injuries. The benefit of AMT is both physical and biological. Physically, AMT improves patient comfort by reducing eyelid friction and also prevents symblepharon formation. Biologic effects of amniotic membrane are due to its expression of TGFB1 and epidermal growth factors, which have roles in wound healing.
- *Limbal stem cell transplantation (LSCT):* Limbal stem transplantation has been employed to replace loss of limbal stem cells which occur due to limbal ischemia following chemical eye injury. Limbal stem cells are responsible for repopulation of corneal epithelial cells and inhibition of conjunctival growth over cornea. In unilateral injury, limbal autografts can be taken from contralateral eye after acute phase of injury. in bilateral cases, limbal grafts can be taken from living related donors after HLA matching or from cadaveric donors which require aggressive immunosuppression therapy.
- *Cultivated oral mucosal epithelium transplantation:* this procedure can be used to reduce inflammation and promote re-epithelization in corneal burns. The cells are harvested from the patient's buccal mucosa which does not require immunosuppressive therapy.
- *Keratoprosthesis:* Keratoprosthesis can be used in severe chemical injury leading to chronic inflammation and scarring where visual recovery becomes challenging. In severely damaged eyes, limbal stem cell transplants and corneal transplants do not survive, and Boston Keratoprosthesis can be used in these cases. Immunosuppression therapy is not necessary on keratoprosthesis as it is independent of stem cell function.

Treatment of Complications

- *Secondary glaucoma:* Anti-glaucoma medication is often required to treat glaucoma. Oral acetazolamide is preferred, as with damage and distortion of trabecular meshwork and uveoscleral pathway, mechanism of action of drugs acting on these pathways may be ineffective. In severe cases of glaucoma, a tube shunt is preferred depending upon the conjunctival health. Phacomorphic glaucoma may need urgent removal of lens with secondary implant later.
- *Dry eye:* The treatment options for dry eye include instillation of artificial tears frequently, punctal occlusion, correction of lid malposition, oral mucous membrane grafts and salivary transplantation.
- *Conjunctival adhesions:* Symblepharon may be released and repaired, and fornix reconstruction can be done with amniotic membrane graft or oral mucous grafts.
- *Lid repair:* Lid repair should be performed early in eyelid tissue loss to prevent exposure with skin grafts or oral mucous membrane grafts. Tarsorrhaphy may be required to prevent exposure and promote healing.
- *Persistent epithelial defect:* Recombinant human nerve growth factor promotes healing of persistent epithelial defects. Nerve growth factor drops can promote corneal nerve regeneration if conjunctival sensation around cornea is preserved. Substrate regenerating eyedrops promote substrate regeneration and coenzyme Q10 promote epithelial healing. Recalcitrant cases may be treated by tarsorrhaphy, amniotic membrane grafts and conjunctival flaps. Limbal stem cell transplantation may be required to treat persistent epithelial defects with total limbal stem cell deficiency.

Difference in Presentation Between Acid and Alkali Injury

- Acids cause damage to the ocular tissue by denaturing and precipitating proteins in tissues of contact. They coagulate protein which acts as a barrier to prevent further penetration and damage.
- Alkalis saponify the fatty acids of cell membranes, penetrate the corneal stroma and destroy the proteoglycan ground substance and collagen bundles leading to deeper penetration of tissues. The damaged tissue secretes proteolytic enzymes, which lead to further damage.

17. Principle of suturing of corneal laceration. (5) (BHU MS 2020)

18. Management of retained intraocular foreign body. (5) (TNMGRMU MS 2018)

Principle of Corneal Wound Repair

Corneal wound should be repaired within 24 hours to reduce the risk of infection and avoid further damage to the eye. The goal of repair is to obtain a watertight closure and restoration of normal anatomy.

The technique of primary corneal wound repair depends on the extent of wound, associated complications like iris prolapse, flat anterior chamber and damage of intraocular contents.

Small corneal wound can be treated with pad and bandage, soft bandage contact lens or with cyanoacrylate or fibrin glue in conjunction with topical antibiotic and cycloplegic.

Medium-sized wound or corneal wound of >2 mm requires suturing as this is often associated with shallow or flat anterior chamber.

Corneal wound with iris prolapse should be sutured meticulously taking care not to incarcerate any uveal tissue into the closure. Prolapsed iris usually needs abscission as repositioning it may introduce infection into the eye, especially in old or infected cases. But in fresh case of corneal injury with iris prolapse with no sign infection, repositioning of iris may be done before suturing to maintain the anatomy of the eye.

Corneal wound with lens damage is treated by suturing the corneal wound meticulously and then removing the lens after reformation of an anterior chamber. Lensectomy with primary or secondary intraocular lens implantation can be performed in conjunction with vitrectomy if associated with vitreous prolapse.

Surgery is usually performed under general anesthesia as giving a block may cause further prolapse of intraocular content. Retrobulbar block with a small volume of fluid may be used if local anesthesia is preferred.

The edged of the wound should be first cleaned thoroughly of debris and foreign bodies. Prolapsed iris should be reposited, but vitrectomy is needed for vitreous prolapse. A 360-degree peritomy is indicated in cases of occult globe rupture in order to view all four quadrants of posterior sclera to identify all rupture sites. Scleral defect can be repaired using either 6-0 to 8-0 Vicryl or 8-0 to 9-0 nylon suture. The first suture may be placed in the middle of the defect and subsequent sutures in the middle of remaining defects.

Corneal wound repair should be watertight while trying to make it as close to normal state as possible. Suturing should be done with 10-0 nylon using interrupted sutures to avoid flattening of cornea. The depth of the suture should be 100% to reduce corneal edema and minimize tissue shift or override. In case of angled wound, the first suture is placed at the angle. If the wound is crosses the whole length of cornea, suturing can be done by using the Rowsey-Hays technique where large bites are first placed at the two ends followed by gradually smaller bites as suturing approach the center of cornea.

Corneoscleral wound is closed by putting the initial suture at the limbus, then suturing the corneal wound before the scleral wound.

Diagnosis

History: To avoid siderosis, a detailed history of the injury must be elicited, and thorough evaluation of anterior and posterior segments are necessary. Slit lamp examination along with Seidel's test, gonioscopy and retinal examination should be performed to rule out intraocular foreign body.

Radiological evaluation: They play a key role to detect IOFB as well as assess damage in ocular siderosis. Imaging modalities that can be used include X-ray, ultrasonography (USG), computed tomography (CT), magnetic resonance imaging (MRI, ultrasound biomicroscopy (UBM) and optical coherence tomography (OCT). Electrophysiological tests like electroretinography (ERG) can be used to assess retinal damage. Other tests like fluorescein angiography (FA), electrooculogram and visual field assessment can be used to assess further damage.

On *plain X-ray,* metallic foreign bodies are seen as radio-opaque foreign bodies but have limitations in localizing and predicting nature of foreign body.

USG can detect both metallic and non-metallic intraocular foreign bodies, which appear as hyperechoic lesion with acoustic black shadowing on B-scan. USG can identify associated ocular injuries such as lens dislocation, vitreous hemorrhage, retinal detachment and choroidal detachment even in the presence of media opacity. Limitations of USG are that it does not provide accurate size of foreign body, may miss foreign bodies lying in the posterior one-third of orbit or within orbital soft tissues, is operator dependent and caution must be exerted in suspected open globe injury.

Non-contrast CT is the gold-standard for identifying IOFBs, providing high accuracy in predicting the nature, location and size of foreign body. Thin scans (1-3 mm) have higher resolutions and are preferred.

MRI has better sensitivity (95%) than CT scan for non-metallic IOFB and visualize soft tissues, optic nerve and orbital apex without radiation exposure but contraindicated on ferromagnetic IOFB due to possible movement within the electromagnetic field.

UBM is useful for imaging foreign bodies located anteriorly like those lodged in the subconjunctival space, cornea, angle, iris, ciliary body but avoided in suspected open globe injury due to increased risk of infection.

OCT is a non-contact, non-invasive ocular imaging investigation tool. Anterior segment OCT can visualize IOFB in the anterior segment, but not beyond the iris due to poor penetrance.

Posterior segment OCT is a useful tool for accurate localization of IOFB in the posterior segment and for quantifying the amount of cystoid macular edema.

ERG is the gold standard electrophysiological test for diagnostic test for subclinical siderosis bulbi. Early phase of the disease shows supernormal response with increase in amplitude of both a and b waves. Subsequently, the amplitude of b-wave decreases with reduction of b/a ratio to less than 1. An extinguished response is seen in ERG in advanced cases with absent a and b waves.

Fluorescein angiography in ocular siderosis may show hyperfluorescent window defects due to capillary non-perfusion, RPE changes and ischemic maculopathy.

Visual field assessment: This may show progressive visual field constriction in ocular siderosis.

Treatment

Prompt removal of IOFB is advocated to avoid the development of endophthalmitis and siderosis. Most intraocular foreign bodies are removed from a new opening unless the entrance wound is large.

Antibiotics are given both by topical and systemic route to combat common pathogen and booster dose of tetanus vaccine administered.

Technique of Removal

- *Magnet:* Magnet can remove ferrous foreign bodies of any size, shape and weight. Removal is performed by making a sclerotomy adjacent to the foreign body, applying magnet to remove it, followed by cryotherapy to the retinal break.
- *Forceps:* Forceps are used to remove non-magnetic foreign bodies or magnetic foreign bodies that cannot be removed safely with a magnet.

Surgical Approach of IOFB Removal

- Anterior segment IOFB should be removed promptly with forceps or intraocular magnet through limbal paracentesis. Anterior chamber foreign body is removed by making a limbal incision over it or an incision 90 to 180 degrees from the object for better access with forceps.
- Intralenticular foreign body may be left as such or may be removed along with the cataract during primary or secondary repair.
- Posterior segment IOFB can be removed with the help of intraocular magnet or forceps after performing pars plana vitrectomy.
- The fibrous capsule of IOFB is released to facilitate its removal and the posterior hyaloid face is detached and removed to prevent tractional detachment.

19. A 12-year-old child sustained injury to right eye while playing with bow and arrow. Discuss the management of corneoscleral perforation with iris prolapse in this patient. (DNB 2020)

Management of Corneoscleral Perforation with Iris Prolapse

Corneoscleral wound and subsequent iris prolapse are complicated by wound in the conjunctiva and should be repaired within 24 hours to reduce risk of infection and avoid further damage to the eye.

Surgical Management

The goal of repair is to obtain a watertight closure and restoration of normal anatomy.

Methods of Repair

- *Repair of wound:* Corneal wound with iris prolapse should be sutured meticulously taking care not to incarcerate any uveal tissue into the closure and prevent further prolapse.
- *Repositioning of iris:* Repositioning of iris is the primary intervention in fresh case of corneal injury with iris prolapse with no sign infection. This may be done before suturing to maintain the anatomy of the eye.
- *Iridectomy:* Prolapsed iris usually needs abscission as repositioning it may introduce infection into the eye, especially in old or infected cases or in cases where damage of iris tissue is beyond repair.
- *Corneoscleral wound* is closed by putting the initial suture at the limbus, then suturing the corneal wound before the scleral wound.

Surgical Procedure

Surgery is usually performed under general anesthesia as giving a block may cause further prolapse of intraocular content. Retrobulbar block with a small volume of fluid may be used if local anesthesia is preferred.

The edged of the wound should be first cleaned thoroughly of debris and foreign bodies. Prolapsed iris should be reposited, but vitrectomy is needed for vitreous prolapse. A 360-degree peritomy is indicated in cases of occult globe rupture in order to view all four quadrants of posterior sclera to identify all rupture sites. Scleral defect can be repaired using either 6-0 to 8-0 Vicryl or 8-0 to 9-0 nylon suture. The first suture may be placed in the middle of the defect and subsequent sutures in the middle of remaining defects.

Corneal wound repair should be watertight while trying to make it as close to normal state as possible. Suturing should be done with 10-0 nylon using interrupted sutures to avoid flattening of cornea. The depth of the suture should be 100% to reduce corneal edema and minimize tissue shift or override. In case of angled wound, the first suture is placed at the angle. If the wound is crosses the whole length of cornea, suturing can be done by using the Rowsey-Hays technique where large bites are first placed at the two ends followed by gradually smaller bites as suturing approach the center of cornea.

Medical Management

- *Antibiotics:* Antibiotics are administered topically (preservative free) or systemically to control infection.
- *Anti-inflammatory:* They are given to reduce inflammation and discomfort in the eye.
- *Cycloplegics:* They help in relaxing the ocular muscles, reduce pain and discomfort and aid in healing process.

Conservative Management

- *Eye shield* is used to protect the eye from further damage.
- *Cyanoacrylate glue and bandage contact lens:* These may be used in small corneal perforation with iris prolapse after repositing the iris.

20. How will you manage a patient with cracker injury? (10) (DNB 2021)

Crackers and fireworks-related injuries can cause serious injuries leading to permanent loss of vision, limb or even life. Common globe injuries cause by crackers include ocular burns, eyelid injuries, subconjunctival hemorrhage, corneal injuries, hyphema, traumatic iritis, vitreous hemorrhage, globe laceration or rupture, retinal injury, lacrimal injury, cataract, glaucoma, orbital fracture or optic neuropathy.

Management of Cracker Injury of Eye

Diagnosis

- *History:* A history of recent injury to the eye by crackers or fireworks will be given by the patient. A complete history is elicited regarding the date and time of injury, mechanism of injury, use of eye protection at the time of injury, the size, weight, velocity, composition of the object and the type of firework.

- *Physical examination:* A detailed examination should be done to document the types of injury including assessment of visual acuity, pupillary examination, extraocular movement, globe malposition, any foreign body, and intraocular pressure. Seidel test is indicated when open globe injury is suspected. Fundoscopic examination should be performed to document posterior segment involvement.
- *Diagnostic procedures:*
  - *CT scan:* CT scan of orbit and face should be taken in case of projectile fireworks to exclude intraocular foreign bodies, preferably with thin cut of 1 mm sections of axial, coronal and parasagittal views.
  - *B-scan ultrasonography and ultrasound biomicroscopy:* They are considered in suspected intraocular foreign body, retinal detachment or in case of poor visualization of fundus.
  - *MRI:* MRI is avoided in suspected cases of metallic foreign bodies.

Primary Prevention

- Stay at a safe distance away from fireworks
- Do not pick up misfires
- Wear eye protection

Treatment

General Treatment

- Treatment of cracker injuries depends on the type of injury present.
- An eye shield is used in open globe injury to protect the eye from further damage.
- Systemic antibiotics and tetanus prophylaxis should be administered.
- Exploration in the operation theater may be required depending on the extent of injury.
- When chemical injury is suspected, copious irrigation is done if found above or below normal pH.

Surgical Treatment

- Exploration of the globe is required in suspected globe rupture or penetrating injury.
- Vitrectomy is indicated in cases of intraocular foreign body or retinal detachment.

SUGGESTED READING

1. Gervasio KA, Peck TJ, Fathy CA, Sivalingam MD, Friedberg MA. The Will's Eye Manual, 8th edition Chapter 3. Lippincott Williams & Wilkins; 2021.
2. Korn BS. 2020-2021 Basic and Clinical Science Course™ (BCSC), Section 07: Oculofacial Plastic and Orbital Surgery. American Academy of Ophthalmology; 2020. pp. 109-22.
3. Salmon JF. Kanski's Clinical Ophthalmology, 9th edition Chapter 22. Elsevier Health Sciences; 2019.
4. Sihota R, Tandon R. Parsons' Diseases of Eye, 23rd edition. Elsevier India; 2019.
5. Weisenthal RW. 2020-2021 Basic and Clinical Science Course™ (BCSC), Section 08: External Disease and Cornea. American Academy of Ophthalmology; 2020. pp. 375-403.

CHAPTER

Community Ophthalmology

Sinjita Dutta

QUESTIONS

1. **Causes and prevalence of corneal blindness in India. What are the prerequisites for arranging eye bank and legislation?** **(10) (TNMGRMU MS 2018)**
2. **Role of NHM and State Blindness Control Society in NPCB.** **(10) (BHU MS 2019)**
3. **Write briefly about Vision 2020.** **(10) (WBHUS MS 2019)**
4. **Write in short about National Programme for Control of Blindness.** **(10) (DNB 2018)**
5. **What are the goals of NPCB? Discuss its strategies.** **(10) (WBUHS MS 2019)**
6. **Describe the organizational structure of NPCB.** **(10) (WBUHS MS 2018)**
7. **Role of NPCB.** **(10) (BHU MS 2019)**
8. **Discuss eye bank in India.** **(10) (BHU MS 2018)**
9. **District Blindness Control Society.** **(10) (WBUHS MS 2018)**
10. **Mention the causes of childhood blindness.** **(5) (TN MGRMU MS 2022)**
11. **Ocular morbidity in school going children.** **(10) (RGUHS MS 2020)**
12. **Discuss the classification, prevention, and management of vitamin A deficiency. Nutritional factors causing ocular morbidity.** **(10) (BHU MS 2021)**
13. **Eye screening in school children.** **(10) (WBUHS MS 2018)**
14. **Discuss in details about School Eye Health Programme.** **(10) (TNMGRMU MS 2021)**
15. **School survey in prevention of childhood blindness.** **(10) (BHU MS 2019)**
16. **Discuss in detail about teleophthalmology, its uses, merits, and demerits in community eye care.** **(15) BHU MS 2022**
17. **Organizing eye camp.** **(10) BHU MS 2018**

1. Causes and prevalence of corneal blindness in India. What are the prerequisites for arranging eye bank and legislation? (10) (TNMGRMU MS 2018)

Causes and Prevalence

Corneal blindness was the fifth leading cause of blindness in the world, following cataracts, glaucoma, refractive error, and age-related macular degeneration. Still, according to the National Blindness and Visual Impairment Survey India 2015–2019, CB has become the third leading cause of blindness. Among 45 million blind people worldwide, 6–8 million are blind due to corneal diseases. About 5.5 million people worldwide are bilaterally blind, and 6.2 million are unilaterally blind due to corneal diseases.

The most common causes include:

- Trauma-the leading cause of corneal blindness in some regions, such as North Telangana and Kurnool. Trauma can be caused by agricultural injuries, and is more common in males due to more outdoor activity
- Infective keratitis-A major risk factor for corneal blindness is contact lens wear.
- Vitamin A deficiency-A common cause of blindness in children
- Pseudophakic bullous keratopathy
- Chemical injuries
- Keratoconus
- Dystrophies

The burden of CB is more in developing countries, in children and young adults. When corneal diseases affect the younger population, the disability-adjusted life years are more significant compared with other causes of blindness such as cataract.

A high prevalence of CB is noted in India (0.88%). The percentage of people affected with corneal diseases in India represents the second highest at 15.8%.

According to the WHO, around 7 million people in India await keratoplasty. India accounts for 20% of the 39 million blind population across the globe. Currently, CB in India is 1.2 million, which is 0.36% of total blindness; about 25,000 to 30,000 people are added every year. Three population-based studies were conducted in India on the burden of CB. In the Andhra Pradesh study, 0.1% suffer from CB; the prevalence is 3.9%; among them, 2.9% are unilaterally blind, 3.7% of CB is prevalent in Northern India, and 13.3% is prevalent in CB in Kurnool. There exists a regional difference in the etiology of CB; ocular trauma is the leading cause of CB in North Telangana and Kurnool (59.3% and 45%, respectively) compared with pseudophakic bullous keratopathy as the leading cause of CB in North India (46.2%).

The highest prevalence of blindness was seen in Bijnor, Uttar Pradesh (UP) (3.7%), and lowest in Thrissur, Kerala (1.1%), and the second most common cause of total blindness was corneal diseases due to infections and trauma.

According to the World Health Organization (WHO) estimates, in 2010, there was a 47% significant reduction in blindness in India through effective measures taken through ongoing NPCB to control blindness and visual impairment.

Prerequisites for Arranging Eye Bank and Legislation (Fig. 1)

"Eye Bank," as described by Rao GN, is a not-for-profit community organization created and managed by members of the community. Its primary function includes harvesting donor corneas, detailed donor tissue and donor blood sample processing, tissue storage, and subsequent distribution to the corneal surgeons.

The eye banking model proposed for India under the NPCB involves a three-tier system consisting of an EB training center (EBTC) at the top, followed by an EB in the middle and eye retrieval centers (ERCs) at the bottom of the pyramid.

ERCs should be affiliated with an EB and perform the function of increasing public awareness about eye donations, coordinating with the community and hospitals, and harvesting, storing, and transporting corneal tissue and blood from donors to the EB.

EBs were assigned the pivotal role of increasing public awareness, harvesting, evaluation, storage, and distribution of corneal tissue in an equitable fashion. The EBs were also assigned to run the Hospital Cornea Retrieval Program (HCRP), which involves retrieving donor corneal tissue from the deceased in major hospitals and medical colleges.

EBTCs are specialized EBs meant to serve additionally as training centers for EB personnel. The functioning of EBTC and EB is governed by a board of directors, a medical director, who should be an ophthalmologist with fellowship training in cornea, and an eye bank manager. The ERC is headed by a director or in charge. Trained and certified EB technicians and eye donation counselors also undergo eye banking and grief counseling training from the rest of the team at all EBTC, EB, and ERC. The EBTC and EB should be equipped with equipment such as slit lamp, specular microscope, and laminar airflow hood and have a functional serology and tissue processing laboratory. EBTC, EB, and ERC

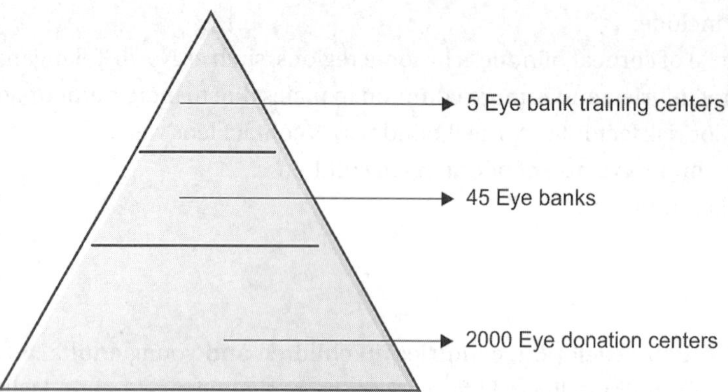

Fig. 1: Organizational pyramid of eye bank.

Legislation

The primary legislation for eye banks in India is the Transplantation of Human Organs Act (THOA) of 1994, which also governs organ donation and transplantation. The act has been amended since 2014.

2. Role of NHM and State Blindness Control Society in NPCB. (10) (BHU MS 2019)

India was the first country to launch the National Programme for Control of Blindness (NPCB) in 1976, as a 100% centrally sponsored Programme. The NPCB funds are released by the Government of India (GOI) to the State Blindness Control Society or State Health and Family Welfare Society based on the Annual Action Plan submitted. India has received technical impetus and financial assistance from World Bank, WHO, DANIDA and other International NGOs for amelioration of blindness program in the country but currently, the program is not dependent on any external funding. The implementation of the said program was subsequently decentralized in 1994–95 with formation of State and District Blindness Control Society.

Role of NHM in NPCB:

1. *Policy and funding support:* NHM integrates NPCB activities into its framework, ensuring funding for blindness control initiatives, infrastructure development, and workforce augmentation.
2. *Program implementation:* Facilitates implementation of NPCB at national, state, and district levels by coordinating with health systems.
3. *Capacity building:* Provides training for healthcare personnel involved in blindness prevention and treatment.
4. *Monitoring and evaluation:* Ensures accountability through regular monitoring, reporting, and performance evaluation.
5. *Public awareness:* Supports campaigns to increase awareness about eye care and preventable blindness.

Role of State Blindness Control Society (SBCS) in NPCB:

- *State-level coordination:* Acts as the nodal agency for implementing NPCB activities within the state, coordinating with district health systems.
- *Service delivery:* Oversees cataract surgeries, distribution of spectacles
- *Planning:* Preparations of state plan based on magnitude and distribution of blind persons and resources available for eye care.
- Implementation of program through utilization of government facilities, involvement of NGOs and community participation.
- Monitoring of program activities and quality control.
- Financial and material management.
- Social mobilization and public awareness.
- Orientation of various functionaries of health and other sectors, formal and nonformal leaders.
- Procurement of good quality refraction sets, drugs, consumables, cataract sets, etc., and maintenance of equipment.

- Arrangement for screening camps, IOL, spectacles, furniture, generator sets, etc.
- Monitoring and financial assistance to eye banks and eye donation centers.

3. Write briefly about Vision 2020. (10) (WBHUS MS 2019)

An estimated 45 million people around the world are blind. Most of them have lost their sight to diseases that are treatable or preventable. 80% of them live in the lesser-developed world in countries where chronic economic deprivation is exacerbated by the added challenge of failing vision.

In response to this global need, the World Health Organization (WHO), Geneva, Switzerland, with the International Agency for the Prevention of Blindness (IAPB), London, England, a partnership of eye care organizations, launched the VISION 2020: The Right to Sight initiative in 1999.

VISION 2020 aims to eliminate avoidable blindness in the world by 2020 and targets the world's leading causes of avoidable visual impairment: cataract, trachoma, onchocerciasis, childhood blindness (including vitamin A deficiency), and refractive error and low vision. The key objectives include:

- Strengthening disease control (e.g., cataract, refractive errors, and trachoma)
- Expanding access to comprehensive eye care
- Promoting human resource development and technology
- Enhancing advocacy and public awareness of blindness prevention

Infrastructure Development

Proposed four-tier structure includes:

1. Centers of Excellence-20
2. Training centers-200
3. Service centers-2000
4. Vision centers-20000

Services at Each Center

Primary level: Vision centers-20000:

- Screening and referral services
- School eye screening program
- Primary eye care
- Refraction and prescription of glasses

Secondary level: Service centers-2000:

- Cataract surgery
- Other common eye surgeries
- Facilities for refraction
- Referral services

Tertiary level:

- Training centers 200—tertiary eye care:
  - Retinal surgery
  - Corneal transplantation
  - Glaucoma surgery
  - Training and CME
- Centers of excellence 20:
  - Professional leadership
  - Strategy development
  - CME
  - Laying of standards and quality assurance Research

This initiative continues to influence global eye health programs today.

4. Write in short about National Programme for Control of Blindness. (10) (DNB 2018)

5. What are the goals of NPCB? Discuss its strategies. (10) (WBUHS MS 2019)

6. Describe the organizational structure of NPCB. (10) (WBUHS MS 2018)

7. Role of NPCB. (10) (BHU MS 2019)

The National Programme for Control of Blindness and Visual Impairment (NPCBVI) was launched in 1976 as a 100% Centrally Sponsored scheme with the goal to reduce the prevalence of blindness from 1.4% to 0.3%. As per Survey in 2001-02, prevalence of blindness is estimated to be 1.1%. A Rapid Survey on Avoidable Blindness conducted under NPCBVI during 2006-07 showed reduction in the prevalence of blindness from 1.1% (2001-02) to 1% (2006-07). Various activities/ initiatives undertaken during the 5-year plans under NPCBVI are targeted toward achieving the goal of reducing the prevalence of blindness to 0.3% by the year 2020.

Goals and Objectives of NPCBVI in the XII Plan

- To reduce the backlog of blindness through identification and treatment of blind at primary, secondary and tertiary levels based on assessment of the overall burden of visual impairment in the country.
- Develop and strengthen the strategy of NPCBVI for "Eye Health" and prevention of visual impairment; through provision of comprehensive Eye Care services and quality service delivery.
- Strengthening and upgradation of RIOs to become center of excellence in various subspecialties of ophthalmology
- Strengthening the existing and developing additional human resources and infrastructure facilities for providing high quality comprehensive Eye Care in all Districts of the country;
- To enhance community awareness on eye care and lay stress on preventive measures;
- Increase and expand research for prevention of blindness and visual impairment
- To secure participation of Voluntary Organizations/Private Practitioners in eye care

Main Activities

1. Cataract surgery and IOL implantation
2. School eye screening
3. Eye banking
4. Eye care education

Strategies

1. Continued emphasis on free cataract surgeries
2. Emphasis on diabetic retinopathy, glaucoma, corneal transplantation, vitreoretinal surgeries, and childhood blindness
3. Active screening of population above 50 years of age
4. Screening of school children for identification and treatment of refractive errors
5. Coverage of underserved areas for eye care through public-private partnership
6. Capacity building of health personnel
7. IEC activities for community
8. Strengthening of Regional Institute of Ophthalmology (RIOs) and Medical Colleges of States and District Hospitals
9. Continuing emphasis on primary eye care
10. Multipurpose District Mobile Ophthalmic Units for better coverage
11. Participation of community and Panchayat Raj Institutions in organizing services in rural areas

Organizational Structure

- *Administration*:
  - *Central:* Ophthalmology section, DGHS, and MOHFW
  - *State:* State ophthalmic cell, directorate of health services, and state health societies
  - *District:* District blindness control societies

- *Service delivery and referral system:*
  - *Tertiary level:* Apex, regional institutes, and medical colleges
  - *Secondary level:* District hospital and NGO eye hospital
  - *Primary level:* Subdistrict level hospitals/CHC mobile ophthalmic units, upgraded PHCs, link worker/panchayats

New Initiatives of the Program

- Provision of free glasses in presbyopia patients.
- Provision of spectacles for school children by conducting eye testing fortnight every year in the month of June
- Provision of Multipurpose District Mobile Ophthalmic Units (MDMOUs) in all districts all over the country.
- To promote eye donation and to urge the eye banks to perform better in the forthcoming years.
- Hospital Cornea Retrieval Programme–inclusion of mandatory required request for eye donation from those who are deceased in the cause of death certificates issued by hospitals need to be firmly put into practice (NPCB quarterly newsletter July–September 2012).

8. Discuss eye bank in India. (10) (BHU MS 2018)

Eye Banking Services in India

A 3-tier community eye banking system has been proposed for India. These are: eye donation centers (EDC), eye banks (EB), and eye bank training centers (EBTC). EBTCs are responsible for tissue harvesting, processing and distribution, creating public awareness as well as training and skill upgradation of eye banking personnel. The middle tier comprises EBs and organizations that comply with all the regulations stipulated by the Eye Bank Association of India (EBAI). EDCs should provide public and professional awareness of eye donation, coordinate with donor families and hospitals to motivate eye donation, to harvest corneal tissue, and collect blood for serology and to ensure safe transportation of tissue to the parent EB.

Presently, there are 435 functional EBs and EDCs in the country involved in collection and distribution of donated eyes as per the National Programme for Control of Blindness (NPCB). This amounts to nearly 1 EB/EDC per 3 million population. However, a majority of these are concentrated in urban regions.

Cornea collection in the country as per the NPCB in 2016–17 was 63 256; Tamil Nadu among the states contributed the maximum of corneas collected. Currently, the utilization rate ranges between 25% and 60%.

Initiatives Under the NPCB

A major proportion of the budget allocation for the NPCB during the 12th five-year plan (2012–17) was allotted to eye banking. Financial support is given to all functional EBs and EDCs in the government/voluntary sector. Full assistance is given to develop new EBs according to quality standards. Training for EB staff, grief counselors and doctors is also provided under the program. Despite continuous increase in the number of eye donations over the past few years, there is a huge gap between demand and supply. To address this gap and to create awareness among people regarding eye donation and related issues, the NPCB celebrates the National Eye Donation Fortnight (25 August to 8 September) every year in India.

Capacity building under the NPCB has been initiated. Reorientation training on eye care of government ophthalmic surgeons, medical officers, paramedical ophthalmic assistants, ophthalmic nursing, school teachers and other general healthcare staff including community link workers and village health volunteers is going on under the NPCB. Training needs to be imparted at all levels and should benefit the farthest and inaccessible regions of the country.

Challenges Ahead

The major challenges include lack of an organized eye banking system, improper regulation and non-supportive legislations. Quality issues such as failure to adopt common medical standards for all EBs, lack of properly trained eye banking personnel and lack of accreditation systems pose additional problems. Other areas of concern are inefficient public awareness programs and lack of motivation among health personnel, need for consent from relatives and no "eventual benefit of pledging eyes before death". All these have aggravated the problems in harvesting an adequate number of quality donor corneas to meet the growing demands, thus creating a gap between demand and supply.

9. District Blindness Control Society. (10) (WBUHS MS 2018)

Goal: "To achieve maximum reduction in avoidable blindness through optimal utilization of available resources".

The program includes:

- Comprehensive eye care
- School eye screening
- Community-based rehabilitation

Composition

The District Blindness Control Society has a maximum of 15 members, consisting of not more than 8 exofficio and 7 other members as follows:

- *Chairman*: District Collector/District Mission Director
- *Vice-Chairman*: Chief Medical & Health Officer/District Health Officer
- *Member Secretary*: Officer of the level of Deputy CMO preferably an Ophthalmologist may be designated as District Programme Manager who would also be the Member Secretary of the society.
- *Technical Advisor*: Chief Ophthalmic Surgeon of District hospital. In districts where Medical Colleges are located, Head of the Department of Ophthalmology may be designated as Technical Advisor to the society.
- *Members*: Medical Superintendent/Civil Surgeon of District Hospital, District Education Officer (IMA, District chapter of AIOS etc.), Representatives from NGOs engaged in eye care services, District Mass media/IEC officer, Prominent practicing eye surgeons

Functions

The primary purpose of the District Blindness Control Society is to plan, implement and monitor blindness control activities in the district as per pattern of assistance approved for the National Programme for Control of Blindness. On the basis of scheme approved for the 11th Plan, important functions of the District Blindness Control Society are:

1. To assess the magnitude and spread of blindness in the district by means of active case finding village wise to be recorded and maintained in Blind Registers
2. To organize screening camps for identifying those requiring cataract surgery and other blinding disorders, organize transportation and conduct of free medical or surgical services including cataract surgery for the poor in Government facilities or NGOs supporting the program
3. To plan and organize training of community level workers, teachers, and ophthalmic assistants/nurses involved in eye care services
4. To procure drugs and consumables including microsurgical instruments required in the Government facilities
5. To receive and monitor use of funds, equipment and materials from the government and other agencies/donors
6. To involve voluntary and private hospitals providing free/subsidized eye care services in the District and identify NGO facilities that can be considered for non-recurring grants under the program
7. To organize screening of school children for detection of refractive errors and other eye problems and provide free glasses to poor children
8. To promote eye donation through various media and monitor collection and utilization of eyes collected by eye donation centers and eye banks
9. The Paramedical Ophthalmic Assistance (PMOAs) shall be doing the regular screening for and other diseases in the outreach camps. They shall be under the direct control of the District Ophthalmic Surgeon/DPM. The TA/DA of the PMOA is for the outreach camps conducted shall be paid by District Blindness Control Society.

10. Mention the causes of childhood blindness. (5) (TN MGRMU MS 2022)

11. Ocular morbidity in school going children. (10) (GUHS MS 2020)

Children usually do not complain of defective vision. They may not even be aware of their problem. They adjust to the poor eyesight by sitting near the blackboard, holding the books closer to their eyes, squeezing the eyes and even avoiding work requiring visual concentration. This evades early detection. Periodic screening of all children helps in early identification of visual defects and prescription/use of corrective spectacles. The prevalence of ocular morbidity in school children varies by location and study, but some common causes include:

- *Refractive errors*: The most common cause of ocular morbidity in children, affecting up to 22% of school children
- *Vitamin A deficiency*: A common cause of ocular morbidity in children, affecting up to 10% of school children
- *Color blindness*: Affects up to 3.3% of school children
- *Eyelid disorders*: Affects up to 1.6% of school children
- *Squint*: Affects up to 2.5% of school children
- *Conjunctivitis*: Affects up to 0.8% of school children

Factors that may be associated with ocular morbidity include:

- *Age*: Ocular morbidity may increase with age, particularly refractive errors and convergence insufficiency
- *Location*: Vitamin A deficiency may be more prevalent in rural areas than urban areas
- *Socioeconomic status*: Ocular morbidity may be associated with socioeconomic status
- *Educational status*: Ocular morbidity may be associated with the educational status of both parents
- *Occupational status*: Ocular morbidity may be associated with the occupational status of both parents
- Regular eye screening programs can help identify and treat preventable and treatable causes of childhood blindness

12. Discuss the classification, prevention, and management of vitamin A deficiency. Nutritional factors causing ocular morbidity. (10) (BHU MS 2021)

Vitamin A deficiency results from a dietary intake of vitamin A that is inadequate to satisfy physiological needs. It may be exacerbated by high rates of infection, especially diarrhea and measles. It is common in developing countries, but rarely seen in developed countries. Vitamin A deficiency is a public health problem in more than half of all countries, especially those in Africa and South-East Asia. The most severe effects of this deficiency are seen in young children and pregnant women in low-income countries.

Vitamin A deficiency can be defined clinically or subclinically. Xerophthalmia is the clinical spectrum of ocular manifestations of vitamin A deficiency; these range from the milder stages of night blindness and Bitot's spots to the potentially blinding stages of corneal xerosis, ulceration and necrosis (keratomalacia). The various stages of xerophthalmia are regarded both as disorders and clinical indicators of vitamin A deficiency. Night blindness (in which it is difficult or impossible to see in relatively low light) is one of the clinical signs of vitamin A deficiency, and is common in children.

Classification

The stages of vitamin A deficiency include:

- *Night blindness*: The first sign of vitamin A deficiency, where it's difficult or impossible to see in low light.
- *Conjunctival xerosis*: The earliest and most benign sign, where the conjunctiva appears dry, dull, thick, wrinkled, and insensitive.
- *Bitot's spots*: Triangular patches of white, opaque deposits on the bulbar conjunctiva.
- *Corneal xerosis*: The cornea appears dry and dull, and there may be corneal haze, punctate epithelial erosions, pannus, and neovascularization.
- *Corneal ulcerations*: Can occur if corneal xerosis is left untreated.
- *Keratomalacia*: The last and most severe sign, where the cornea softens, and the eyeball may perforate, leading to blindness.

Prevention

- *Promoting consumption of vitamin a rich food*:
  - Regular dietary intake of vitamin A rich foods by pregnant and lactating mothers and by children under 5 years of age to be promoted.
  - The mothers attending antenatal clinics and immunization sessions as well as mothers and children enrolled in the ICDS program are to be made aware of the importance of preventing vitamin A deficiency.

   - Breastfeeding, including feeding of colostrums, to be encouraged.
   - Feeding of locally available B-carotene (precursor of vitamin A) rich food such as green leafy vegetables and yellow and orange vegetables, and fruits such as pumpkin, carrots, papaya, mango, oranges along with cereal and pulse to a weaning child to be promoted widely. In addition, whenever economically feasible, consumption of milk, cheese, paneer, dahi (yogurt), ghee, eggs, liver, etc., is to be promoted.
   - For increasing availability of vitamin A rich food, growing of vitamin A rich food, growing of vitamin A rich foods in home gardens and consumption of these must be promoted.
- *Administering supplemental dose of vitamin A*:
   - Unlike most other micronutrients, vitamin A is stored in the body for prolonged periods and hence periodic administration of massive doses ensures adequate vitamin A.
   - Administration of supplemental doses of vitamin A to preschool children at periodic intervals is a simple, effective and most direct intervention strategy. This is a short term strategy. Under this strategy, every infant 6–11 months and children 1–5 years is to be administered vitamin A every 6 months. The recommended schedule is as follows:
      - 6–11 months—one dose of 100,000 IU
      - 1–5 years—200,000 IU/6 months
      - A child must receive a total of 9 oral doses of vitamin A by its fifth birthday
   - The contact with an infant during administration of the measles vaccine between the age of 9–12 months is considered a practical time for administering the vitamin A supplement—100,000 IU for infants.
   - A biannual approach may be used for administering vitamin A to children 1–3 years and 3–5 years. However, the DPT/OPV booster in mid-second year to a child is a suitable time for the second dose of vitamin A (200,000 IU). Wherever, ICDS Program is functioning, AWW should be involved in the distribution and administration of vitamin A.
   - The joint Mother-Child Health Card should be used to record and monitor the administration of vitamin A dose to children under two years.
   - In addition, records of under-lives maintained under the MCH Services and the ICDS program are recommended to be used for identifying as well as monitoring children for administration of a total of 9 oral doses of vitamin A per child.
   - Communication strategy for creating awareness about Vitamin A must be in place.

Management

All children with clinical signs of vitamin A deficiency must be treated as early as possible. Treatment schedule is to administer 200,000 IU of vitamin A immediately after diagnosis. This must be followed by another dose of 200,000 IU 1–4 weeks later. Vitamin A concentrate is available at primary health centers and sub health centers in the form of flavored syrup at a concentration of 100,000 IU/mL. Vitamin A syrup should be administered using the 2 mL. Spoon/dispenser provided with each bottle of vitamin A. A marked level full 2 mL spoon of vitamin A contains 200,000 IU vitamin A. Vitamin A solution must be kept away from direct sunlight. It should be stored in a cold dark room temperature stable for a minimum of 1 year. Vitamin A solution bottle once opened must be utilized within 6–8 weeks.

Children with eye lesions must be treated immediately with vitamin A even if they are being referred for special care. Infants and young children suffering from diarrhea, measles, or acute respiratory infection must be monitored closely and encouraged to consume vitamin A rich food. In case, early signs of vitamin A deficiency are observed, the above treatment schedule must be followed.

13. Eye screening in school children. (10) (WBUHS MS 2018)

14. Discuss in details about School Eye Health Programme. (10) (TNMGRMU MS 2021)

15. School survey in prevention of childhood blindness. (10) (BHU MS 2019)

School children represent a needy and big target group requiring identification and treatment of refractive errors. They are a "captive" group and can be reached through the organized educational system. Reading and writing are their felt needs for which good eyesight is required. Many children, their teachers and parents realize this. The teachers see their pupils daily. It is possible for them to observe the behavior of their students to facilitate early detection of vision defects. School teachers can insist on the children, who are provided spectacles, to use them regularly while reading, writing or working.

Objective: Cover all school going children in the district

Strategy: Utilize school teachers to identify children with poor vision

Milestones:
- Training of teachers
- Procurement and distribution of the required materials Screening by teachers
- Examination of referred children by ophthalmic assistants
- Provision of spectacles to needy children
- Use of spectacles by children

Outcome:
- Screening of all school children
- Provision and use of spectacles by children with Refractive errors

The ultimate impact of the program will be on the performance of children with improved eyesight. But this cannot be easily assessed. The improvement in the performance of the children in academic studies and in their work is a strong motivational tool for the school teachers and the parents to continue their interest in the program. Monetary or material incentives for the teachers must be avoided and this activity should be perceived as a regular activity of the identified teachers. In the long run vision screening should become a routine activity linked to school entry or shoal health checkup.

Steps of eye screening in school children are shown in **Flowchart 1**.

Flowchart 1: Steps of eye screening in school.

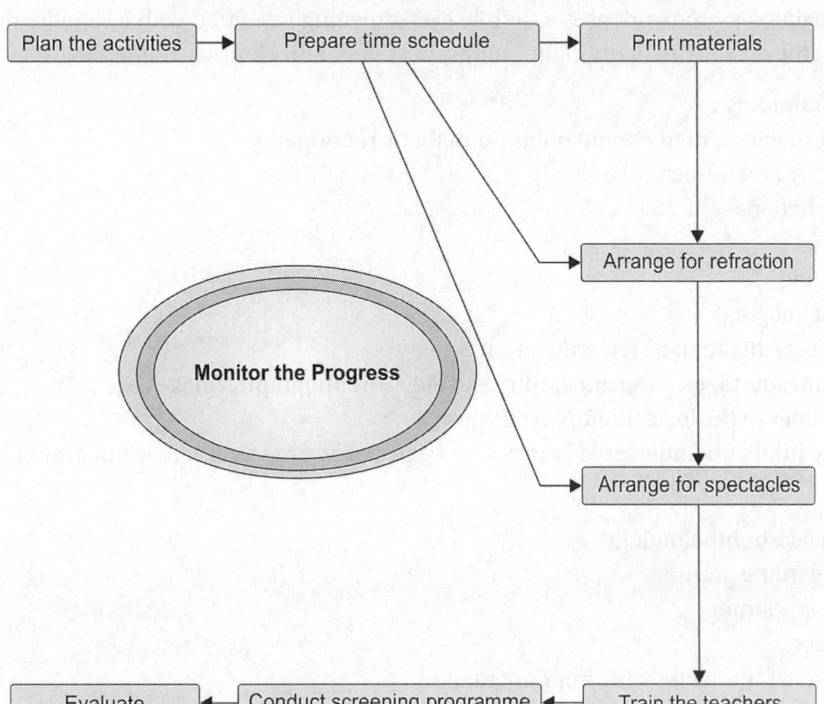

16. Discuss in detail about teleophthalmology, its uses, merits, and demerits in community eye care. (15) (BHU MS 2022)

The World Health Organization (WHO) defines telemedicine as "The delivery of healthcare services, where distance is a critical factor, by all healthcare professionals using information and communication technologies for the exchange of valid information for diagnosis, treatment and prevention of disease and injuries, research and evaluation, and for the continuing education of health care providers, all in the interests of advancing the health of individuals and their communities."

Teleophthalmology has special significance to India considering its vast geographical spread and predominant rural population where medical care is neither available nor accessible. While 72% of India's population live in rural areas, over 70% of the doctors practice in urban areas.

Technology and Technical Support

To support telemedicine activities within the country, the Department of Information Technology has defined the Standards for Telemedicine Systems, and the Ministry of Health and Family Welfare has constituted the National Telemedicine Task Force. The ISRO has coupled its prowess in satellite communication technology with medical science and information technology to project specialty healthcare to the doorsteps of the remote, rural, and underserved populations across the country.

Examples of Teleophthalmology Projects in India

1. MDRF/WDF Rural India Diabetes Prevention Project by Madras Diabetic Research Foundation (MDRF), Chennai, in collaboration with the World Diabetes Foundation (WDF): This rural community outreach program serves a cluster of 42 villages in Kanchipuram District, Tamil Nadu. Screening is carried out for diabetes and its complications especially diabetic eye diseases by using a mobile telemedicine van with satellite connectivity.
2. The teleophthalmology project conducted by Sankar Nethralaya Medical Research Foundation at Chennai uses a customized mobile van with an in-built ophthalmic examination facility having satellite connectivity provided by ISRO, along with a social worker and an optometrist. Patients undergo a preliminary screening for ophthalmic diseases at camps organized at these villages.
3. Aravind Teleophthalmology Network uses a mobile eye-screening van fitted with a satellite that has been specially designed to screen the diabetic patients in the camps, hospitals, and clinics of diabetologists.

Benefits of Teleophthalmology

1. Diagnosis and formulation of treatment plans for diabetic retinopathy
2. Visual acuity testing and refraction
3. Low vision consultations
4. Cataract screening
5. Glaucoma screening
6. Anterior segment imaging
7. Continuing medical education by tele-education
8. Transferring of ultrasound, electrooculography and electroretinography images
9. Employment facilities to the local unemployed youth
10. Can reach remote rural and underserved areas where specialized medical care is not available

Barriers

1. Unfamiliarity with tele-ophthalmology
2. Patient concern regarding accuracy
3. High cost of initial investment
4. Poor quality of images
5. Lack of dedicated staff for telemedicine implementation
6. Policy barriers

7. Privacy and security concerns
8. Software and hardware of the equipment needs to be regularly updated.
9. Teleconsultation using mobile apps or video calls is possible only when reliable high speed internet is available.

Advantages of Teleconsultation

1. Extensive outreach
2. Timely intervention in emergency situation
3. Avoiding unnecessary referrals
4. Saves cost, time, and effort
5. Health education
6. Professional opinion
7. Protection against infection

17. Organizing eye camp. (10) (BHU MS 2018)

Community outreach is taking healthcare to that part of the community which has no access and awareness of such services. In the field of ophthalmology, it is providing eye care service to eliminate needless blindness at the patients' doorstep. Community outreach in eye care is a practice of conducting eye camps involving the local community as partners, thereby creating ownership by the community.

Planning of outreach is best done in an organized manner. Planning of an outreach camp has to be conducted by considering the following factors: the target group, the approach to the camp, the timing of the camp, the correct place for the camp and the methodology to be adopted.

The Target Group for Outreach

First, determine the specific group or audience being targeted:

- Patients with cataract, glaucoma, or diabetic retinopathy
- Patients with refractive error
- Elderly, children or general population
- An industrial sector
- Rural unreached or urban/suburban unreached
- Specific neighborhoods or geographic areas

The Best Approach to be Adopted

The next step is to determine what approach will meet the needs of stakeholders:

- A short-term event or a longer-term initiative?
- A temporary set-up or a permanent facility?
- Provision of primary eye care or secondary eye care?
- Screening program? (Surgical camp only in parts of the world where absolutely necessary)
- How much of an educational component should be included?
- What will be its impact from other outreach activities, both geographically and chronologically?

The Timing of the Camp

First, outreach can be used to increase the uptake of services at the eye care institution, eye clinic or ophthalmology practice. But to do this successfully necessitates the introduction of demand management strategies into outreach planning. That means structuring service management and scheduling outreach activities to meet the variations of daily, weekly and seasonal peaks in demand, to reduce patient waiting time and to keep staff work schedules running smoothly.

The Selection of a Suitable Place for the Camp

A macro and micro location of the outreach program must both be considered. On the macro level, where the outreach activity will take place depends on the target audience, the size and attributes of the catchment area (population, area, access to public transportation) and proximity to the base hospital. There are several factors to keep in mind when choosing where to hold or place an outreach activity or initiative on the micro level:

- Is the location free or cheap (educational institution on weekends, community center, church premises, factory owned by the sponsor)?
- Is it clean and hygienic?
- Is there access to the proper equipment and furniture (benches, chairs, tables)?
- Is reliable electricity available?
- Is it centrally located or located near public transportation?
- Is internet connectivity available (for vision centers)?

The Methodology in Conducting Outreach

In short, this is how outreach programs are planned:

- Assign dedicated outreach staff to coordinate programs.
- Estimate the unmet need in the catchment area.
- Set achievable targets.
- Do annual planning for meeting target outcomes, with monthly distribution for the year (keeping holidays and festivals in mind).
- Develop detailed action plans and determine how to meet those targets.
- Engage the community leaders, taking advantage of their knowledge of the host community.
- Use community resources as much as possible to keep costs down.
- Develop micro level planning on a weekly basis.
- Plan and execute effective publicity campaigns
- Monitor and evaluate regularly

SUGGESTED READING

1. Agrawal D, Sahu A, Agrawal D. Prevalence of ocular morbidities among school children in Raipur district, India. Indian J Ophthalmol. 2020;68(2):340-4.
2. Anitha V, Tandon R, Shah SG, Radhakrishnan N, Singh S, Murugesan V, et al. Corneal blindness and eye banking: Current strategies and best practices. Indian J Ophthalmol. 2023;71(9):3142-8.
3. Chaurasia S, Dureja R, Roy A, Das S. The expanding roles of eye banks in India: Past, present, and future. Indian J Ophthalmol. 2024;72(Suppl 4):S542-S552.
4. Government of India. National Programme for Control of Blindness in India. New Delhi: Ministry of Health and Family Welfare.
5. Government of Punjab. District Blindness Control Society. [online] Available from https://patiala.nic.in/district-blindness-control-society/. [Last accessed March, 2025].
6. Government of Tripura. National Programme for Control of Blindness (NPCB). [online] Available from https://health.tripura.gov.in/national-programme-control-blindness-npcb). [Last accessed March, 2025].
7. Gupta N, Vashist P, Ganger A, Tandon R, Gupta SK. Eye donation and eye banking in India. Natl Med J India. 2018;31(5):283-286.
8. Kishore J. National Health Programs of India: National Policies & Legislations Related to Health, 9th edition. New Delhi: Century Publication; 2011.
9. Ministry of Health and Family Welfare. (2004). Vision Screening in School Children. [online] Available from https://npcbvi.mohfw.gov.in/Douments/Training_Manuals/2004_Vision_Screening_in_School_Children_A_Training_Module_OCR.pdf. [Last accessed March, 2025].
10. Ministry of Health and Family Welfare. Vitamin A and IFA Supplementation. [online] Available from https://nhm.gov.in/images/pdf/programmes/child-health/guidelines/goi_vit_a.pdf. [Last accessed March, 2025].
11. National Programme for Control of Blindness and Visual Impairment. Eye Banking Standards of India 2020. New Delhi: National Programme for Control of Blindness and Visual Impairment; 2020.
12. National Programme for Control of Blindness and Visual Impairment. (2009) Guidelines for State Health Society and District Health Society. New Delhi: National Programme for Control of Blindness and Visual Impairment; 2009.
13. Pizzarello L, Abiose A, Ffytche T, Duerksen R, Thulasiraj R, Taylor H, et al. VISION 2020: The Right to Sight A Global Initiative to Eliminate Avoidable Blindness. Arch Ophthalmol. 2004;122(4):615-620.

14. Prathiba V, Rema M. Teleophthalmology: a model for eye care delivery in rural and underserved areas of India. Int J Family Med. 2011;2011:683267.
15. Sarkar A, Medhi GK, Bhattacharyya H, Pala S, Gogoi S. Pattern of ocular morbidities: A cross-sectional study on school-going children in Shillong city. J Family Med Prim Care. 2019;8(6):2124-8.
16. Sharma M, Jain N, Ranganathan S, Sharma N, Honavar SG, Sharma N, et al. Tele-ophthalmology: Need of the hour. Indian J Ophthalmol. 2020;68(7):1328-38.
17. Singh V, Malik KPS, Malik VK, Jain K. Prevalence of ocular morbidity in school going children in West Uttar Pradesh. Indian J Ophthalmol. 2017;65(6):500-8.
18. Sundaram RM. Reaching the Unreached: Community-Based Eye Care Outreach in Developing Nations. [online] Available from https://aravind.org/wp-content/uploads/2019/05/How-to-organise-a-camp.pdf. [Last accessed March, 2025].
19. World Health Organization. (2009). Vitamin A deficiency. [online] Available from https://www.who.int/data/nutrition/nlis/info/vitamin-a-deficiency. [Last accessed March, 2025].

CHAPTER

Ocular Therapeutics and Laser

Shashwat Bhattacharyya, Tanweesha Chakraborty, Oindrila Chakraborty

QUESTIONS

1. **Drug delivery systems utilized in ophthalmology.** **(5 + 5) (WBUHS MS 2020)**
2. **Mention briefly about the drug delivery systems in ophthalmology.** **(5) (DNB 2023)**
3. **Botulinum toxin use in ophthalmology—mechanism of action, indications, and complications.** **(2 + 4 + 4) (DNB 2019, MS 2020)**
4. **Classify pharmacological agents available to treat glaucoma. Mechanism of action of topical agents. Adverse effects and contraindications of systemic agents.** **(4 + 3 + 3) (DNB 2019)**
5. **Discuss the mechanism of action of local anesthetic agents used in ophthalmology. What are the various routes of administration? What are the complications of peribulbar anesthesia?** **(6 + 4) (DNB 2020, MS 2021)**
6. **Enumerate the various types of lasers used in ophthalmic practice. Uses of lasers in ocular disorders.** **(4 + 6) (DNB 2023)**
7. **Short note on: Topical low dose atropine.** **(5) (DNB 2021)**
8. **Cyclodestructive procedures.** **(10) (RGUHS MS 2020)**
9. **Interferons use in ophthalmology.** **(5) (MS 2019, DNB 2022)**
10. **Discuss the risk factors, clinical features, evaluation, and management of ethambutol toxicity.** **(2 + 2 + 4 + 2) (DNB 2021)**
11. **Role of antimetabolites and immunosuppressives drugs in ophthalmology.** **(5 + 5) (DNB 2019)**
12. **What are antiviral drugs? Describe mechanism of action of acyclovir and dosages in different viral affection in the eye.** **(3 + 4 + 3) (DNB 2022)**
13. **Classify antifungal drugs. Briefly describe the various route of administering antifungal drugs in mycotic keratitis.** **(5 + 5) (MS WBUHS 2021)**
14. **Different stains used for diagnostic and therapeutic purposes in ophthalmology and their uses.** **(10) (MS WBUHS 2019)**

1. Drug delivery systems utilized in ophthalmology. (5 + 5) (WBUHS MS 2020)

2. Mention briefly about the drug delivery systems in ophthalmology. (5) (DNB 2023)

Topical Drug Delivery

- *Instillation of liquid formulations:*
  - Most favored for targeting ocular surface and anterior segment
  - Least invasive and least expensive method
  - Inadequate drug concentration achieved in posterior segment disorders
  - Lesser systemic adverse effects

- *Sprays:*
  - Less irritating than solutions
  - Stinging sensation is an indicator of presence of drug in precorneal tear film
  - Risk of contamination is negligible
  - High patient acceptability, especially in pediatric age group
- *Extraocular irrigation:*
  - Required in acute chemical burns or foreign body removal
  - In patients requiring continuous irrigation, a polyethylene tube is inserted into the lower fornix through lid and fixed with sutures and/or tapes
- *Lid scrubs:*
  - Directly applied to lid margins with cotton tipped applicator
  - Used in blepharitis
- *Filter paper strips:*
  - Used to instill ophthalmic dyes such as fluorescein sodium, rose bengal, lissamine green, etc.
  - The strips can be moistened with a drop of saline and touched to the inferior fornix or inferior bulbar conjunctiva
  - This avoids risk of contamination
- *Cotton pledgets:*
  - Used for prolonged delivery of mydriatics in slow dilating pupil to break posterior synechiae
  - These are soaked with the drug and placed in inferior fornix
  - Can cause foreign body sensation
- *Contact lenses:*
  - Useful in treatment of dry eyes, bullous keratopathy
  - Extent of drug permeation into the lens material depends upon the size of pores within it, molecular size of drug, water content of leas, thickness of lens, soaking time, etc.

Conventional Drug Delivery System in Anterior Segment

- *Aqueous solutions:*
  - Manufactured by combination of active and inactive ingredients along with preservatives
  - Corneal penetration can be enhanced by increasing corneal contact time, by increasing solution concentration or adding viscosity enhancers
- *Suspensions:*
  - Suitable for delivery of lipophilic ophthalmic drugs with limited water solubility
  - These contain suspending agents, wetting agents, preservatives, etc.
- *Ointments:*
  - Applied to inferior fornix
  - In case of co administration with solutions, ointments should be applied later as they prevent the former from reaching precorneal tear film
  - May lead to blurring of vision due to spreading of a thick film of ointment
  - Has an advantage of prolonged corneal contact time
- *Gels:*
  - Contains drug with gelling agent with high water binding affinity
  - These melt at body temperature to release active ingredients
  - The chances of blurring of vision are lesser compared to ointments

Nonconventional Drug Delivery System in Anterior Segment

- *Polymeric gels:*
  - These can again be subdivided into two types:
    1. Preformed gels
    2. In situ forming gels

- *Preformed gels* form strong noncovalent bonds with the mucin layer of tear film and prolong corneal contact time
- *In situ forming gels* transition from solution to gel due to change in temperature, pH or electrolyte concentration in the ocular surface and facilitate accurate administration

- *Colloidal solutions:*
  - These systems contain colloids complexed with active drug suspended in aqueous solution
  - These can be subdivided into several types:
    - *Liposomes:* Consist of lipid bilayer made up of phospholipid, in the form of vesicles that trap the active drug. Hydrophobic drugs are more compatible for this formulation
    - *Nanoparticles:* Polymeric colloidal particles, in the form of nanospheres and nanocapsules. Active drugs can either be incorporated into the matrix of nanospheres or adsorbed on their surface, however, they are located inside nanocapsules
    - *Niosomes:* Physically similar to liposomes but are made up of nonionic surfactant. They are chemically more stable and suitable for both lipophilic and hydrophilic drugs.
    - *Discomes:* Larger particle size as compared to niosomes and are made up of Solulan C24, a nonionic surfactant that has lesser chances of systemic absorption
    - *Microemulsions:* These are oil-in-water formulations because of presence of surfactant and co-surfactant that can achieve sustained release of drugs
- *Cyclodextrins:*
  - These are used for administration of poorly soluble, unstable, irritating and difficult to formulate substances
  - These are homologous cyclic oligosaccharides with hydrophilic outer surface consisting of glucose units
  - They also have a hydrophilic cavity in the center
- *Inserts:*
  - These are erodible or nonerodible substances that contain the drug and start releasing it at a steady rate once in contact with ocular surface
  - Commonly used inserts include *Ocusert* (containing pilocarpine), *Lacrisert* (hydroxypropyl methyl cellulose without preservative)
- *Prodrug (chemical delivery system):*
  - These ensure selective and site-specific drug delivery system
  - It is an inactive drug derivative that may undergo specific enzymatic alterations via inactive intermediates to deliver the active drug

Posterior Segment Drug Delivery Systems

- *Iontophoretic devices:*
  - These can be of various types, some of which have been described as under:
  - *Coulomb controlled iontophoresis (CCI):* It produces and maintains a constant electrical field across the conjunctival epithelium, that aids in dang delivery during trans scleral iontophoresis
  - *Mini-ion iontophoretic unit:* It is portable and can be battery operated and uses disposable drug delivery electrode probes
  - *EyeGate:* Made up of soft silicone rubber, to fit human eye palpebral opening. The vision is not affected as the dang solution does not cover the corneal surface
- *Scleral implants:*
  - Sustained release biodegradable or nonbiodegradable devices that elude drug through a polyvinyl alcohol membrane
  - These are especially useful in treatment of chronic ocular diseases
- *Photodynamic therapy:*
  - Used in treatment of neovascular age-related macular degeneration
  - There is intravenous administration of verteporfin, which is activated by light of 689 nm wavelength and generates free radicals that cause death of abnormal new vessels

3. Botulinum toxin use in ophthalmology—mechanism of action, indications, and complications. (2 + 4 + 4) (DNB 2019, MS 2020)

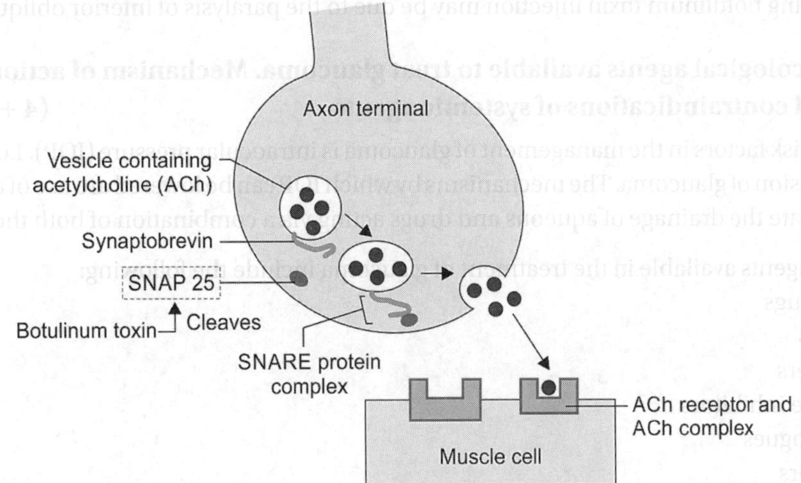

Fig. 1: Mechanism of action of botulinum toxin.

- Botulinum toxin blocks neuromuscular transmission at cholinergic nerve terminals.
- It is an exotoxin produced by *Clostridium botulinum* .
- Acetylcholine (ACh) vesicles are released into the synaptic cleft due to the presence of a protein aggregate known as SNARE protein complex.
- ACh release results in binding to specific receptors that open up sodium channels, resulting in depolarization and contraction of the muscle.
- Presence of action potential at nerve terminal results in opening of calcium channels that bind to SNARE proteins, consisting of synaptobrevin, SNAP 25, etc., and result in activation of SNARE complex that aids in docking of vesicles and release of acetylcholine into synaptic cleft.
- Botulinum toxin molecules at nerve terminals cleave specific SNARE protein, hence preventing release of ACh into synaptic cleft **(Fig. 1)**.

Indications of Botulinum Toxin

- Benign essential blepharospasm
- Hemifacial spasm
- Strabismus
- Cosmetic use—to treat periorbital wrinkles
- Upper eyelid retraction in thyroid eye disease
- Congenital and acquired ectropion
- Lacrimal gland hypersecretion
- Facial palsy leading to incomplete eyelid closure

Complications of Botulinum Toxin

- *Eyelid ptosis:*
  - Piercing of orbital septum during botulinum toxin injections may lead to eye lid ptosis. Apraclonidine eye drops may be used to enhance Müller muscle action and improve ptosis.
- *Bruising and hemorrhage:*
  - It is commonly seen at the injection site and can be minimized by discontinuation of anticoagulants.
- *Headache, mild pain, and flu-like symptoms:*
  - May be associated with administration of botulinum toxin injection and can be treated by systemic NSAIDs.

- *Dry eye and disruption of eye closure reflex:*
  - Paralysis of orbicularis oculi may result in incomplete closure of the eye leading to dry eye.
- *Diplopia:*
  - Diplopia following botulinum toxin injection may be due to the paralysis of inferior oblique muscle.

4. Classify pharmacological agents available to treat glaucoma. Mechanism of action of topical agents. Adverse effects and contraindications of systemic agents. (4 + 3 + 3) (DNB 2019)

One of the modifiable risk factors in the management of glaucoma is intraocular pressure (IOP). Lowering of the IOP may help to stall the progression of glaucoma. The mechanisms by which IOP can be lowered are use of aqueous suppressants, use of drugs that facilitate the drainage of aqueous and drugs acting via a combination of both the pathways.

The pharmacological agents available in the treatment of glaucoma include the following:

- Cholinomimetic drugs
- Sympathomimetics
- Sympathetic blockers
- Carbonic anhydrase inhibitors
- Prostaglandin analogues
- Rho kinase inhibitors
- Systemic hyperosmotic agents

Cholinomimetic Drugs

- *Drugs:* Pilocarpine and carbachol
- *Mode of administration:* Topical
- *Mechanism of action:* Acting on M3 muscarinic receptors → release of acetylcholine → pupillary constriction → widening of angle of anterior chamber → increased drainage of aqueous

Sympathomimetics (Alpha Agonists)

- *Drugs:* Apraclonidine, brimonidine, and dipivefrine
- *Mode of administration:* Topical
- *Mechanism of action:* Acting on alpha 2 presynaptic receptors in ciliary body → results in decreased release of catecholamines → leading to decreased production of aqueous humor

Sympathetic Blockers (Beta Blockers)

- *Drugs:*
  - Nonselective beta blockers—timolol, levobunolol, and carteolol
  - Beta 1 selective blockers—betaxolol
- *Mode of administration:* Topical
  - *Mechanism of action:* Inhibition of beta 1 receptors postsynaptically in the ciliary body → decreases release of catecholamines → decreases aqueous production

Carbonic Anhydrase Inhibitors

- *Drugs:*
  - Systemic: Acetazolamide and methazolamide
  - Topical: Dorzolamide and brinzolamide
- *Mode of administration:* Systemic and topical
- *Mechanism of action:* Carbonic anhydrase catalyzes the formation of bicarbonate and hydrogen ions from water and carbon dioxide in nonpigmented ciliary epithelium of ciliary body. Bicarbonate is the main anion and sodium ions are the main cations of the nonpigmented ciliary epithelium. Sodium ions are brought inside the cells with the help of Na^+- H^+ exchanger. Na^+ and HCO_3^- are transported into the lateral intercellular space with the help of Na^+ - K^+ - ATPase. They also bring water with them due to osmosis. As these cannot traverse the blood aqueous barrier towards the stromal side, they are released into the posterior chamber, hence forming aqueous.

Carbonic anhydrase inhibitors inhibit this whole process, thus decreasing aqueous humor production.

- *Adverse effects:*
  - Tingling and numbness of fingers, toes, and perioral region
  - Malaise, fatigue, and weight loss
  - Games, nausea, and diarrhea—due to gastrointestinal irritation
  - Alkaline urine and metabolic acidosis
  - Calcium phosphate precipitation in urine
  - Blood dyscrasias—thrombocytopenia, agranulocytosis, and aplastic anemia
  - Myopic shift in refractive error
  - Topical dorzolamide may cause burning and foreign body sensation
- *Contraindications:*
  - Hypersensitivity to sulfonamides
  - Impaired renal and hepatic function
  - Patients with severe chronic obstructive pulmonary disease
  - Patients with aqueous outflow obstruction
  - Pregnant women
  - Patients taking thiazide diuretic may develop hypokalemia

Prostaglandin Analogs (PGF2 Alpha Analogs)

- *Drugs:* Latanoprost, bimatoprost, and travoprost
- *Mode of administration:* Topical
- *Mechanism of action:* Acting through prostanoid receptors in ciliary muscle, circular muscle of iris and aqueous outflow pathways → leads to extracellular matrix remodeling via activation of matrix metalloproteinases → reduced collagen in ciliary muscle and adjacent sclera → reduced resistance to outflow via uveoscleral pathway

Rho Kinase Inhibitors

- *Drugs:* Ripasudil, netarsudil, and fasudil
- *Mode of administration:* Topical, intracameral (proposed recently, helps to heal the corneal endothelium by anterior chamber injection with cultured endothelial cells)
- *Mechanism of action:*
  - Rho kinase inhibitors act through various pathways
  - These drugs inhibit phosphorylation of myosin light chain (a function of Rho kinase) → reduces the resistance and diastolic pressure of trabecular cells → enhancing outflow of aqueous.
  - These drugs also decrease reactive oxygen species-related damage to the trabecular meshwork.
  - Rho kinase inhibitors also promote vasodilation and improve perfusion to optic nerve head.
  - Rho kinase inhibitors were also shown to have a role in corneal wound healing and progression of cell cycle along with cell proliferation and migration of corneal cells.
- *Indications:* Fuchs endothelial corneal dystrophy, ocular hypertension, and primary open angle glaucoma
- *Adverse effects:* Conjunctival hyperemia, conjunctival hemorrhage, and corneal verticillata.

Hyperosmotic Agents

- *Drugs:* Systemic—glycerol and mannitol; topical—hypertonic saline
- *Mode of administration:* Systemic and topical
- *Mechanism of action:* These drugs act by increasing osmolality of intravascular fluid → draws out fluid from other compartments to intravascular compartment → draws out fluid from vitreous → reduces vitreous volume → reduces IOP
- *Adverse effects:*
  - Nausea and vomiting
  - Diuresis

   - Dehydration
   - Acidemia
   - Anaphylactic shock
   - Cardiovascular overload
   - Pulmonary edema
- *Contraindications:*
   - Patients with compromised cardiac function
   - Diabetic patients for risk of hyperglycemia
   - Hyper sensitivity reactions
   - Frank pulmonary edema

5. Discuss the mechanism of action of local anesthetic agents used in ophthalmology. What are the various routes of administration? What are the complications of peribulbar anesthesia?

(6 + 4) (DNB 2020, MS 2021)

Mechanism of Action

Voltage gated sodium channels located at the membrane of neurons of striated muscles are significant in action potential conduction. These channels have three states that maintain the polarity of the cells: Inactive, active, and resting states → in the active state Na^+ ions move from extracellular to intracellular compartment → changes the resting membrane potential of cells from –90 mV to +40 mV, that transmits the action potential → this is succeeded by inactive state when no more entry of Na^+ ions is allowed → outward flow of K^+ ions result in repolarization of membranes that brings these channels into resting state → local anesthetics have highest affinity of binding Na^+ channels at the inactive state → this increases the refractory period, where the channels remain in inactive state for a long time, without going back to the resting state, to receive the next impulse.

Routes of Administration

There are five main types of routes of administration of local anesthetics:

1. Retrobulbar
2. Peribulbar
3. Sub-Tenon's
4. Topical
5. Local infiltration

Retrobulbar

Suitable for: Cataract surgery, glaucoma filtering surgeries, iris surgeries, trans pars plana posterior segment procedures, and orbital exploration

Target nerves: Oculomotor nerve, abducens nerve, intraorbital part of ophthalmic division of trigeminal nerve, ciliary nerves, and ganglion

Location: Intraconal space posterior to the globe

Amount of anesthetic required: 2–4 mL

Technique: Needle (22 G, 35 mm) inserted parallel to orbital floor just above the inferior orbital margin in the inferotemporal quadrant

Complication: Retrobulbar hemorrhage and optic nerve damage

Peribulbar

Suitable for: Same as retrobulbar

Target nerves: Oculomotor nerve, abducens nerve, trochlear nerve, and intraorbital part of ophthalmic division of trigeminal nerve

Location: Outside the muscle cone

Amount of anesthetic required: 4–5 mL

Technique: Needle (23 G 1 inch) injected just above the lateral one third of inferior orbital rim

Complication: Orbital hemorrhage and globe perforation

Sub-Tenon's Block

Suitable for: Same as retrobulbar; relatively safer

Target nerves: Traversing sensory and motor nerves (ciliary nerves)

Location: Sub-Tenon's space between Tenon's capsule and sclera

Amount of anesthetic required: 2–5 mL

Technique: Peritomy over inferonasal quadrant 5–10 mm away from limbus → blunt dissection to separate Tenon's capsule → cannula (21G Rycroft cannula) passed along the curvature of the globe → injected after passing the equator

Complication: Subconjunctival hemorrhage and swelling

Local Infiltration

Suitable for: Eyelid surgeries

Target nerves: Superficial nerves supplying the skin, subcutaneous tissue, and muscles in the ocular adnexa

Amount of anesthetic required: Variable; as per the area to be anesthetized

Technique: Injected along the area required avoiding any vasculature with a 26 G needle

Complication: Hematoma formation

Topical

Suitable for: Applanation tonometry, gonioscopy, superficial foreign body removal, suture removal, and phacoemulsification

Target nerves: Conjunctival nerves

Amount of anesthetic required: One drop of topical anesthetic solution

Technique: Instilled into conjunctival fornix

Complication: Persistent epithelial defects on prolonged use

Complications of Peribulbar Anesthesia

- Globe perforation
- Transient blindness
- Periorbital ecchymoses
- Orbital hemorrhage
- Optic nerve damage
- Oculocardiac reflex activation
- Brainstem anesthesia (low incidence)
- Allergic reaction

6. Enumerate the various types of lasers used in ophthalmic practice. Uses of lasers in ocular disorders. (4 + 6) (DNB 2023)

The acronym for LASER is light amplified stimulated emission of radiation. It makes use of stimulated emission of photons to produce a light beam that is coherent, collimated and monochromatic.

A laser system consists of:

- Gain medium
- Reflective optical cavity
- Pump source

Laser-tissue Interaction

- *Photothermal:* Damage to tissues is due to increased temperature
    - Photocoagulation:

    Rise in temperature within target tissue causes denaturation of proteins.
    Examples: Argon, krypton, diode (810), frequency doubled Nd:YAG laser
    - Photovaporization:

    Laser beam leads to vaporization of intracellular and extracellular water.
    Examples: Carbon dioxide laser with far-infrared wavelengths
- *Photochemical:* Light-induced chemical reactions cause damage to target tissue
    - Photoradiation:
      After injecting a photosensitive intravenous agent, laser is applied that generates cytotoxic free radicals that inflict damage
      Example: Photodynamic therapy
    - Photoablation:
      Laser induces breakage of long chain polymers into small volatile fragments
      Example: Excimer laser
- *Photoablation (photoionizing):* Laser strips electron from target tissue → creating a shockwave → damaging tissue

Classification

Based on the physical state of the gain medium of the lasers, these can be divided into various types.

- *Solid state lasers:*
    - Ruby
    - Nd:YAG
- Gas lasers:
    - Argon laser
    - Krypton laser
    - Carbon dioxide laser
- Liquid lasers:
    - Dye laser
- Semiconductor lasers:
    - Diode lasers

Common Lasers Used in Ophthalmology

- *Argon laser:*
    - *Wavelength:* 488–514 nm
    - *Gain medium:* Gas
    - *Damage mechanism:* Photothermal and photochemical
    - *Uses:* Trabeculoplasty, iridotomy, iridoplasty, and panretinal photocoagulation

- *Carbon dioxide laser:*
  - *Wavelength:* 10,600 nm
  - *Gain medium:* Gas
  - *Damage mechanism:* Photothermal
  - *Uses:* Oculoplastic surgery and sclerostomy
- *Excimer laser:*
  - *Wavelength:* 193 nm
  - *Gain medium:* gas
  - *Damage mechanism:* Photochemical
  - *Uses:* PRK, LASIK, and LASEK
- *Nd:YAG laser:*
  - *Wavelength:* 532 nm (green), 1,064 nm (near infrared)
  - *Gain medium:* Solid
  - *Damage mechanism:* Photoionization and photothermal
  - *Uses:* Capsulotomy, iridectomy, trabeculoplasty, and cyclophotocoagulation
- *Diode laser:*
  - *Wavelength:* 620–895 nm (red and infrared)
  - *Gain medium:* Solid
  - *Damage mechanism:* Photothermal
  - *Uses:* Panretinal photocoagulation, iridoplasty, trabeculoplasty, and cyclophotocoagulation
- *Dye laser:*
  - *Wavelength:* 310–1,200 nm (UV to visible to infrared spectrum)
  - *Gain medium:* Fluorescent dye
  - *Damage mechanism:* Photothermal and photochemical
  - *Uses:* Photodynamic therapy, iridotomy, and sclerostomy

Uses of Lasers in Ocular Disorders

Diagnostic uses:

- *Confocal scanning laser ophthalmoscope:* For optic nerve head evaluation
- *Optical coherence tomography:* To evaluate retinal and anterior segment pathologies
- *Laser retinal Doppler flowmetry:* To evaluate optic nerve head perfusion

Therapeutic uses:

- *Cornea:*
  - LASIK
  - PRK
  - Phototherapeutic keratectomy
  - LASEK
- *Glaucoma:*
  - Peripheral iridotomy
  - Laser iridoplasty
  - Laser pupilloplasty
  - Argon laser trabeculoplasty and selective laser trabeculoplasty
  - Cyclophotocoagulation
  - Laser vitreolysis
- *Cataract:*
  - Femtosecond laser-assisted cataract surgery (FLACS)
  - Posterior capsulotomy after cataract surgery

- *Retina:*
  - Pan retinal photocoagulation
  - Endolaser for retinal tears and retinal detachments
  - Argon laser photocoagulation for choroidal neovascularization
  - Argon or Krypton laser for retinoblastomas, melanomas, and retinal angiomas
  - Focal laser treatment of retinal microaneurysms and Coat's disease

7. Short note on: Topical low dose atropine. (5) (DNB 2021)

Topical low dose atropine finds its place in prevention of childhood myopia. This has been established in various studies such as: ATOM 1, ATOM 2 (atropine for treatment of myopia), and LAMP studies.

Mechanism of Action of Atropine in Myopia Prevention

Atropine *inhibits signal transmission* from retina via RPE and choroid into the sclera → this signal leads to gene expression → cell proliferation → scleral matrix remodeling → axial length elongation and myopia.

Atropine also decreases vitreous chamber depth → decreased elongation of eyeball → myopia prevention.

ATOM 1 trial:

- Conducted in 2006 among 400 children (6–12 years) divided into two groups; observed for 3 years
- Randomized, double-blind, placebo-controlled trial
- Treatment group received 1% atropine topically once nightly in one eye for 2 years
- The mean increase in axial length remained unchanged in the treatment group, compared to the placebo group, which showed significant elongation
- During washout period of 1 year when atropine was withdrawn, myopia progression was greater in the treated group in comparison to the placebo group

ATOM 2 trial:

Phase 1:

- Conducted in 2012 among 400 children to test the action of lower concentration of atropine, namely - 0.5%, 0.1%, and 0.01% for prevention of myopia progression
- The children were randomly allocated as 2:2:1 where they received the different concentrations of atropine
- Once nightly administration of atropine to one eye of the children was continued for 2 years
- It was observed that 0.01% atropine was as effective in prevention of myopia progression as the 0.5% and 0.1% atropine, with minimal pupillary dilation or accommodation loss.

Phase 2:

- Atropine was stopped and children were observed for 1 year
- In this wash out period, lower doses (0.01%) of atropine showed lesser rates of myopia progression

Phase 3:

- This is known as the re-treatment phase where children with >–0.5 D of myopia progression were started on 0.01% atropine and observed for 2 years
- Fewer children in the 0.01% atropine group of phase 1 required re-treatment in this phase

Thus, it was established after 5 years of ATOM 2 study that 0.01% atropine was more efficacious in prevention of myopia progression when compared to higher doses of atropine.

LAMP Study:

- 438 children aged 4–12 years with myopia of at least –1.0 D were recruited into the study
- It was a randomized, double-blinded, placebo controlled trial
- The children were randomly allocated the following groups: 0.05%, 0.025%, 0.01% atropine and placebo
- Once nightly administration of the drug to one eye of the children for 1 year
- At the end of this period, 0.05% atropine was found to be most effective in controlling myopia progression.

8. Cyclodestructive procedures. (10) RGUHS MS 2020

Cyclodestructive procedures are used to reduce aqueous secretion and thus lower IOP in a painful eye with low visual potential by selective destruction of ciliary body.

Lasers, cyclodiathermy, cyclectomy, and cryotherapy are used to perform cyclodestructive procedures, either transsclerally or endoscopically.

Indications

- Elevated IOP with low visual potential
- Failed incisional glaucoma surgeries
- Patients in whom glaucoma filtration surgeries are contraindicated
- Pain relief in no vision

Contraindications

- Uveitic glaucoma
- Uncooperative patient

Transscleral Cyclophotocoagulation

- The laser is delivered through sclera to the ciliary body
- The melanin in ciliary body absorbs laser energy → coagulative necrosis of ciliary body → reduction of aqueous secretion
- Laser also induces ciliary muscle contraction → posterior movement of scleral spur → increased aqueous outflow through trabecular meshwork
- The procedure is performed under local anesthesia
- Laser used: Nd:YAG, semiconductor diode laser
- Location: 1–1.5 mm posterior to surgical limbus over 270–360 degrees avoiding 3- and 9-O'clock positions, to avoid damage to long ciliary nerves
- Nd:YAG laser can be performed as *contact* (with sapphire probe attached to fiber optic system) and noncontact (at the slit lamp) procedures
- Semiconductor laser acts like contact Nd:YAG laser

Endocyclophotocoagulation

- Semiconductor diode laser (810 nm) is used by limbal or pars plana route
- Endoscope can be helpful in visualization of ciliary processes, thus preventing collateral damage to ciliary muscle and associated stromal tissues
- Ciliary processes are destroyed for 270–360 degrees at laser power of 150–300 mW, nitrated till the processes blanch and shrink
- *Complication:* Risk of endophthalmitis

Other Available Procedures

- High intensity focused ultrasound → delivering ultrasound energy by piezoelectric transducers → thermal necrosis of ciliary epithelium
- Transpupillary cyclophotocoagulation → argon laser is used to perform cyclodestruction through a well dilated pupil, or in a patient of aniridia

Complications

- Hyphema
- Inflammation
- Cystic macular edema
- Loss of vision
- Hypotony

- Sympathetic ophthalmia
- Phthisic bulbi

9. Interferons use in ophthalmology. (5) (MS 2019, DNB 2022)

Interferons (IFN) are natural proteins of the cytokine family that have a significant role in innate immunity.

On the basis of the cell that produces the interferon, they can be divided into:

- Type I interferons—produced by almost every cell; impart resistance to host cells
  These can further be subdivided into alpha, beta and gamma based on their amino acid sequence
- Type II interferons—produced by natural killer cells and T-lymphocytes; responsible for cytotoxic and antiproliferative properties

Mechanism of Action

Interferons bind to cell surface proteins → initiate intracellular signaling pathways → induction of protein kinases → phosphorylation of protein synthesis factors

Interferons also activate oligoadenylate synthetase → activatès specific RNAase → cleaves viral RNA → inhibit viral replication

Indications

Interferons are used in a variety of ocular disorders. Some of which have been are as follows:

- *Behcet's disease:* Interferon alpha was initially introduced, which showed improvements in visual acuity and posterior uveitis score. This was beneficial even for its extraocular manifestations. IFN alpha-2a was found superior to placebo in ocular flare reduction. IFN alpha-2a was found to be better at treating Behçet's disease when compared to IFN alpha-2b.
- *Intermediate uveitis:* IFN beta-1a when used in the treatment of intermediate uveitis associated with multiple sclerosis, refractory to corticosteroid therapy, appeared to improve visual acuity, inflammation, and macular edema.
- *Inflammatory macular edema:* IFN alpha-2a has been shown to improve uveitic cystoid macular edema, especially in those showing poor response to corticosteroid therapy.
- *Severe posterior and panuveitis:* IFN alpha-2b has shown significant results in the treatment of severe posterior and panuveitis.

10. Discuss the risk factors, clinical features, evaluation, and management of ethambutol toxicity. (2 + 2 + 4 + 2) (DNB 2021)

Ethambutol is a key antitubercular drug, which has a major adverse effect of causing optic neuritis, which can lead to significant visual loss. Ethambutol toxicity has to be assessed after initiation of antitubercular medications with pretreatment assessment of:

- Visual acuity
- Fundoscopy
- Diagnostic modalities

Risk factors for ethambutol toxicity are mostly systemic derangements.

- Studies suggest that optic neuritis incidence ranges from 0.5% to 6% among ethambutol users, with older age, renal impairment, and daily dose >15 mg/kg implicated as potential risk factors.
- The concomitant use of other anti-tuberculosis drugs, such as isoniazid, has been suggested as a contributing factor.
- Ethambutol is excreted through kidneys, so any renal disease affecting the kidneys or the glomerular filtration is going to induce ethambutol toxicity.

Clinical Features

The symptoms of ethambutol toxicity can occur at any duration after initiation of treatment regimen, but usually 3-5 months is commonly the duration.

Majority of patients (>60%) present:

- Bilateral, painless, and symmetric loss of central visual acuity
- Central visual field (central/centrocecal scotoma)
- Dyschromatopsia
- The visual acuity loss may vary from minimal (20/25) to severe (no light perception) and the severity of the visual loss at onset is often mild and insidious.
- Color vision loss may be the first sign of toxicity and usually involves loss of red and green color perception, but loss of blue and yellow is also possible, but rare.
- Central vision loss is the most common visual field defect, including central or centrocecal scotoma (intra-axial form) on formal visual field testing. However, other possible visual defects include bitemporal hemianopsia due to optic chiasm involvement and peripheral field constriction (extra-axial form).
- Pupil responses may be normal initially but then patents develop sluggish pupillary light reflex bilaterally with preservation of the near response (light near dissociation of the pupils).
- A relative afferent pupillary defect may not be seen due to the bilateral and symmetric nature of involvement but if there is any asymmetry RAPD may be visible on careful assessment.
- Initially, the optic nerve may be normal on fundoscopy, but optic disc pallor may eventually develop as the visual loss progresses. Severity of the optic nerve involvement may be variable over the period of evaluation.

Diagnosis and Evaluation

- Ideally the patient who is planned for initiation of ATD regimen with fixed drug combination, baseline visual examination in the clinics and diagnostic tests have to be done to record the pre-treatment visual status.
- The dosage of ethambutol is preferably to be <15 mg/kg to reduce the adverse effects.
- The baseline evaluation should include visual acuity, color vision, contrast sensitivity, and visual field test. Additionally, if the facility is available, baseline OCT RNFL and VEP should be documented.

The biomarkers that can help detect ethambutol toxicity at the subclinical stage include a change in average RNFL thickness, most seen in the temporal quadrant with an initial increase followed by decrease and GCC thinning on OCT, reduction in visual field index, presence of visual field defect on the pattern standard deviation plot, and prolonged VEP latency.

Visual field testing most often reveals central or centrocecal scotoma, though bitemporal breakout of the visual field defect with optic chiasma involvement has also been reported. Baseline automated perimetry is thus a good option for screening and follow-up purposes.

The optical coherence tomography of the peripapillary nerve fiber layer has proven to be a useful tool for the detection of toxic optic neuropathy and changes may be seen in the retinal nerve fiber and ganglion cell layers. While changes on the OCT are not conclusively specific to toxic optic neuropathy, they may help in the prognosis and follow-up.

VEP may show abnormalities in the amplitude or the latency of the observed waves which may point to the progression if any.

ERG and EOG have been also tried in diagnosis but the results are nonspecific and definitive interpretation is lacking. Multifocal ERG is now being studied to detect occult macular changes in subclinical neuropathies.

Management of Ethambutol Toxicity

- Currently there is no effective treatment for ethambutol toxicity, so multiple experts suggest focus on primary prevention more.
- However, if the condition is detected early and the drug is discontinued promptly, before the development of irreversible optic atrophy, any proportion of between 30 and 64% of patients have been reported to show visual improvements over a course of several months.
- Though full recovery is rarely seen, average improvement is about two lines on Snellen chart. Older patients above 60 years have lesser chances of improvement.

- Zinc and copper deficiencies have been associated with ethambutol toxicity, so careful regulated supplementation may help.
- Vitamin B complex, vitamin E supplements can also be thought of.

11. Role of antimetabolites and immunosuppressives drugs in ophthalmology. (5 + 5) (DNB 2019)

Ocular inflammation is a significant cause of ocular morbidity and visual impairment. Topical, periocular, intraocular and systemic steroid s have been long used in the treatment. However there is usage is constrained by the local and systemic side effects in the long term therapy. Immunosuppressive agents thus were introduces and are widely accepted in various ocular pathologies as potent line of treatment.

The four categories of agents used in treatment are:

1. *Antimetabolites:* Methotrexate, azathioprine, mycophenolate mofetil, 5-FU, mitomycin C
2. *T cell inhibitors:* Cyclosporine, tacrolimus, sirolimus, and voclosporin
3. Alkylating agents: Cyclophosphamide and chlorambucil
4. *Biologics:*
   - *TNF inhibitors:* Adalimumab, infliximab, and etanercept
   - Interferons 2a
   - IL-1 antagonist—anakinra
   - IL-2 antagonist—daclizumab
   - Lymphocyte inhibitors—rituximab and abatacept
   - Anti-VEGFs—ranibizumab, aflibercept, and bevacizumab

The primary goals of immunosuppressive therapy are:

- To control inflammation when corticosteroids fail to do so
- To prevent corticosteroid-induced toxicity when the necessary corticosteroid dosage exceeds the desired or safe level (corticosteroid sparing)
- To treat specific high-risk uveitis syndromes known to respond poorly to corticosteroids alone

Growing evidence shows the effectiveness of immunosuppressive drugs in achieving these goals, as well as improved visual function, prevention of ocular complications, and in some cases even disease remission.

Immunosuppressive therapy is to be considered in the following scenarios:

- Sight-threatening ocular inflammation
- Unacceptable/intolerable side effects due to steroids
- Inadequate response to corticosteroids
- Long-term dependence on steroid therapy, if >5–10 mg/day of prednisolone is required to keep the disease in control-steroid-sparing alternatives is indicated.
- Contraindications of steroid therapy/allergy to steroid

When the ocular inflammation becomes stable and immunosuppressives begins to take effect, the steroid is gradually tapered and these drugs are continued long-term in these diseases. These diseases include:

- Vogt-Koyanagi-Harada syndrome (VKH)
- Sympathetic ophthalmia (SO)
- Behçet disease (BD)
- Ocular cicatricial pemphigoid (OCP)
- Necrotizing scleritis (NS) associated with systemic vasculitis (granulomatosis with polyangiitis, polyarteritis nodosa)
- Serpiginous choroiditis (SC)

Other indications for early initiation of these drugs include:

- Birdshot chorioretinopathy (BSCR)
- Uveitis associated with juvenile idiopathic arthritis, ankylosing spondylitis
- Autoimmune retinopathy (nonparaneoplastic)

- Necrotizing scleritis and peripheral ulcerative keratitis associated with
- Rheumatoid arthritis
- Granulomatosis with polyangiitis (formerly known as Wegener's)
- Relapsing polychondritis

Role of Antimetabolites in Ophthalmology

To understand the role of antimetabolites that are used in ophthalmology, the mechanism of action is vital. The antimetabolites are basically inhibitors of cell cycle and cellular division by interfering in DNA and RNA replication and proliferation.

Methotrexate:

- Inhibits dihydrofolate reductase enzyme-prevents synthesis of purine nucleotides and thymidylate → interferes with DNA synthesis, repair, and cellular replication
- Anti-inflammatory actions may be related to extracellular release of adenosine
- Inhibition of T-cell activation and production of cytokines and intercellular adhesion molecules
- Inhibition of purine metabolism
- Inhibition of IL-1β receptor binding

Azathioprine: Purine analog, incorporates in the DNA at sites of purine bases and derange DNA replication.

Mycophenolate mofetil: Inhibits Inosine-5'-monophosphate dehydrogenase-alters purine metabolisms.

Mitomycin C: Inhibits DNA synthesis and cross-links DNA at the N6 position of adenine and at the O6 and N2 positions of guanine. In addition, single-strand breakage of DNA is caused by reduced mitomycin C

Various ophthalmological scenarios where antimetabolites are used:

Ocular Inflammation:

- Uveitis associated with arthritis: JIA, AS, RA, psoriatic arthritis, and reactive arthritis
- Ocular cicatricial pemphigoid
- VKH
- Sympathetic ophthalmia
- Serpiginous choroidopathy
- Pars planitis
- Uveitis in sarcoidosis and SLE
- Scleritis
- *Trabeculectomy with antimetabolites:* The success of trabeculectomy in an eye with prior surgery—either prior cataract or glaucoma surgery—is much lower than in a patient without prior eye surgery. Frequently, the success of such complicated surgery may be <50%. Failure is due to postoperative scarring. Antimetabolite medications prevent postoperative scarring. They have been shown to improve the success of glaucoma surgery in these complicated eyes. Mitomycin C and 5-fluorouracil have been used in GDD and trabeculectomy to prevent the exaggerated cellular reaction that leads to fibrosis. The adjunctive administration of these drugs intraoperatively and postoperatively has resulted in a lower rate of the hypertensive phase, and possibly a better long-term success rate in Ahmed valve surgeries.

Role of Immunosuppresives in Ophthalmology

T cell inhibitors: They are calcineurin receptor inhibitors which prevent chemoattraction of T cell to reduce immune response.

Used commonly in:
- Behçet's disease
- Sarcoidosis
- Pars planitis
- VKH
- Multiple sclerosis-related optic neuropathy idiopathic posterior uveitis
- PUK
- Scleritis with GPA
- Corneal graft rejection

Anti-VEGF agents: The action of these medications is by preventing abnormal vascular proliferation in the ocular tissues due to prevailing ischemia. VEGF is a key factor in the process of angiogenesis by promoting proliferation and vascular endothelial cell migration. It increases vascular permeability and vasodilation required in physiological processes like lesion healing, but is also involved in pathological neovascularization found in ocular diseases with irreversible vision loss. Anti-VEGFs stop this highly leaky fragile vessels to form and prevent complications.

Usage of anti-VEGF:
- *Wet age-related macular degeneration:* AMD is the most common form of vision loss in elderly patients in developed countries. Neovascularization secondary to wet AMD is responsible for most AMD-related severe vision loss. Intravitreal injections with anti-VEGF aim to stop the growth of these abnormal vessels and improve sight.
- *Diabetic retinopathy (DR):* DR affects around 28 million people in the world. About one in three patients with diabetes have DR. From the forms of DR, the proliferative one and diabetic macular edema (DME) are among one-third of the patients with DR. 5% of the mild, 20% of the moderate and 50% of the severe forms of non-proliferative DR can progress in one year into the proliferative form.
- Retinal vein occlusion (RVO)
- *Other anti-VEGF indications:*
    - Myopic choroidal neovascularization
    - Retinopathy of prematurity
    - Central serous chorioretinopathy
    - Neovascular glaucoma
    - Corneal neovascularization

Role in Ocular Tumors

OSSN: When surgical excision is difficult or recurrence is possible topical mitomycin C, cyclosporine is used to prevent recurrence.

12. What are antiviral drugs? Describe mechanism of action of acyclovir and dosages in different viral affection in the eye. (3 + 4 + 3) (DNB 2022)

Antiviral drugs are the antimicrobials which are directed against viral affections. The arsenal of such drugs which are used in ophthalmology is still limited but vital.

Antivirals can be divided based on the targets which can be either host or viral factors. Virus-directed agents bind viral proteins or nucleic acids involved in viral entry, transcription, replication of the viral genome, assembly, and release of infectious viral particles. Host-directed antivirals modulate the activity of host factors and pathways involved in the synthesis, processing, and transport of viral building blocks, as well as in the development of antiviral and inflammatory responses.

Flowchart 1: Classification of human antiviral drugs.

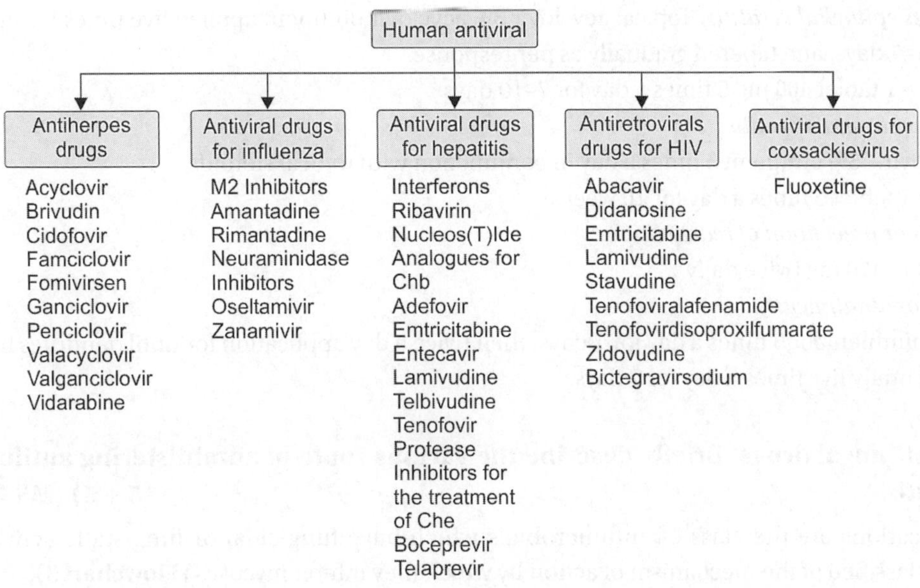

Flowchart 1 shows the broad classification of antiviral drugs that are clinically used in various systemic infections. The mechanism of action of the various classes of antiviral drugs is given in the **Flowchart 2**.

Flowchart 2: Mechanism of action of the different antiviral agents.

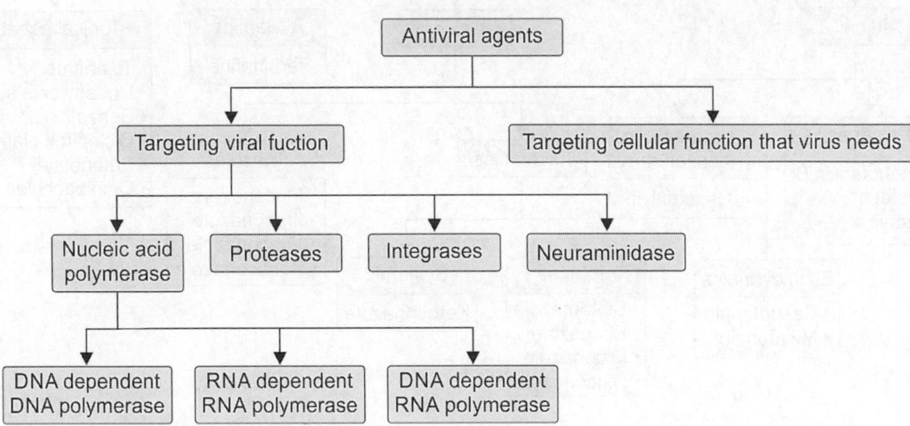

Mechanism of Action of Acyclovir

- Acyclovir is a new antiviral drug that acts as a specific inhibitor of herpesvirus DNA polymerase. It shows good in vitro activity against herpes simplex and varicella-zoster viruses. The drug may be administered topically to the skin, intravenously, orally, or topically to the eye.
- Acyclovir [9-2-hydroxymethyl)guanine] is a nucleoside analogue that selectively inhibits the replication of herpes simplex virus types 1 and 2 (HSV-1, HSV-2) and varicella-zoster virus (VZV). After intracellular uptake, it is converted to acyclovir monophosphate by virally-encoded thymidine kinase. This step does not occur to any significant degree in uninfected cells and thereby lends specificity to the drug's activity. The monophosphate derivative is subsequently converted to acyclovir triphosphate by cellular enzymes.
- Competitively inhibits viral DNA polymerase by acting as an analog to deoxyguanosine triphosphate (dGTP). This abnormal base results in chain termination.

Dosage of Acyclovir in Various Ocular Viral Affections

- *Simplex herpes epithelial keratitis:* Topical acyclovir 3% acyclovir ointment applied five times locally for 7 days, then for three times 7 days, and tapered gradually as per response.
  Systemic oral—1 tablet 400 mg 5 times a day for 7–10 days.
- *Herpes simplex stromal keratitis:*
  Topical acyclovir—3% ointment 5 times a day in conjunction with topical steroids
  Oral—400 mg 1 tablet 5 times a day for 10 weeks
- *In prophylaxis or prevention of reactivation:*
  Oral—1 tablet of 400 mg twice daily
- *Herpes zoster ophthalmicus:*
  Topical—3% ointment for 5 times a day for 7 days, then twice a day application for until dendrites have resolved.
  Oral—800 mg orally five times a day for 7 days.

13. Classify antifungal drugs. Briefly describe the various route of administering antifungal drugs in mycotic keratitis. (5 + 5) (MS WBUHS 2021)

Antifungal medications are the class of antimicrobials which have fungicidal or fungistatic activities. Antifungal medications are classified of the mechanism of action by which they inhibit mycoses **(Flowchart 3)**.

Flowchart 3: Classification of antifungal drugs.

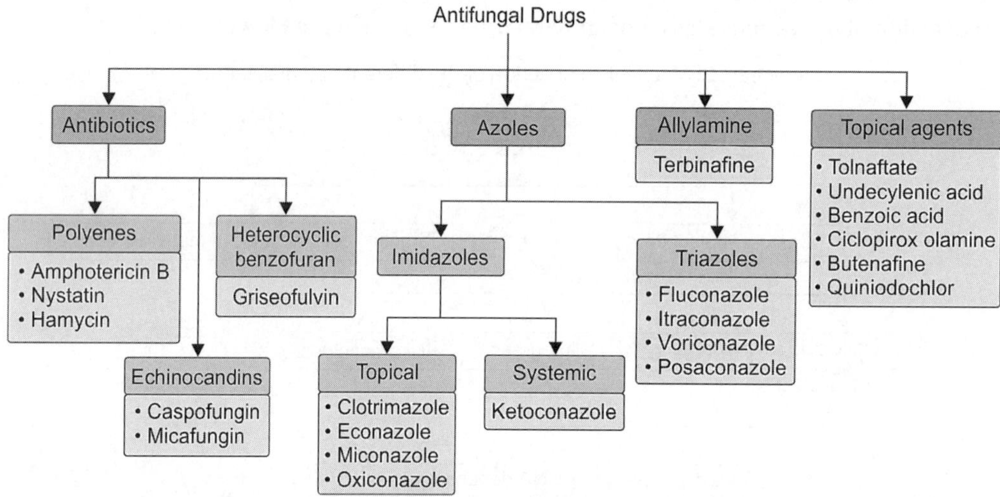

- *Loss of cell membrane integrity:*
  - *Polyenes:* Amphotericin B deoxycholate, liposomal amphotericin B, amphotericin B lipid complex, nystatin
  - *Azoles:* Ketoconazole, miconazole, clotrimazole, itraconazole, isavuconazonium sulfate (isavuconazole), fluconazole, voriconazole, posaconazole
  - *Allylamines:* Terbinafine
- *Loss of cell wall integrity:*
  - *Echinocandins:* Anidulafungin, caspofungin, and micafungin
- *Mitotic inhibitors:* Griseofulvin
- *Antimetabolites:* Flucytosine
- Ciclopirox
- *Quinoline derivatives:* Iodoquinol and clioquinol
- *Potassium Iodide:* Saturated solution of potassium iodide (SSKI)

- *Zinc pyrithione:* In patients of mycotic keratitis, the commonly used antifungal agents are polyenes (e.g., natamycin, amphotericin B), azoles (e.g., voriconazole, itraconazole, miconazole, ketoconazole, and fluconazole), and fluorinated pyrimidines (e.g., flucytosine). Amphotericin B is the drug of choice in fungal keratitis caused by yeasts. Natamycin has a broad spectrum of activity against filamentous organisms. Oral fluconazole and ketoconazole should be considered in the management of deep fungal keratitis.

Routes of Administration

Topical:

- *Natamycin eye drop:* Natamycin is the only antifungal formulation that has been US-FDA approved for treating ocular fungal infections. Natamycin 5% eye drop is commercially available.
- *Amphotericin B:* Reconstituted 0.15% drops are also used in yeast like fungi.
- *Voriconazole:* 2% voriconazole eye drops is available with limited availability and has to be reconstituted at store. AuroLab manufactures in India, and the shelf life is usually 5–7 days.
- *Itraconazole:* 1% eye ointment is now commercially available for multidrug regimen

Intrastromal Therapy

Intrastromal corneal injection of antifungal medications, e.g., voriconazole and amphotericin B may result in steady-state drug levels within the corneal tissue and prevent intervals of decreased antifungal dosing below its therapeutic level, ensures antifungal penetration in cases presented with the involvement of deep layers of the corneal stroma.

Amphotericin B 3–5 µg in 0.1 mL or voriconazole 50 µg/0.1 mL is used or both drugs in combination voriconazole 0.05 mg/0.1 mL + amphotericin B 0.01 mg/0.1 mL.

The procedure is performed in the operation theater under complete aseptic measurements using topical, with or without peribulbar anesthesia. The reconstituted solution is loaded in a disposable 1 mL insulin syringe with a 30-gauge needle. Using an operating microscope, the needle is inserted bevel-down obliquely in a clear unaffected cornea to mid-stromal level. Up to five divided doses are injected to form a barrage of intrastromal drugs around the ulcer till corneal hydration is achieved.

Intracameral Therapy

Intracameral injection of antifungal agents may be effective in severe cases of fungal keratitis where there is deep stromal involvement with unsatisfactory response to treatment. It provides a high drug delivery level into the anterior chamber. Injection should be done in an operating room under strictly aseptic conditions. Anterior chamber wash may also be performed to remove exudates and hypopyon, but care must be taken if the infection involves the anterior lens capsule to avoid capsular injury and cataract formation.

Most of the studies used Amphotericin B in a dose of 5–10 µg in 0.1 mL, some used voriconazole 50–100 µg in 0.1 mL.

Systemic Therapy

Oral or parenteral antifungal medications may be indicated if large corneal ulcers are reaching the limbus, severe deep keratitis or if the ulcer is associated with scleritis or endophthalmitis. Systemic antifungal therapy must be continued for 6–8 weeks.

- Oral voriconazole 200 mg twice daily exhibits excellent ocular penetration and can reach minimal inhibitory concentration and provide consistent drug levels.
- Oral ketoconazole 600 mg/day. Liver functions must be monitored every 2 weeks after its use.
- Oral itraconazole 200 mg/day.
- Oral fluconazole 200 mg/day.
- Intravenous miconazole.

Intravitreal Injections

Used in cases of severe keratitis with anterior chamber fungal infiltrates or posterior segment spread. Amphotericin B and Voriconazole are the two drugs used here.

14. Different stains used for diagnostic and therapeutic purposes in ophthalmology and their uses. (10) (MS WBUHS 2019)

Various stains and dyes are used in ophthalmology for a wide array of diagnostic and therapeutic purposes. From ocular surface staining dyes to posterior segment surgeries, stains, and dyes are available from commercially available dye impregnated paper strips to complex injections.

- *Sodium fluorescein:*
  - Available as sterile prepacked dye impregnated strips with 1% of 0.6–1 mg dye OR as IV injection of 10% in 5 mL or 20% in 2 mL.
  - Orange water soluble dye, adheres to basement membrane and highlights areas of epithelial breakdown.
  - The fluorescence property is utilized in fundus fluorescent angiography, where it is 70% protein bound.
  - The ocular surface is examined in cobalt blue filter light of slit lamp.
  - For retinal imaging, the photographs are taken with special filters to study the vasculature and pathologies of retina.
  - Diagnostic uses for identifying corneal epithelial breach, keratitis, dry eye, in applanation tonometry, Seidel's test, Jones dye test, and retinal vascular disorders
  - Therapeutic—canalicular repair in traumatic lacerations and contact lens fitting.
- *Lissamine green:*
  - Available as 1.5 mg dye impregnated sterile strips or 1%–3% liquid formulations.
  - High affinity for ocular surface staining in dead and devitalized tissue, outlining the area of disrupted cell junction.
  - Peak absorption at red-end of light. Red free filter absorbs transmitted wavelength, stained areas appear black.
  - Preferred dye to stain bulbar conjunctiva.
  - Therapeutic purpose is limited but Diagnostic purpose is better than fluorescein dye.
  - *Uses:* In dry eye disease to rule out Keratoconjunctivitis Sicca, to ascertain proper fitting of contact lens. Also used for assessment of lid margins for lid wiper epitheliopathy.
- *Rose bengal:*
  - Available as 1.3 mg dye impregnated sterile prepacked strip.
  - Stains dead and devitalized tissue cells on ocular surface
  - Taken up wherever there is deficiency of preocular tear film protection.
  - Visualization of dendritic viral keratitis and fungal bulbs in mycotic keratitis is better.
  - *Uses:* Conjunctival staining in dry eye disease and metaplastic cells in conjunctival neoplasm. Corneal staining for herpetic dendrites and SPKs. Also aids in diagnosis of meibomian gland dysfunction.
- *Trypan Blue:*
  - Available as liquid formulations of various concentration as per the need and surgery to be done.
  - 0.06% dye is used in staining of the anterior capsule of the lens for capsulorhexis during cataract extraction surgery. Very useful when the fundal glow is not prominent or there is weak zonules.
  - Same concentration is used to stain the Descemet membrane for DSEK surgeries.
  - Aid in stripping the corneal endothelium from donor button in DALK.
  - 0.06% dye is also used in staining of Tenon's capsule before enucleation surgery.
  - 0.15% dye is used in posterior segment surgery to stain the ERM after fluid or air exchange.
- *Indocyanine green:*
  - Has high affinity for collagen type 4 and laminin, which are in high concentration in ILM.
  - 90% of it remains plasma protein bound on IV injection, and this property is used to visualized choroidal circulation and help in diagnosis of choroidal pathologies.
  - Better tolerated than FFA, and also preferred in eyes with media opacities where FFA imaging may be difficult, since infrared rays can penetrate ocular pigments and give clear image.
  - Available as 40 mg in 2 mL for IV injection, 0.05–0.5% for posterior segment surgeries, 0.5% (25 mg in 5 mL solvent) for anterior lens capsule staining.

- *Uses:* Choroidal angiography in cases of suspected choroidal vascular disorders, neovascular membranes, and choroidal polyps.
- For staining of ILM before peeling in vitreo-retinal ERM staining is also concurrent

▪ *Brilliant blue G:*
- Has strong affinity for ILM without staining ERM or vitreous.
- Used in macular ERM where ILM takes the dye and ERM is visible against the blue background (negative staining)
- FDA approved

▪ *Triamcinolone acetonide:*
- Very commonly available as 40 mg in 1 mL vial for intralesional injections or intravitreal injections.
- For vitreous staining, 0.1–0.3 mL/40 mg per mL drug.
- It has got both diagnostic and therapeutic purposes.
- TA binds avidly to acellular tissue and gives good contrast between those areas of cleared and persistent vitreous.
- Used to detect PC rent and vitreous strand in AC
- IVTA injections are given for treatment of macular edema in cases of RVO and DR.
- Intralesional injections are used for chalazion treatment.

▪ *Other dyes:*
- *Bromophenol blue:* 0.13–0.2% for chromovitrectomy due to high affinity for ILM and ERM
- *Patent blue:* Highly selective affinity for ERM with lesser toxicity to retinal than ICG. Used as 0.25% for chromovitrectomy.

SUGGESTED READING

1. Chamberlain PD, Sadaka A, Berry S, Lee AG. Ethambutol optic neuropathy. Curr Opin Ophthalmol. 2017;28(6):545-51.
2. Han J, Byun MK, Lee J, Han SY, Lee JB, Han SH. Longitudinal analysis of retinal nerve fiber layer and ganglion cell-inner plexiform layer thickness in ethambutol-induced optic neuropathy. Graefes Arch Clin Exp Ophthalmol. 2015;253(12):2293-9.
3. Hoffman J. Overview of antiviral medications used in ophthalmology. Community Eye Health. 2020;33(108):85-8.
4. Hornbeak DM, Thorne JE. Immunosuppressive therapy for eye diseases: Effectiveness, safety, side effects and their prevention. Taiwan J Ophthalmol. 2015;5(4):156-63.
5. Ianevski A, Ahmad S, Anunnitipat K, Oksenych V, Zusinaite E, Tenson T, et al. Seven classes of antiviral agents. Cell Mol Life Sci. 2022;79(12):605.
6. Karachrysafi S, Sioga A, Komnenou A, Karamitsos A, Xioteli M, Dori I, et al. Histological Effects of Intravitreal Injection of Antifungal Agents in New Zealand White Rabbits: An Electron Microscopic and Immunohistochemical Study. Pharmaceuticals (Basel). 2020;13(10):267.
7. Saxena R, Singh D, Phuljhele S, Kalaiselvan V, Karna S, Gandhi R, et al. Ethambutol toxicity: Expert panel consensus for the primary prevention, diagnosis and management of ethambutol-induced optic neuropathy. Indian J Ophthalmol. 2021;69(12):3734-9.
8. Sharma P, Sharma R. Toxic optic neuropathy. Indian J Ophthalmol. 2011;59(2):137-41.
9. Thomas RE, Crichton A, Thomas BC. Antimetabolites in cataract surgery to prevent failure of a previous trabeculectomy. Cochrane Database Syst Rev. 2014;2014(7):CD010627.
10. Tripathy K. (2023). Immunomodulatory Therapy (IMT) for Ocular Inflammation. [online] Available from eyewiki.org/Immunomodulatory_Therapy_(IMT)_for_Ocular_Inflammation. [Last accessed March, 2025].

CHAPTER

Ocular Manifestations of Systemic Diseases

Smiti Rani Srivastava, Rajkumari Bigyabati, Rituparna Sarkar

QUESTIONS

1. **Ocular manifestations of HIV infection.** **(10) (MS 2023)**
2. **What is AIDS? Describe the management of ocular manifestation of AIDS.** **(3 + 7) (DNB 2022)**
3. **Ocular tuberculosis: Clinical features and management.** **(5 + 5) (MS 2019/DNB 2023)**
4. **Discuss the management of a case of pulmonary tuberculosis who develop sudden decrease of vision.** **(10) (DNB 2022)**
5. **Ocular manifestation of mucormycosis.** **(10) (DNB 2021)**
6. **Ocular manifestation of sarcoidosis.** **(10) (DNB 2023)**
7. **Ocular manifestation of neurofibromatosis.** **(10) (DNB 2023, 2024)**
8. **Ocular manifestations of Hansen's disease. How will you manage a case of eyelid involvement in leprosy?** **(10) (WBUHS MS 2024, 2022)**

1. Ocular manifestations of HIV infection. (10) (MS 2023)

Human immunodeficiency virus (HIV), an RNA retrovirus causes a multisystem disease known as acquired immunodeficiency syndrome (AIDS). Transmission of HIV occurs by sexual contact with infected person, exposure to contaminated blood or blood products through needles sharing with infected person, transfusion of infected blood and vertical spread from infected mother.

Ocular involvement of HIV can be due to opportunistic infection, vascular abnormalities, neoplasms, neuro-ophthalmic conditions and from side effect of medications. Ocular manifestations of HIV infection can occur in various ways according to the severity of disease.

Ocular Manifestation of HIV

- *Ocular infections:* They cause more severe infection is AIDS patients in comparison to healthy patients and include Herpes simplex infections, Herpes zoster ophthalmicus, toxoplasmosis, ocular tuberculosis, fungal corneal ulcers, and syphilis.
- *Opportunistic infection of eye:* They are caused by microorganisms that do not normally affect normal individual, but affect people who are immunosuppressed by immunodeficiency diseases such as HIV and leukemia. These include *Cytomegalovirus* retinitis, *Pneumocystis carinii* infection, *Candida* endophthalmitis, and cryptococcal infections.
- *Retinal microvasculopathy:* This develops from vaso-occlusion of retinal vasculature which may develop either due to toxic effects of virus on vascular endothelium or due to immune complex deposits on precapillary arterioles.
- *Unusual neoplasms:* These include Kaposi sarcoma and Burkitt's lymphoma.
- *Neuro-ophthalmic lesions:* Infections of the brain may result in neuro-ophthalmic lesions such as cranial nerve palsies, loss of nerve supply to eye and optic nerve involvement leading to loss of vision.

Anatomical Categorization of Ocular Manifestations

Eyelid

- *Blepharitis:* Blepharitis has been found to be more common and serious in HIV-infected individuals and may be due to reduced ability to control the normal flora of the eye or because of changes that occur in the lid glands that occur with immunosuppression. Ocular herpes simplex can cause blepharitis and symptoms of blepharitis in patients with AIDS are more severe when there is concurrent dry eye disease.
- *Kaposi sarcoma:* This is a slow-growing malignant vascular tumor which typically occurs in patients with AIDS. It is caused by infection of the vascular endothelium with Kaposi sarcoma virus which is same as Human herpesvirus 8 (HH-8) and occur when the CD4+ cells are ≤ 150 cell/μ. It presents in adult life with irritation or painless swelling that is deep red or purple in color and appears as multiple nodules on eyelid, conjunctiva or rarely the orbit. There is proliferation of spindle-shaped cells, vascular channels, mitotic figures and inflammatory cells on histological examination.
- *Molluscum contagiosum:* This is a dermatitis caused by poxvirus and appears as a multiple small, painless, umbilicated papules of about 1 to 3 millimeters on the skin of eyelid.
- *Herpes zoster ophthalmicus (HZO):* HZO is a vesicobullous dermatitis presenting as crusted, painful vesicles in the course of ophthalmic division of trigeminal nerve caused by Varicella zoster virus infection.
- *Herpes simplex virus:* Herpes simplex virus can cause blepharitis and blepharoconjunctivitis with crusting of periorbital skin in patients with AIDS.

Orbit

- *Orbital cellulitis:* Orbit can become infected due to contiguous sinus disease, Aspergillosis being the most common.
- B-cell lymphoma

Conjunctiva

- *Conjunctival microvasculopathy:* This is characterized by segmental dilatation and narrowing of blood vessels, comma shaped vascular segments, narrowing of blood vessels and microvasculopathy.
- *Conjunctival intraepithelial neoplasia (CIN):* CIN occurs typically at the junction of conjunctiva and cornea as a swelling, causing mild redness and foreign body sensation and may mimic pterygium or *Pinguicula.*
- *Squamous cell carcinoma:* This presents as an elevated lesion with a rough surface and feeder vessel and is invasive.
- *Conjunctival lymphoma:* These lymphomas have a characteristic salmon-patch appearance.
- Conjunctiva Kaposi sarcoma

Cornea

- *Bacterial keratitis:* Bacterial keratitis is due to opportunistic infection of avascular corneal stroma initiated by breakdown in epithelial barrier. Common pathogens causing bacterial keratitis are *Staphylococcus epidermis, Staphylococcus aureus* and *Pseudomonas aeruginosa* which cause severe bacterial keratitis and may lead to blindness.
- *Herpes simplex keratitis:* Recurrence of Herpes simplex keratitis is more common in AIDS. Herpes simplex keratitis is characterized by painful, recurrent corneal ulcerations dendrites with terminal end bulbs. Herpes simplex keratitis can cause superficial punctate keratitis, stellate epithelial lesions, microdendrites, dendritic ulceration or geographic ulceration.
- *Herpes zoster keratitis:* Herpes zoster keratitis occurs in <5% of HIV positive individuals leading to permanent loss of vision. Following infection by the virus, they become latent and reactivation occurs when the host's immune response is compromised. The lesions contain live virus and may progress to form dendrite with tapered ends.
- *Fungal keratitis:* Fungal infection occurs in HIV positive individuals due to immunosuppression and severity of disease is greater in these individuals. Most common fungal organism causing keratitis in HIV positive individuals is *Candida* species. *Fusarium* and *Aspergillus* species also cause keratitis.
- *Superficial punctate keratitis:* This is caused by the protozoal parasite microsporidia. This infection is may cause keratoconjunctivitis and stromal keratitis.

Iris and Ciliary Body

- *Iritis:* Iritis may be seen with HIV infection only or may accompany bacterial or viral keratitis.
- *Mild iridocyclitis:* This is often associated with retinitis due to Cytomegalovirus and Herpes zoster.
- *Severe iridocyclitis:* This is associated with tuberculosis, toxoplasmosis, syphilis, and bacterial and fungal retinitis.
- *Drug-induced iritis:* Drugs that cause iritis are rifabutin used in treatment of mycobacteria infection and Cidofovir used in treatment of cytomegalovirus retinitis. Cidofovir has been associated with side effects such as granulomatous anterior uveitis. The increased number of CD4+ T cells following HAART can lead to an inflammatory response resulting in uveitis.

Retina

- *Neuroretina:* HIV associated neuroretinal disorder occurs in some AIDS patients in which there is loss of nerve fiber layer and manifests as abnormal color vision, decrease in contrast sensitivity, and loss of visual field.
- *Retinal microangiopathy:* Microangiopathy is the most common ocular manifestation of HIV infection and presents in the retina as cotton wool spots.
- *Infectious disease of retina:*
    - *Cytomegalovirus (CMV) retinitis:* CMV retinitis is the most common ocular opportunistic infection in AIDS patients prior to HAART therapy. The incidence of this disease has reduced with the advent of HAART therapy. Mode of is spread by contact with body fluid. As the virus is endotheliotropic, the lesions follow vascular distribution. Depending upon the size of the vessels infected, the retinitis can be indolent type with mild granular opacity and few punctate hemorrhage or fulminant type with exudation and retinal hemorrhage along the retinal vascular arcade that may involve the optic head. Clearing occurs within the lesions as slow replication of the virus allows central healing.
    - *Progressive outer retinal necrosis (PORN):* PORN occurs predominantly in AIDS. It is a rare but devastating necrotizing herpetic retinitis caused by Varicella zoster virus. The disease presents with rapid visual loss and is characterized by rapid progression to a full thickness retinal necrosis.
    - *Toxoplasma retinochoroiditis:* Toxoplasma retinitis is caused by Toxoplasma gondii in immunocompetent individual like AIDS patients. The disease manifest with uveitis, retinal lesions and vitritis. Preexisting scar may be less common in AIDS patients and they are more prone to progression if left untreated.
    - *Syphilitic chorioretinitis:* Syphilis is an uncommon cause of uveitis in HIV infected patients but cause more aggressive disease. Ocular manifestations of syphilis include iridocyclitis, intermediate uveitis, chorioretinitis, periphlebitis and neuroretinitis giving rise to secondary optic atrophy. The chorioretinitis is characterized by large, placoid pale-yellowish subretinal lesions.

Choroid

- *Choroiditis: Pneumocystis carinii* choroiditis was common before the advent of effective prophylaxis against the organism characterized by deep orange lesions. They usually resolve with antimicrobials such as Trimethoprim-sulfamethoxazole.
  Cryptococcus neoformans choroiditis can occur from systemic dissemination or spread from cryptococcal meningitis via optic nerve, but has become less common in the HAART era.
- *Ocular tuberculosis:* HIV infection can cause ocular tuberculosis though rare.
  Granulomas can occur in the anterior uvea or choroid. Extensive diffuse choroiditis may occur in patients with AIDS.

2. What is AIDS? Describe the management of ocular manifestation of AIDS. (3 + 7) (DNB 2022)

Acquired immunodeficiency syndrome (AIDS) is a multisystem disease caused by human immunodeficiency virus (HIV) which is an RNA retrovirus.

Mode of Infection

Transmission of HIV occurs by:

- Sexual contact with infected person
- Exposure to contaminated blood or blood products through needles sharing with infected person

- Transfusion of infected blood
- Vertical spread from infected mother transplacentally or via breast milk

Pathogenesis

HIV targets CD4+ T-helper lymphocytes, which play a vital role in initiation of immune response. The number of CD4+ T lymphocyte decline steadily causing interference with the mechanism of production of immune bodies, resulting in immunodeficiency, particularly of cell mediated immunity. Immunodeficiency renders the individual prone to various infections and tumors involving multiple systems.

Progression of HIV Infection

- *Acute seroconversion phase:* This occurs a few weeks after HIV infection and sometimes causes constitutional symptoms such as fever, malaise, headache, maculopapular rashes and generalized lymphadenopathy. Anti-HIV antibodies start appearing soon after this.
- *Asymptomatic phase:* This phase may last many years, during which there is steady depletion of CD4+ T lymphocytes.
- *Symptomatic phase:* HIV infection (AIDS) become manifest, characterized by opportunistic infections, tissue damage and neoplasm as a result of HIV infection.

Clinical Diagnostic Criteria of AIDS

The WHO recommends the presence of at least two major and one minor systemic manifestation for diagnosis of AIDS.

- *Major signs:* These include loss of body weight, chronic diarrhea, and fever.
- *Minor signs:* These include chronic cough, itchy dermatitis, oropharyngeal candidiasis, recurrent herpes zoster, generalized lymphadenopathy.

Clinical Features

Systemic Features

- Opportunistic infections
- Tumors such as Kaposi sarcoma, non-Hodgkin B-cell lymphoma, and squamous cell carcinoma of conjunctiva, cervix, and anus
- HIV encephalopathy

Management of AIDS

Diagnosis

Serological testing for HIV infection: This should be performed after obtaining informed consent after proper counseling. ELISA and Western Blot tests are used to confirm HIV infection by demonstration of anti-HIV antibodies in the serum. Serial testing may be necessary as seroconversion may take 3 months or longer following exposure to HIV.

CD4+ T lymphocyte count is measured every 3 months after establishment of HIV positivity and high risk of HIV related disease is implicated by CD4+T lymphocyte count <200/mm^3.

Treatment

AIDS has no cure, but the progress of the disease can be slowed down by a number of drugs by reducing the viral load.

Indication for antiretroviral therapy:

- Symptomatic HIV disease
- Viral load > 10,000/mL of plasma
- Rapidly falling CD4+ T lymphocyte count

Drugs treatment for HIV:

Highly active antiretroviral therapy (HAART) is used to treat HIV infection by using two nucleoside reverse transcriptase inhibitors with either one non-nucleoside reverse transcriptase inhibitor or one or two protease inhibitors.

- *Nucleoside reverse transcriptase inhibitors:* These include zidovudine, lamivudine, and zalcitabine.
- *Non-nucleoside reverse transcriptase inhibitors:* They include nevirapine and efavirenz.
- *Protease inhibitors:* Include amprenavir, indinavir, and nelfinavir.

Management of Ocular Manifestations of AIDS

- *Treatment of Cytomegalovirus (CMV) retinitis:*
    - CMV retinitis is treated with intravenous ganciclovir with induction dose of 5 mg/kg twice daily for 2 weeks, followed by long term maintenance therapy of 5 mg/kg once daily.
    - Oral valganciclovir can be used as an alternative treatment with an induction dose of 900 mg twice daily for 21 days followed by 900 mg once daily.
    - Intravenous foscarnet can be used for cases resistant to ganciclovir with an induction dose of 90 mg/kg every 12 hours for 2 weeks, followed by long term maintenance therapy of 90 to 120 mg/kg daily.
    - Intravitreal injection of 2.0 mg ganciclovir in 0.05 mL once per week can be as maintenance therapy.
    - Intravitreal foscarnet can be used as a substitute or combined with ganciclovir in the dose of 1.2 mg in 0.05 mL.
- *Treatment of progressive outer retinal necrosis (PORN):* PORN can be treated with intravitreal antiviral treatment of combined intravenous ganciclovir and foscarnet with HAART.
- *Treatment of toxoplasma retinochoroiditis:* Toxoplasma retinochoroiditis is treated with standard antitoxoplasmosis regimen with comprising of systemic prednisolone (1 mg/kg) in conjunction with one or more of the following agents: Clindamycin (300 mg qid for 3–4 weeks), sulfadiazine (1 g qid for 3–4 weeks), pyrimethamine (loading dose of 50 mg followed by 25–50 mg for 4 weeks), co-trimozole (960 mg for 4–6 weeks), atovaquone (750 mg tid), and azithromycin 500 mg.
- *Treatment of syphilitic chorioretinitis:* Treatment of syphilitic chorioretinitis is with one of the following regimens: Intravenous penicillin G (12–24 mega units for 10–15 days, intramuscular procaine penicillin (2.4 mega unit for 10–14 days), oral amoxicillin (3 g bd for 28 days).
- *Treatment of ocular tuberculosis:* Treatment is with systemic antitubercular therapy with rifampicin, isoniazid, pyrazinamide, ethambutol or streptomycin along with HAART.
- *Treatment for molluscum contagiosum:*
    - Molluscum contagiosum can be treated with HAART, conservatively with topical phenol, trichloroacetic acid or liquid nitrogen.
    - It can also be treated by excision, incision and curettage.
- *Herpes zoster ophthalmicus (HZO):* HZO is treated by induction with acyclovir 10 mg/kg intravenously, and maintenance with acyclovir 500 mg orally 5 times/day or oral valacyclovir 1 g thrice daily. Resistant cases can be treated with famciclovir or foscarnet.
- *Herpes simplex keratitis:*
    - This can be treated with acyclovir eye ointment five times daily.
    - Systemic therapy with acyclovir 400 mg five times daily or Valacyclovir 500 mg twice daily is used in severe cases.
- Treatment of *Kaposi sarcoma:*
    - Treatment is indicated for cosmetic purpose, bleeding or infection.
    - Treatment depends on the site and extension of Kaposi sarcoma with focal radiotherapy and excision, with or without adjunctive cryotherapy and systemic chemotherapy.
    - HAART can treat AIDS-related primary Kaposi sarcoma as well as reduce need for other methods of treatment like chemotherapy or radiotherapy.
- *Treatment of ocular surface squamous neoplasia (OSSN):*
    - OSSN can be treated by surgical excision with wide clear margin of about 4 millimeters with adjuvant cryotherapy or chemotherapy along with amniotic membrane grafting.
    - Medical management of OSSN can be done using topical mitomycin-C or 5-fluorouracil for a week, followed by drug holiday and repetition of same cycle until lesion regresses.
    - Interferon can be used as eye drops or weekly subconjunctival injection.
- *Treatment of drug-induced uveitis:*
    - Most cases of drug induced uveitis respond well to topical corticosteroid and cycloplegic agents.
    - Inciting drug should be discontinued to treat refractory cases.

3. Ocular tuberculosis: Clinical features and management. (5 + 5) (MS 2019/DNB 2023)

4. Discuss the management of a case of pulmonary tuberculosis who develop sudden decrease of vision. (10) (DNB 2022)

Tuberculosis (TB) is a chronic granulomatous infection caused by the tubercle bacilli *Mycobacterium tuberculosis* which is transmitted by inhalation of respiratory droplets containing the bacteria. The lung is the site of primary tuberculosis, but extrapulmonary sites are lymph nodes, pleura, central nervous system and the eye.

Ocular tuberculosis may not be associated with clinical evidence of pulmonary tuberculosis and may be the initial presentation of extrapulmonary TB.

Mycobacterium tuberculosis can affect the eye by the following ways:

- Hematogenous spread from pulmonary or extrapulmonary sites
- Direct ocular infection from adjacent structures
- Hypersensitivity reaction in ocular structure following exposure to *Mycobacterium* antigen.

The most common route of ocular involvement is by hematogenous spread from pulmonary tuberculosis which occur by inhalation of aerosolized droplets containing mycobacteria.

Ocular manifestation of mycobacteria can vary depending on the mode of infection. Primary ocular infection due to direct contact with the eye leads to involvement of eyelids and adnexa, sclera, conjunctiva, cornea or lacrimal system.

Hematogenous spread from pulmonary or extrapulmonary sites commonly affects the uveal tract leading to uveitis. Choroid, which receives the highest unit of blood flow in the eye, is susceptible to deposition of mycobacteria-laden macrophages, leading to posterior uveitis. The bacilli multiply inside the choroid, causing local inflammation which manifests as choroidal tubercle. Tuberculomas are tubercles that coalesce or become enlarged. These lesions involve all layers of choroid and may liquefy into a subretinal abscess. Retinal pigment epithelium may become disrupted as the disease advance, leading to retinal detachment. The lesion may resolve with early intervention or may lead to an atrophic scar.

Hypersensitivity reactions of the bacilli involving the eye include phlyctenular keratoconjunctivitis and Eales disease, which result from an immunological response to nonviable mycobacteria in ocular tissue.

Clinical Features of Ocular Tuberculosis

Symptoms: The disease can affect various ocular tissues and may be asymptomatic or cause a wide range of symptoms such as:

- Headache
- Flashes and floaters
- Red eyes
- Photophobia and dimness of vision when tubercles involve the macula

Signs: Ocular involvement of tuberculosis may show clinical signs according to the anatomical location as discussed here.

Extraocular Tuberculosis

- *Eyelid TB:* Eyelid TB is quite common, especially in children. The disease occurs as a result of spread of infection from face and lymph nodes or by hematogenous route. Eyelid TB begins as a red papule that becomes indurated, enlarges to form a nodule or plaque that ulcerates which is chronic and painless. The skin lesion can become popular and hyperkeratotic, though rare. Lupus vulgaris of the face may spread to the eyelid which is characterized by reddish brown apple jelly nodules, chronic blepharitis, lid abscess or atypical chalazion. TB of the tarsal plate can simulate recurrent chalazion. Tuberculids of eyelid present as small, multiple popular, and chronic lesions. Tubercular lid involvement by spread from underlying bone or lacrimal sac manifest as a red, fluctuant nodule with induration that ulcerates leading to formation of a fistula surrounded by granulation tissue.
- *Lacrimal gland TB:* Tubercular involvement of the lacrimal system is unusual. Lacrimal gland TB may present as asymptomatic dacryoadenitis or lacrimal gland abscess. TB dacryoadenitis usually develop from hematogenous

spread and occasionally from direct spread from conjunctival and corneal disease presenting as a gradually enlarging painless swelling that may lead to abscess formation and chronic fistula in the upper lid. Regional lymphadenopathy is usually associated with TB of lacrimal system.

- *Conjunctiva TB:* Tuberculosis can involve the conjunctiva primarily manifesting as conjunctival TB and lupus vulgaris or secondarily as tuberculids and phlyctens. Primary tuberculous conjunctivitis present with discomfort and redness of eyes, mucopurulent discharge and unilateral nodular or ulcerative conjunctivitis with regional lymphadenopathy. TB infection of conjunctiva may also present with phlycten, ulcers, subconjunctival nodules, tuberculomas and polyps. Conjunctival tuberculomas begin insidiously and develop regional lymphadenopathy in 3–4 weeks. Conjunctival TB can very rarely acute purulent or mucopurulent cause conjunctivitis presenting with fever and malaise.
- *Corneal TB:* Corneal involvement of TB present with phlyctenular keratoconjunctivitis or interstitial keratitis. Phlyctenular keratoconjunctivitis is an inflammatory nodule found at the limbus and is due to hypersensitivity reaction to tubercular antigen. Tubercular interstitial keratitis presents with peripheral stroma infiltrate with vascularization. TB of cornea can also cause corneal erosion and ulcer and disciform keratitis.
- *Scleral TB:* Tuberculous scleritis is rare and may occur by direct spread from conjunctival or choroidal lesions. It may present as nodular or necrotizing lesion usually anteriorly and rarely posteriorly. It is difficult to diagnose and does not respond to anti-inflammatory treatment. Tuberculous scleritis can also cause nodular and diffuse anterior scleritis, sclerokeratitis, sclerouveitis, and scleromalacia.
- *Orbital TB:* Tuberculosis may involve the orbit commonly in children presenting with headache, epistaxis, decreased vision, epiphora, proptosis, eyelid swelling, periorbital swelling, chemosis, Marcus Gunn pupil, and visual field abnormalities. Orbital TB may also cause soft tissue tuberculoma, cold abscess, orbital periostitis, bony destruction, extraocular muscle involvement and orbital apex syndrome.

Intraocular Tuberculosis

- *Anterior uveitis:* Tubercular anterior uveitis may present as acute nongranulomatous iridocyclitis, but is usually as granulomatous anterior uveitis which may in turn be in form of miliary tubercular iritis conglomerate granuloma. Features of iris granulomas include mutton fat keratic precipitates, Koeppe and Busacca nodules, broad based posterior synechiae or complicated cataract.
- *Intermediate uveitis:* Presentation is usually with unilateral or bilateral pars planitis characterized by mild to moderate vitritis with snowballs, snow banking, peripheral vascular sheathing, peripheral retinochoroidal granuloma and cystoid macular edema.
- *Posterior uveitis or choroidal tuberculosis:* Posterior uveitis is the most common presentation of ocular tuberculosis and usually results from hematogenous dissemination. It may occur as a solitary tubercle, multiple miliary choroidal tubercles, multifocal choroiditis, diffuse choroiditis in chronic disease, tuberculoma, tubercular subretinal abscess or rarely as a large solitary granuloma and are due to direct infection of mycobacteria. Choroidal tubercles appear as round, yellow-while nodules, about one-sixth to two half disc diameter found in the posterior pole. Multifocal choroiditis may progress to diffuse, contiguous choroiditis. Ocular tuberculosis can also cause serpiginous-like lesion that spares the fovea leading to vitreal inflammation. Choroiditis and tuberculoma may be associated with choroidal neovascular membrane.
- *Retinal tuberculosis:* Retinal involvement in tuberculosis is secondary to choroidal disease and rarely from hematogenous spread. Tubercular lesions of retina include focal tubercle or retinitis, diffuse retinitis and subretinal abscess. Occlusive retinal vasculitis or Eales' disease result from hypersensitive reaction to tuberculoprotein. It is characterized by retinal periphlebitis and capillary non-perfusion that result in hypoxia which leads to neovascularization either on retinal surface or on optic nerve head. These vessels are very fragile and tend to bleed into vitreous. Intraocular TB can cause exudative retinal hemorrhagic periphlebitis with uveitis.
- *Endophthalmitis and panophthalmitis:* These may ensue following rupture of tubercular subretinal abscess into the vitreous cavity. TB endophthalmitis can be sight threatening if there is delay in diagnosis and treatment.

- *Cranial nerves:* Optic neuropathy may result from direct infection of tubercular bacilli or as a hypersensitive to the infectious agent or due to secondary disease. They present as papillitis, papilledema, neuroretinitis, optic nerve tubercle and neuroretinitis. TB meningitis can involve cranial nerves, particularly abducens nerves. Tuberculosis can cause third, fourth, or sixth cranial nerve palsies.

Management of Ocular Tuberculosis

Diagnosis

- *Tuberculin skin test (Mantoux test):* This test is useful in the diagnosis of latent TB and is performed by intradermal injection of purified protein derivative of *Mycobacterium tuberculosis.*
    - *Positive result* is characterized by development of an induration of 10–14 mm within 48 hours.
    - Negative result is implicated when the induration is <5 mm and excludes TB, but may occur in advanced disease.
    - *Weakly positive result* does not distinguish between active disease and prior exposure as most individuals have received BCG vaccination leading to a hypersensitive response.
    - *Strongly positive result* shows an induration >15 mm indicates an active disease.
- *Sputum examination:* Sputum examination for acid-fast bacilli using Ziehl–Neelsen stain is diagnostic
- Chest X-ray
- Interferon-Gamma release assay
- Culture

Treatment

- Ocular tuberculosis is treated according to the guidelines for treatment of pulmonary and extrapulmonary tuberculosis with standard anti-tubercular treatment (ATT) of 6 months.
    - *First 8 weeks:* rifampicin, isoniazid, ethambutol and pyrazinamide. Ethambutol may be replaced with fluoroquinolone like moxifloxacin or levofloxacin.
    - *Next 18 weeks:* Rifampicin and isoniazid
- Drug resistant cases are treated with alternate regimen based on culture report.
- *Corticosteroids:*
    - Topical or oral corticosteroids may be used to control inflammation and tapered over 6–12 weeks.
    - Intravitreal steroids may be used in management of ocular tuberculosis
- *Immunosuppressive therapy:* This may be used in conjunction with ATT or corticosteroid to treat ocular tuberculosis.

5. Ocular manifestation of mucormycosis. (10) (DNB 2021)

Mucormycosis also called Rhino-orbito-cerebral mucormycosis (ROCM) is caused by filamentous fungi of family Mucoraceae.

It causes opportunist infection in patients with severe weakening of both innate and humoral immunity.

Route of Spread

- The fungal invasion occurs through the nasal mucosa into the paranasal sinuses such as maxillary and ethmoid sinuses.
- From the sinuses it enters into the orbit by eroding the medial orbital wall.
- Inside the orbit, it rapidly involves the orbital apex leading to complete ophthalmoplegia, ptosis and vision loss.
- From the orbital apex, it reaches the brain causing ischemic necrosis of brain parenchyma leading to severe debilitation and death.

Risk Factors

- Diabetes
- Any prior organ transplantation
- HIV infection
- Neutropenia
- Immunosuppressant therapy
- IV drug users

Spectrum of Clinical Presentation from High to Low Incidence

- Ptosis
- Proptosis
- Complete ophthalmoplegia
- Cellulitis
- Central retinal artery occlusion (CRAO)
- Disc edema
- Optic atrophy
- Necrosis of adnexal tissue
- Dentopalatal involvement

Systemic features include fever and malaise.

Symptoms

- Sinusitis-inflammation of the paranasal sinuses
- Nasal discharge
- Nasal bleeding
- Hallmark–blackish eschar over the skin of nasal mucosa, palate and orbit

Signs

- *Eyelids:*
  - Ptosis-drooping of the eyelid due to 3rd cranial nerve involvement
  - Proptosis secondary to periorbital edema or orbital cellulitis
  - Swelling of the eyelids secondary to inflammation
  - Eyelid gangrene
- *Orbit and ocular adnexa:*
  - Sinusitis-inflammation of the paranasal sinuses
  - Periocular edema-inflammatory edema in the periorbital space
  - Orbital cellulitis
  - Orbital compartment
- *Lacrimal system:* Presents with epiphora due to inflammation of the conjunctiva.
- *Conjunctiva:*
  - Acute conjunctivitis-presenting with redness, ocular irritation, tearing with mucoid discharge, congestion, and chemosis.
  - Keratoconjunctivitis-conjunctival injection, follicles on the palpebral conjunctiva, transient pseudodendritic lesions on the cornea with subepithelial infiltrates.
  - Hemorrhagic conjunctivitis
  - Pseudomembrane formation seen after admission in intensive care unit.
- *Sclera/episcleral:*
  - Unilateral and nodular episcleritis may be seen at the start of symptoms.
  - Necrotizing anterior scleritis can occur as late as 3 weeks after infection.
- Anterior chamber may have cells and flare in cases of anterior uveitis.
- *Retina and choroid:*
  - Exudative RD secondary to inflammation
  - CRAO/CRVO-these occur due to complement induced prothrombotic and inflammatory state resulting in endothelial injury.
  - Acute macular neuro retinopathy/paracentral acute middle maculopathy-due to ischemia in the deep retinal capillary plexus.
- Optic nerve gets affected due to direct neuronal invasion, endothelial dysfunction, or an inflammatory reaction.
  - Optic neuritis cases present with vision loss, RAPD, pain with eye movement, and optic disc edema.

- Neuromyelitis optica
- Papilledema can occur due to raised intracranial pressure due to cerebral sinus thrombosis.

- Extraocular motility due to involvement of cranial nerves 3, 4 and 6. Ocular cranial neuropathies may be associated with diplopia. Ocular myasthenia gravis is a postinfectious complication due to the cross reaction of the acetylcholine receptors with the antibodies targeting SARS-CoV-2 protein in COVID-associated mucormycosis. This can be managed with immunoglobulins and pyridostigmine.
- *Pupils:*
    - Mydriasis
    - Tonic pupils due to cholinergic supersensitivity
- *Nystagmus presents with:*
    - Oscillopsia
    - Central vestibular nystagmus with nausea and vomiting
- *Visual cortex:* Homonymous visual field defect due to bilateral posterior cerebral artery involvement.

Diagnosis

- Direct visualization of the nasal mucosa show blackish necrotic tissue.
- *Imaging of the sinuses will guide in diagnosis:*
    - Contrast-enhanced CT scan of the orbits and paranasal sinuses show hypodense soft tissue thickening of the involved sinuses.
    - In MRI, there is T2 isointense or hypointense soft tissue thickening with heterogeneous post-contrast enhancement.
    - Diffusion-weighted images show increased intensity in the affected areas.
- *Biopsy:* The signs and symptoms of mucormycosis are nonspecific, hence direct histopathological examination of scrapings and tissues are diagnostic. The specimen are stained with:
    - Calcofluor white
    - Periodic acid–Schiff
    - Grocott-Gomori methenamine silver stains showing broad, irregular, nonseptated hyphae branching at right angles are pathognomonic.

Management

General measures:

- To correct the underlying metabolic derangements such as diabetes and ketoacidosis.
- The dose of preexisting corticosteroids should be tapered
- The dose of preexisting immunosuppressives should be reduced.

Medical treatment: The mainstay of therapy is intravenous antifungals, lipid-soluble amphotericin-B at dose of 5–7 mg/kg/day.

- Second-line of treatment–posaconazole
- Use of transcutaneous retrobulbar amphotericin B injections (5 mL of 1 mg/mL daily for 7 days) can be used in addition to intravenous therapy

Surgical:

- Early surgical debridement of the involved tissue must be undertaken in cases of extensive tissue necrosis.
- Debridement must be done till fresh bleeding occurs is the accepted norm as there is no clear guideline to the extent of debridement.
- Intraoperative frozen sections can also be used.

Complications of Mucormycosis

- Cavernous sinus thrombosis
- Carotid artery obstruction

- CNS infarction secondary to mycotic intravascular thrombosis, presenting with hemiparesis, hemiplegia, coma and death.
- CNS inflammation, hemorrhage, and abscess
- Blindness
- Airway obstruction from head and neck infections

6. Ocular manifestation of sarcoidosis. (10) (DNB 2023)

Sarcoidosis is a multisystem granulomatous disorder of unknown etiology. It primarily involves:

- Lungs
- Lymph nodes
- Skin
- Eyes
- CNS
- Bones and joint
- Liver
- Heart

Prevalence

- Ocular involvement is seen in 50% of patients with systemic disease
- It accounts for 10% of all cases of uveitis.

Ocular manifestations involve:

- *Intraocular features:*
  - Uveitis presenting as anterior, intermediate, posterior involvement, or panuveitis
  - Bilateral anterior uveitis presenting with pain, redness, and photophobia
  - Granulomatous keratic precipitates
  - Iris nodules
  - Anterior/posterior synechiae
  - Intermediate uveitis–blurry vision and floaters, snowballs, and snow banking
  - Posterior uveitis—bilateral or asymmetric
  - Choroidal granulomas
  - Periphlebitis
  - Candle wax drippings—scattered whitish perivascular exudates along the retinal veins.
- *Ocular surface manifestations:*
  - Acute follicular conjunctivitis
  - Conjunctival nodules
  - Chronic cicatricial conjunctivitis
  - Scleritis (non-necrotizing) is rare, mostly in older age groups
  - Corneal involvement–keratoconjunctivitis sicca
  - Superficial punctate keratitis
  - Interstitial keratitis
  - Peripheral ulcerative keratitis
  - Calcific band keratopathy
- *Adnexal and orbital manifestations:*
  - Lacrimal gland inflammation
  - Epiphora
  - Cicatricial entropion
  - Eyelid swelling
  - May present with ptosis, proptosis, and pain

- Neuro-ophthalmic manifestations:
    - Cranial nerve involvement—commonly facial and optic nerves
    - Neuro sarcoidosis presenting with papilledema, nystagmus, and visual field defects

Revised International Workshop on Ocular Sarcoidosis (IWOS) Criteria for the Diagnosis of Ocular Sarcoidosis (OS)-2017

I. *Other causes of granulomatous uveitis must be ruled out.*

II. *Intraocular clinical signs suggestive of OS:*
- Mutton-fat keratic precipitates (KPs) (large and small) and/or iris nodules at pupillary margin (Koeppe) or in stroma (Busacca).
- Trabecular mesh work nodules and/or tent-shaped peripheral anterior synechiae.
- Snowballs/string of pearls vitreous opacities.
- Multiple chorioretinal peripheral lesions (active and atrophic).
- Nodular and/or segmental periphlebitis (candle wax drippings) and/or macroaneurysm in an inflamed eye.
- Optic disc nodule(s)/granuloma(s) and/or solitary choroidal nodule.
- Bilaterality (assessed by ophthalmological examination including ocular imaging showing subclinical inflammation).

III. *Systemic investigation results in suspected OS:*
- Bilateral hilar lymphadenopathy (BHL) by chest X-ray and/or chest computed CT scan.
- Negative tuberculin test or interferon-gamma releasing assays.
- Elevated serum angiotensin-converting enzyme (ACE).
- Elevated serum lysozyme.
- Elevated CD4/CD8 ratio (>3.5) in bronchoalveolar lavage fluid.
- Abnormal accumulation of gallium-67 scintigraphy or 18F-fluorodeoxyglucose positron emission tomography imaging.
- Lymphopenia
- Parenchymal lung changes consistent with sarcoidosis, as determined by pulmonologists or radiologists.

IV. *Diagnostic criteria:*
- *Definite OS:* Diagnosis confirmed by biopsy with compatible uveitis.
- *Presumed OS:* Diagnosis not confirmed by biopsy, but BHL present with two intraocular signs.
- *Probable OS:* Diagnosis not confirmed by biopsy and BHL absent, but three intraocular signs and two systemic investigations selected from two to eight are present.

Complications of chronic uveitis:
- Cataract formation
- Glaucoma
- Cystoid macular edema

Complications of orbital masses secondary to sarcoidosis can lead to CRAO and permanent blindness.

Diagnosis

1. *Clinical assessment:*
    - History and physical examination—essential for understanding the patients' symptoms and identifying potential signs of the disease.
    - Exclusion of other diseases—ruling out conditions such as tuberculosis and syphilis, which also cause granulomas.
2. *Imaging:*
    - Chest X-ray—common screening tool for pulmonary involvement.
    - CT scan—more sensitive than X-ray but typically reserved for cases with high suspicion and negative X-ray findings.

3. *Laboratory tests:*
    - Serum ACE may be elevated in some cases
    - Calcium levels can be raised
    - ESR may be raised as a marker of inflammation
4. *Tissue biopsy:* Considered the gold standard for diagnosis, allowing for histopathological examination of affected tissues to confirm the presence of granulomas.
5. Ocular sarcoidosis IWOS criteria

Management

- Uveitis is the most common manifestation of sarcoidosis.
- Corticosteroids are the cornerstone of treatment for both ocular and systemic sarcoidosis.
- The choice of steroid delivery (topical, regional, and systemic) depends on the severity and location of the ocular inflammation.
- Immunosuppressive agents are considered when steroids are ineffective or have significant side effects.
- Biologic agents like TNF-α inhibitors are promising options for severe and refractory cases.
- Treatment of manifestations of conjunctivitis, scleritis, and orbital involvement requires a tailored approach based on specific presentation.
- *Patient education:* They should be informed about their condition, treatment options, and the need for regular eye examinations.

7. Ocular manifestation of neurofibromatosis. (10) (DNB 2023, 2024)

Neurofibromatosis is a neurocutaneous syndrome which affects organs originating from the ectoderm. It mainly affects:

- Central nervous system
- Eyes
- Skin

Neurofibromatosis is of two types:

1. *Neurofibromatosis type 1:* Due to mutation in *NF1* gene, in chromosome 17q. This gene codes for the protein neurofibromin, which is highly expressed in the peripheral nervous system. Hence, peripheral nerve sheath tumors and gliomas are more common.
2. *Neurofibromatosis type 2:* Due to mutation in *NF2* gene in chromosome 22q. This gene codes for protein merlin which regulates various mitogenic signaling pathways.

Common clinical features of NF1:

- Plexiform neurofibromas—benign peripheral nerve sheath tumors arising on or underneath the skin
- Café au lait spots—hyperpigmented macules in different parts of the body
- Freckles—these are hyperpigmented areas in the axillary and inguinal regions
- Sphenoid wing dysplasia

Ocular features are more commonly seen in NF1:

- Lisch nodules in the iris—(<1-2 mm) small pigmented hamartomas (pathognomonic)
- Optic nerve gliomas
- Glaucoma

Clinical features of NF2:

- Bilateral acoustic neuromas
- Seizures
- Spinal and cerebral tumors like meningiomas or ependymomas

Ocular features of NF2:

- Early onset bilateral cataract.

- Optic nerve sheath meningiomas
- Hamartomas of retina and RPE
- Strabismus
- Amblyopia
- Extra-ocular movement abnormalities

The criteria to diagnose NF1 and NF2 are mentioned in **Tables 1 and 2** respectively.

TABLE 1: Diagnosis of NF1.

Must have ≥ 2 of the following:
1. ≥6 café au lait macules >5 mm in prepubertal, 15 mm in postpubertal patients
2. ≥2 neurofibromas of any type or 1 plexiform neurofibroma
3. Freckling in the inguinal or axillary region
4. ≥2 Lisch nodules
5. Optic glioma
6. Osseous lesion-sphenoid wing dysplasia, thinning of long bone cortex
7. Family history of NF in first-degree relative

TABLE 2: Diagnosis of NF2.

Must have any 1 of the following:
1. Bilateral vestibular schwannoma before age 70 years
2. Unilateral vestibular schwannoma before 70 and first-degree relative with NF2
3. Any 2 of these: Nonvestibular schwannoma, meningioma, neurofibroma, glioma, cerebral calcification, cataract and either: - First-degree relative with NF2 or - Unilateral vestibular schwannoma and negative LZTR1 testing
4. 4 multiple meningiomas and - U/L vestibular schwannoma or - Any 2 of the following: Nonvestibular schwannoma, meningioma, neurofibroma, glioma, cerebral calcification, and cataract
5. Constitutional or pathogenic NF2 mutation from blood or by identification of similar mutation from 2 distinct tumors in the same individual.

- Apart from clinical testing, genetic testing may be needed to diagnose neurofibromatosis. This is required in those who lack a positive family history or bilateral vestibular schwannoma are present.
- Detailed imaging of the brain and spina cord is necessary for diagnosing schwannomas on the peripheral nerves.

Management

- Regular eye examinations—annual ophthalmologic evaluation is critical for early detection and management
- Imaging—MRI for optic pathway glioma and orbital tumors
- Multidisciplinary approach—collaboration with neurology, oncology, and geneticist for systemic management
- Intervention—surgery or chemotherapy or radiotherapy for optic pathway gliomas if symptomatic
- Cataract surgery for visually significant lens changes
- Removal of neurofibromas can also be tried if they cause significant disfiguration or impair quality of life

8. Ocular manifestations of Hansen's disease. How will you manage a case of eyelid involvement in leprosy? (10) (WBUHS MS 2024, 2022)

Leprosy (Hansen's disease) is a multisystem bacterial disease caused by *Mycobacterium leprae*. It primarily affects the skin, peripheral nerves causing chronic granulomatous inflammation.

Ocular involvement in leprosy is around 70–75%, with 10–15% patients suffering from severe ocular symptoms and 5% patients progressing to blindness.

Pathology

The range of clinical manifestations in leprosy depends on the immune status of the individual. It ranges from:

- Tuberculoid type—in this type, patients suffer from cellular immune response to the *Mycobacterium* having few lesions on the skin and nerve trunks.
- Borderline
- Lepromatous type—here there is no specific immune response to the bacteria, hence it proliferates. There are multiple skin and nerve trunk lesions with the presence of systemic signs.

  Acute immune complications can occur before or after treatment with antibiotics. These are known as lepra reaction. It is of two types:

  1. Type 1 lepra reaction—characterized by sudden painful loss of nerve function. This is due to delayed hypersensitivity.
  2. Type 2 lepra reaction—characterized by erythema nodosum leprosum, which are deposition of immune complex in skin and organs. These are painful and are seen in borderline lepromatous and lepromatous leprosy.

  Ocular pathogenesis of leprosy:

  - *M. leprae* mostly invades the anterior segment of the eye.
  - The entry into the eye occurs through the blood vessels of the ciliary body and then enters the iris.

Ocular clinical features:

- *Eyelid:*
  - Madarosis—loss of eyebrows and eyelashes. This occurs due to direct involvement of the hair follicles by *M. leprae* with subsequent atrophy.
  - Ectropion
  - Entropion
  - Trichiasis
  - Blepharochalasis
  - Lagophthalmos
  - Reduced blinking
  - Eyelid nodules
- *Conjunctiva:*
  - Conjunctivitis is caused by *M. leprae* eye infection
  - Conjunctival scarring
  - Pterygium
  - Conjunctival crystalline deposits are side effects of consuming clofazimine
- *Cornea:*
  - Thickened corneal nerves
  - Superficial stromal keratitis
  - Corneal anesthesia
  - Exposure keratopathy
  - Interstitial keratitis
  - Band shaped keratopathy
  - Corneal leproma
- *Iris:*
  - Acute iritis—synechiae, seclusion pupillae, and secondary glaucoma. These are commonly seen in multibacillary leprosy.
  - Chronic iritis—iris pearls, iris atrophy, miosis, corectopia, and polycoria
  - Iris leproma
- *Ciliary body:*
  - Loss of accommodation

    - Hypotonia (low intraocular pressure)—this occurs due to destruction of the ciliary body
    - Phthisis
- *Sclera:*
    - Episcleritis
    - Scleritis
    - Nodules
    - Staphyloma
- *Lens:* Cataract
- Glaucoma is an uncommon complication which can happen.
- *Posterior segment:*
    - Retinal vasculitis
    - Papillitis
    - Peripheral choroidal lesions
- *Lacrimal system:*
    - Acute dacryocystitis
    - Chronic dacryocystitis

Diagnosis is made clinically:
- Presence of hypopigmented skin lesions with loss of sensation
- With or without the presence of thickened peripheral nerves
- Presence of acid-fast bacilli on skin smears and biopsy samples

Based on skin smears:
- Patients with skin smear negative on all sites are called paucibacillary leprosy.
- Patients with at least 1 positive skin smear are called multibacillary leprosy

Based on number of skin lesions:
- Paucibacillary—lesions are 1–5 in number
- Multibacillary—more than five lesions

Management

Treatment is mainly pharmacological with oral antibiotics. It requires multidrug therapy with the duration depending on whether it is pauci- or multi-bacillary.

First-line drugs—rifampicin, dapsone, and clofazimine

WHO recommendations for leprosy:
- Multibacillary leprosy—standard regimen has 12 months duration
    - Rifampicin 600 mg once a month
    - Dapsone 100 mg daily
    - Clofazimine 300 mg once a month
- Paucibacillary leprosy—standard regimen of 6 months
    - Rifampicin 600 mg once a month
    - Dapsone 100 mg daily
- If only one skin lesion present:
    - Rifampicin 600 mg
    - Ofloxacin 400 mg
    - Minocycline 100 mg

Treatment of uveitis in leprosy requires topical and oral corticosteroids.

The risk factors of severe visual impairment in leprosy include:
- Multibacillary disease
- Active disease for 10 years or more
- Lepra reaction type 2
- Lagophthalmos
- Corneal hypoesthesia or anesthesia
- Scleritis
- One eyed patient
- Facial skin lesion
- Coexisting conditions like diabetes or glaucoma

Management of eyelid involvement in leprosy:
- Ectropion correction—surgical correction of everted eyelid margin.
- Entropion correction—surgical procedure correcting inversion of eyelids.
- Lateral canthoplasty—a procedure which reduces sagging of the eyelids.
- *Lagophthalmos:*
  - Tarsorrhaphy—a reversible procedure which reduces the opening of eyelids by suturing them together.
  - Static eyelid slings are considered in patients with lower corneal changes. The orbital fissure is permanently narrowed.
  - Somerset's operation is the procedure of running silk/nylon suture round the lid margins. It has higher chances of infection.
  - Temporalis transfer is the procedure of passing a strip from temporalis muscle through the eyelid and connecting it to the inner canthus.

SUGGESTED READING

1. www.eyewiki.org.
2. Gervasio KA, Peck TJ, Fathy CA, Sivalingam MD, Friedberg MA. The Wills Eye Manual: Office and Emergency Room Diagnosis and Treatment of Eye Disease, 8th Edition. Philadelphia: Lippincott Williams & Wilkins; 2021.
3. Salmon JF. Kanski's Clinical Ophthalmology: A Systematic Approach, 9th edition. Amsterdam: Elsevier; 2019.
4. Sen HN, et al. 2020-2021 Basic and Clinical Science Course (BCSC), Section 09: Uveitis and Ocular Inflammation. San Francisco, California: American Academy of Ophthalmology; 2020.

CHAPTER

Miscellaneous

Smiti Rani Srivastava, Rituparna Ghosh, Rituparna Sarkar

QUESTIONS

1. **Sterilization in ophthalmology.** **(10) (DNB 2019)**
2. **Artificial intelligence in ophthalmology.** **(10) (MS WBUHS 2023)**
3. **Discuss about AS-OCT.** **(10) (WBUHS MS 2020)**
4. **What is amniotic membrane transplantation? Describe its role in ophthalmology.** **(4+6) (DNB 2022)**
   Mechanism of action amniotic membrane. **(4) (DNB 2023)**
5. **What is post-traumatic hyphema?** **(5) (DNB 2023) (DNB 2021)**
   Discuss etiopathogenesis and management of post-traumatic hyphema. **(5+5) (DNB 2023)**
6. **Define the term steroid responder. Various drugs which are used as an alternative to corticosteroids in different ophthalmological disorders.** **(2+8) (MS 2023)**
7. **What are the various types of tonometry? Describe the optics and sterilization of Goldmann tonometer. What are the sources of error and how to overcome?** **(3+4+3) (DNB 2021)**
8. **Discuss the role of gene therapy in ophthalmology.** **(10) (WBUHS MS 2024)**
9. **Discuss the role of nanotechnology in ophthalmology.** **(10) (WBUHS MS 2024)**

1. Sterilization in ophthalmology. (10) (DNB 2019)

Sterilization is defined as a process that eliminates all forms of microorganism including spores through various physical and chemical means.

Disinfection is the removal of pathogenic bacteria from objects in the environment to prevent diseases.

Sterilization is having aseptic surgical techniques that has a remarkable reduction in the incidence of postoperative infection in ophthalmology. The other terminologies to understand sterilization include:

- Asepsis—the state of being free from living pathogenic organisms
- Cleaning—removal of all contaminants by washing/scrubbing
- Sterile—anything which is free from living microorganism
- Sterilize—complete elimination of all living forms
- Sterilizer—equipment which sterilizes
- Fumigation—the process of disinfecting an area with chemical/gaseous fumes
- Biologic indicator—a preparation made of bacterial spores which is standardized for checking effective sterilizing conditions.
- Chemical indicator—these are agents or devices which are used to confirm one or more parameters required for satisfactory sterilization.

Sterilization in ophthalmology can be discussed under:

- OT sterilization

- Surveillance of OT sterilization
- Sterilization of instruments
- Surveillance of instrument sterilization

Operation theater layout: The operation theater must be planned in such a manner that it is away from noise, dust, crowd, with proper lighting and ventilation. It is divided into 4 zones:

1. *Protective zone:*
   - Changing room for doctors and OT staff
   - Storage and record maintenance
   - Storage rooms for keeping sterilized objects
   - Transferring passage for patients and materials
   - Pre- and postoperative area
2. *Clean zone:*
   - Storage room for equipment
   - Emergency exit
3. *Aseptic zone:*
   - Operating room
   - Scrub area
4. Disposal zone—for disposal of OT waste

Autoclave room:

- Located in a clean zone, away from operating room
- Room has exhaust fan to remove the excess moisture.

Operation theater:

- Minimum size should be 6.5 m × 6.5 m × 3.5 m
- Sliding doors are preferred to reduce the generation of air currents during surgery.
- The width of the OT doors should be 1.2–1.5 m.
- The length of operation table 1.8 m and operation trolley 0.9 m.
- Workspace of 1.2 m around the operation table and trolley.
- There should be no crowding, maximum of 5–7 people should be posted at a time.
- Parameters are given in **Table 1**.

TABLE 1: Parameters.

Parameter	*NABH standard*
Humidity	40–60%
Air exchange	20–30 cycles/h 10–20% fresh air changes/hour
Temperature (degree)	21 ± 3
Positive pressure (Psi)	2.5
Occupancy	5–8 persons
Area	260 square feet, height 10 feet
Air velocity (FPM)	25–35
Air movement	From clean to less clean areas
Equipment load (KW)	5–7

Modular operation theater is a concept that divides a system into smaller parts that can be created separately nd can be used to create a system, e.g., the parts of OT are manufactured in a company and brought to the build site for assembly.

OT sterilization:

Fumigation:

Fumigation kills microorganisms and prevents growth of microorganisms in air and surface. Formaldehyde used is prepared by boiling 40% formaldehyde or by adding potassium permanganate to it.

- For 10 × 10 × 10 feet room, 150 g of potassium permanganate is added to 280 mL of formaldehyde or 250 mL of formalin is added to 3,000 mL of tap water and put in auto mist for 2 hours with doors and windows closed, OT sealed overnight.

Fogging:

In this process, a chemical (N-alkyl-dimethyl-benzalkonium chloride) is dispelled using a fogger.

- All the OT appliances are covered.
- Fogger placed in one corner, diagonally at 45° angle.
- It is used for 20 minutes.
- Room sealed for 2 hours. After 2 hours the fogger is removed.

Other agents used:

- Bacillocid-containing (formaldehyde, glutaraldehyde, benzyl-C12-18-alkyldimethyl ammonium chloride)
- Bacillol-ethanol, 2-propanol and 1-propanol.

Heating, ventilation, and air conditioning:

- *Vertical:* In this type, air passes through HEPA filters from the ceiling downwards at 0.3 m/s. This system provides clean air for surgeries and minimizes infection though it requires costly maintenance.
- *Horizontal:* This type forms part of a wall. Adequate clean zone is not possible with this.

TABLE 2: Cleaning protocol of operation theater.

Cleaning schedule	*Cleaning protocol*
Daily cleaning of OT	Mopping floor, microscope, trolley and chairs
Weekly cleaning of OT	Cleaning of ceiling, AC filters, items on walls
Monthly cleaning of OT	All OT equipment is taken out and cleaned

*Daily cleaning protocol **(Table 2)**:*

- First the operating room is cleaned, then sterilization area and common corridor.
- Operating microscope head to be cleaned first with Bacillocid solution.
- Antiseptic solution is used to clean chairs, operating tables and trolleys and IV stands.
- Door handles to be cleaned separately.
- The floor to be mopped last using 2 bucket technique:
  - First bucket containing antiseptic solution
  - Second bucket containing warm water

Surveillance of OT sterilization—microbiological surveillance is done by 2 methods:

1. *Swab method:*
   - Done once a month
   - Swabs taken from 6 sites—walls, floor, OT table, trolley, microscope, AC filter
   - 1 control swab also taken.
2. *Air sampling is done to quantify the microbial count.*
   - Settle plate method
   - Slit sample method

Instrument sterilization

1. *Cleaning of instruments:*
   - Gloves to be worn before washing.
   - All instruments are washed under running tap water then rinsed using distilled water/RO water.

- Instruments cleaned using toothbrush and soaked in (Ortho-Phthalaldehyde) solution for 15 minutes.
- Then they are washed again with distilled water/RO water.

2. *Cleaning of cannulas:*
   - Using automated cleaners or manually flushed 3 times with distilled water and 3 times with air.
   - Dried using dryer or ambient air
   - Autoclaved
3. *Cleaning of tubing:*
   - Tubings are pressure dried to remove all particulate matter.
   - Tubings are then dried at room temperature.
   - Then subjected to ETO/autoclaved
4. *Moist heat sterilization:* The method is called autoclaving

   Autoclave
   - Works under the principle of steam under pressure
   - **Parameters used: 121°Celsius at pressure of 15 psi/775 mm Hg for 15–30 minutes.**
   - It is the most reliable method of sterilization
   - There is irreversible loss of microbial activity due to coagulation of proteins.

   Types of autoclaves:
   i. Pressure cooker type/laboratory bench autoclave—N type
   ii. Horizontal type
   iii. Gravity displacement type
   iv. Positive pressure displacement type
   v. Negative pressure displacement type
5. *Dry heat sterilization:*
   - In this process, heat is absorbed by the surface and transferred through the whole device till target temperature is reached.
   - Dry heat oxidizes molecules killing pathogens
   - E.g.: hot air oven, flaming, glass bead sterilizers
6. *Gaseous sterilization:*
   - Ethylene trioxide (ETO), an alkylating agent
   - Used for heat-sensitive materials like plastic tubings and fiber optics.
   - The objects must be completely dry before ETO.
7. *Plasma sterilization:*
   - Hydrogen peroxide is used.
   - Special polypropylene packaging is required.
   - Suitable for those which cannot withstand high temperature and moisture.
   - Expensive method.
8. *Irradiation using gamma rays, X-rays, and electron beams are used.*
   - *Advantages:* Heat-sensitive material can be sterilized.
   - Very quick effect
   - Reaches all parts of the object
   - Disadvantages: Carcinogenic
   - Process requires monitoring.
   - Special equipment is needed.
9. *Ultrasonic sterilization:*
   - Used for cleaning curved instruments
   - Works on the principle of sound waves
   - Bacteria disintegrate due to coagulation of proteins

Surveillance of instrument sterilization is done by monitoring 3 parameters:

1. Time
2. Temperature
3. Pressure

Type of indicator used:

- Chemical indicator
  - Helps distinguish between sterilized and unsterilized instruments
  - They have been divided into 6 classes **(Table 3)**

TABLE 3: Classes of clinical indicators.

Class	*Name*	*Use*
Class 1	Process indicator	E.g.: Autoclave tape used externally
Class 2	For specific tests	Bowie–Dick type tests checking sterilizer performance
Class 3	Single variable indicators	Designed to react to a single variable, e.g., time/temperature
Class 4	Multivariable	• Designed to react to 2/more variables • Used in ETO
Class 5	Integrating indicators	• Designed to react to all variables • Comparable to biological indicators
Class 6	Emulating indicators	Designed to react to all variables for specified sterilization cycle

- *Biological indicator:* This type of indicators directly helps confirm the sterility of autoclaved items. Heat-resistant bacterial spores are used.
  - Bacillus stearothermophilus for autoclave
  - Bacillus subtilis for ETO.

Hand hygiene—is the most important technique of reducing the risk of infections in OT.

- Watches and jewelry to be removed.
- Warm, RO water is used for handwashing.
- Hands and forearms to be washed 5 cm above the elbow.
- Antiseptic agents should be used while washing.
- Lathering should be done from the fingertips up to 5 cm above the elbow.
- Rubbing should be done for a minimum period of 3–5 minutes.

2. Artificial intelligence in ophthalmology. (10) (MS WBUHS 2023)

Definition

Artificial intelligence is a software that mimics cognitive functions such as learning and problem solving.

The term "artificial intelligence" (AI) was coined by John McCarthy at the Dartmouth conference in 1955. The simplified meaning of AI is to accomplish tasks using advanced computers with minimum human contribution. It aims to simulate human behavior.

Artificial intelligence is a broad term comprising of multiple components. The institute of Electrical and Electronics engineers (IEEE) divides AI into 3 fields.

1. Artificial neural networks (ANN), which are based on connectionist models, trying to function like the human brain.
2. Evolutionary algorithms which use bioinspired methods of optimization.
3. Fuzzy logic which uses the natural language in humans, modifying the classical logic.

Computational intelligence (CI) is the numerical representation of the knowledge compared to the symbolic representation of the AI.

Vapnik and Chervonenkis proposed models that could learn from data and were called Machine Learning (ML).

Advanced neural networks with the addition of layers to the ANN models were called Deep Learning (DL). It is currently the most popular method to solve problems in image processing.

AI in health is a subspecialty, which makes use of different methods and techniques to address different challenges in areas associated to health sciences. The expectations are as follows:

- Outperform doctors
- Help diagnose what is difficult to diagnose
- Help treat what is difficult to treat
- Identify on images what is difficult to identify
- Decrease misdiagnosis
- Decrease patient harm
- Reduce hospital admissions
- Reduce workflow inefficiency
- Increase medication adherence
- To predict and classify in medical science what has not been done so far.

Machine learning: It is defined as the area of study where the computers have the ability to extract relation and features of the data as a learning process without being programmed. The automatic analysis of the images in ophthalmology as a tool to predict the diagnosis has been a challenge in terms of using the best model with the lowest cost.

Types of learning models for ML: The algorithms used in ML are based on the type of learning used by them. Supervised and unsupervised learning are widely used with ocular imaging and videos while reinforcement learning is studied to perform ocular surgery.

- *Supervised learning:* Here, the algorithm is given inputs and outputs and has a function which finds a relationship between the input and the desired output.
- *Unsupervised learning:* The algorithm is given inputs and according to the similarity among them, it is clustered into N-groups.
- *Reinforcement learning:* The algorithm is given actions and states and it learns how to act in a given state.

Deep learning is a branch of ML that consists of a whole family of algorithms with a common feature: an architecture organized by hierarchical levels. DL works on the principle of deep neural networks modeled after the human brain which are used to recognize a pattern. DL learns the pointing features by itself in order to classify a disease or grade its severity, using the entire images with their clinical diagnosis.

Types of DL programs are:

- *Convolutional neural network (CNN):* For image-based diagnosis, a CNN algorithm self teaches by analyzing pixel or voxel intensities in a labeled training set of expert graded images and then provides an output at the top layer.
- M*assive-training artificial neural network (MT-ANN):* Here, the convolutional operations are carried on outside the network.

CNN and MT-ANN are structured like the human brain consisting of multiple interconnected layer of neurons designed to "THINK". An input is given into first layer whose output becomes the input for the next layer. The output from each layer is sent to the network until final outcome is formed.

Applications in ophthalmology:

- AI in diabetic retinopathy
    - *FDA-approved systems:* Several AI systems like IDx-DR, EyeArt, and AEYE-DS have received FDA approval for DR screening.
    - *High sensitivity and specificity:* These systems demonstrate high accuracy in detecting DR, often surpassing human clinicians in sensitivity.
    - AI can also assess the severity of DR and identify clinically significant macular edema.

- AI in retinopathy of prematurity:
  - *i-ROP DL system:* This AI tool can effectively distinguish features like "plus disease" in ROP, showing comparable or superior performance to expert diagnosis.
- AI in age-related macular degeneration:
  - *Differentiating AMD types:* AI can help differentiate between exudative and nonexudative AMD.
  - The development of AI for AMD screening faces unique challenges, which organizations like the CCOI group are actively addressing.
- *AI in glaucoma:* AI is revolutionizing the field of glaucoma diagnosis and management.
  - Deep learning algorithms have demonstrated impressive accuracy in detecting glaucomatous optic nerve changes.
  - AI systems analyze various diagnostic data like OCT images, color fundus photographs, VF test results, IOP and corneal thickness measurements.
  - AI is also being used to identify individuals at high risk for glaucoma, enabling earlier intervention and preventing vision loss.
- *AI in cataract:*
  - *Cataract detection and grading:* ML algorithms like ResNet can effectively identify the presence and severity of cataracts including congenital cataracts. Systems like CC-Cruiser can identify the location and density of cataract.
  - *Surgical planning and postoperative care:* ML models assist in planning cataract surgery by assessing the patient suitability and predicting the risk of complications like PCO.
  - *IOL power calculation:* ML methods like Hill-RBF formula can accurately calculate the power of intraocular lenses needed for cataract surgery by analyzing various eye measurements.
- *AI in oculoplasty:*
  - *Automated facial measurements:* AI, particularly schematic segmentation networks, can accurately measure facial dimensions from images. This can streamline pre- and postoperative assessments.
  - *Clinical decision support:* AI helps non-ophthalmologists in deciding whether to refer the patient for oculoplastic evaluation. This enhances the quality of referral.
  - AI can analyze patient progress after eyelid surgery, providing standardized evaluations.
- *AI in ocular oncology:*
  - *Predicting the course of periocular reconstruction:* A decision tree model was formed to predict surgical course for patients with basal cell carcinoma.
  - ANNs were used to analyze oncologic history to predict outcomes for patients with choroidal melanoma.
  - A multispectral imaging system was developed to detect ocular surface squamous neoplasia. It can identify the areas of neoplastic changes helping in decision making about treatment.
- *AI in pediatric ophthalmology:*
  - Timely ocular management in children is crucial for preserving vision.
  - AI-powered screening for various eye conditions like strabismus and high myopia.
  - AI-based strabismus assessment can be integrated into tele-ophthalmology, expanding access to care.
  - Different AI systems utilize DL, eye tracking and retinal birefringence scanning for diagnosing eye conditions.
  - The Van Eenwyk et al. system combines multiple imaging techniques (Bruckner pupil red reflex imaging and eccentric photorefraction) to detect amblyogenic features associated with strabismus and high refractive errors.

3. Discuss about AS-OCT. (10) (WBUHS MS 2020)

- It is a noninvasive imaging procedure which contributes both quantitative and qualitative reports about cornea, anterior chamber angle, iris, and lens.
- It also measures anterior chamber depth, anterior chamber angle, and corneal thickness.
- High-resolution multiple cross-sectioned images are taken to provide details of the anterior segment.

Principle:

- Michelson interferometer principle is followed in AS-OCT.

- It is based on the measurement of delay in light which is reflected from various anterior chamber structures.
- Low coherence infrared light is split by beam-splitter in Michelson interferometer.
- It has two components—where a movable mirror in the reference arm and the object of interest in sample arm.
- The two components are superimposed at interferometer.
- The strength of the signal reflects the depth of each scan.
- It has longer wavelength (1,310 nm).
- The anterior segment images are taken within 0.125 sec with 18 μm resolution.
- As posterior part of iris is pigmented, it prevents light penetration.

Characteristics:

1. Anterior segment spectral-domain OCT:
   - Spectralis SD-OCT captures high-resolution cornea, sclera and anterior chamber angle images.
   - Lateral scan have two patterns:
     1. Single
     2. Raster
   - It ranges from 8 to 16 nm.
   - It assesses:
     i. Thickness of cornea
     ii. Corneal opacities
     iii. Scar
     iv. Postkeratoplasty evaluation
     v. Lamellar keratopathies
     vi. Refractive surgeries
     vii. Detection of *acanthamoeba* disease
     viii. Cytomegalovirus-associated keratitis
   - It also assesses—scleral and conjunctival neoplasia, i.e., OSSN.
   - Post-glaucoma surgery with filtering bleb
2. *Anterior segment swept source OCT (SS-OCT):*
   - At a high speed, the AS-OCT (SS) sends 1,300 nm wavelength light which causes high-resolution images of anterior segment.
   - The detailed images of anterior segment are captured by AS-OCT.
   - The structures between anterior part of cornea to posterior part of lens and anterior chamber angle are registered to proceed for cataract surgery, glaucoma surgery and refractive surgeries.
   - The images of cornea are taken within 8 mm of corneal diameter.

Applications of AS-OCT:

- *Anterior chamber angle:* In primary angle closure, anterior chamber angle is an important measurement to treat as an angle closure. The angle opening distance and trabecular-iris-angle are the parameters of angle closure which help to evaluate angle closure. TIA is an angle which is formed by apex at the iris recess and an arm passes by the point on the trabecular meshwork 500 μm or 700 μm from the scleral spur to the opposite point in iris perpendicularly. Anterior chamber depth and anterior chamber volume are prime parameters to diagnose primary angle closure.
- *Filtering bleb in post-trabeculectomy eye:* The formation of bleb after trabeculectomy is determined by AS-OCT. As it is a non-contact procedure, it can study the healing and remodeling process of bleb. The images of diffuse to flat blebs are captured by AS-OCT and the function of bleb is determined by slit lamp appearance. The bleb wall structure is recognized by SD-OCT but the internal ostium or flap could not be determined by bleb wall.
- Glaucoma drainage devices are monitored by AS-OCT. The position, patency, and course of drainage tubes are computed by AS-OCT.
- *Ocular surface squamous neoplasia:* It is an epithelial lesion which is determined by AS-OCT. It has 94% sensitivity and 100% specificity. It detects thickening of OSSN, hyper-reflective epithelial layer and transitional zone are well demarcated.

- *Conjunctival melanoma:* It is seen as hyper-reflective basal layer with hyper-reflective subepithelial lesion. Thickened hyper-reflective epithelium suggests atypical melanocytes.
- *Conjunctival lymphoma:* Conjunctival lymphoma is characterized by normal epithelium with hyporeflective subepithelial lesion which has smooth and discrete borders along with stippled monomorphic infiltrates.
- *Pterygium:* In AS-OCT, hyper-reflective areas are denoted between epithelium and Bowman's layer of cornea. High-resolution AS-OCT is important to differentiate between pterygium and OSSN. Epithelial layer is looked for OSSN and subepithelial layer is looked for pterygium in AS-OCT.
- *Conjunctival nevus:* Nevi show normal epithelium with well-circumscribed subepithelial lesion along with cysts.
- *Conjunctival amyloidosis:* In AS-OCT, it shows normal epithelium with homogenous, hyporeflective subepithelial lesion with irregular diffuse borders and hyper-reflective linear material.
- *Keratoconus:* AS-OCT shows changes in corneal microarchitecture and epithelial changes in early keratoconus and postoperative corneal ectasia. AS-OCT is a useful tool to find out the position and depth of intracorneal ring.
- *Corneal dystrophy:* Salzmann dystrophy shows hyper-reflectivity between anterior stroma and Bowman's layer.

    Band-shaped keratopathy shows hyper-reflective material at Bowman's layer with posterior shadowing.

    Thiel Behnke dystrophy shows hyper-reflective material as sawtooth pattern deposition present in Bowman's layer extends under the epithelium layer.
- *Infective keratitis:* Hyper-reflective material in corneal stroma which is an indicator of infective material. Corneal thinning, scarring, and the level of corneal opacities are denoted with AS-OCT.
- *Anterior segment surgery:* It is an important tool for DSEAK, DMEK, LASIK, and K-Pro before taking decision for anterior segment surgery.

Disadvantages:

- It cannot visualize the structures posterior to iris like ciliary body, zonules, and peripheral lens.
- Acute angle closure glaucoma and lens-induced glaucoma are nonvisible by AS-OCT. As it needs clear media, it does not show the angular structures.
- It is limited to cross-section of images.
- Only 20–30% sclera spur is seen.
- As it is a noncontact procedure, it cannot indent to show beyond the posterior structures.

4. What is amniotic membrane transplantation? Describe its role in ophthalmology. (4+6) (DNB 2022)

Mechanism of action amniotic membrane. (4) (DNB 2023)

Amniotic membrane transplantation (AMT): Amnion is the deeper layer of the placenta with a thick basement membrane and avascular structure. At sterile condition, it is collected from elective cesarean section. Donors are screened for any transmissible infections. After collection, AM is treated with broad spectrum of antibiotics. Epithelium, stroma, and basement membrane are three layers of AM. It acts like physical barrier which promotes healing of ocular surface disorder. It stimulates epithelial growth cell migration, adhesion and differentiation and inhibits apoptosis.

Role in ophthalmology:

- For reconstruction of ocular surface, AMT is helpful.
- In chemical injury, melting cornea is reformed by AMT as a graft.
- In persistent epithelial defects or ocular surface disorders, AMT is used to rejuvenate the cornea.
- Used to cover conjunctival defect in pterygium surgery.
- In infective or sterile ulcer, AMT is used to prevent ulcer.
- To prevent scarring over burnt area, AMT is used as a graft over periorbital area.
- Amnion-assisted conjunctival epithelial redirection procedure is used along with SLET to reduce the inflammation in limbal cell deficiency.
- In lid mass cases, AMG and mucosal graft is used to cover the defect after excision of lid mass.

- Recently AMT is used for macular hole surgery which shows complete closure of macular hole.
- In cases of repeat-trabeculectomy surgeries, the lost conjunctiva is replaced by AMG.
- In benign and malignant tumors of conjunctiva is excised and graft reposition is done with AMG.
- In adhered muscle or fibrosed muscle is repaired by AMG in strabismus cases.
- In symblepharon or cicatricial eyelid is repaired by AMG.

Mechanism of action of amniotic membrane:
- Basement layer of amniotic membrane has similar property like conjunctiva.
- It supports epithelial cells, limbal stem cells, and corneal transient amplifying cells.
- Further AM stimulates goblet cells and non-goblet cells differentiation and it inhibits the inflammatory cells and protease activities.
- It inhibits TGF-β signal transduction which has anti-scarring properties.
- It has inter-α-trypsin and hyaluronan/pentraxin-3(HC-HA/PTX-3) which promotes anti-angiogenic, anti-inflammatory, anti-scarring and anti-fibrotic factors.
- Lubricin acts as a lubricant to reduce inflammation and friction.
- Reduction of IL-6 and TNF-α level can be seen due to presence of IL-10.
- It secretes elafin and secretory leukocyte proteinase inhibitor which have antimicrobial activity.
- EGF, KGF, and neurotrophic factors cause healing, regeneration of corneal epithelium, and prevention of apoptosis.

5. What is post-traumatic hyphema? (5) (DNB 2023) (DNB 2021)

Discuss etiopathogenesis and management of post-traumatic hyphema. (5+5) (DNB 2023)

Introduction
- Collection of red blood cells within the anterior chamber is referred to as a hyphema.
  - Small amount of blood when it is evident only under microscope is called microhyphema.
  - Incidence: 0.52 in one lakh population.

Etiology
- Most common cause—blunt trauma
- Less common traumatic cause
  - Iatrogenic—more common with ACIOL causing secondary iris neovascularization
- Spontaneous:
  - Juvenile xanthogranuloma

Pathogenesis
- Compressive force during blunt trauma globe causes injury to the iris, ciliary body, trabecular meshwork, and their associated vasculature.
- Shearing forces lead to tear these vessels causes accumulation of red blood cells within the anterior chamber.

Clinical Features
Symptoms:
- Blurring of vision
- Pain
- Headache
- Photophobia
  - History
    - History of ocular trauma or surgery
    - Risk factors:
      - Bleeding diathesis or anticoagulant therapy
      - Sickle cell disease—higher risk of glaucoma

- Ocular examination:
  - *Visual acuity:* Daily evaluation to look for improvement
  - *IOP:* Daily monitoring
  - *Gonioscopy to be avoided for first 5 days:* High risk of rebleed due to undue pressure from gonioscopy. PAS or angle recession is noted.
  - Grading of hyphema is mentioned in **Figure 1**.

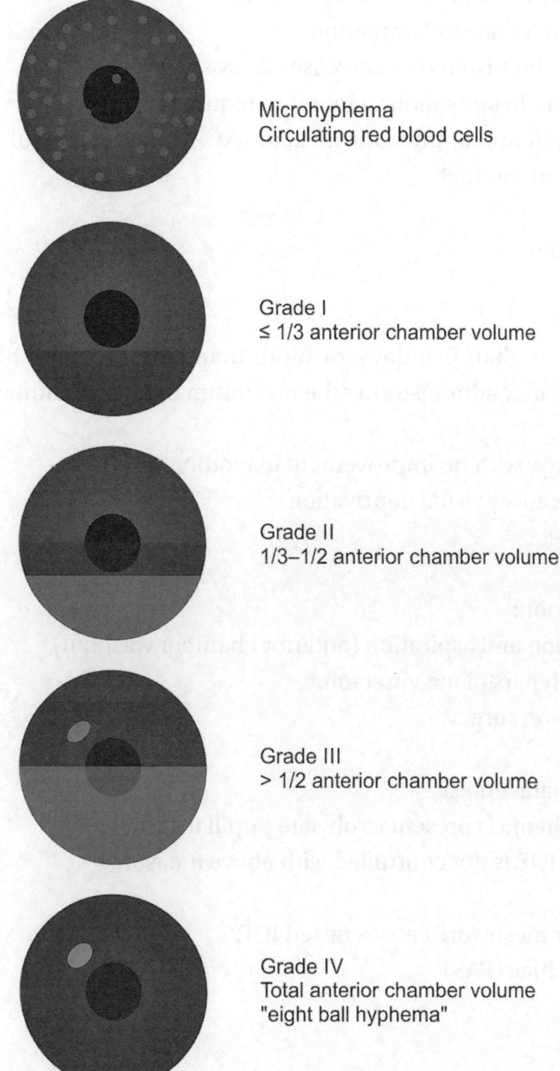

Fig. 1: Grading of hyphema. *(For Color version, See Color Plate 11)*

- Investigations:
  - B scan to look for concurrent vitreous hemorrhage or retinal detachment
  - Look for any sickle cell trait or sickle cell disease—confirmed by Hb electrophoresis
- Management:
  - *General measures:*
    - Observation for first week (highest risk of rebleeding)
    - Maintaining head elevation at 45°—helps to settle down hyphema inferior part of AC.
    - Pain control—avoid NSAIDs like aspirin—increased risk of rebleed

- The patient should stop taking all antiplatelet medications including aspirin as these drugs increase the risk of rebleeding in the eye due to their blood thinning properties.
- *Medical management:*
  - Isolated hyphema—topical medications suffice
  - Topical steroid to reduce inflammation and synechiae formation
  - Topical anti-glaucoma medications: Prefer beta-blockers or alpha-agonists
    - Avoid carbonic anhydrase inhibitors—favor sickling
    - Avoid PG analogs—exacerbate inflammation
  - Topical cycloplegics are administered to decrease ciliary spasm.
  - Systemic CA inhibitors and hyperosmotic agents are required.
  - Various studies show systemic aminocaproic acid (ACA) may be useful for secondary hemorrhages for fibrinolysis. It is rarely used routinely.
- *Surgical management:*
  - Often postponed till 5th day
  - Indications:
    - IOP not under control
      - ≥50 mm Hg for more than five days, or more than 25 mm Hg for >24 hours in patients with sickle hemoglobinopathy after administering the maximum medical treatment.
    - Persistent hyphema:
      - Lasting beyond 5 days with no improvement in grading
      - In younger patient causes visual deprivation.
    - Corneal blood staining
- *Methods*
  - Tickling the blood collection:
  - Anterior chamber irrigation and aspiration (anterior chamber washout)
  - Removal of hyphema with pars plana vitrectomy
  - Clot irrigation with filtration surgery
    - For controlling IOP:
      - Anterior chamber paracentesis
      - YAG PI (if total hyphema is present to obviate pupillary block)
      - Trabeculectomy: If IOP is not controlled with above measures
- Complications
  - Obstruction of trabecular meshwork causes raised IOP.
  - Peripheral anterior synechiae (PAS)
  - Posterior synechiae
  - Corneal bloodstaining
  - Rebleeding:
    - Risk factors:
      - Hypotony or elevated IOP
      - 50% or greater hyphema
      - Systemic hypertension
      - Use of aspirin
  - Mechanism:
    - When the initial clot retracts and lyses allowing for a second episode of bleeding.
    - More severe than the initial bleed, more likely to lead to glaucoma, corneal blood staining, and synechiae formation.

- Pupillary Block
  - Amblyopia (in pediatric individuals):

Prognosis: Early stages hyphema resolves with proper treatment. Hyphema along with complications leads to poor visual outcomes.

6. Define the term steroid responder. Various drugs which are used as an alternative to corticosteroids in different ophthalmological disorders. (2+8) (MS 2023)

The normal population can be divided into 3 groups on the basis of their IOP response to a 6 week course of topical steroids (dexamethasone).

1. High responders exhibit a marked elevation of IOP (>30 mm Hg)
2. Moderate responders display a moderate elevation of IOP (22–30 mm Hg)
3. Nonresponders manifest no change in IOP. There is a marked increase in myocilin production by the trabecular meshwork cells after treatment with dexamethasone but the exact mechanism which results in the rise of IOP is unclear. It has been seen that in a high or intermediate steroid responder, the strong steroids (dexamethasone, prednisolone, betamethasone) are potent in their ability to raise IOP, while fluorometholone has a lesser propensity to raise IOP. Fluorometholone raises IOP half as much as betamethasone.

Mechanism of action of steroid:

- Glucocorticoids have anti-inflammatory effects which bind with glucocorticoid receptor (GR) present in cytoplasm.
  - Corticosteroid–GR complex travels to nucleus which modulates genomic expression of proteins.
  - The corticosteroid–GR complex increases the release of anti-inflammatory mediators and suppresses the pro-inflammatory cell mediators.
- Elevated concentration of lipocortin is essential. Lipocortin inhibits phospholipase A2 and histamine synthesis in mast cells. Phospholipase A2 inhibition prevents the conversion of phospholipids to arachidonic acid which is important to induce inflammatory pathway.

Rest see conjunctiva.

7. What are the various types of tonometry? Describe the optics and sterilization of Goldmann tonometer. What are the sources of error and how to overcome? (3+4+3) (DNB 2021)

Classification of tonometry (Flowchart 1):

Types of tonometry:

- Indentation tonometry:
  - Indentation tonometry works on principle that plunger will indent a soft eye more than a hard eye, e.g., Schiotz tonometry
- Applanation tonometry:
  - Variable area and (fixed force) applanation tonometer. E.g., Goldmann applanation tonometry

Variable area fixed force tonometer:

Maklakov tonometer:

- Measures the area of cornea that is flattened by a known force
- Other variable area fixed force tonometer:
  - Applanation tonometer—ceramic end plates
  - Disposable end plates
  - Barraquer tonometer: Plastic tonometer used in operating rooms
  - Ocular tension indicator—uses Goldmann prisms and standard weight for screening
  - Test-screening tonometer with multiple end plates for selecting different pressure cut off.

Flowchart 1: Classification of tonometer.

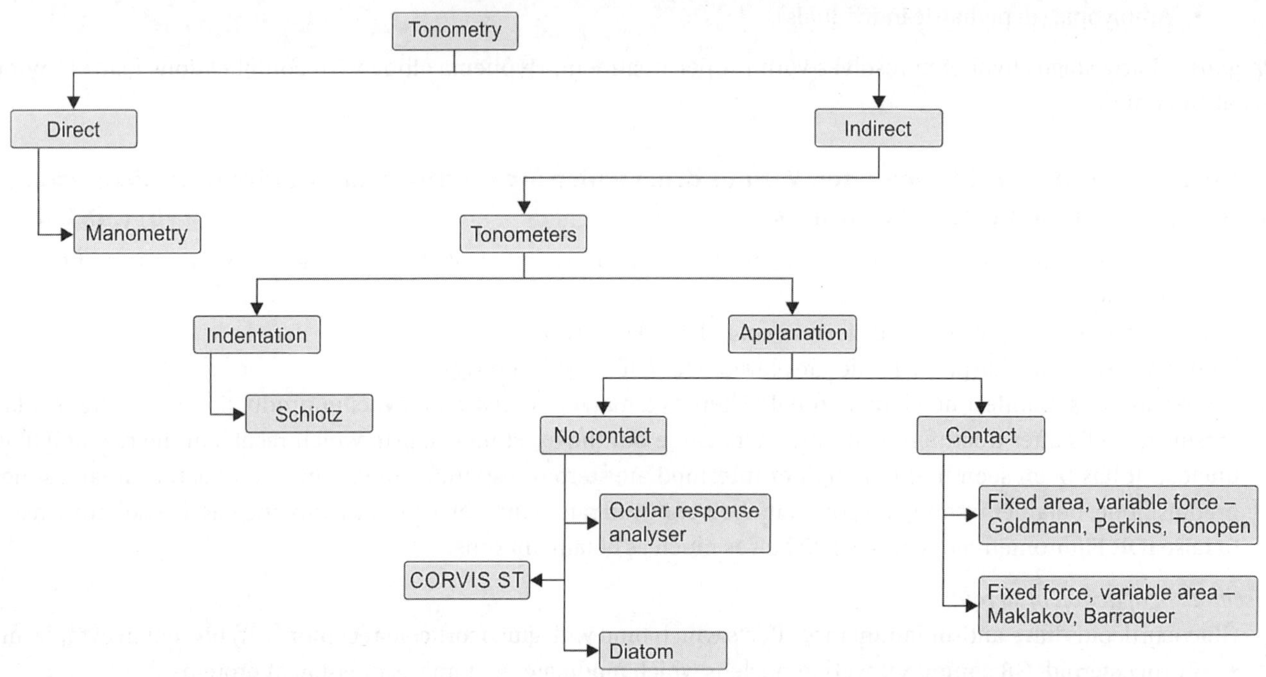

Variable force fixed area tonometer:

This type of tonometer measures the force that is required to applanate a standard area of corneal surface. The method of tonometry is far more accurate than indentation tonometry since in this technique a very tiny area of cornea is applanated so the ocular rigidity does not interfere with the readings.

a. *Goldmann applanation tonometer:* Described below
b. *Hand-held Goldmann type tonometer:*
   - *Perkins applanation:*
     - Hand-held tonometer uses the same biprism as in the Goldmann tonometer
     - Small, easy to carry and does not require slit lamp applanation tonometer.
     - Light source is powered by a battery and forces is varied manually.
   - *Draeger applanation:* Similar to Perkins tonometer but uses a different biprism and has an electric motor that varies the force.
c. *Air based tonometer:*

   Air puff tonometer:
   - It is a non-contact type of tonometer
   - Central part of cornea is flattened by a jet of air
   - Useful for mass screening.

   Pulse air tonometer—can be used for patients in any position.
d. *Mackay Marg tonometer:*
   - Principle:
     - The original Mackay Marg tonometer consisted of 1.5 mm plunger affixed to rigid spring that extends 10 microns beyond the plane of surrounding rubber sleeve. Movement of the plunger is electronically monitored by a transducer and recorded on a moving paper slip.
     - Interpretation:
       - At 1.5-mm area of corneal applanation, tracing reaches peak and the force applied equals to the IOP and the force required to deform the cornea.

- At 3-mm flattening force required to deform the cornea can be transferred from plunger to swooning sleeve creating a dip in tracing corresponding to IOP. Other Mackay Marg type tonometer-
  - *Tonopen:* Hand-held instrument with a stain gauge that creates an electrical signal as the foot plate flattens the cornea.
  - *Pneumometer:* In this, the cornea is applanated by touching its apex by a sialistic diaphragm covering sensory nozzle.

e. *Newer tonometer:*
- Pascal dynamic contour tonometer:
  - Working:
    - Uses miniature pressure sensors embedded within a tonometer tip contour matched to the shape of cornea.
    - Tip rests on the cornea with a constant appositional force of 1 g.
    - When the sensors are subjected to change in pressure the electrical resistance is altered and Pascal's computer calculates a change in pressure in concordance with change in resistance.
- Diatom transparalleled tonometer:
  - Based on processing the rod acceleration time resulting from its free fall constant height and interaction with the eye through the eyelid.
- Reichert's ocular response analyzer:
  - It measures corneal hysteresis.
- iCare rebound tonometer:
  - Consists of a pair of coil coaxial with the probe, shaft, solenoid coil and sensing coil.
  - A light-weighted probe is propelled towards the cornea by the solenoid and sensing coil monitors the movement.
- Smart lens:
  - It has a contact lens that incorporates an electric pressure sensor which is able to measure IOP and ocular pulse.
- Previewed pressure phosphene tonometer:
  - Self-monitoring device utilizes a psychophysical technique based on the phenomenon of pressure phosphene.

f. *Others (invasive type):*
- Implantable IOP sensors
- IOL IOP probe
- Contact lens sensor
- Choroid IOP sensor

Goldmann applanation tonometry:

Principle

Imbert-Fick law **(Fig. 2):**
- Not ideal in applying to cornea
- Surface should be perfectly spherical, dry, perfectly flexible, and infinitely thin to apply this principle.
- The cornea fails to satisfy any of these requirements.
- The moisture creates a surface tension (S), and the lack of flexibility requires a force to bend the cornea (B), which is independent of the internal pressure. In addition, because the cornea has a central thickness of approximately 550 μm, the outer area of flattening (A) is not the same as the inner area (A1).
- When A1 equals 7.35 mm^2, S balances B and W equal P_t.

Design/arrangement:
- Mounted on a standard slit lamp **(Fig. 3)**
  - Examiner's view is directed through the center of a plastic biprism, which is used to applanate the cornea.
- The biprism is attached by a rod to a housing, which contains a coil spring and series of levers that are used to adjust the force of the biprism against the cornea

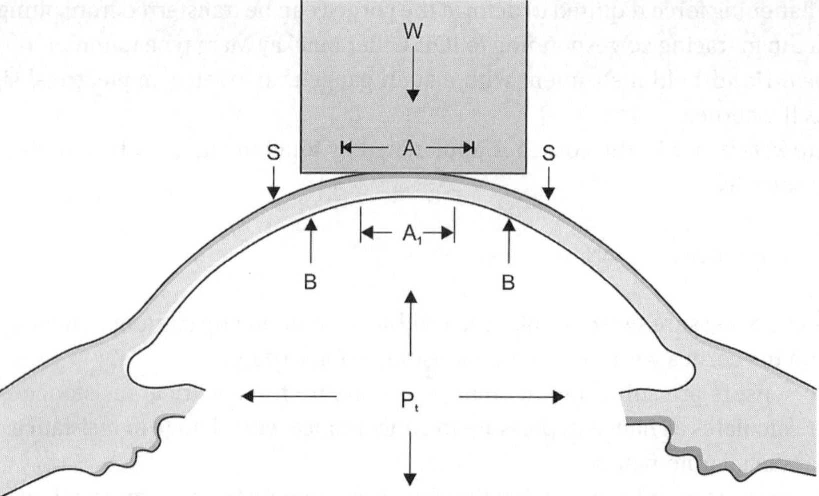

Fig. 2: Imbert–Fick principle.

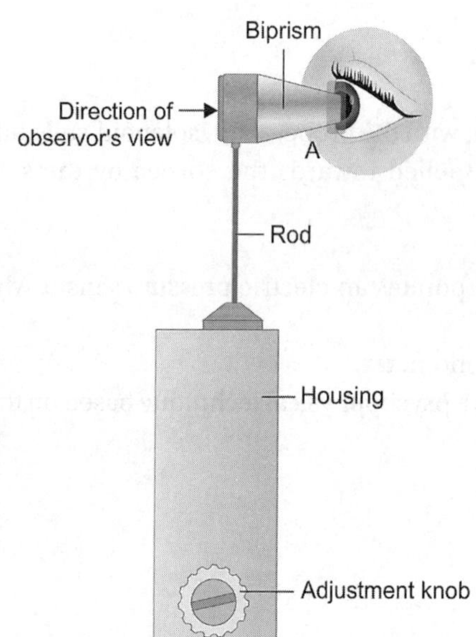

Fig. 3: The parts of applanation tonometer.

- Two beam-splitting prisms within the applanating unit split the circular area of corneal contact into semicircles.
  - Inner margins of the semicircles are made to overlap when 3.06 mm of cornea is applanated.

Technique:

- Topical anesthetic drops are used, and the tear film is stained with sodium fluorescein. Using a cobalt blue light from the slit-lamp, the biprism is brought into contact with the corneal apex.
- The **fluorescence of the stained tears** facilitates visualization of the tear meniscus at the margin of contact between cornea and biprism.
- Semicircles are viewed through the biprism, then force against the cornea is adjusted until the inner edges overlap **(Fig. 4)**.
- The influence of the ocular pulsations is seen when the instrument is properly positioned, and the excursions must be averaged to give the desired endpoint. The IOP is then read directly from a scale on the tonometer housing.

Sources of error:

- Quantity of fluorescein is important—the width of the semicircle meniscus influences the reading.

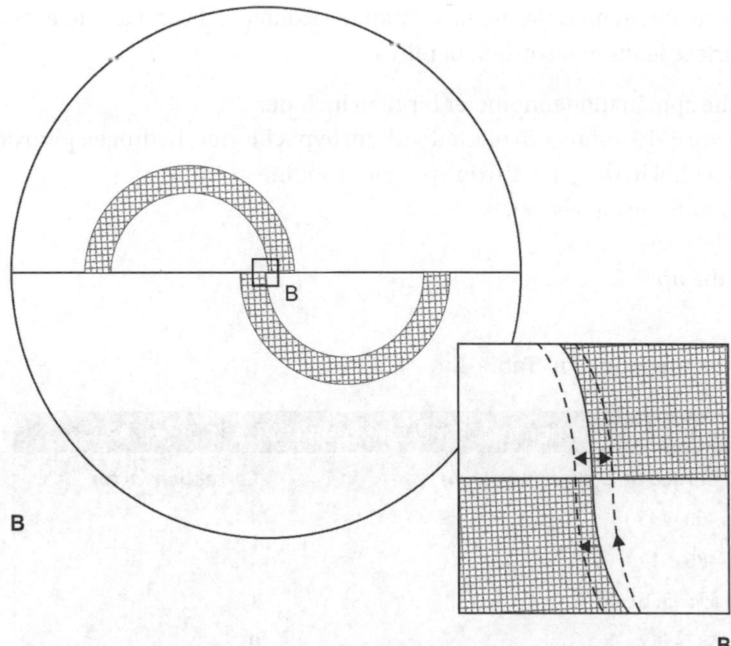

Fig. 4: The overlap of semicircular beams in AT.

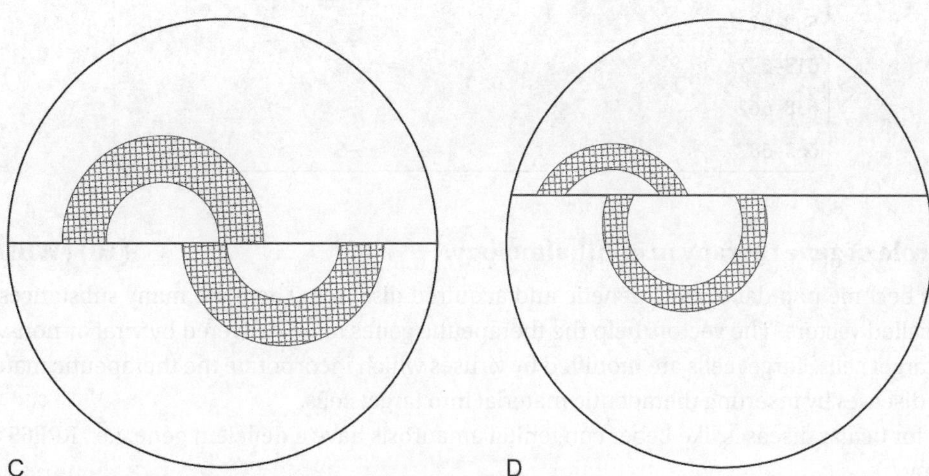

Fig. 5: Sources of error.

- Wider menisci falsely show (C) higher-pressure estimates **(Fig. 5)**.
- Improper vertical alignment (D) (one semicircle larger than the other) will also lead to a falsely high IOP estimate.

- Calculation for Goldmann applanation tonometry:
  - Presumed average CCT of 520 µm.
  - Falsely higher-pressure readings with thicker corneas and falsely lower ones with thinner corneas.
  - After refractive surgery (LASIK), thin cornea → Lower IOP
- Deviations of corneal curvature:
  - 1 mm Hg for every 3 diopters (D) of increase in corneal power (180).
  - IOP is underestimated for with the rule and overestimated for against the rule astigmatism, with approximately 1 mm Hg of error for every 4 D of astigmatism.
  - With the rule astigmatism underestimates while against the rule astigmatism overestimates the IOP. To minimize this, tonometer biprisms should be rotated so that axis of least corneal curvature is opposite the red mark on the biprism. This results in the separation of 43 and an applanation area of 7.35 mm^2.

- The other method is to obtain measurements in both horizontal and vertical and average the readings.
- Irregular corneal surface leads to distortion of mires

Methods used to sterilize the applanation tonometer biprism include:
- Soaking applanation tip for 5–15 minutes in diluted sodium hypochloride, hydrogen peroxide 3% or isopropyl alcohol 70% or by wiping with alcohol hydrogen peroxide povidone iodine.
- 10 minutes of rinsing in running tap water
- Soap water wash
- Disposable film covers the tip
- Expose to UV light

Correction factors for IOP are mentioned in **Table 4**.

TABLE 4: Correction for IOP measured using GAT.

Cornea thickness (in microns)	*Correction factor*
460–485	+3
486–512	+ 2
513–536	1
537–562	0
563–587	–1
588–612	–2
613–637	–3
638–662	–4
663–687	–5

8. Discuss the role of gene therapy in ophthalmology. (10) (WBUHS MS 2024)

Gene therapy has become popular to treat genetic and acquired diseases. There are many substances used to deliver genes which are called vectors. The vectors help the therapeutic genes to be delivered by viral or non-viral vectors and take them to the target cells. Target cells are modified by viruses which incorporate the therapeutic material into nuclei. It treats acquired diseases by inserting therapeutic material into target cells.
- Gene therapy for ocular diseases like Leber congenital amaurosis have a deficient gene, i.e., RPE65 which is treated by gene therapy.
- Viral vectors like adenovirus, HSV and retrovirus are used for gene transfer.
- The limiting factor is activation of proto-oncogenes while genetic material inserted via transduction.
- The delivery systems have different modalities like suprachoroidal, subretinal or intravitreal injection which may cause inflammation and immunological responses.
- Normal gene is added to episome and the extrachromosomal DNA leaves the defective gene.

Different approaches for gene therapy:
- *Gene replacement therapy:*
  - It is a direct approach in which functional copy of a damaged or non-functional gene produces functional protein.
  - Without changing the damaged gene role gene therapy treats it.
- *Gene silencing:*
  - Gene associated with siRNA or miRNA which targets VEGF to treat ARMD, NVG and ocular diseases.
- *Gene editing:*
  - Mutation of gene or expression of gene is corrected in gene editing approach.

- Multiple editing techniques are there like—CRISPR/Cas-9, zinc finger nuclease homing endonucleases and transcription activator-like effector nucleases (TALENs).
- CRISPR/Cas9 has two components one is involved with RNA specific gene interest and another modulates gene by endonuclease.

▪ *Modifier gene therapy:*
  - It may affect in gene expression. It modifies the mutated genes rather than healthy one.

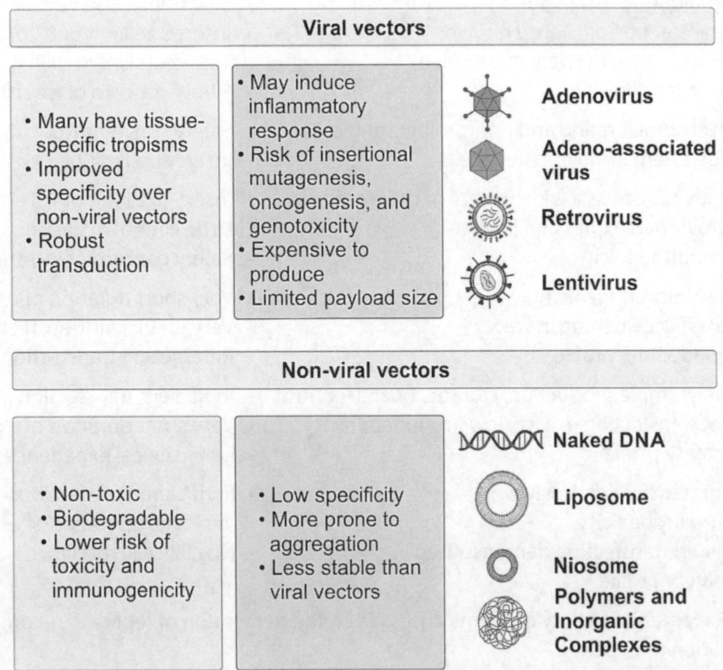

Fig. 6: List of viral and nonviral factors. *(For Color version, See Color Plate 12)*

Viral vectors are given in **Figure 6** and **Table 5.**

▪ Adenovirus:
  - It is a DNA virus producing high protein which inserts into the cell forming multiple genes.
  - It is used in broad spectrum of tissue tropism in both anterior and posterior segment diseases.
  - Currently, it is only used in retinoblastoma trial.
  - As side effects, it causes fever, liver diseases and adenoviral infection sequelae.

▪ Adeno-associated virus:
  - AAV2 is introduced for subretinal injection to transduce RPE in gene trials.
  - It is the first gene which is FDA approved gene therapy, i.e., voretigene neparvovec-rzyl (Luxturna) for Leber congenital amaurosis.
  - AAV8 virus is delivered in subretinal artery which causes efficient photoreceptor transduction.
  - AAV is rapidly eliminated by the body by reducing capsids number and cell-mediated T cell immune response.

▪ Lentivirus:
  - It is a SS-RNA virus causes stable transduction in dividing and non-dividing cells in target organs.
  - It is used in Stargardt's disease and Usher syndrome.

▪ Non-viral gene therapy:
  - Non-viral vectors are utilized for large DNA like plasmid transfer, small DNA, and RNA molecules.
  - By chemical methods, it forms nano-complexes with genetic material which are transduced into the outer retina to prevent premature degeneration in the subretina.
  - Zimura is a complement C5 protein inhibitor which is used in Stargardt's disease 1 and geographic atrophy.

TABLE 5: Features of gene transfer.

Vector	*Advantages*	*Disadvantages*
Adenovirus	• Very high transfection efficiency ex vivo and in vivo • Transfects proliferating and non-proliferating cells • Substantial clinical experience acquired • Efficient retargeted transfection demonstrated	• Repeat dosing ineffective owing to strong immune response • Insert-size limit of 7.5 kb • Short duration of expression
Retrovirus	• Fairly prolonged expression • High transfection efficiency ex vivo • Substantial clinical experience ex vivo • Low immunogenicity	• Low transfection efficiency in vivo • Insert-size limit of 8 kb • Transfects only proliferating cells • Safety concern of insertional mutagenesis
Lentivirus	• Transfects proliferating and non-proliferating cells • Transfects hematopoietic stem cells	• Safety concerns from immunodeficiency virus origins • Insert-size limit of 8 kb
AAV	• Efficiently transfects a wide variety of cells in vivo • Very prolonged expression in vivo • Low immunogenicity	• Insert-size limit of 4.5 kb • Little clinical experience • Safety concern of insertional mutagenesis
Naked DNA	• Very low immunogenicity • Clinical efficacy demonstrated • Very good safety profile	• Very short duration of expression in most tissues • Very inefficient transfection ex vivo and in vivo • Retargeting transfection very difficult
Cationic lipids	• Relatively simple production, storage, quality control • Efficient transfection ex vivo, low immunogenicity • Good safety profile	• Inefficient transfection in vivo • Very short duration of expression • Little clinical experience
Condensed DNA particles	• Efficient transfection ex vivo • Low immunogenicity • Retargeted transfection demonstrated • Good safety profile	• Inefficient transfection in vivo • Very short duration of expression • No clinical experience
All viral vectors share the disadvantage of safety concerns arising from the generation of replication-competent virus during production or after administration to patients.		

TABLE 6: Gene therapy in posterior segment diseases.

Ocular site	*Disease*	*Vector*	*Drug*	*Route*	*Development*
Cornea	Herpes simplex keratitis	CRISPR/Cas-9 mRNA instantaneous gene ending product	BD111: In adult single dose	Intracorneal injection	Phase I/II
Glaucoma	Ocular HTN and open angle glaucoma	siRNA	SYL040012	Topical instillation	Phase I and II
Retinal diseases	X-linked retinoschisis	AAV (AAV8)	AAV8-scRS/IRBPhRS	Intravitreal injection	Phase I/II
Optic nerve diseases	LHON	AAV (AAV 2)	scAAV-2–P1ND4v2	Intravitreal injection	Phase I
Tumors	Recurrent retinoblastoma	Adenovirus	Oncolytic adenovirus VCN-01	Intravitreal virus	Phase I

Applications of gene therapy **(Tables 6 and 7)**:

- *Corneal diseases:* Corneal diseases, i.e., dry eye, Sjogren's syndrome, corneal graft rejection, and mucopolysaccharides are applied by gene therapy.
- *Glaucoma:* Primary open glaucoma is hereditary disease. In phase 1 study, gene therapy along with siRNA is introduced which suppresses β-adrenergic receptor synthesis lowers the IOP in glaucoma patients.

TABLE 7: Side effects of injection.

	Invasiveness	*Sustainable outer retinal transduction*	*Immune response*	*Antibody production*	*Severity of inflammation*
Intravitreal	+	+	±	++++	++
Subretinal	++++	++++	+++	+	+
Suprachoroidal	+	+	−	++	+

- *Retinal diseases:*
  - *Stargardt's disease:* ABCA4 mutations cause accumulation of lipofuscin pigment in RPE and photoreceptors. EIAV-vector carrying the ABCA4 gene is administered via subretinal route.
  - *Retinitis pigmentosa:* It is an heterogeneous autosomal disease. RPGR genes associated with viral and non-viral vectors are injected via subretinal and intravitreal injections to assess RP.
  - *Leber congenital amaurosis:* RPE65 associated LCA is suitable for retinal diseases. No adverse effect is noted during treatment in LCA.
  - *AMD:* Intravitreal injection of AAV along with aflibercept gene treats neovascular AMD and shows promising results. EIAV expressing endostatin and angiostatin for neovascular AMD is treated.
  - *Diabetic retinopathy:* Suprachoroidal delivery of an AAV vector carries anti-VEGF. Fab segment is treated in DR without DME.

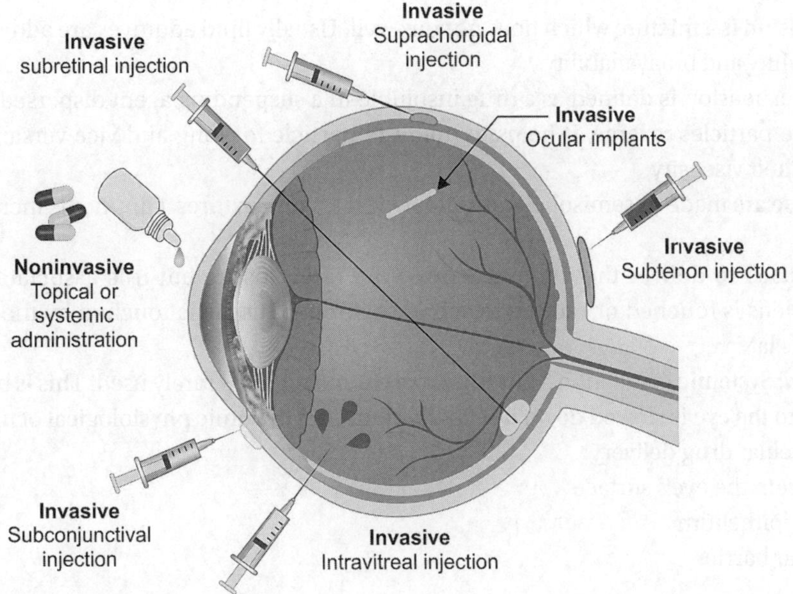

Fig. 7: Route of administration of gene therapy. *(For Color version, See Color Plate 12)*

Figure 7 lists out the routes of administration of gene therapy.

Electrotransfection: It is a non-viral gene therapy which uses high electric pulses, increasing cell membrane permeability. But there is no data on side effects, safety measures, anatomical and physiological toxicities.

Conclusion

- It is an on-going process to grow more developed vector system to improve efficacy of gene therapy.

9. Discuss the role of nanotechnology in ophthalmology. (10) (WBUHS MS 2024)

Nanotechnology is the discipline that studies, designs and operates various materials and devices at the size of intracellular structures and molecules in the order of <100 nm. One significant application is in medicine, particularly diagnosing, treating and managing diseases, which is referred to as nanomedicine.

In ophthalmology, nanotechnology has advanced significantly, leading to nano-systems for eye treatments. These systems enhance drug bioavailability, prolong drug contact time and reduce the need for eye removal procedures.

The eye is a biologically closed compartment and there are different methods of drug delivery for the treating ocular diseases but only a minute amount of drug reaches the aqueous humor. Topical drug application is the most common due to the ease of installation and efficacy. Drug installation to the anterior and posterior segments depends on the natural barriers namely, the blood-aqueous barrier and the blood-retinal barrier.

- *Conventional methods of ocular treatment:*
  - Eye drops are the easiest to use, most effective and safe method of medication but the transfusion and absorption of the solution into the eye is difficult. Hence, additives such as chelators are used which enhance permeability of the drug.
  - *Periocular implants:* Subtenon, subconjunctival, retrobulbar, posterior sclera are the popular sites for administration of drugs. It treats retinal disorders but ocular barriers prevent the absorption of drugs.
  - *Subtenon injections:* Subtenon area is an avascular zone where drug is injected and stays for long time. It devoid lens penetration or cataract formation like complications. It delivers anterior and posterior segment diseases.
  - *Suprachoroidal injections:* This route provides the drug in posterior segment of eye. The drug reaches retina and choroid area. The complications like choroidal detachment and suprachoroidal hemorrhages are noted frequently.
  - *Emulsion:* Emulsion is a mixture which does not mix well. Usually lipid additives are added to emulsions for easy ocular permeability and bioavailability.
  - *Suspension:* A suspension is defined as a drug insoluble in a suspending agent dispersed on a liquefied solvent. If the size of the particles is large, it helps to hold the particle for long and vice versa. The only drawback to suspensions is their viscosity.
  - *Ointments:* These are made of semisolid and solid hydrocarbon mixtures. Ointments increase the bioavailability of the drug.
  - Injections are used to deliver the drug directly to the target tissue but it is associated with complications like, cataract if lens is touched or retinal detachment if retinal tissue is touched by the needle and can cause endophthalmitis later.
  - *Systemic method:* Systemic instillation by oral and parenteral routes is rarely used. This is because the rate of drug administration to the eye is slowed down due to the static and dynamic physiological ocular barriers.
- The challenges in ocular drug delivery:
  - Drug washout from the eye's surface
  - Role of corneal epithelium
  - The blood-ocular barrier
  - Tear turnover
  - Nasolacrimal drainage
  - Drug binding to tear proteins
  - Melanin binding
  - Drug metabolism
- Several nano-based treatments for eye diseases include:
  - Nanoparticle-filled contact lenses with acetazolamide for glaucoma.
  - Biodegradable subconjunctival implants for xerophthalmia
  - Diclofenac eye-release nano-colloid systems using hydrogels
  - Polymer nano-colloid systems for inflammatory diseases
  - Nanostructured lipid transporters for controlled ocular drug delivery.
- Role of nanotechnology in ocular drug delivery is to help in drug transportation to the site of effect. The different challenges which arise in drug delivery can be attenuated using nanotechnology. Nanomaterials include:

- *Nanoemulsions:* These are mixture of 2 phases: water in oil or oil in water. A surfactant is used to stabilize them. The components of nanoemulsion are oil or lipid droplets, surfactants and cosurfactant. A lipophilic medicine can be given with the help of nanoemulsion in oily phase. If these compounds are not stabilized then they separate over time.
- *Nanosuspension:* These are clarified drugs which are insoluble in water and suspended on a dispersion medium. It is used for giving hydrophobic drugs as the medicines are readily absorbed.
- *Nanoparticles:* Particles with a diameter below 1 mm are called nanoparticles. They are made of lipids, polymers, phospholipids and metals, e.g., chitosan, albumin, gelatin, and polylactides (PLAs). These are particularly used for giving medications directly into the eye due to these benefits:
    - Small size
    - Eye irritation is less
    - No frequent instillation
    - Has the property of sustained release
- *Liposomes:* These are tiny vesicles made of artificial substances, e.g., lipid bilayers. Over time, these liposomes can inject medication directly into the eye. Their size ranges from 0.8–10 micrometers. The vesicles are tiny, big, or polymeric. Liposomes can carry hydrophobic and hydrophilic drugs. They also have drawbacks. They are not well stable and have short half-lives.
- *Dendrimers:* These are tiny particles in the nanometer range with high branching pattern. The molecular weight varies from each other by their functional group. Dendrimers act as carrier to administer the drug directly into the eye. Due to the high branching pattern, they can carry a large number of drugs. Along with hydrophobic, it can also transfer hydrophilic and lipophilic drugs by joining the medication to the exterior of the dendrimer or by closing and compressing the medicines inside the cage of dendrimers.
- *Nanomicelles:* These are aggregated amphiphilic particles with the properties of surfactant or polymer quality. The advantages of using nanomicelles include:
    - High drug-holding capacity
    - Simple preparation method
    - Tiny in the nano range

  These increase the bioavailability and penetration of drugs in the eye tissues.
- *Niosomes:* These are bilayered structure like liposomes. They act as surfactants without ions. They are capable of entrapping both water and oil soluble medications. The features why niosomes are preferred are:
    - They have better chemical stability
    - Can transport both hydrophobic and hydrophilic drugs
    - Less toxic as they do not contain ions
    - Handling surfactant surfaces easily

Nanopreparations used for the treatment of eye diseases:

- *Nanosuspension—refer to text above*
- *Contact lenses:* Contact lenses are hard or soft polymer lenses which correct the refractive anomalies of the cornea. The use of drug-coated contact lenses is an effective way to prolong drug delivery. The drugs are incorporated by printing, simple immersion, and colloidal nanoparticles.
- *Intraocular implant:* This is a new treatment method for the controlled release of drugs by reducing the dose and increasing the drug load. The systemic side effects are less as the drug is closer to the target site. There are 2 types of implants—biodegradable and nonbiodegradable. The nonbiodegradable implants have to be removed or filled at appropriate intervals. The latest biodegradable implant system is ENV705 implant Envisia therapeutic implant and Zordera, nanoporous membrane device. This device when injected into the vitreous is only 40 micron in diameter and the drug release order is close to 0. After the entire drug has released, the polymer degrades.

Applications of nanotechnology in various ocular diseases **(Table 8)**:

TABLE 8: Common eye diseases and treatment application.

Pathology	*Drugs/devices*	*Therapeutic target*	*Associated nanoparticles*	*Mechanism of NP action*
Keratitis	Ofloxacin, colirios, aciclovir	• Fluoroquinolone. Inhibition of topoisomerase II and IV • Herpes polymerase DNA inhibitor	• Polyethylene glycol oxide and Eudragit® in the form of microspheres • Acyclovir drug encapsulated by polylactic acid microspheres	Improve the bioavailability and controlled release of antibiotics. Delay the degradation of acyclovir prodrug
Conjunctivitis	Tobramicina, colirios	Inhibit the synthesis and binding of polypeptides in ribosomes	Solid lipid NP	They increase the bioavailability of the corneal surface and help retain it in the conjunctival sac
Dry keratoconjunctivitis	Ciclosporin A, colirios	Immune modulators that prevent T lymphocyte activation	Chitosan	Sustained release carrier
Uveitis	• Nanosuspension of prednisone • Subconjunctival prednisolone injection • Intravitreal injection of infliximab	Prostaglandin and leukopenia monoclonal antibody synthesis inhibitors that inhibit TNF-α activity	Submicron colloidal carrier of hydrophobic drugs in surfactant stabilized medium	Sustained release and controlled release of drugs, as well as higher bioavailability and lower toxicity
Cataract	Lithium with metabolic activity	Inhibit ROS activity and regulate the level of H_2O_2 and lipid peroxidation in the surrounding environment	Deposition of platinum nanoparticles by magnetron sputtering	Inorganic catalytic antioxidant
Glaucoma	• Nanotransporters: Pilocarpine, timolol, carbonic anhydrase inhibitor, acetazolamida, dorzolamida, brinzolamide and brimonidina • Silicone and hydrogel contact lenses hydrogel contact lenses containing thymolol • Thymolol-containing contact lenses • Wireless sensors	• Traditional treatment of nonselective β-blockers to reduce aqueous humor • Continuous intraocular pressure monitoring	Dendrimers, liposomes, nanocapsules, nanospheres, hydrogels PGT (triglyceride) NP gold	Drug sustained release increases the loading and absorption of the thymus
Wet DMRE	• Hyaluronic acid implant: Bevacizumab • Nanopore devices: ranibizumab biodegradable	Humanized monoclonal antibody against vascular endothelial growth factor	Chitosan NA	• Sustained release vehicle • Drug release through nanopores

Contd...

Contd...

Pathology	***Drugs/devices***	***Therapeutic target***	***Associated nanoparticles***	***Mechanism of NP action***
Diabetic retinopathy	Reservoir stimulation response device: Nintedanib	Vascular kinase inhibitor, blocking VEGF receptor, platelet-derived growth factor receptor, fibroblast growth factor receptor	Polylactic acid glycolic acid microspheres and nitrobenzene monomer	UV stimulates drug release
Retinitis pigmentosa	Vitreous fluorooctane sulfonate	Microglia activity attenuation	Polyamide dendritic molecule	Drug-sustained release
Retinoblastoma	• Subconjunctival carboplatin • Photodynamic therapy and verteporfin	Alkylating agent, inhibiting DNA replication, RNA transcription, nano protein synthesis, selective neovascular endothelial cells, inducing apoptosis and autophagy	NP dendritic polyamidoamine nonthermal laser activated liposome vertebral body	• Sustained release and controlled release of drugs • Reactive oxygen species production and cell death in tumor cells
Optic neuromyelitis	Biosensor	NA	Carbon nano-tubes	AQP4 antibody detection
Endophthalmitis	dapamycin, cholinesterase	Anti-gram-positive natural lipopeptide antibiotics, including SAMR	Chitosan	Promote the penetration of antibiotics by opening the connection between corneal cells

(AQP4: antithrombin 4; ARMD: age-related macular degeneration; ERK: extracellular signal-regulated kinase; IOL: intraocular lens; NA: not applicable; NP: nanoparticles; IOP: intraocular pressure; ROS: reactive oxygen species; MRSA: methicillin-resistant *Staphylococcus aureus*; VEGFR-2: vascular endothelial growth factor receptor 2)
Source: Gomez-Garzon M, Martínez-Ceballos MA, Gómez-López A, Rojas-Villarraga A. Application of Nanotechnology in Ophthalmology: Where Are We?" Charact Appl Nanomater. 2022;5(1):66-78

Conclusion
- Nanotechnology-based therapeutic drugs are used to treat the ocular diseases.
- The development of nanoscale clinical drug delivery vehicle should be a target to cure various diseases.
- Active target ligands enhance the penetration of drug to reach in the posterior segment of eye.

SUGGESTED READING

1. Chen EJ, Fasiuddin A. Management of Traumatic Hyphema and Prevention of Its Complications. Cureus. 2021;13(6):e15771.
2. Delhi Ophthalmology Society. An overview of Artificial Intelligence in ophthalmology. DOS Times. 2020; 25(5).
3. Ghoraba HH, Akhavanrezayat A, Karaca I, Yavari N, Lajevardi S, Hwang J, et al. Ocular Gene Therapy: A Literature Review with Special Focus on Immune and Inflammatory Responses. Clin Ophthalmol. 2022;16:1753-71.
4. Gupta R, Bawankule PK. Operation theatre sterilisation and modular operation theatre. Delhi J Ophthalmol. 2023;33:266-76.
5. Zarbin MA, Montemagno C, Leary JF, Ritch R. Nanomedicine in ophthalmology: the new frontier. Am J Ophthalmol. 2010;150(2):144-162.e2.

Index

Page numbers followed by *f* refer to figure, *fc* refer to flowchart, and *t* refer to table.

A

Ab externo trabeculectomy 263, 264*f*
Aberrations, peripheral 39
Acanthamoeba 177
  disease 506
Accessory lacrimal glands 157
Acetazolamide 464
Acid 434, 441
  acetic 434
  amino 8
  ascorbic 7, 437, 440
  hydrochloric 434
  nitric 434
  sulphuric 434
Acquired immunodeficiency syndrome 484
  diagnostic criteria of 485
  management of 485
Acquired pendular nystagmus 378
Acute posterior multifocal placoid pigment epitheliopathy 271, 345, 346*f*
Acute retinal screening examinations, termination of 309
Acyclovir 477
  dosage of 478
  mechanism of action of 476, 477
  therapy, long-term 177
Address squint correction 409
Adduction, partial deficiency of 380
Adenovirus 517, 518
  keratoconjunctivitis 141
    management of 141
    signs of 141
    symptoms of 141
Adie's pupil, signs of 409
Adie's syndrome 411
Adie's tonic pupil 410, 411
Adjunctive therapy 147
Adrenalin 210
Aflibercept 310, 348, 353, 356, 365
Agricultural accidents 434
Ahmed glaucoma valve 258, 259
  adverse effects of 257
  build of 258*fc*
  design of 258*fc*
  patented trapezoidal valve mechanism of 259*f*
Air
  based tonometer 512
  conditioning 501
  puff tonometer 512
  sampling 501
Alkali 434, 441
Allergic conjunctivitis, seasonal 143
Allergy 384
Allylamines 478
Alpha-agonists 464
Alternate cover test 91
Alternative surgical techniques 409
Ambisome-leishmaniasis 323
Amblyopia 370, 371, 511
  component 374
  development 375
  mixed 370
  reverse 370
  therapy 197
  types of 370
Amiodarone 394
Amniotic membrane
  grafting 147
  mechanism of action of 507, 508
  transplantation 164, 438, 441, 507
Amphotericin B 479
Amsler grid 41, 42*f*, 94, 339, 340*f*
  test, types of 95*f*
Amsler sign 236
Analgesics 427
Analogue scale 439
Anderson's procedure 379
Anesthesia 247
  examination under 261
  intraoperative 384
Aneurysm 277
Angiogenesis 476
Angioid streaks 364
Aniridia 262
  traumatic 420
Aniseikonia 56
Anisocoria 390, 410
  causes of 410
  management of 410
Anisometropia 55
Annular detachment 250
Annulus of Zinn 24
Anomalies, developmental 328
Anomalous retinal correspondence 20, 369
  advantages of 368
  types of 369
Anterior chamber 233, 432
  angle 233, 506
    neovascularization 235*t*
  depth 204
  maintenance of 249
  placement 267
  silicone oil 321
Anterior segment optical coherence tomography 240
  applications of 506
Anterior segment surgery 507
Antiangiogenic therapies 348
Antibiotics
  broad spectrum of 507
  systemic 429
Antibody production 519
Anti-elevation syndrome 383, 385
Antifungal drugs 478
  classification of 478*fc*
Antifungal medications 478
Anti-glaucoma agents 236
Anti-inflammatory drugs 160, 427
  role of 160
Antimetabolites 475, 478
  role of 474, 475
  use of 249
Antioxidants 228, 349
Antiretroviral therapy, indication for 485
Anti-suppression technique 377
Antithrombin 523
Anti-tumor necrosis factor 281
Anti-vascular endothelial growth factor 309, 309*t*, 310, 353*t*, 356, 356*t*
  agents 348, 476
  doses 356*t*
  indications 476
Antiviral agents 477*fc*
Aphakia 267
  implantation in 211
  management of 197, 212*fc*
Aphakic bullous keratopathy 186
Apical compression 121*f*
Apoptosis 507
Applanation 13
  tonometer 275
    parts of 514*f*
Apraclonidine 391, 464
  test 410
Aqueous formation, steps of 7
Aqueous humor, formation of 7
Aqueous misdirection syndrome 238, 251

Aqueous solutions 461
Arc
diagnostic procedures for 369
evaluation of 369
features of 368
Arden gratings 46
Argon
laser 468
trabeculoplasty 243, 246
pretreatment 244
Argyll Robertson pupil 19
Arterial blood pressure 10
Arterial changes 303
Arterial thrombosis 277
Artificial intelligence 503
Asepsis 499
Aspergillus 483
Asteroid hyalosis 332
Asthenopia 403
Astigmatism 49, 54
against rule 49
investigations 54
management 54
mixed 49
signs 54
symptoms 54
types 54
Astrocytic hamartoma 335
Atonic pupil 192
Atropine 240, 440
mechanism of action of 470
topical low dose 470
Augmented Anderson procedure 379
Augmented Knapp's 384
Autoclave
room 500
types of 502
Autoimmune
disease 180
disorder 119
optic neuritis 388
Autologous serum 437, 440
Automated facial measurements 505
Automated perimetry 222
Automated refraction, principles of 67
Autonomic nerve dysfunction 409
Axial system 26
Azathioprine 122, 149, 274, 475
Azoles 478

B

Back vertex distance 68, 68*f*
Bacterial keratitis 483
Baerveldt implant 237
Bagolini striate lenses 368
Balloon catheter 139*f*
dilatation 132, 138
Balloon dacryoplasty 132, 138
Band keratopathy 356
Basal skull fracture 418, 419
Basement membrane 507
Bayonetting sign 229
Bean pot cupping 229
Behçet's disease 275, 276, 472, 474
clinical features 275
etiology 275
management 275
Berger's space 328
Bergmeister's papilla 328
Berlin's edema 415
Bernoulli's principle 258
Beta-blockers 464
Beta-carotene, exclusion of 349
Bevacizumab 302, 310, 348, 353, 356, 365
B-Hex pupil expander 193*f*
Bicarbonate 8
Bielschowsky phenomenon 381
Bifocals 69
Bimatoprost 465
Binocular indirect ophthalmoscopy 85
Binocular single vision 19
Binocular vision 79, 367
grades of 19, 19*f*
Biochemical properties 327
Biometry, challenges in 196
Biopsy 491
Birmingham eye trauma terminology
classification, modified 414, 414*fc*
system 413
Bitemporal hemianopia 407
Bitemporal superior quadrantanopia 407
Bitot's spots 453
Bleb leak 250
Blebitis 265
Bleeding, mild 245
Blepharitis 483
Blepharoptosis 102
Blepharospasm 435
Blood
aqueous barrier 8, 10*f*
cholesterol 299
dyscrasias 331
extravasation of 424, 427
pH 11
pressure 299
retinal barrier 16, 16*f*
Blood-aqueous barrier 9
Blowout fracture 426
impure 424
investigations of 427
mechanism of 426
types of 426
Blue limbal zone 5
Blunt trauma 364, 415
accidental 425
effect of 415, 419
signs of 238
Bone placed back 125*f*
Boresch gauge 191
Borrelia burgdorferi 388
Boston KPRO type 1 keratoprosthesis 187
Boston sign 120
Botulinum toxin
chemodenervation with 379
complications of 463
indications of 463
mechanism of action of 463*f*
use 463
Bowman's layer 4
Bowman's probe 134*f*, 139
Brachytherapy 294
Brainstem lesions 18
Brimonidine 232, 464
Brinzolamide 464
topical 379
Brolucizumab 356
Bromophenol blue 481
Bruch's membrane 347, 416
Bruising 463
B-scan ultrasonography 240, 445
Bubble, persistence of 208
Buckling theory 424
Bullous keratopathy 175, 193
Buoyancy 321
Buphthalmos 269, 269*t*

C

Calcium channel blockers 228
Calcofluor white 182
Canalicular injury 135
causes of 136
repair of 137*f*
Canalicular obstruction 134*f*
Canalicular slitting 140
Canalicular system 134*f*
Canaliculus, superior 139*f*
Cancer-associated cone dysfunction 296
Candida endophthalmitis 482
Cannulas, cleaning of 502
Capillary hemangioma 118
Capsular bag support 207*fc*
Capsular block syndrome 204
Capsular tension ring 207
Carbachol 464
Carbidopa 371
Carbon dioxide laser 469
Carbonic anhydrase inhibitors 464
Cardiac arrest 384
Cardinal points 35
Carotid artery, internal 28, 410
Cataract 356, 469, 505, 522
anterior capsular 195
blue dot 198*f*
complicated 209
coronary 195, 198*f*
detection 505
formation 193, 245, 280, 321
nuclear 195, 198*f*
punctate 195
sunflower 433
surgery 192, 203, 216, 466

sutural 198*f*
traumatic 420
types of 195
zonular 195, 198*f*
Cationic lipids 518
Cat-scratch disease 388
Causative organism, infective 271
Cavernous sinus 28, 28*f*
anatomy of 27
applied importance of 28
relations of 27, 27*f*
Cavitation, force of 207
Cell
gelatinization of 439
membrane integrity, loss of 478
wall integrity, loss of 478
CEMAS classification 378
Central corneal thickness 204, 220
Central fundus, stereo-photography of 221
Central Horner's syndrome 410
Central retinal
artery 25, 30
vein occlusion 305, 364
classification of 305
Central scotoma 361
Central serous chorioretinopathy 344, 359
Central vestibular imbalance 378
Chalcosis 432
Charleaux sign 179
Chelating calcium 440
Chemical delivery system 462
Chemical injuries, Dua's classification of 439
Childhood blindness
causes of 452
prevention of 454
Chin elevation 369
Chloramphenicol 394
Chloride 7
Chloroquine 394
Cholesterol 301
Choriocapillaris 25, 348
Chorioretinal degenerations 314, 315*t*
Chorioretinitis sclopetaria 416
Choroid 415, 484, 490
complex 347
detachment 241, 265
hemangioma 345*f*
Choroidal melanoma
classification of 292
clinical features of 292
diagnosis of 292
management of 292
types of 293*t*
Choroidal neovascularization 360, 363
Choroidal rupture 415
Choroidal tuberculosis 488
Choroidal tumors 345
Choroiditis 484
Chromatic aberration 38, 38*f*
Cicatricial ectropion 105, 107, 108, 110*f*
Ciliary arteries
anterior 15
posterior 25
long 15, 25, 30
short 15, 25, 30
Ciliary body 420, 484, 496
disorders 231
layers 15
Ciliary ganglion, lesions of 18
Ciliary nerves 30, 466, 467
Ciliary process 328
ultrastructure of 16
Ciliary shock 420
Ciliary veins, anterior 15
Ciliary zonules 15
Cionni toric axis marker 191*f*
Citicoline 371
Clarity toric marker 191
Classic grid 231*f*, 351, 351*t*
Clofazimine 497
Cloquet's canal 328
Clostridium botulinum 463
Coagulation disorders 331
Coagulative laser 244
Coagulopathy 364
Coats' disease 277, 284, 298
Cobalt alloy 129
Cocaine test 410
Cogan syndrome 177
Collaborative corneal transplantation study 185
Collagen
cross-linking 179
types of 327
Colloidal solutions 462
Color
blindness 453
desaturation 407
fundus picture 355
Color vision 44
methods of evaluation of 44
testing 41, 339
theories of 44
Commotio retinae 415
Community ophthalmology 446
Computational intelligence 503
Concentric atrophy 228
Confocal laser microscopy 83
optic of 83*f*
Confocal optics 83
Confocal scanning laser ophthalmoscope 363*f*
Congenital cranial dysinnervation disorder 380
Congenital hereditary endothelial dystrophy 186
Congenital nasolacrimal duct obstruction 131, 145
causes of 133
management of 133
Congenital ptosis 102
management of 102
Conjunctiva 141, 142, 149, 234, 263*f*, 419, 435, 483, 490, 496, 511
keratinization of 149
states of 267
TB 488
Conjunctiva-DCR 134, 135*f*
complications 134
contraindications 134
indications 134
Conjunctival adhesions 438, 441
Conjunctival amyloidosis 507
Conjunctival autograft 147
Conjunctival closure 249
Conjunctival epithelium, hyperplasia of 150
Conjunctival flap
fornix-based 247
limbal-based 247
procedure, double-sliding 147
Conjunctival foreign body 418
Conjunctival fornix 467
Conjunctival incision 385
Conjunctival injection 99
Conjunctival intraepithelial neoplasia 483
Conjunctival lymphoma 483, 507
Conjunctival melanoma 507
Conjunctival microvasculopathy 483
Conjunctival nerves 467
Conjunctival nevus 507
Conjunctival peritomy 186
Conjunctival scarring 385
Conjunctival transposition 438, 441
Conjunctival wounds 422
Conjunctival xerosis 453
Conjunctivitis 453, 522
allergic 143
chemical 146
chronic 132
mild 146
severe 146
Consciousness, loss of 224
Consensual light reflex 409
Conservative treatment 152
Contact lens 50, 52, 197, 461, 521
assisted CXL 179
bandage 444
clinical uses of 74
sensor 14
soft 250
uses of 73
Contracted socket
management of 130
morphological classification of 129, 130, 130*t*
Contrast sensitivity
recording of 46
test 43, 45
types of 45
Contusion 413
Conventional drug delivery system 461
Conventional glaucoma surgeries 262
Convergence insufficiency 59, 375, 376

Convolutional neural network 504
Copious irrigation 440
Corectopia 236
Cornea 142, 148, 170, 184, 234, 419, 423, 430, 432, 435, 439, 469, 483, 496, 518
  artificial 187
  histological structure of 4
  perforated 182
  peripheral 248*f*
  thickness 516
Cornea-based procedures 52
Corneal allogenic intracorneal ring segment implantation 179
Corneal astigmatism, computing total 191
Corneal blindness 446
  causes of 446
  prevalence of 446
Corneal causes 49
Corneal collagen cross linking 170
Corneal compensation, enhanced 222
Corneal curvature, deviations of 515
Corneal decompensation 193, 236
Corneal diseases 518
Corneal dystrophy 507
Corneal ecstatic disorders 189
Corneal edema 175, 204, 419
  primary 184
Corneal endothelial
  blood staining 419
  cell
    loss of 192
    peripheral 180
    proliferation 228
  function 267
Corneal endothelium 3
  cross-section of 3*f*
Corneal erosion, recurrent 419
Corneal foreign body 418
Corneal graft rejection 184
Corneal hydration, control of 5
Corneal incisions 208
Corneal inlays 61
Corneal intraepithelial neoplasia 153
Corneal laceration, suturing of 442
Corneal layers 4
Corneal matrix turnover 180
Corneal nerve supply 4
Corneal scar 419
Corneal staining 100
Corneal surgeries 203
Corneal tear 419
Corneal thickness 171
Corneal thinning 179, 182
Corneal tomography
  maps, examination of 172
  uses of 173
Corneal topography
  techniques 171
  types of 171*t*
  uses of 173
Corneal transparency 5
Corneal tuberculosis 488
Corneal ulceration 146, 453
Corneal vascularization 173
  types of 173*t*
Corneal wound 422
  complicated 422
  repair 442, 444
    principle of 442
  small 442
  with iris prolapse 442
Corneal xerosis 453
Corneoscleral wound 443, 444
Correct refractive errors 408
Corticosteroids 144, 160, 280, 489, 511
  sparing agents 143
Corticotropic adenoma 407
Cosmetic
  blemish 381
  lenses 75
  measures 410
Cotton pledgets 461
Cotton-wool spots 303
Coulomb controlled iontophoresis 462
Cover test 91, 92*f*, 92*fc*, 93, 93*f*
Cranial nerve 489
  examination 117
  palsy, causes of 403
Crawford technique 104, 104*f*
Crigler massage 134*f*
Cryotherapy 356
Cryptococcal meningitis 388
Cryptococcus neoformans 484
Crystalline lens, loss of 211
Cultivated oral mucosal epithelium transplantation 438, 441
Curve of Goniolens, anterior 80
Cyanoacrylate
  adhesive 182
  glue 444
Cyclodestructive procedure 237, 471
Cyclodextrins 462
Cyclopentolate 440
Cyclophosphamides 274
Cycloplegic refraction 371, 374
Cyclosporine 149, 274, 281
  side effects of 144
  systemic side effects of 145
Cystoid bodies 303
Cystoid degeneration, peripheral 314-316
Cystoid macular edema 280, 350
Cytomegalovirus
  associated keratitis 506
  retinitis 482, 484
    treatment of 486

D

Dacryocystocele, congenital 132
Dalfampridine 392
Dalrymple's sign 120
Dandruff 233
Dapsone 497
DCR, contraindications of 137
Deep anterior
  chamber 238
  lamellar keratoplasty 180
Deep neural networks 504
Deep tendon reflexes 411
  loss of 411
Deferoxamine 432
Degenerative disorder 346
Degenerative retinoschisis 315
Degenerative vitreous syndrome 333
Deliberate chemical attacks 434
Demyelination 391, 392
Dendrimers 323, 521
Depression 369
Dermoid cyst 118
Descemet membrane tear 4, 174, 419
Destroy extracellular matrix 180
Dexamethasone 354, 511
Diabetes mellitus 192
Diabetic macular edema 303, 349, 352*fc*
  treatment of 304, 354, 354*t*
Diabetic maculopathy 303, 349
Diabetic retinopathy 299, 309*t*, 364, 476, 519, 523
  classification of 299*t*, 300*t*
  clinical research network 301, 352, 352*fc*
  management of 299
  prevention of 299
  risk factors of 301
Diabetic vitreopathy 328
Dichoptic therapy 371
Digenesis, anterior segment 192, 262
Digital tonometry 13
Dilated choroidal vessels 360
Diode laser 469
  ablation 348
Dipivefrine 464
Diplopia 224, 367, 368, 385, 403, 424, 427, 464
  awareness technique 377
  vertical oblique 391
Direct gonioscopy 80
  optic of 80*f*
Direct ophthalmoscope 84, 85*f*
  optical principle of 84*f*
Disc edema 406
  causes of true 406
  mechanical signs 406
Dispersion syndrome 231
Dissociated vertical divergence 381
  management of 381
  measurement of 381
  signs of 381
  symptoms of 381
District Blindness Control Society 452
Dizziness 224
Domestic accidents 434

Donders' reduced eye 35, 36*f*
Donor
  and tissue, evaluation of 183
  cornea, criteria for 183
  corneoscleral button 186
  graft 184
Dorzolamide 464
Double linear echo sign 317
Double-layer sign 361
Doxycycline 437, 440
Drug
  antiviral 476
  cholinomimetic 464
  immunosuppressive 474
Drug delivery systems 75, 460
  posterior segment 462
Dry eye 157, 160, 438, 441, 464
  management of 160, 161
  severity scale 163, 163*t*
Dry eye disease
  pathogenesis of 161*fc*
  pathophysiology of 162*fc*
  treatment of 160*t*
Dry heat sterilization 502
Dua's classification 439
Dua's layer 4
Duane retraction syndrome 380
Dye laser 469
Dysautonomia, generalized 409
Dyschromatopsia 388
Dysthyroid optic neuropathy 120

E

Eales disease 331
Ectatic corneal disorders 173
Ectopia lentis 238
Ectropion
  classification of 108
  involutional 108, 109
  surgical management of 108
  types of 108
Eculizumab 394
Edema 388
  persistent 354
Efferent pathway defects 18
Efferent pupillary defects, causes of 18
Electrodes 88
Electron beams 502
Electroretinogram 88
Elliot Nankin's recession 383
Embryonic mesenchymal cells 327
Emmetrope 65
Emmetropia 87*f*
Endocyclophotocoagulation 471
Endolaser 356
Endonasal DCR 137
Endophthalmitis 193, 356, 482, 488, 523
  comparable risk of 325
Endoscopic sinus surgery 119
Endothelial cell
  abnormalities 233
  surface 348
Endothelial damage 245
Endothelial decompensation 174
Endothelial fluid pump 5
Endothelial folds 175
Endothelial keratoplasty 185
Endothelial mosaic 174
Endothelial transport properties 5
Endothelium-single layer 4
Enlarged recti muscles 121*f*
Enophthalmos 126, 126*f*, 424, 427
  pathophysiology of 126*t*
  surgical management of 127
Enroth's sign 120
Entopic imaging 43, 339
Entropion 105
  congenital 105
  grade of 106
  surgical management of 105
Enucleation 292
Epiphora 131, 132, 435
Epiretinal membranes 314, 324, 362
Episclera 165
Episcleral veins 7
Epithelial bullae 175
Epithelial damage 419
Epithelial edema 174
Epithelial growth cell migration 507
Epithelial keratoconjunctivitis, progression of 142*f*
Epithelial layer, anterior 12
Epithelial microcyst 175
Epithelial rejection 185
Epithelial transport properties 5
Epithelium 4, 507
Equatorial subconjunctival space 266
Erggelet's space 328
Erythema 418
Erythromycin eye ointment 440
Esodeviations, types of 372
Esotropia 372, 373
  cyclic 372
  infantile 374
  types of 374
Essential infantile esotropia 372
Ethambutol 394, 472
  toxicity
    management of 472, 473
    risk factors of 472
    symptoms of 472
Ethmoid sinus 29
EW nucleus damage 410
Excimer laser 469
Excitotoxicity 228
Exenteration, types of 129*t*
Exophthalmometry 116
Exotropia 376
  basic 375
  classification of 376, 376*t*
  nonspecific 375
  small residual 377
Extended depth of focus, principle of 215*f*
Extensive papillae 151*f*
Extracellular signal-regulated kinase 523
Extralenticular theory 60
Extraocular foreign bodies 418
  types of 418
Extraocular irrigation 461
Extraocular tuberculosis 487
Extraretinal fibrovascular proliferation 308
Extrascleral extension 295
Exudates 303
Eye
  abduction of 392
  angle of anterior chamber of 6
  anterior chamber of 6
  aphakic 267
  blunt trauma of 413-415, 419
  chemical injury 413, 433, 434
  closure reflex, disruption of 464
  drops 175
  involvement, severity of 148, 148*t*
  irrigation 437, 440
  opportunistic infection of 482
  optical aberrations of 37
  optical system, mathematical models of 36
  posterior
    segment of 413
    surface of 30
  post-vitrectomy 354*t*
  power of 36
  right 443
  screening 454
    steps of 455, 455*fc*
  shield 444
  vitreous 267
  watering in 131
  white 236
Eye bank 451
  organizational pyramid of 448*f*
  prerequisites of arranging 447
  services 451
Eye disease 522*t*
  age-related 349
  allergic 143
  treatment of 520, 521
Eyeball 233
  formation, embryological steps of 2
  posterior surface of 30, 31*f*
Eyegate 462
Eyelid 23, 97, 148, 419, 435, 483, 490, 496
  anatomy of 97
  bruit over 120
  coloboma 113
    classification of 113*t*
  development of 97
  disorders 453
  ecchymosis of 150
  edema of 142, 418
  emphysema of 424, 427
  in leprosy, management of 498

laceration 418
ligaments of 24*f*
management of 498
margin keratinization, posterior 149
ptosis 463
reconstruction techniques 112*t*
redness of 99
skin 134*f*
surgeries 467
tuberculosis 487
tumor excision, principle of 112

F

Failed dacryocystorhinostomy, prevention of 138
Faricimab 353, 356
Fascicles, lesion of 389
Fascicular third nerve lesions 18
Fasudil 465
Fat-adherence syndrome 383
Femtosecond laser-assisted cataract surgery 207
principle of 209*f*
Fenofibrate 304
Fever 490
Fibers
afferent 18
internuncial 18
parasympathetic 18
superficial 98
zonular 328
Fibrous capsule 216
Field loss, pattern of 222, 223*f*
Field of vision 85
Filmy vision 99
Filter paper strips 461
Filtration surgery 237
Fine central grid 42
Fine vision intraocular lens 77
Fink's recession 383
Fixation behavior 47
Flap
handling 248
size 247
Floaters, cause of 330
Flu symptoms 393, 463
Fluid
currents 314
movement 314
Fluocinolone acetonide 354
Fluorescein 182
angiography 302, 364, 431, 443
staining 436
Fluorescence 514
dye disappearance test 132
Focal atrophy 228
Focal grid 351*t*
Focal subcapsular cataract 238
Fogging 501
Forced duction test 429
Forceps 443
Foreign body
lacrimal 418
palpebral 418
sensation 99
Formaldehyde 501
Foveal cyst 357
Foveal edema 303
Fox pentagon frontalis sling surgery 104*f*
Fresnel prism optics 72*f*
Fuchs' endothelial dystrophy 174, 186
Fuchs' heterochromic iridocyclitis 236, 278
Full tendon transposition 383
Full thickness macular hole
evaluation of 357
management of 357
pathology of 357
Fumigation 499, 501
Fundoscopy 472
Fundus
autofluorescence 272, 273, 293, 338, 355
examination 221, 224, 273, 275
fluorescein angiography 272, 273, 300, 306, 331, 334, 342, 342*f*, 355
principle of 335*f*
peripheral 279
Fungal corneal ulcer 182
Fungal keratitis 483
Fusarium 483
Fused bifocals 70*f*
Fusional amplitudes 374
Fusional control, gradual loss of 377

G

Gabapentin 379
Galilei 171
Ganglion 466
Gas
expansion of 319*f*
injection 358
lasers 468
tamponade 319*f*, 362
Gaseous sterilization 502
Gene
editing 516
regulating natural production of collagen 188
replacement therapy 516
silencing 516
transfer, features of 518*t*
Gene therapy 311, 516, 518*t*
applications of 518
modifier 517
role of 516
route of administration of 519*f*
General anesthesia 139
Genetic 220, 408
testing 290
Germline mutation 290
Giant cell arteritis 389
Giant retinal tear 316, 320
management of 316
Giemsa stain 182
Gifford's sign 120
Ginkgo biloba
extracts 228
influences intracellular signaling 228
Glass, optic of 72*f*
Glaucoma 219, 222, 223*f*, 224, 226*fc*, 227, 228, 321, 464, 469, 497, 505, 518, 522
acute angle closure 236
angle closure 253
angle recession 237
aphakic 262
congenital 132, 262
drainage devices 237
classification of 257*fc*
exfoliative 224
filtering surgeries 258, 466
formation 280
juvenile 262
low tension 224
management of 226, 228
pathogenesis of 242
pathophysiology of 226
pigmentary 231
postpenetrating 241*t*
pre-perimetric 221
primary angle closure 244
pseudoexfoliation 232
pseudophakic 262
pupillary block 241, 321
secondary 438, 441
angle closure 321
open angle 321
to uveitis 262
shunt procedures 266
silicon oil-associated 356
surgeries 257, 262
micro-invasive 253
treatment of 464
unilateral chronic 238
uveitic 236, 253
variants of 224*t*
Glaucomatous 230
damage 233
diagnostic criteria for 224
field loss 222
hemifield test 224
Glaucomatous optic atrophy 229, 230*t*
disc patterns of 228
vascular signs of 229
Glaukos iStent 251, 251*f*
Glial tissue overlying pit 363*f*
Glioma 395
Globe injury, zone of 416
Globe rupture 421
Glutaraldehyde 501
Glycerol 465
Glycosaminoglycan 327

Goldmann applanation tonometer 512, 513, 515
Gomori methenamine silver 182
Gonioscopes 80
Gonioscopy 82, 230, 231, 238, 509
- examination 6
- indirect 81
- types of 80

Gonioscopy-assisted transluminal trabeculotomy 255
Goniotomy 260
- complications of 261
- principles of 261

Gonococcal infection 146
Gopal Krishna classification of contracted socket 130, 130*t*
Gore synthetic cornea device 187
Graft
- detachment 186
- failure 183, 184
- inversion 186
- melting of 182
- rejection 183
  - signs of 185

Gram's stain 182
Granulocytic sarcoma 118
Granulomatous 166, 168
- uveitis, causes of 493

Grave's disease 119
Griffith's sign 120
Grove sign 120
Guttae on Descemet's membrane 175

H

Haidinger's brushes 43, 341
Haller's layer 25
Hand hygiene 503
Hand-held Goldmann type tonometer 512
Hansen's disease 495
- ocular manifestation of 495

Haploscopic principle 79*f*
Hardy–Rand–rittler test 45
Head tilt 369
Headache 224, 391, 405, 407, 463, 508
- ophthalmological causes of 405
- severe 388

Hematoma 417, 418
- formation 467

Hemorrhage 383, 463
- choroidal 356, 415
- dense subconjunctival 421
- orbital 467
- retinal 302, 422
- retrobulbar 466
- subarachnoid 331
- subconjunctival 467
- submacular 363
- suprachoroidal 241, 251
- vitreous 317, 330, 415, 422

Herniation 428
Herpes simplex 177
- epithelial keratitis 175
- infection 146
- keratitis 483
- stromal keratitis 478
- virus 177, 483

Herpes zoster
- keratitis 483
- ophthalmicus 478, 483, 486

Herpetic eye disease study 177
Hess chart 93, 94*f*, 374
Hess screen 93
Heterochromia 423
Hirsberg test 381
Holmes-Adie
- pupil 409
- syndrome 409

Holmgren's wool test 45
Horizontal gaze
- centers 392*f*
- palsy 392

Horner's muscle 29
Horner's pupil 391
Horner's syndrome 390, 390*t*, 391, 410, 411
- postganglionic 410
- preganglionic 410

Hourglass pattern 224
Human antiviral drugs, classification of 477*fc*
Human immunodeficiency virus
- infection 485
  - ocular manifestation of 482
  - progression of 485
- ocular manifestation of 482
- transmission of 484
- treatment of 485

Hummelsheim procedure 383
Hyalocytes 327
Hyaloid artery 328
Hyaloid canal 328
Hyaloideocapsular ligament of Weigert 328
Hyaluronan 327
Hydraulic forces 312
Hydro dissection 216
Hydrogel 323
- soft lenses, extended wear 74

Hydrophilic tube 256
Hydrops, acute 179, 180
Hydroxyamphetamine 391
- test 410

Hydrus device 255*f*
Hyperbaric oxygenation 352
Hypercapnia 11
Hyperfluorescence, causes of 335
Hyperglycemia 307
Hypermetrope 65
- retinoscopy of 65*f*

Hypermetropia 50, 51, 51*f*, 87*f*
- causes of 50
- types of 50

Hyperopia 50
Hyperosmotic agents 165
Hyperreflective membrane 363*f*
Hypersensitivity reaction 204
Hypertension 301
- idiopathic intracranial 396

Hyperthyroidism 119
Hyphema 213, 265, 420
- grading of 425, 509, 509*f*
- management of post-traumatic 424, 508
- post-traumatic 508
- total 425
- traumatic 424

Hypochromic heterochromia 390
Hypocyanescent patches 345*f*
Hypofluorescence, causes of 336
Hypoosmolar riboflavin 171
Hypotony 265
- chronic 321

Hypoxia 11

I

Iatrogenic brown syndrome 385
Ideal bleb position 247
Imbert–Fick law 513
Imbert–Fick principle 514*f*
Immobile hypopyon 275
Immune
- response 519
- system, drugs targeting 311

Immunologic rejection 186
Immunomodulators 122
Immunosuppresives, role of 475
Immunosuppressants, indications of 143
Immunosuppressive agents 281
Immunosuppressive therapy 474
Implant displacement 265
In vitro staining 182
Inadequate gas bubble size 320
Indentation gonioscopy, optic of 81*f*
Indirect ophthalmoscope
- optic of 86*f*
- optical principle of 85

Indocyanine green 480
- angiography 272, 336, 342, 342*t*, 273, 355, 359, 364

Inebilizumab 394
Infection 180, 193
- mode of 484
- ocular 482
- transmissible 507
- viral 388

Infectious optic neuritis 388, 389
Inferior oblique
- muscle, attachment of 30
- overaction 382, 382*t*
- weakening procedures, indications for 382

Inflammation 168
- severity of 519

Inflammatory cells 330

Inflammatory disease 330
Inflammatory macular edema 472
Infraorbital nerve anesthesia 424, 427
Inherent deficiencies 184
Inhibits deoxyribonucleic acid synthesis 475
Initial visual factor 417
Injury
 adnexal 413
 alkali 441
 canalicular 135
 cracker 444
 mechanical globe 413
 mechanism of 419
 open globe 413, 416, 421
 orbital 413
 penetrating 422
 perforating 414, 421, 422
 thermal 413
Inner blood retinal barrier 16
Inosine-5'-monophosphate dehydrogenase 475
Instrument
 cleaning of 501
 sterilization 501
  surveillance of 503
Integumentary signs 288
Interferons 472
Intermediate uveitis 279, 472, 488
 management of 280
Intermittent exotropia 374-376
Internal limiting membrane
 changes 362
 peeling 362
Interstitial keratitis 177
Intra-arterial chemotherapy 292
Intracameral lidocaine 192
Intracameral lignocaine 203
Intracameral phenylepinephrine 192
Intracameral therapy 479
Intracorneal ring segment implantation 179
Intraocular features 492
Intraocular foreign body 283, 423
 injury 414
 management of retained 442
Intraocular gas 319
 bubble 320
  migration of 320
 indications of 320
Intraocular implant 521
 placement of 324
Intraocular inflammation 283
 severe 211
Intraocular lens 523
 implantation, criteria for 196
 power calculations 76
  formulae for 75
Intraocular pressure 5, 117, 320, 435, 523
 diurnal variation in 11
 elevation of 186, 320
 factors influencing 10
 measurement 437
Intraocular silicone oil 258
Intraocular steroid implants 323*t*
Intraocular tuberculosis 488
Intraocular tumors 324
Intraretinal degenerations 314, 314*t*
Intraretinal microvascular abnormalities 303
Intrastromal therapy 479
Intravenous chemotherapy 291
Intravenous steroids, bilateral involvement 389
Intravitreal anti-VEGF agents 351
Intravitreal chemotherapy 292
Intravitreal dexamethasone delivery system 352
Intravitreal implants 322, 322*t*
Intravitreal injections 330, 479
Intravitreal triamcinolone 304, 352
Iontophoretic devices 462
Ipsilateral epistaxis 424, 427
Iridectomy 444
 peripheral 248
Iridocorneal endothelial syndrome 236
Iridocyclitis
 mild 484
 severe 484
Iridodialysis 213, 420
Iridodonesis 238
Iridoplegia 420
Iridoschisis 192, 238
Iridotomy 243
Iris 231, 233, 234, 235*t*, 245, 420, 423, 431, 432, 435, 484, 496
 anteflexion of 420
 anterior surface of 11
 atrophy 236
 cross-section of 12
 fixated intraocular lens 212
 heterochromia 236
 microscopic structure of 11, 12
 nodules 285*f*
 pigment epithelium, disruption of 231
 posterior surface of 12
 repositioning of 444
 retroflexion of 420
 sphincter tear 238
 stroma 12
 stromal tear 420
 surgery 466
Iritis 484
 drug-induced 484
Ischemia 303
 anterior segment 385
Ischemic CRVO 305, 305*t*
Ischemic disease 390
Ischemic dysfunction 303
Ischemic maculopathy 303
Ischemic necrosis, stages of acute 436
Ischemic optic neuropathy, anterior 387, 387*t*
Ischemic theory 226
Ishihara test 44
Isolated orbital floor fracture 127
 repair of 127*t*
Isoniazid 394
Isotonic riboflavin 171
iStent 251, 254*f*
 advantages of 252
 disadvantages of 252
 in glaucoma, complications of 251
 inject 252, 254*f*
 second-generation 252*f*
 supra 252, 256
Itraconazole 479

J

Jackson cross cylinder 61
Jaw-wink 408
 classification of 408
 mild-to-moderate 409
 phenomenon 408
 severe 409
Jellinek's sign 120
Jensen's procedure 383
Jones procedure 107, 107*f*
Juvenile idiopathic arthritis 281
 ocular manifestation of 282
Juvenile xanthogranuloma 284
Juxtacanalicular trabecular meshwork 251

K

Kahook blade 255*f*
Kaposi sarcoma 483
 treatment of 486
Kaye's dots 185
Kayser-Fleischer ring 432
Keratitis 132, 522
 infective 507
Keratoconjunctivitis, dry 522
Keratoconus 178, 507
 progression of 170
Keratomalacia 453
Keratopathy 153, 322
Keratoplasty 180
 penetrating 241
  failed 186
 types of 241
Keratoprosthesis 438, 441
Kestenbaum procedure 379
Knapp's procedure 384
Kocher's sign 120
Kronlein's operation 29
Kuglen hooks 192

L

Laceration 413
Lacrimal apparatus 131
Lacrimal bone 134*f*
Lacrimal gland 157, 158*f*

anatomy of 21, 22
tuberculosis 487
Lacrimal sac 134f, 139f
Lacrimal system 490, 497
Lacrimation 174, 181
Lactophenol cotton blue 182
Lactotrophic adenoma 407
Lagophthalmos 101, 498
Lamellar dot sign 229
Lamellar graft, posterior 108f
Lamellar keratoplasty 241
Lamellar laceration 413
Lamina cribrosa 26
Lantern test 45
Large vein thrombosis 277
Laser 348, 355
augmentation 332
cyclophotocoagulation 240
interferometry 43, 341
iridotomy 232, 243
adverse effect of 243
parameters 304
photocoagulation 174, 304, 351, 354
refractive surgery 61
retinopexy 318, 331
therapy 354
trabeculoplasty 232
types of 468
uses of 469
Laser-tissue interaction 468
Lashes, matting of 132
Latanoprost 465
Lateral orbitotomy 124, 124f
steps of 124
Lateral rectus, Y-split of 381
Latest technique 147
Lattice degeneration 315
Leber congenital amaurosis 519
Lee and Hirst classification 153t
Lens 189, 233, 420, 423, 431, 433, 497
dislocation of 245, 420
overcorrecting minus 377
spherocylindrical 61
subluxation 345
thickness 204
traumatic absorption of 420
trifocals 77
vesicle, formation of 2
wound of 422
Lensectomy 317
role of 317
Lenticular causes 49
Lenticular theory 60
Lentivirus 517, 518
Leprosy 495
ocular pathogenesis of 496
Lesion
etiology of 390
types of 415
Leukemia 283
Leukocoria 297
differential diagnosis of 297, 297fc
Levator muscle 23
Levator palpebrae superioris muscle 24, 389
Levodopa 371
Lid 234, 418
lacerations 418
repair 438, 441
scrubs 461
signs 120
tumor excision 112
Ligamentum hyaloideocapsular 328
Limbal border, anterior 5
Limbal ischemia 439
Limbal stem cell transplantation 438, 441
Limbal vernal disease 151f
Limbus 247t
anatomy of 5
Linear scar 110f
Lipid layer 22
Liposomal amphotericin 323
Liposomes 462, 521
Liquefied vitreous gel 329
Liquid
formulations, instillation of 460
lasers 468
Lissamine green 480
Listing's reduced eye 37f
Local anesthetic agents, mechanism of action of 466
LogMAR chart 40, 40f
Low vision aids 78
types of 78
Lower eyelid
anatomy of 99f
retractors 24
Lumbar puncture 400
Lutein 349
Lyme disease 388
Lysozyme activity 145

M

Machine learning 504
Mackay-Marg tonometer 13, 512
Macula 363f
diseases of 334
hole, stages of 357, 358
Macular degeneration
age-related 346, 347t, 349, 363, 523
wet 476
Macular diseases, evaluation of 334
Macular edema 281, 362
management of 301
nerve fiber layer, clinically significant of 303
Macular function tests 40, 338
Macular hole
impending 357
management of 357
size of 358
surgery 320
principles 357
Macular inflammation 388
Macular neurosensory detachment 363f
Macular serpiginous choroiditis 273
Macular translocation 365
Maculopathy 361
Maddox rod 62
test 43, 340
working of 62f
Maddox wing 63f
test 63
measurement for 64f
Magnesium hydroxide 434, 435
Maklakov tonometer 511
Malaise 490
Mannitol 465
Mantoux test 167, 489
Marcus Gunn Jaw-winking
phenomenon 102
syndrome 102
Martegiani space 328
Masquerade syndrome 283
Maxillary process, visceral mesoderm of 2
Maxwell's spot 43, 341
Means sign 120
Measles 388
Mechanical ectropion 109
Medial canthal plication 110f
Medial palpebral ligament, anterior part of 23
Medial rectus, ligament of 29
Medial wall fracture, surgical repair of 428
Medical therapy 402
end point of 371
Medroxyprogesterone 437, 440
Megalocornea 269, 269t
Meibomian gland dysfunction 99
stages of 100t
Melanoma 111
related retinopathy 296
Menace reflex 47
Mendez gauge 191
Merkel cell carcinoma 111
Mesenchymal structures 3
Mesoderm 2
Metamorphopsia 348, 361
Metastatic diseases 295
Methazolamide 464
Methicillin-resistant *Staphylococcus aureus* 523
Methotrexate 281, 394, 475
Microaneurysms 302
Microemulsions 462
Microfine vision 77
Microperimetry 43
Micropulse diode laser 304
Microsphincterotomies 210
Microtropia 372
Mid-limbal line 5
Migraine
attack, phases of 398
types of 398

Mini sphincterotomy 194*f*
Mini-ion iontophoretic unit 462
Miosis, traumatic 420
Mitomycin C 475
Mitotic inhibitors 478
Mittendorf's dot 328
Modular operation theater 500
Mohs micrographic surgery 112*f*
Moist heat sterilization 502
Molecular viscoelastic substances 192
Molecular weight 319
Molluscum contagiosum 483
  treatment of 486
Molteno implant 237
Monocular vision 379
Motor adaptations 367, 368
Motor nerves 467
Mucopurulent reflex 132
Mucormycosis
  complications of 491
  ocular manifestation of 489
Mucous membrane grafting 149
Mucus layer 22
Multibacillary leprosy 497
Multifactorial disease 224
Multimodal imaging 360*f*
Multiple evanescent white dot syndrome 345, 345*f*
Multiple sclerosis 392
Mumps 388
Munson's sign 179
Muscle 467
  cone 32
  palsy, vertical 384
  system of 24
  transposition 383
Myasthenia gravis 389
Mycobacterium
  leprae 495
  tuberculosis 487
Mycophenolate mofetil 281, 475
Mycotic keratitis 478
Mydriasis 238, 423
  traumatic 420
Mydriatics 240, 440
Myectomy 383
Myelinated optic nerve fibers 388
Myelitis, acute 393, 394
Myope 65
Myopia 65*f*, 66*f*, 87*f*, 330
  high 51
  pathological 52
  prevention 470
Myotomy 383

N

Nagel's anomaloscope test 45
Nanoemulsions 521
Nanomicelles 521
Nanoparticles 462, 523
Nanosuspension 521
Nanotechnology
  applications of 521
  role of 519
Nasal bleeding 138
Nasolacrimal duct 139*f*
Natamycin eye drop 479
National Blindness and Visual Impairment Survey 446
National Programme for Control of Blindness and Visual Impairment 450
Necrotic and contaminated tissue, debridement of 438, 440
Necrotizing scleritis 167, 168, 474
Neodymium-doped yttrium aluminum garnet laser 469
Neoplasms 234
Neovascular glaucoma 234, 244, 253, 266
  differential diagnosis of 236
  stages of 235*t*
  treatment of 236*fc*
Neovascular tissue 348
Neovascularization 280, 306, 360
Nerve
  abducens 28, 466
  axons, ischemic disruption of 303
  fiber layer 303
  maxillary 28
  oculomotor 28, 466
  palsy 383, 384
  pphthalmic 28
  target 466, 467
  trochlear 28, 466
Netarsudil 465
Neural pathway 157
Neuritis, retrobulbar 388
Neurofibromatosis 494
  diagnosis of 495*t*
  ocular manifestation of 494
Neurological diseases 288
Neurological symptoms 224
Neuromyelitis optica 393
  clinical features of 393
  investigations of 393
  treatment of 393
Neuron, composed of 26
Neuronal cell death, stages of 227, 227*fc*
Neuronal death 227*f*
  pathophysiology of 226
Neuronal debris, accumulations of 303
Neuro-ophthalmic
  lesions 482
  manifestations 493
Neuro-ophthalmology 386
Neuropathic tonic pupil 410
Neuropharmacological treatment 371
Neuroprotection 227
Neuroretina 484
Neuroretinitis 388
Neurosarcoidosis 388
Neurotrophic keratopathy 436
Neurotrophic ulcers, nonhealing 176
Newcastle score 376*f*
Newer tonometry techniques 14
Next generation therapeutics 310*t*
Night blindness 453
Niosomes 462, 521
Nishida procedure 383
Nitric oxide synthetase inhibitors 228
N-methyl-D-aspartate antagonists 228
Non-arteritic anterior ischemic optic neuropathy 387*t*
Noncontact tonometer 14
Nonconventional drug delivery system 461
Non-glaucomatous optic atrophy 228, 230*t*
Nonischemic central retinal vein occlusion 305, 305*t*
Non-neoplastic masquerade syndromes 283
Non-nucleoside reverse transcriptase inhibitors 485
Nonpenetrating glaucoma surgery 262
  classification of 262*fc*
Non-pigmented ciliary epithelium, passive transport across 8
Nonpupillary block mechanism 244
Nonvalved devices 266
Non-viral gene therapy 517
Normal tension glaucoma 224
  differential diagnosis of 225, 225*t*
Nucleoside reverse transcriptase inhibitors 485
Nucleus, lesion of 389
Nuijts-Solomon bubble marker 191, 191*f*
Nutritional deficiency 394
Nystagmoid conditions 378
Nystagmus 378, 379, 491
  pathologic 378

O

Occlusion 370
Occult globe rupture 421
Ocular adnexa 467, 490
Ocular chemical injury
  Dua's classification of 439*t*
  Rooper-Hall classification of 439*t*
Ocular cicatricial pemphigoid 474
Ocular clinical features 496
Ocular damage 424, 427, 430
Ocular diseases 476, 521
Ocular disorders 468, 469
Ocular examination 331, 374, 509
Ocular features 494
Ocular fluid antibody assessment 286
Ocular hypertension 220
  clinical features 220
  management 220
Ocular inflammation 234, 474, 475
Ocular injury 412, 417
  Betts classification of 413*fc*

Ocular ischemic syndrome 283
Ocular malignancy 183
Ocular manifestations
  anatomical categorization of 483
  management of 147, 486
Ocular morbidity 452, 453
Ocular motility 392
  defective 424, 427
Ocular movement 374
Ocular oncology 505
Ocular penetrating 422
Ocular recovery, phases of 436, 436*t*
Ocular response analyzer 14
Ocular sarcoidosis 285*f*
Ocular surface
  disorder 507
  manifestations 284, 492
  staining 162
Ocular surface squamous
    neoplasia 153, 506
  clinical features of 153
  etiopathogenesis of 153
  histopathology of 153
  management of 153, 155
  treatment of 486
Ocular symptoms 286
Ocular therapeutics 460
Ocular tissue 476
  cells 415
  mechanical tearing of 415
Ocular trauma 317, 331, 413
  classification of 413
  score 416
Ocular treatment 149
  conventional methods of 520
Ocular tuberculosis 484, 487, 489
  clinical features of 487
  management of 487, 489
  treatment of 486
Ocular tumors 290, 476
Ocular vascular pathology 224
Ocular viral affections 478
Oculo-cardiac reflex 384
Oculodigital sign 379
Oculoplasty 505
Ointments 461, 520
Omega-3 fatty acids 349
Omidria 192
Onchocerciasis 177
One-and-a-half syndrome 392
Operation theater 500
  cleaning protocol of 501*t*
Ophthalmia
  neonatorum 145
  sympathetic 474
Ophthalmic B-scan ultrasonography 433
Ophthalmic migraine, management of 398
Ophthalmic neonatorum 145
Ophthalmic veins 27
Ophthalmic viscosurgical devices 202
Ophthalmological disorders 511
Ophthalmology 73, 474, 475, 507
  sterilization in 499
Ophthalmoplegia 123
  differential diagnosis of painful 399
  internuclear 391
Opponent color theory 44
Optic atrophy 407
  causes 404
  classification 404
  clinical features 404
  management 404
Optic cup 3*f*
  formation of 3
Optic disc 328, 363*f*
  cupping 269
  hemorrhages 229
  hyperemia 388
  pallor 296
  pit 362, 363*f*
    maculopathy 361
Optic nerve 30, 416, 490
  avulsion 416
  blood supply of 25, 26, 26*f*
  damage 466
  diseases 518
  fenestration surgery 401, 402
  glioma 118
  parts of 26
Optic neuritis 388, 393
  acute 394
  causes of 388
  clinical signs of 388
  demyelinating 388
  non-infectious 388, 389
  sign of 388
  sinus-related 388
  symptoms of 388
  treatment of 388
  types of 388
Optic neuromyelitis 523
Optic neuropathy 416
  causes of traumatic 401
  chronic 222, 226
  classification of traumatic 401
  traumatic 401
Optic vesicle
  conversion of 3*f*
  formation of 2, 2*f*
Optical aberrations, types of 37
Optical biometry 75, 204, 205*fc*
  advantages of 204
Optical coherence tomography 300, 306,
    314, 331, 337, 348, 350, 355, 359,
    361, 364
  angiography 337, 355
  applications of 337
  multimodal imaging 361*f*
  principle of 337*fc*
  spectral domain 363*f*
Optical correction 60, 377
  types of 51
Optical principle 84, 84*f*, 85,
Optokinetic nystagmus test 47
Ora serrata 328
Oral acetazolamide 240
Oral corticosteroids 497
Orbicularis
  muscle 23
  oculi muscle 24
    orbital part of 23
  paralysis of 464
Orbit 115, 418, 483, 490
  apex of 29
  base of 29
  blowout fracture of 424
  bones 30*f*
    forming wall of 28
  enlargement of 126
  inferior wall of 29
  lateral wall of 29
  magnetic resonance imaging of 121*f*
  medial wall of 28
  role of 29
  surgical spaces of 32, 33*f*
  vault of 29
Orbital apex syndrome 122, 122, 123
  causes of 123*t*
Orbital apex, anatomy of 122, 123*f*
Orbital blowout fracture 424
Orbital cellulitis 118, 119, 119*f*
  complications of 119*t*
  management of 118
Orbital computed tomography 429
Orbital contents
  contracture of 126
  reduction of 126
Orbital decompression 122, 122*t*
Orbital exenteration 294
  types of 129
Orbital floor 428
  fracture 126*f*, 419
Orbital foreign 418
Orbital implants
  after evisceration 128*f*
  clinical importance 127
  types of 127*t*
Orbital manifestations 492
Orbital mass, excision of 125*f*
Orbital pseudotumor 389
Orbital roof fracture 418
Orbital tuberculosis 488
Orbital wall fracture 128*t*
Organizing eye camp 457
Orthoptic exercises 377
Oscillations 378
Oscillopsia 379
Osteo-odonto keratoprosthesis 187

P

Pachychoroid neovasculopathy 359
Pachychoroid pigment
    epitheliopathy 359, 360

Pachychoroid spectrum 358, 359
Pachymetry 179
Pachyvessels 360
Pain 177
  mild 463
  severe 435
Palpebral fissure changes 385
Palpebral type 151
Palpebral vernal disease 151*f*
Palsy, cause of 390
Panophthalmitis 488
Panoptix trifocal intraocular lens 77
Panretinal photocoagulation 237, 331
Panum's fusional area 21, 21*f*
Panuveitis 472
Papilledema 406, 407, 407*t*
Papillitis 388, 407, 407*t*
  bilateral 388
  causes of 395
Paracentral scotoma 348
Parainfectious optic neuritis 388, 389
Paralytic ectropion 108
Paralytic strabismus 383
Paraneoplastic syndromes 295, 295*t*
Paraneoplastic vitelliform maculopathy 296
Park's 3-step test 403
Park's modification of Kestenbaum 379
Park's point 383
Pars plana vitrectomy 281, 304, 317, 352, 356, 357, 362
  enumerate indications of 318
  indications 323
  technique 323
Partial retinal detachment 308
Pascal dynamic contour tonometer 14
Patella fossa 327, 328
Paucibacillary leprosy 497
Paving stone degeneration 315, 316
Pediatric cataract 195, 298
  management of 199, 202*fc*
  morphological classification of 198*fc*
  types of 195, 197, 197*fc*, 198*f*
Pediatric ophthalmology 505
Pegaptanib 348, 356
Penalization 371
PentaCam 171, 173
  advantages of 172
Perennial allergic conjunctivitis 143
Periaxial system 26
Peribulbar anesthesia 210
  complications of 467
Periocular hematoma 419
Periocular implants 520
Periocular steroid 280
Periodic acid Schiff 182
Periorbital edema 424, 427
Peripapillary atrophy 229
Peripheral retinal
  degenerations 314, 315
    classification of 314
  drusen 315
  tears 315
Periphlebitis 279
Permanent punctal occlusion 163
Persistent epithelial
  defect 438, 441, 467
  edema 175
Persistent fetal vasculature 298
Persistent hyphema 510
Petrosal sinus
  inferior 27
  superior 27
Phacodonesis 238
Phacoemulsification 217
Phakic intraocular lens implantation
  complications of 192
  risks of 192
Phakonit 194
Pharmacological agents 464
Pharmacological testing 409
Phenocaine injection 192
Phenylephrine 391
Phlebitis 277
Photodynamic therapy 174, 348, 462
Photophobia 174, 177, 181, 508
Photoreceptor outer segment 300
Photostress rest 41, 339
Phototherapeutic keratectomy 171
Physiologic adhesion 312
Physiologic antiscarring agents 249
Physiological anisocoria 410
Pigment
  epithelial detachment 360
  epithelial layer, posterior 12
  management of 231
Pigment dispersion syndrome 193, 231, 283
  stages of 232*t*
Pilocarpine 464
  test 409
Pinealoblastoma 290
Pinholes 83
Pituitary adenoma
  management of 407
  types of 407
Pituitary gland 28
Placido disc technique 172
Placoid lesions 346*f*
Plasma
  osmolarity 11
  sterilization 502
Plastic prism 72*f*
Plus disease 308
Pneumatic displacement 320, 365
Pneumatic retinopexy 320, 355
Pneumocystis carinii infection 482
Polar cataract, posterior 196, 198*f*
Polyarteritis nodosa 169
Polyenes 478
Polymerase chain reaction 143, 286
Polymeric gels 461
Polypoidal choroidal vasculopathy 331, 344, 359, 360
Posterior hyaloid
  surface 328
  traction 350
Posterior segment diseases 518*t*
Postganglionic nerve, functioning 391
Post-gas injection 320
Postpenetrating keratoplasty glaucoma 241
  management of 243*fc*
Post-trabeculectomy eye, filtering bleb in 506
Postuveitic cataract, management of 209
Potassium 7
  hydroxide 182, 434
  iodide 478
Potential visual acuity meter 43, 341
Preferential looking test 47
Prelaminar region 26
Premacular cortex, contraction of 357
Pre-perimetric glaucoma 221
  diagnosis of 221*fc*
Preplus disease 308
Presbyopia 60
  management of 60
Primary angle closure glaucoma 244
  natural course of 230*f*
Prism
  clinical uses of 72
  optic of 71, 71*f*
  test 93*f*
Prismotherapy 377
Progressive outer retinal necrosis 484
  treatment of 486
Prolactin-secreting adenoma 407
Prolene suture 125*f*
Proliferative diabetic retinopathy 302-304, 330
Proliferative retinopathy
  traumatic 416
  treatment of 304
Proliferative sickle cell retinopathy 331
Prophylactic procedure 243
Proptosis 116, 120, 291
  examination of 116
  unilateral 115*t*
Prostaglandin analogs 232, 465
  alpha analogs 465
Protease inhibitors 485
Prototype 13
Pseudo disc edema, causes of 406
Pseudoexfoliation
  material 232
  syndrome 192, 216, 232
Pseudofluorescence 335
Pseudoisochromatic plates, function of 44
Pseudomonas aeruginosa 483
Pseudophakia, management of 197
Pseudophakic bullous keratopathy 186
Pseudopolycoria 236
Pseudoxerontoxon 151
Pterygium 146, 507
  surgical treatment of 146

Ptosis 102, 123, 391
mild 390
sling surgery of 103
surgery 409
principles of 102
unilateral 408
Pulmonary tuberculosis 487
Pulse air tonometer 512
Punctal atresia 132
Punctal dilatation 139*f*
Punctate keratitis, superficial 483
Pupil 355, 420, 423, 431, 435, 491
appearance 409
enlargement 210
small 193*f*, 194*f*
Pupillary border movements 409
Pupillary defect 18
Pupillary light reflex pathway 18, 18*f*
Pupillary margin rupture 420
Pupillary membranes, removal of 210
Pupillary pathway 17
Pupillary reactions, abnormal 17
Pupillary reflexes, abnormal 18
Pupillary relaxing incision 210
Pupillary zone 11
Pure blowout fracture 424

Q

Quickert procedure 107
Quinine 394
Quinoline derivatives 478

R

Radiation treatment 292
Radiotherapy 295, 408
Ranibizumab 302, 310, 348, 353, 356, 365
Reactive oxygen species 523
Rebleeding 425
Rebound compression wave force 415, 419
Rebound macular events 356
Rebound tonometer 14
Recurrent vitreous hemorrhage, management of 330
Red blood cells, collection of 508
Red filter test 368
Red glass test 381
Reflected compression wave force 415, 419
Reflex, light 409
Refraction 34
subjective 67
Refractive abnormalities 187
Refractive amblyopia 370
Refractive challenges 52
Refractive error 84, 453
correction of 373, 377
Refractive surgery 52, 183
Regression formulae 76
Regular eye examinations 495
Reinforcement learning 504
Relapsing polychondritis 169
Residual exotropia 377
Restrictive myopathy 120
Retina 312, 415, 423, 431, 433, 470, 484, 490
diseases of 299
infectious disease of 484
neurosensory 329
Retinal adaptation 89
Retinal adhesion, normal 312
Retinal angiomatous proliferation 343
Retinal arterial
attenuation 296
macroaneurysm 331
Retinal blood vessels, tortuosity of 229
Retinal breaks 314, 330, 356
Retinal correspondence, abnormal 368
Retinal damage, pathogenesis of 364
Retinal degeneration, sites of 328
Retinal detachment 88, 193, 280, 283, 312, 316, 320, 328, 330, 356, 416
management of post-traumatic 317
mechanism of 313*f*
recurrent 322
repair 237
total 308
traumatic 318
types of 316, 316*t*
Retinal diseases 309, 518, 519
Retinal findings, abnormal 327
Retinal hole 315
Retinal imaging technique 350
Retinal inner layers 300
Retinal ischemic causes 234
Retinal microangiopathy 484
Retinal microvasculopathy 482
Retinal pigment epithelial
detachment 358
hyperplasia 316
hypertrophy 316
Retinal pigment epithelium 17, 312, 347, 360, 363
Retinal tear 315, 416, 422
Retinal thickening, diffuse 350
Retinal thickness 204
Retinal tuberculosis 488
Retinal tufts 315
Retinal vascular occlusions 88
Retinal vasculitis 331
Retinal vein occlusion 331
Retinal vessel 317
avulsion 331
Retinitis pigmentosa 88, 283, 519, 523
clinical features of 358
Retinitis proliferans 416
Retinoblastoma 284, 298, 523
Retinopathy
cancer-associated 296
of prematurity 505
aggressive 308
management of 307
Retinoschisis 362, 363*f*
Retinoscopy 65, 65*f*, 66*f*
optics 65
prerequisites of 66
principles of 64
procedure of 66
Retrobulbar space 32
Retrobulbar tumors palpation 29
Retrolaminar region 26
Retrovirus 518
Revised International Workshop on Ocular Sarcoidosis Criteria for Diagnosis of Ocular Sarcoidosis 493
Rhabdomyosarcoma 118
Rhegmatogenous retinal detachment 329
Rheumatoid arthritis 169
Rhino-orbito-cerebral mucormycosis 489
Rho-kinase inhibitor 175, 228, 465
Riesman's sign 120
Rifampicin 497
Ripasudil 465
Road traffic accident 417
Rooper-Hall classification 439, 439*t*
Rosenbach's sign 120
Rotational flap, lateral semicircular 113*f*
Rundle's curve 120*f*
Ruptured retinal artery macroaneurysm 364

S

Saccadic intrusions 378
Salivary gland auto-transplantation 164
Sarcoidosis 177
ocular manifestation of 284, 492
Sattler's layer 25
Scheimpflug law 172
Scheimpflug technique 172
Schiotz tonometer 13
Schirmer's strip test 159*f*, 162
Schisis cavity 361, 363*f*
Schlemm's canal 7, 8, 251, 256, 263*f*
inner wall of 263*f*
School Eye Health Programme 454
Schwalbe's line 6
Sclera 165, 248*f*, 420, 432, 467, 490, 497
flap, superficial 264
Scleral buckling 318, 355
Scleral fixation intraocular lens 214*fc*
Scleral flap 248*f*
rectangular 248*f*
Scleral implants 462
Scleral perforation 356, 384
Scleral rigid gas permeable lenses 74
Sclerectomy, deep 263*fc*, 265
Scleritis 165
classification of 165, 165*fc*
clinical features of posterior 165
diagnosis of posterior 165
investigations of posterior 165
management of posterior 165

posterior 166
systemic association of 169
Scleromalacia perforans 166, 168
Scotoma, junctional 407
Sebaceous gland carcinoma 111
Secretion 7
Seidel's test rules 250
Selective laser trabeculoplasty 243, 245
Self-inflicted chemical injuries 434
Semicircular beams, overlap of 515*f*
Senile 115
miosis 192
retinoschisis 314, 315
sclerotic group 224
Sensory
adaptations 367
esotropia 372
Sepsis 307
Septum orbitale 29
Serous retinal detachment 361, 362
Serpiginous choroiditis 273, 474
Serum eye drop 163
Shield's classification 277
Short acting mydriatics 211
Short vertex distance 69*f*
Sickle cell disease 364
Siderosis 430
bulbi 423
causes 430
evaluation 430
management 430
direct 430
indirect 430
oculi 430
Silicone oil
complications of 320, 321
overfill of 321
physical properties of 320
principles of 320
use, indications of 321
uses of 320
Silver wiring 303
Simmon's shell 250
Simple excision technique 146
Simplex herpes epithelial keratitis 478
Sinskey's hook 192
Sinuses 491
Sirius 171
Sjogren's etiopathogenesis 159
Sjögren's syndrome 159
pathogenesis of 159*fc*
Skin
lesions, number of 497
smears 497
Slipped muscle 385
Slit scanning technique 172
Slit-lamp
biomicroscopy 166, 175, 293
evaluation 238
examination 181, 183, 230, 239, 274, 284
mounted 13
Small incision trabeculectomy 247
Small pupil surgery, irregular 211
Small-gauge sutureless pars plana vitrectomy
advantages of 325
disadvantages of 326
Snail track degeneration 315
Snowballs 285*f*
Snowbanking 279
Snowflake degeneration 314, 315
Sodium 7
citrate 437, 440
fluorescein 334, 480
Soft shell technique 203
Solid bifocals 71*f*
Somatic extraocular muscle dysfunction 389
Somatotrophic adenoma 407
Spaeth grading 250*t*
Spasmus Nutans syndrome 379
Spatial contrast sensitivity 45
Spectacles 51, 52
Spectrographic test 45
Specular microscopy 82
contraindications of 82, 83
Sphenoethmoidal sinusitis 388, 389
Sphenoid wing meningioma 395
Sphenoidal air cells 28
Spherical aberration 38, 38*f*
Spherical power calculation 191
Sphincter tears 420
Split bifocals 70*f*
Spring catarrh 150
Sputum examination 489
Squamous cell carcinoma 111, 483
Squint 453
Staphyloma optical biometers, posterior 204
Stargardt's disease 519
State Blindness Control Society, role of 448
Stellwag's sign 120
Stem cell 311
Stent, third-generation 252*f*
Sterile 499
Sterilize applanation tonometer biprism 516
Sterilizer 499
Steroid 274, 322
complicated diseases 281
eye drops 437, 440
implants 323
intravitreal 280
mechanism of action of 511
regimen 389
responder 511
side effects of 323
sparing agent 281
Steven-Johnson syndrome 147
Stiles-Crawford phenomena 39
Stimulus
light 88
types of 89
Stitchless trabeculectomy 248
steps of 249*f*
Stocker method 147
Stoploss Jones tube 135*f*
Strabismic amblyopia 370
Strabismus 367, 409
surgery, complications of 384
Streptomycin 394
Striated muscle, layer of 23
Stroke 391
Stroma 4, 507
Stromal edema 175
Stromal filtrates, active transport of 7
Stromal pool, formation of 7
Stromal rejection 185
Stromal scar 175
Stromal structure 5
Sturge-Weber syndrome 262
Sturm's conoid 47, 48*f*, 49*f*
etiology of 49
focal interval of 47
Subcutaneous tissue 467
Subepithelial infiltrates 185
Subfoveal choroidal thickness 300
Subfoveal neurosensory detachment 300
Subluxated lens, management of 205
Subluxation 420
Submacular hemorrhage 363
causes of 363
pneumatic displacement of 320
Submacular surgery trials 365
Subperiosteal space 32
Subretinal fluid 350, 358, 360
management of 354
Subtenon injection 280, 520
Sub-Tenon's
block 32, 467
space 467
Subthreshold diode laser 304
Subtle retinal arteriolar dilatation 303
Sulfonamides 394
Sulfur hexafluoride 319
Sump syndrome 137, 138, 138*f*
prevention of 138
Superficial fibers 98
Superficial nerves supplying skin 467
Superior oblique muscle, attachment of 30
Superior oblique palsy, clinical features of 403
Superior orbital fissure 31, 31*f*
Suprachoroidal injections 520
Suprachoroidal shunts 256*f*
Surface nerve fiber layer 26
Surgery
contraindications of 402
indications of 377
timing of 373
types of 375
Surgical site related complication, postoperative 385
Surgical technique 259, 397, 402

Suture granuloma 385
Suture-based modifications 248
Swab method 501
Swelling 467
Swinging flashlight test 18
Symblepharon 436
Sympathetic blockers 464
Synaptophore 368
  clinical uses of 79
Synechiolysis 210
Synoptophore, working principle of 78
Syphilis 388
  congenital 177
  serology 409
Syphilitic chorioretinitis 484
  treatment of 486
Systemic agents, contraindications of 464
Systemic diseases, ocular manifestation of 482
Systemic immunosuppressive therapy 169
Systemic steroids 119, 281
  side effects of 144
Systemic therapy 479
Systemic venous pressure 10

T

Tacrolimus 281
Tarsal fracture 107*f*
Tarsal strip, lateral 107
Tarsorrhaphy 149, 498
T-cell
  activation 159
  inhibitors 144, 160, 475
Tear
  artificial 437, 440
  break-up time 162
  film 22, 158
    function of 23
    layer of 22
  secretion 157
Teleconsultation, advantages of 457
Teleophthalmology, benefits of 456
Teller's acuity cards 47
Temporal contrast sensitivity 46
Temporal lobe 28
Tenon's capsule 467
Tenon's dissection 247
Tenon's transposition 438, 441
Tenoplasty 438, 441
Teprotumumab 122
Terson syndrome 331
Therapeutic contact lenses 75
Thermal argon 348
Thermal burn, prevent 194
Third cranial nerve palsy 410, 411
Thoracic sympathectomy 410
Thromboembolic events, risk of 356
Thyroid associated orbitopathy 389
Thyroid eye disease 119
  management of 122*t*
Thyroid ophthalmopathy
  clinical features of 119
  investigations of 119
  treatment of 119
Tissue
  disruption 418
  plasminogen activator 365
Titmus fly test 96
Tobacco dusting 415
Tocilizumab 122
Tonic pupil 19
  etiologies of 410
Tonometer 513
  classification of 511, 512*fc*
  types of 13, 511
Tonopen tonometer 13
Topical agents, mechanism of action of 464
Topical carbonic anhydrase inhibitors 232
Topical corticosteroid 280, 497
  side effects of 144
Topical drug delivery 460
Topical lubricants, combination of 181
Topography guided cross-linking 171
Toric intraocular lens 190*f*
  implantation 189
Toric version 77
Torsion assessment 403
Toxic optic neuropathy 394
  causes of 394
  management of 394
Toxic retinopathy 88
Toxoplasma
  retinochoroiditis 484
    treatment of 486
  serology 286
Toxoplasmosis 286, 298
Trabectome 255*f*
Trabecular meshwork 6, 254, 285*f*, 423, 430
  anterior 246
  nodular involvement of 285*f*
Trabecular outflow 8
Trabeculectomy 232, 247, 249, 268, 375
  discuss advances in 247
Traction suture 247
Tractional retinal detachment 350
Traditional myopia correction 51
Trans pars plana posterior segment procedures 466
Transscleral cyclophotocoagulation 237, 471
Trauma 330, 418
Travoprost 465
Treponema pallidum 388
Triamcinolone 280
  acetonide 280, 481
Trichiasis 101
Trichoepithelioma 111
Trichromatic theory 44
Trigeminal nerve, ophthalmic division of 466
Trypan blue 480
Tube
  placement 260
  shunt 266
    implantation 266
Tuberculin skin test 489
Tuberculosis, scleral 488
Tumor 395, 518
  recurrence 295
Two-point discrimination test 43, 339

U

Ulcerative keratitis, peripheral 180
Ultrasonic sterilization 502
Ultrasonography 318
Ultrasound biomicroscopy 240, 318, 445
Uncover test 91, 92*fc*
Upper eyelid
  anatomy of 98*f*
  coloboma, congenital 114*f*
Upper respiratory tract 169
Uvea 271
Uveal lymphoma, primary 283
Uveal melanocytic proliferation, bilateral diffuse 296
Uveal tissue 15
  arterial supply of 15
  blood supply of 15, 15*f*
  venous drainage of 15
Uveitic eye 209
  unilateral intermediate 280
Uveitic phase, acute 288
Uveitis 132, 192, 283, 522
  acute 266
  anterior 274, 282, 488
  complications of chronic 493
  drug-induced 486
  masquerade syndrome 283
  non-infectious 281
  posterior 488
  treatment of 497
Uveoscleral outflow 8

V

Valsalva
  maneuver 117
  retinopathy 331
Valved devices 266
van Buskirk theory 245
Varicella zoster 388
  virus infection 388
Vascular endothelial
  cell migration 476
  growth factor
    inhibition 304
    inhibitors block 348
    receptor 309, 523
Vascular siderosis 430
Vascular signs 229, 406
Vascularization, types of 173

Vector 518
Venae verticosae 15
Venolymphatic malformation 118
Ventilation 501
Vernal disease 153
Vernal keratoconjunctivitis 143, 150, 151*f*
  medical management 150
  surgical management 150
Vertigo 391
Vessels, nasal shifting of 229
Vestibular imbalance, peripheral 378
Vestibular mechanisms, instability of 378
Videokeratoscopes 172
Vigouroux sign 120
Vincristine 394
Viral vectors 517
Viscoanesthesia 203
Viscocanalostomy 264, 264*fc*
Viscosity 321
Viscous mucopolysaccharide substance 312
Vision 348
  2020 449
  blurring of 508
  degrading myodesopsia 330
  diminished 166
  diminution of 123, 374
  gains 301
  in one eye, loss of 395
  loss 476
  stabilization of 371
Visitech chart 46
Visual acuity 306, 375, 388, 435, 472, 509
  assessment of 379
  best corrected 358
  category 417*t*
  indicators of 46
  measurement of 46
  test 41, 47, 338
Visual behavior 379
Visual cortex 491
Visual deprivation amblyopia 370
Visual evoked potential 90, 121
  uses of 90
  waveforms 90*f*
Visual field 327
  analysis 242
  assessment 431, 443
  defects 407
  loss 222
  testing 473
Visual fixation, disorders of 378
Visual hallucination 398
Visual impairment, risk factors of severe 498
Visual loss 361
  pathogenesis of 364
  severe 389
Visual recovery, spontaneous 389
Visual rehabilitation 197
Visual symptoms 407
Visual system copes 367
Vitamin
  A deficiency 88, 453
    management of 453
  A, supplemental dose of 454
  promoting consumption of 453
Vitrectomy 318, 354, 362
  large-gauge 325
Vitreomacular traction 324, 357, 361, 362
Vitreoretinal degenerations 314, 315*t*
Vitreoretinal interface 329
Vitreoretinal surgeon 206
Vitreoretinal surgery 319*f*, 320
Vitreoretinal traction forces 313
Vitreous 328, 433
  anatomy 329*f*
  base 328, 329
  body 328
  cavity 317
  cells, anterior 279
  cortex 329
  disorders 327
  fluid 327
  haze, grading of 279*t*
  hemorrhage, nonclearing 324
  humor 327
  opacities 333
  prolapse 213, 415
  removal, effective 326
  surface 328
  surgical anatomy of 328
  syneresis 330
  traction 313
Vitreous degeneration 332
  age-related 328
  causes of 333
  types of 333
Vitreous detachment 415
  posterior 330, 332
Vitreous floaters 330
  benign 333
  management of 330
  symptomatic 333
Vogt striae 179
Vogt-Koyanagi-Harada
  disease 287-289, 346, 346*f*
  syndrome 287, 474
von Graefe's sign 120
Voriconazole 479
Vortex veins 30

W

Water-soluble dye 334
Waveform 90
Wegener granulomatosis 169
Weiss and Gold classification 235*t*
Weiss procedure 106*f*
Wernicke's hemianopic pupil 18
White dot syndrome, differential diagnosis of 273
White limbal zone 5
White pupillary reflex 291
White-without-pressure 314, 315
White-with-pressure 314, 315
Whooping cough 388
Wide-field retinal photography 293
Wieger's ligament 328
Wilson releasable suture 248*f*
Wilson technique 248
Window defect 335
Windshield wiper keratopathy 248
Worth four dot test 48*f*, 57, 57*f*, 368
Wound
  construction, traumatic 325
  dehiscence 110
  leak 265
  medium-sized 442
  repair of 444
  scleral 422

X

Xen gel stent 256*f*
Xeroderma pigmentosa 154
X-rays 502

Z

Zeaxanthin 349
Zhongshan angle closure prevention trial 231
Zinc 349
  dosage, adjustment of 349
  pyrithione 479
Zonular dehiscence 211
Zonular dialysis 420
Zonular laxity 233
Zonular tractional retinal tuft 315
Z-plasty 110*f*
Zygomatico-sphenoid suture 29